PRACTICAL THERAPEUTICS

of

TRADITIONAL CHINESE MEDICINE

Yan Wu

Warren Fisher

Edited by Jake Fratkin

Paradigm Publications   *1997*   *Brookline, Massachusetts*

Practical Therapeutics of Traditional Chinese Medicine
Yan Wu
Warren Fischer

Jake Fratkin, Editor

Copyright © Paradigm Publications
44 Linden Street
Brookline, Massachusetts 02146 USA

Library of Congress Cataloging-in-Publication Data:
Wu, Yan, 1944-
    Practical therapeutics of traditional Chinese medicine / Yan Wu,
    Warren Fischer ; Jake Fratkin, editor.
    p. cm.
    Includes bibliographical references and index.
    1. Medicine, Chinese. I. Fischer, Warren, 1963- .
    II. Fratkin, Jake, 1948- . III. Title.
    R601.W768 1997
    610'.951--dc21   97-4808
                              CIP

Library of Congress Number: 97-4808
International Standard Book Number (ISBN): 0-912111-39-9
Printed in the United States of America

TABLE OF CONTENTS

ACKNOWLEDGEMENTS

We are highly gratified that *Practical Therapeutics of Traditional Chinese Medicine* has finally made it into the hands of the readers. It has been only through the close cooperation and concerted efforts of the authors, editors and publishers that this has come to fruition.

We would like to extend our most heartfelt thanks to Mr. Robert Felt and Ms. Martha Fielding of Paradigm Publications for their wisdom, skills, patience and freindship. This book would not be possible without their hard work and untiring efforts. We are also deeply indebted to the editor, Mr. Jake Fratkin, for his inspiring suggestions and encouragement in helping to get this project started. We greatly appreciate his enthusiasm, guidance, energy and the time spent on this project. We wish to thank Mr. Nigel Wiseman, one of our most respected scholars, for his valuable opinions concerning traditional Chinese medical terminology, and Mr. Keviin Ergil, Dean of the Pacific Institute of Oriental Medicine, for his kindness and effort in support of this project. We are grateful to all those involved in the editing, research, publishing and distribution of this book, including Mrs. Marnae Ergil, Mrs. Deborah Chiel and Mr. Henry Dreher, for their contributions in helping to make this book a reality.

At the same time, we would like to extend our respects to former Minister of Health of the People's Republic of China, now president of the Red Cross Society of China and president of China National Chinese Medicine Association, Mr. Cui Yue-Li, as well as to professor Meng Shu, former principal of the Acupuncture College of Beijing Pei-Li University. Their commentaries and recommendation for this book have honored us twice over.

Finally, we thank both our wives, Mrs. Li Yan-Hua and Mrs. Heather Fischer. It was only through their love, understanding and support that we were ultimately able to finish this work.

FOREWORD

In recent years, there has been a significant increase of English-language resources for learning the clinical practice of traditional Chinese medicine. However, these all have had limitations in some essential aspect. There are problems in the quality of translation, the breadth of topics, or the organization of materials. The work presented here by Yan Wu and Warren Fischer has overcome these problems and offers readers, be they clinicians or scholars, the first readily accessible and comprehensive presentation of a standard and informed perspective on the Chinese medical approach to a wide array of clinical problems.

The attention to traditional perspectives in the organization of topics is apparent from an examination of the Table of Contents which lists topics by traditional clinical category. More importantly, the sections on conditions are titled using traditional, rather than biomedical nomenclature. Atony patterns *(wěi zhèng)* and strangury patterns *(lín zhèng)* are presented, as are other conditions less familiar to the Western reader, such as snake cinnabar *(shé dān)* and ox-hide tinea *(niú pí xiǎn)*. This retains the broader, more inclusive approach to clinical issues that typifies the practice of Chinese medicine.

This care in presentation is continued in each section where clinicians and students alike will be pleased to find a wide range of patterns discussed in association with each condition. Beyond the immediately apparent excellence of this book in terms of its coverage, accessibility and usefulness, is its fundamental concern with linguistic transparency and systematic translation. This allows the user to understand the relations to Chinese language source materials and the clinical thinking of Chinese practitioners, issues critical to the full development of Chinese medicine in countries where the native clinical language is not Chinese. Such a systematic approach places readers in close relation to the clinical approaches of the Chinese tradition. It protects them from imprisonment by presentations that substitute an author's idiosyncratic interpretation for faithful description of clinical practice, or that obscure the meaning of Chinese ideas with a biomedicalized vocabulary.

The approach adopted here allows the reader to enter the sophisticated world of Chinese medical therapeutics as a participant rather than as a recipient of second-hand or mislabeled information. The use of a systematic method of translation also provides practitioners and students with ownership of the language and concepts that constitute their medicine. Although for some there may be a momentary difficulty adjusting to terms such as "repletion" and "vacuity," this adjustment is more than repaid with clarity and assurance. Knowing that each and every technical term is related by reference to its Chinese counterpart and that the use of this vocabulary represents definitive knowledge, rather than rough approximation, inspires confidence.

Although this book will be of substantial value to the physician of Chinese medicine, its value to the student of Chinese medicine is even greater. As someone who began their learning in between the period of there being "no books" in

English and this present period of relative abundance, I can still remember the anxiety of studying in the absence of good supporting texts. We copied our teachers words with the clear sense that this was our sole opportunity to gather information about the treatment of a specific condition. If we, as students, failed to write it down, there was no other place to go to remedy the situation. Later, as more materials became available, there were new problems imposed by varying translational standards and differing approaches to the presentation of clinical materials. This text furnishes a single comprehensive reference for the core practice of internal medicine as well as supporting other areas of clinical endeavor. The student may now go to a single well-written and well-translated source as a core reference; and faculty now have a reliable foundation upon which to build their clinical discussions.

Practical Therapeutics of Traditional Chinese Medicine also has a unique feature that emerges from its textual origins and the collaborative nature of its authorship. Yan Wu is a senior clinician and educator, and in compiling the materials presented here he has brought to bear years of experience working with both Western and Chinese students, as well as decades of clinical experience. Beyond that he has had the opportunity to test and refine this material in an American classroom over more than three years as a professor at the Pacific Institute of Oriental Medicine in New York. In sum, this work represents his perspective as a very informed clinician, scholar and teacher of the clinical practice of Chinese medicine. Warren Fischer's contribution as a North American practitioner who has devoted years of study in China and practice in Canada provides a lens which focuses the content on what is relevant for the Western practitioner. Thus this work is neither a compilation of clinical interventions uninformed by clinical practice, nor is it a single perspective on clinical methodologies. It is a powerful expression of the synergy of study and clinical practice and as such is of enormous value to our community.

This book lives up to many of my concepts concerning the nature of an ideal book in the field. It results from the collaboration of two experienced and educated individuals, both trained clinicians who have grappled with the issues that surround the cultural transposition of Chinese medicine. In addition, they have been willing to receive assistance and guidance from two individuals who are highly conversant with the issues surrounding Chinese medical text translation and who are both translators in their own right: Nigel Wiseman, a specialist in linguistics, and Marnae Ergil, an anthropologist and specialist in education in traditional Chinese medicine. The willingness of both authors to engage the technical issues that emerged from discussions with both these consultants exemplifies their commitment to providing a text that offers rock-solid technical information with fidelity to source materials. The collaboration links clinical expertise in China with clinical experience in the West and does so on the foundation of definitive knowledge of the tradition of practice in China acquired through study and experience.

As an observer and occasional helper in the process of bringing this book into being I would like to thank Yan Wu and Warren Fischer for their enormous act of generosity in bringing this book into existence. The time that they have expended on it and the attention to detail are the product of a conscientious concern and love for Chinese medicine that will be manifest to every reader.

Kevin V. Ergil, M.S., L.Ac., FNAOOM.
Dean, Pacific Institute of Oriental Medicine

EDITOR'S PREFACE

In the fall of 1987, I participated in an advanced herbal training program at Xi Yuan Hospital, in Beijing, China. During that time, I had the pleasure of meeting Dr. Yan Wu, an associate professor at Beijing University of Traditional Chinese Medicine. I was impressed with his personal charm, his excellent command of English, and his knowledge of Chinese herbal medicine. We discussed possible writing projects in English on T.C.M., and I encouraged him to write a treatment of disease based on the main teaching texts at the Beijing University. Of all the texts that were required in the West, a thorough organization of disease, with differential diagnosis and emphasis on herbal therapy, was certainly needed.

In June of 1988, I returned to Beijing as organizer of a group of American acupuncturists. During this trip, I again met with Dr. Wu, and was happy to hear that he indeed had started his book. He introduced me to his co-author, a Canadian student finishing the program at Beijing University of T.C.M. Warren Fischer was the first foreigner I had met who was able to proceed through the entire five year program at Beijing University of T.C.M., and of course, he did it in Chinese. I felt that Warren would be an excellent co-author, understanding T.C.M. as taught in China, yet with a native command of the English language. I heartily encouraged them to continue the project, which I would edit and organize. Over the next several years, the 100 or so chapters that comprise this book were mailed to me. The manuscript was converted to computer, from which I edited, organized and formatted the material.

Our goals, in producing this book, were two-fold. First, we wished to create a standard reference work on the treatment of disease which most closely followed the educational standards at advanced institutions such as the Beijing University of Traditional Chinese Medicine. Towards this end, Dr. Wu and Dr. Fischer researched the top medical books used at Beijing and Shanghai Universities of T.C.M. (see Bibliography). These books, in turn, were created by a panel of T.C.M. experts empowered to organize the traditional medical material. Here, I am quite certain we achieved our objective: *Practical Therapeutics* represents the highest standards of traditional medicine being taught to T.C.M. students in China.

Our second goal was to make the book easy for the practitioner to use in a busy clinical situation. Our format reflects our desire for ease and practicality of use. Categories within each chapter make it easy to target specific differentiations. Extensive indexing also makes it easy to find specific chapters based on common symptoms or Western diagnosis, English or Pinyin drug and formula names, etc.

We chose common diseases that were known to be effectively treated with traditional Chinese medicine. Each disease is divided into its most representational differentiations, and each differentiation offers treatment using both herbal formulas and acupuncture. Herbal and acupuncture prescriptions are modified depending on variations within a particular differentiation. Where effective, indications for supportive therapies are indicated, including ear acupuncture, electroacupuncture, plum-blossom needle, qigong exercise, tuina massage, diet and lifestyle recommendations.

Of particular usefulness to the clinician are the opening statements, etiology and pathogenesis, and the closing remarks. These provide not only a useful overview, but in many cases offer important points affecting treatment that need to be considered The glossary and extensive cross-referencing index will also be useful to many readers.

As far as our choice of English vocabulary for Chinese medical terms, our publisher encouraged the authors and myself to utilize Nigel Wiseman's *Glossary of Chinese Medical Terms and Acupuncture Points,* with the intention of having one English word for one Chinese term. This prompted Dr. Wu to seriously examine the English terms he had chosen for *Practical Therapeutics*.

Dr. Wu enlisted the help of Kevin Ergil, director of the Pacific Institute of Oriental Medicine, New York City, and Marnae Ergil, a Ph.D. candidate with a strong background in Chinese linguistics. Together, they spent long hours analyzing and discussing the T.C.M. terms, deciding upon what they felt to be the best translations for the Chinese medical vocabulary. Mr. Wiseman also participated via fax, phone and letter, giving valuable suggestions and opinions.I would like to thank those who generously gave their time and effort in contributing to this project: Anne Peacocke, for her laborious transcription of the original text to computer; Marnae Ergil, who read through the final version, verifying pinyin tones, Chinese characters, and glossary choices; David Cohen, professor at T.C.M. University, Los Angeles, who read the manuscript for clarity, consistency and accuracy in both traditional Chinese and Western medical terminology; and Sally Rudich, who helped edit the text in its earlier stages. Also, Jay Nelson who made valuable suggestions concerning format, and Jack Boyce for our beautiful cover. I also would like to thank Charles Chace for his early encouragement to adopt Mr. Wiseman's *Glossary,* and of course Bob Felt, for his guidance and encouragement throughout the project, and his insistence on strenuous academic standards so that our text can emerge as an important, accurate and clinically valuable reference work on Chinese medical therapeutics.

It is our hope that *Practical Therapeutics of Traditional Chinese Medicine* will endure.

Jake Paul Fratkin, O.M.D.
Boulder, Colorado, June, 1995

AUTHORS' PREFACE

Traditional Chinese medicine, with its two-thousand year history, unique theoretical systems and satisfying clinical results, is receiving increasingly greater attention worldwide. Acupuncture and moxibustion, which form a major part of traditional Chinese medicine, first spread to the West during the 1950's. Since then, medical practitioners involved in the study, research and therapeutic use of acupuncture have steadily increased.

Related academic exchange has also become more and more frequent and brisk. In 1979, acupuncture and moxibustion therapy received the attention of the World Health Organization. Currently, acumoxa therapy is playing an ever more important role in medicine and health care in more than 100 countries and territories around the world. Beginning in the 1980's, traditional Chinese herbal medicine has also gradually become a worldwide trend. Its unique diagnostic and therapeutic techniques and its favorable clinical results have captured the interest of many.

Although our family roots in China and Canada are quite distant, we have taken advantage of our common interest and profession to compile and translate *Practical Therapeutics of Traditional Chinese Medicine* to meet the needs of academic study and clinical research around the globe. We believe it to have several distinct characteristics as outlined below:

1. Authority

This work is the first treatise published in English on traditional Chinese medical therapeutics to use the teaching materials of the superior schools and colleges of the People's Republic of China as its foundation. These teaching materials are the product of the collective compilation, examination and approval of the special assembly of Chinese medical specialties organized by the Chinese government during the 1980's specifically for that purpose. These teaching materials are currently serving as the standard texts for the training of high-level traditional Chinese medical doctors and acupuncturists in the superior traditional Chinese medical schools and colleges in the People's Republic of China. This work therefore reflects the present academic standard of higher education in traditional Chinese medicine in mainland China.

2. Practicality

This work introduces more than 100 illnesses from the fields of internal medicine, surgery, dermatology, gynecology, obstetrics, pediatrics, ophthalmology, otorhinolaryngology, stomatology and emergentology in a clear and systematic manner. All the illnesses selected are commonly observed or frequently occurring conditions that definitely respond favorably to traditional Chinese medical techniques. To aid in the use of this book in a practical setting, in addition to expounding the etiology and pathogenesis of each illness, we have introduced various Chinese therapeutic techniques including herbal medicine, acupuncture, plum blossom needle therapy, electroacupuncture, fire cupping and auricular and scalp acupuncture, as well as various external therapies. All prescriptions cited (apart from commercially prepared formulas) include information on the addition and deletion of constituents according to symptom variations. To the end of increasing the clinical effectiveness of acupuncture and moxibustion therapy, this work has set Chinese herbal medicine, acupuncture and moxibustion in parallel as unified treatments following a single differential diagnosis and treatment plan. This unification of needles and medicinals, as well as the emphasis on differential diagnosis and selection of acupoints, maintains the distinctive characteristics of traditional Chinese medical therapeutics. The text also contains a glossary, bibliography, and indices of Chinese medicinals, herbal prescriptions, acupoints and Chinese and Western medical terms to assist the reader in further research.

3. Standardization

The chapter titles in this book utilize the traditional Chinese names for the conditions. The Western medical disease names, Western medical terms and the names of Chinese medicinals appearing in all parts of the text were, without exception, translated into English according to dictionaries of international authority. The English names, abbreviations and Pinyin names of the fourteen channels and acupoints, as well as the extra acupoints and scalp acupoints, use the channel and acupoint nomenclature according to the international standardization program set down by the WHO Ri-Nei-Wa conference in 1979 as the standard reference, with additional reference to the People's Republic of China national standard GB-123456-90, "Channel and Point Location," distributed by the national technology control bureau in 1990.

As concerns the English translations of Chinese medical terminology, this book has followed the principles of fidelity, meaning and smoothness. Every effort was made to provide the reader with information that is veritable, accurate, understandable and which explains the profound in a simple fashion.

Practical Therapeutics of Traditional Chinese Medicine developed through several different writings and numerous manuscript changes during the compilation and translation process. The Chinese teaching materials mentioned earlier served as the foundation for the contents and design of this book. Some further additions and deletions, amendments and revisions were implemented based on the author's years of teaching and clinical experience to suit it to current English language educational and clinical demands.

Traditional Chinese medicine is a great treasurehouse. We hope that in publishing *Practical Therapeutics of Traditional Chinese Medicine*, new opportunities are made available for the understanding and study of Chinese medicine. We also hope that traditional Chinese medicine will soon spread on a global scale and that it will become the common wealth of all people.

DESIGNATION

Paradigm Publications is a participant in the Council of Oriental Medical Publishers and supports their effort to inform readers of how works in Chinese medicine are prepared. *Practical Therapeutics of Traditional Chinese Medicine* is an original work prepared from the studies and clinical practice of Dr. Yan Wu, building upon the Text Series for Medical Colleges and Universities published by the Shanghai Science and Technology Publishing House (see Bibliography).

Unless noted, the translation follows (for Chinese speakers) Wiseman, N. *English-Chinese Chinese-English Dictionary of Chinese Medicine.* Hunan, China: Hunan Science and Technology Press, 1995; and for English speakers, Wiseman's *Glossary of Chinese Medical Terms and Acupuncture Points* (see Bibliography), and Wiseman, N. *Clinical Dictionary of Chinese Medicine.* Brookline, MA: Paradigm Publications, 1997.

AUTHORS' INTRODUCTION

GUIDE TO THE USE OF THIS BOOK

I. Disease and Disease Patterns

This book introduces more than 100 diseases of internal medicine, surgery, dermatology, gynecology, obstetrics, pediatrics, ophthalmology, otorhinolaryngology, emergentology and stomatology as regards their diagnoses and various treatments. The classification of disease in this book is mainly based on the traditional Chinese medical perspective, which is different from the meaning of disease in Western medicine. In Western medicine, disease refers to a disorder with a specific cause and recognizable symptoms and signs designated by its etiological and pathological characteristics. In T.C.M., however, many disease names are actually names of symptoms and signs of illness. For example, lower back pain that is considered as a disease entity in T.C.M. is recognized by a Western doctor as only a clinical symptom.

For the translation of some traditional Chinese diseases, a corresponding Western terminology is provided. However, this may not precisely reflect the way in which it is understood in Western medicine. For example, according to Western medical perspective, depression is a mental state characterized by excessive sadness. Activity can be agitated and restless or slow and retarded. Behavior is governed by pessimistic and despairing beliefs, and sleep, appetite and concentration are disturbed. In T.C.M., depression is known as *yù zhèng* and refers to a class of patterns brought on by emotional disturbance as a resultant stagnation of qi, blood, phlegm, dampness, heat and food. Hence the Chinese term "six depressions" obviously covers a wider range of clinical implications. To avoid misunderstanding and confusion, a Pinyin transliteration supplements the English name of each disease.

Because factors such as age, sex, constitution, diet, lifestyle and emotional tenure vary from one person to the next, the clinical manifestations of the same disease may differ for each patient. T.C.M. diagnosis, therefore, includes not only the differentiation of disease, but more important to the process, the differentiation by disease patterns. Neither can be dispensed with and, because each complements the other, both are necessary for diagnosis.

This book includes under each disease the basic disease patterns most commonly encountered in clinic. These basic patterns can appear in various combinations such that they may be transformed into another pattern. Clinical manifestation is thus both complex and changeable, and the process of pattern differentiation is based not only on set patterns, but also various combinations of patterns. Practitioners must therefore avoid approaching diagnosis in a mechanical fashion. The basic patterns must be studied and understood, but students and practitioners must not be rigidly bound by them.

As mentioned, differentiation of disease in T.C.M. is based on the primary symptoms. For example, when a patient's chief complaint is lateral costal pain, the disease will be differentiated as "lateral costal pain." Although simple, easy and practical, this method is not scientifically rigorous. Therefore, when modern T.C.M. practitioners diagnose and treat patients, they often refer to a Western medical concept. For example, "bi patterns" is a general term that includes several disorders known in Western medicine as osteoarthritis, rheumatoid arthritis, rheumatic arthritis, fibrositis, gout and sciatica. Each of these types has its own etiological and pathological characteristics. Thus, in the treatment of arthritis, in addition to the differentiation of traditional Chinese disease (bi patterns) and a further pattern differentiation (wind bi, cold bi, dampness bi or heat bi), practitioners may also take into account the Western disease entity by consulting objective indices such as laboratory tests and other examinations. The herbal or acupuncture formula prescribed will depend primarily on the disease pattern. In addition, other medicinals or acupoints may be added to treat the specific disease.

For example, in cases of rheumatoid arthritis, because it is an autoimmune disorder, *xiān líng pí* (epimedium) and *lù fēng fáng* (hornet's nest) may be added to regulate the body's immune functions. For gout, a metabolic disorder causing an excess of uric acid to be produced and insufficiently discharged, *tǔ fú líng* (smooth greenbrier root) and *bì xiè* (fish poison yam) may be added to reduce production of uric acid. Osteoarthritis is a degenerative pathologic change of the cartilage that produces bone spurs. *Gǔ suì bǔ* (drynaria) and *lù hán cǎo* (pyrolae) may be added to slow the degenerative process and prohibit the growth of bone spurs. For spurs of the cervical vertebrae, *gé gēn* (pueraria root) may be added, and for spurs of the lumbar vertebrae, *xù duàn* (dipsacus root) may be added. The application of those particular medicinals is based on the experience of many practitioners over years of practice, and the efficacy of some of these medicinals has already been proven through modern scientific research.

II. Etiology and Pathogenesis

In each section of this text, before discussing the different disease patterns, there is a general discussion of the etiology and pathogenesis of each disease. This will be helpful and important in understanding the basic process of diagnosis and treatment in traditional Chinese medicine.

For example, the main etiological agent of the common cold is wind evil. Thus, the common cold is known as *shāng fēng* in T.C.M., meaning "attacked by wind." Hence, dispelling wind is a very important part of treating the common cold. In T.C.M., jaundice may be classified either as yang jaundice, which is caused by damp-heat evils, or yin jaundice, which is caused by cold-dampness evils. The dampness evil is the main cause of jaundice, so the treatment should always include the elimination of dampness. For lower back pain, note that the discussion is grouped as lower back pain caused by external evils, of which dampness is always considered to be the primary factor, or by internal damage, which is always related to a kidney vacuity, or by traumatic injury, which is always related to stagnation of qi and blood. The appropriate treatments for lower back pain are therefore given based on the understanding of these patterns.

Thus, disease etiology and pathogenesis can serve as guides to the differentiation of the patterns and their treatment.

III. Balancing Prudence with Flexibility

In the diagnosis and treatment of patients, the practitioner must understand and employ two techniques: prudence and flexibility. When the precise pattern is determined, care should be taken to use the specific medicinal or acupuncture formula designated for that pattern. But the practitioner must also be sensitive to changing conditions. When the patient's condition changes, the medicinals or acupoints should also be changed accordingly. These changes, however, should be undertaken with caution, rather than easily and indiscriminately – hence the emphasis on balancing prudence with flexibility.

After the administration of medicinal formulas or acupuncture, the patient may exhibit one of three responses:

1. *The symptoms may be alleviated.* In such a situation, the use of the basic formula should be continued, although a very subtle change in dose or an adjustment of one or two of the medicinals may be necessary.

2. *There may be an absence of marked improvement, but no worsening of the symptoms.* Less experienced practitioners are often too eager to alter the formula because they are not confident of a positive result. Despite any possible reluctance to continue with the basic formula, in most cases it is wise to maintain the treatment because a greater period of therapy may be required to be effective. In some cases, however, the dose of the medicinals – especially that of the principal medicinals – may need to be increased, or more acupoints may be added with a stronger stimulation.

3. *The symptoms are aggravated, and the patient's condition worsens.* Practitioners may be confused and opt to use a different formula without fully considering the patient's condition. If they are convinced that their diagnosis is correct, they should not be misled by the aggravated symptoms, which may signal that the treatment is working, and that the evil is being dispelled. The basic formula can be maintained, with possible changes. The key is to be patient and attend further results. Since the cooperation of patients is very important, they must, of course, be informed of this possibility, so that they don't lose heart before the treatment has been completed.

IV. Principles of Treatment and Clinical Manifestations

In T.C.M., there are four general principles of treatment:

1. Treat the root of the disease.

2. Reinforce the correct qi and eliminate the evil.

3. Regulate yin and yang

4. Treat according to the season, weather conditions and geographic region, and the individual's conditions, as noted above.

The principle of treatment for each pattern of a disease is closely linked to, and should be consistent with, the pattern of differentiation.

The clinical manifestations of each pattern mentioned in this book, including the conditions of the tongue and pulse, are general and typical symptoms and signs commonly seen by most practitioners. However, each and every patient will not necessarily exhibit all the typical symptoms and signs. The differentiation of the patterns are therefore based on the principal symptoms and signs. The clinical manifestations are sometimes very complicated and confusing. Students and practitioners who fail to pay attention to the principal symptoms and signs, and who do not differentiate what is primary from what is secondary, will find it difficult to make an accurate and precise diagnosis.

The terminology regarding some of the symptoms of clinical manifestations mentioned in the text has a different meaning in T.C.M. than it does in Western medicine. For example, "high fever" is defined in Western medicine as a body temperature above 102.2° F. In T.C.M., high fever covers a wider range of temperatures and more general meanings. The definition of high fever in T.C.M. is not only based on body temperature, but also on other pronounced heat signs such as flushed face, severe thirst, red or crimson tongue and rapid surging pulse.

This is but one of many illustrations of how T.C.M. practitioners pay more attention to qualitative rather than quantitative measures of diagnosis. Another example in diagnostic technique would be determination of a "floating pulse" as opposed to a "deep pulse," a difference with clinical implications. There is no precise way to determine whether a pulse is in fact floating or deep; it depends upon a qualitative determination by an experienced practitioner who has learned to detect such differences.

V. Medicinal and Acupunctural Formulas

Sometimes, when less experienced practitioners or recently graduated students prescribe medicinal formulas, they apply medicinals or acupoints without regard to the necessary hierarchy set forth in the formulas. Sometimes, they use too many medicinals or too many acupoints because they are overly concerned with treating each and every one of the symptoms the patient manifests. The patient's symptoms must be examined as a whole, rather than being analyzed into many different components. The medicinals and acupoints should not be applied symptom by symptom, but rather to the principal symptoms and the essential nature of the disease. Some clinical situations are very complicated because the patient has many different symptoms and signs. But such situations do not necessarily call for a more complex or voluminous use of medicinals or acupoints. To the contrary, the more severe the condition, the more specific the selection must be.

Hundreds of medicinal and acupuncture formulas are described in this book. These formulas have been proven effective through long-term clinical practice. To aid in the use of this book in clinical settings, the ingredients for each of the formulas are listed in English, Latin and Pinyin transliteration. In the text, the dose given for each medicinal is a general adult dose that must be adjusted to the age, gender and constitution of the individual patient. The following doses are standard according to the 1985 edition of the pharmacopoeia of the People's Republic of China, as adjusted for age and based on fractions of the adult dosages:

New-born infants to one month old	1/18 to 1/14
One month old to six months old	1/14 to 1/7
Six months old to one year old	1/7 to 1/5
One year old to two years old	1/5 to 1/4
Two years old to four years old	1/4 to 1/3
Four years old to six years old	1/3 to 2/5
Six years old to nine years old	2/5 to 1/2
Nine years old to fourteen years old	1/2 to 2/3
Fourteen to eighteen years old	2/3 to full dosage
Eighteen to sixty years old	full dosage
Over sixty years old	3/4 dosage

Chinese medicinals are generally safe, but there are toxic medicinals that must be used with great caution, especially in regard to dose. There is sometimes only a small difference between an effective treatment dose and an amount of the drug that can be harmful. Thus, with poisonous medicinals it is very important to begin with a small dose and increase it gradually to the appropriate level. If any sign of toxicity occurs, stop treatment immediately and take the measures necessary to counteract that toxicity.

Because the names of formulas are sometimes literal and sometimes allusions, the Pinyin is also given for each formula. It is helpful for practitioners to become familiar with the names of the formulas, because the name of a formula may signify the ingredients or the functions of that formula. For example, *"bàn xià bái zhú tiān má tāng"* (Pinellia, Ovate Atractylodes and Gastrodia Decoction) tells you the principal constituents of the formula; *"bǔ zhōng yì qì tāng"* (Center-Supplementing Qi-Boosting Decoction) tells you the function of the formula.

Since the time of ancient China, acupuncture and herbal medicine have been commonly used together to treat patients. To increase clinical effectiveness, this book treats medicinals and acupuncture as parallel, placing them together as a unified treatment, following a single differential diagnosis and principle of treatment. This unification serves to maintain the distinctive characteristics of traditional Chinese medicine.

VI. Herbal Decoction and Needle Manipulation

Herbal decoction is a very common form of Chinese pharmaceutical preparation. It is a liquid preparation made by boiling medicinals with a proper amount of water. When preparing a decoction, medicinals are put into a clean vessel of which the material's chemical property is comparatively stable (such as an earthenware, glass or enamel cooking vessel, but never an iron, aluminum, tin or copper pot). Then, clean cold water is added (to one inch above the medicinals) to submerge all the medicinals. After the medicinals are soaked for 30 to 60 minutes, the pot with the medicinals is placed on a fire, first quickboiled (with a strong fire), and then simmered (the heat is turned down). The medicinals should be decocted for a certain period of time according to the different requirements and then the liquid decoction decanted and strained out. After that, water can be added to the same level and then the medicinals boiled again in the same way. Usually from the same pack of medicinals we can obtain two cups of liquid decoction, which should be mixed and then divided into two portions (two cups) and taken two or more times a day, generally in the morning and in the evening.

The amount of water, the boiling time and heat intensity all depend on the types of medicinals used. Sweat-inducing medicinals should be decocted in a relatively small amount of water and boiled for a short period of time, usually 5 to 10 minutes after boiling. Supplements should be decocted with more water (one more cup) for a longer period, usually 30 to 40 minutes after boiling.

Some precious medicinals such as *rén shēn* (ginseng) should be decocted separately. The decoction obtained can be taken separately or mixed with the finished decoction to avoid waste of these precious medicinals. Precious medicinals that are unsuitable for decoction should be ground into fine powder and infused with warm water or the decoction prepared from other medicinals. Liquid medicinals such as bamboo juice and ginger juice should be taken in the same way.

Some of the gluey and very sticky medicinals, for example, *ē jiāo* (ass hide glue) or *yí táng* (malt sugar) should be melted or dissolved in boiling water or a hot prepared decoction for oral administration. Some other special medicinals, such as minerals and shells, should be smashed and decocted 10 to 20 minutes after boiling before adding other medicinals. Some toxic medicinals such as *zhì wū tóu* (prepared aconite root) and *zhì fù zǐ* (prepared aconite accessory tuber) should also be decocted first for 30 to 60 minutes to reduce their toxicity. Those medicinals with fragrance or a volatile oil such as *bò hé* (mint) and *shā rén* (amomum fruit) should be decocted only for about five minutes. Some medicinals such as *chē qián zǐ* (plantago seed), *chì shí zhī* (halloysite) and *xuán fù huā* (inula flower) should be wrapped in a piece of cloth before decocting with other medicinals because they may either cause the decoction to become turbid or irritate the throat. Notes on decocting each of the special medicinals are given in the text.

As regards the method of administration, usually one pack of decoction is given daily. For mild and chronic illnesses, the decocted medicinals should be taken twice daily, in the morning and in the evening; for severe and acute cases, two packs once every four hours may be appropriate. Supplements should be taken before meals (with an empty stomach), while stomach- or intestine-irritating medicinals should be taken one to two hours before or after meals. Sedatives and tranquilizers should be taken before bedtime. Some medicinals can be infused with boiling water in a vessel with a lid and taken frequently as tea. Medicinal decoctions are usually taken while warm. Pills, boluses, powders or granules should be taken with warm boiled water, if no special direction is given. Some medicinals may be taken in the form of medicated wine, which refers to a transparent medicated liquid obtained by using wine as a solvent to soak the medicinals. Medicated wine is suitable for the treatment of general weakness, rheumatic pain and traumatic injury.

The methods of making and taking a decoction are closely related to the effectiveness of a medicinal formula.

Special attention must also be paid to the manipulation of acupuncture needles. Treatment results are very dependent on proper needle technique. The general principles for needle manipulations are as follows: draining manipulations are performed in the case of repletion patterns, supplementing manipulations are used in the case of vacuity patterns. Even draining, even supplementing manipulations are applied for patterns complicated by both repletion and vacuity. Traditionally, there are nearly 100 different needling techniques based on these principles.

Through the many dynasties, Chinese acupuncture practitioners have emphasized the importance of these various techniques and accumulated a wealth of experience in this matter. T.C.M. students and practitioners must therefore pay close attention to the study of needling techniques to raise the level of their acupuncture practice to meet the high standards of traditional Chinese medical practice through the ages.

PART I

INTERNAL MEDICINE

COMMON COLD

Găn Mào

1. Invasion of Wind-Cold - 2. Invasion of Wind-Heat - 3. Invasion of Summerheat-Dampness - 4. Colds in Cases of Qi Vacuity - 5. Colds in Cases of Yin Vacuity

The common cold is a frequently observed external illness that may be contracted in any of the four seasons; it is most prevalent in winter and spring. Mild cases of the cold are commonly known as *shāng fēng* (attacks of wind) and severe cases as *zhòng shāng fēng* (strong attacks of wind). If, during a certain period, many cases are observed over a large area and the symptoms are very similar, then it is known as *shí xíng găn mào* (epidemic cold), or, in Western medicine, as flu.

The major symptoms of a cold are stuffy nose, sore throat, runny nose, cough, aversion to cold, fever and headache. Symptoms persist for five to seven days. These are generally not severe and seldom develop secondary conditions. Epidemic cold, characterized by chills of sudden onset, high fever and aching of the entire body, is highly contagious and can develop into secondary conditions.

ETIOLOGY AND PATHOGENESIS

External wind is the main cause of the common cold and is usually combined with cold, heat, summerheat or dampness. Wind-cold is most common in autumn and winter; wind-heat in spring and summer and wind accompanied by summerheat-dampness in late summer, that is, the last month of summer. The pathology of colds varies with the exterior evils. Wind-cold, wind-heat and summerheat-dampness types are commonly seen.

1. INVASION OF WIND-COLD

Clinical Manifestations: Strong aversion to cold, slight fever, no perspiration, headache, aching joints and limbs, stuffy nose, runny nose, scratchy throat, cough with thin white phlegm, without sensation of excessive thirst.

Tongue: Thin white moist coating.

Pulse: Floating, tight.

Treatment Method: Dispel wind, dissipate cold, resolve the exterior.

PRESCRIPTION

Schizonepeta and Ledebouriella Toxin-Vanquishing Powder
jīng fáng bài dú săn

jīng jiè	schizonepeta (abbreviated decoction)	Schizonepetae Herba et Flos	6 g.
fáng fēng	ledebouriella [root]	Ledebouriellae Radix	6 g.
qiāng huó	notopterygium [root]	Notopterygii Rhizoma	6 g.
dú huó	tuhuo [angelica root]	Angelicae Duhuo Radix	6 g.
chái hú	bupleurum [root]	Bupleuri Radix	6 g.
qián hú	peucedanum [root]	Peucedani Radix	6 g.
chuān xiōng	ligusticum [root]	Ligustici Rhizoma	6 g.
zhǐ shí	unripe bitter orange	Aurantii Fructus Immaturus	6 g.
fú líng	poria	Poria	6 g.
jié gěng	platycodon [root]	Platycodonis Radix	6 g.
gān căo	licorice [root]	Glycyrrhizae Radix	3 g.

MODIFICATIONS

In cases where cold evil is predominant, the prescription is modified to reinforce the cold dispersing actions. Add:

má huáng	ephedra	Ephedrae Herba	6 g.
guì zhī	cinnamon [twig]	Cinnamomi Ramulus	4.5 g.

ACUPUNCTURE AND MOXIBUSTION

Main points: Needle with draining; moxibustion may follow.

LU-07	*liè quē*
LI-20	*yíng xiāng*
SI-07	*zhī zhèng*
BL-12	*fēng mén*
GB-20	*fēng chí*
LI-04	*hé gǔ*

Auxiliary points:

With headache, add:

M-HN-3	*yìn táng* (Hall of Impression)
M-HN-9	*tài yáng* (Greater Yang)

With upper backache, apply cupping to:

BL-13	*fèi shū*

2. INVASION OF WIND-HEAT

Clinical Manifestations: Slight aversion to cold, prominent fever, perspiration, headache, cough with thick yellow phlegm, dry or sore swollen throat, stuffy nose with turbid yellow mucus, thirst.

Tongue: Thin yellow coating.

Pulse: Floating, rapid.

Treatment Method: Dispel wind, clear heat, resolve the exterior.

PRESCRIPTION

Lonicera and Forsythia Powder *yín qiào săn*

jīn yín huā	lonicera [flower]	Lonicerae Flos	9 g.
lián qiào ké	forsythia [fruit]	Forsythiae Fructus	9 g.
dàn dòu chǐ	fermented soybean (unsalted)	Glycines Semen Fermentatum Insulsum	6 g.
niú bàng zǐ	arctium [seed]	Arctii Fructus	9 g.
bò hé	mint (abbreviated decoction)	Menthae Herba	6 g.
jīng jiè suì	schizonepeta [spike] (abbreviated decoction)	Schizonepetae Flos	6 g.
jié gěng	platycodon [root]	Platycodonis Radix	6 g.
gān cǎo	licorice [root]	Glycyrrhizae Radix	6 g.
lú gēn	phragmites [root]	Phragmititis Rhizoma	9 g.
zhú yè	black bamboo [leaf]	Bambusae Folium	6 g.

MODIFICATIONS

With severe headache, the prescription is modified to soothe the headache. Add:

sāng yè	mulberry [leaf]	Mori Folium	9 g.
jú huā	chrysanthemum [flower]	Chrysanthemi Flos	9 g.

For coughing with excessive phlegm, the prescription is modified to transform phlegm and relieve coughing. Add:

zhè bèi mǔ	Zhejiang fritillaria [bulb]	Fritillariae Verticillatae Bulbus	9 g.
qián hú	peucedanum [root]	Peucedani Radix	9 g.
xìng rén	apricot [kernel] (abbreviated decoction)	Armeniacae Semen	9 g.

For coughing with thick yellow mucus, the prescription is modified to clear heat and transform phlegm. Add:

huáng qín	scutellaria [root]	Scutellariae Radix	9 g.
zhī mǔ	anemarrhena [root]	Anemarrhenae Rhizoma	9 g.
guā lóu pí	trichosanthes [rind]	Trichosanthis Pericarpium	9 g.

For red sore swollen throat, the prescription is modified to remove heat-toxin and disinhibit the pharynx. Add:

tǔ niú xī	native achyranthes [root]	Achyranthis Radix	12 g.
xuán shēn	scrophularia [root]	Scrophulariae Radix	9 g.

In cases where symptoms of epidemic heat-toxin are evident, the prescription is modified to clear heat and disperse toxin. Add:

dà qīng yè	isatis [leaf]	Isatidis Folium	12 g.
pú gōng yīng	dandelion	Taraxaci Herba cum Radice	9 g.

If the lung contains chronic heat and the body surface is invaded by external wind-cold, causing the obstruction of heat by cold with symptoms of fever, aversion to cold, little perspiration, dyspnea, cough with thick yellow phlegm and hoarseness, the prescription is modified to clear heat and diffuse the lung. Add:

shí gāo	gypsum (extended decoction)	Gypsum	18 g.
má huáng	ephedra	Ephedrae Herba	6 g.

In cases of wind-heat producing dryness that dehydrates fluids, or illnesses caused by external warm-dryness in autumn with symptoms of coughing with scanty phlegm, dry throat, lips, mouth and nose, red tongue with thin coating and little saliva, the prescription is modified to clear the lung and moisten dryness. Add:

běi shā shēn	glehnia [root]	Glehniae Radix	12 g.
tiān huā fěn	trichosanthes [root]	Trichosanthis Radix	12 g.
lí pí	pear [skin]	Pyri Exocarpium	6 g.

ACUPUNCTURE AND MOXIBUSTION

Main points: Needle with draining.

LU-05	*chǐ zé*
GB-20	*fēng chí*
LI-11	*qū chí*
LI-04	*hé gǔ*
GV-14	*dà zhuī*
TB-05	*wài guān*

Auxiliary points:

For cases with sore swollen throat, bleed at:

LU-11   *shào shāng*

For infantile convulsions from high fever, use a filiform needle which should just penetrate the skin and then be quickly removed. After removal of the needle a drop of blood can be squeezed from the points:

GV-26   *shuǐ gōu*
M-UE-1-5   *shí xuān* (Ten Diffusing Points)

3. INVASION OF SUMMERHEAT-DAMPNESS

Clinical Manifestations: Unsurfaced fever,* slight aversion to cold, little perspiration, headache with a sensation of heaviness (as though the head were tightly bandaged), aching and heaviness of the limbs and joints, coughing with sticky phlegm, greasy feeling in the mouth, no thirst or thirst with a preference for hot drinks, nausea, dark scanty urine, oppression in the chest, distention and fullness of the epigastrium and abdomen, loose stools.

Tongue: Yellow, slimy coating.

Pulse: Soft, rapid.

Treatment Method: Clear summerheat, transform dampness, resolve the exterior.

PRESCRIPTION

Newly Supplemented Elsholtzia Beverage *xīn jiā xiāng rú yǐn*

xiāng rú	elsholtzia	Elsholtziae Herba	6 g.
biǎn dòu huā	lablab [flower]	Lablab Flos	9 g.
hòu pò	magnolia [bark]	Magnoliae Cortex	6 g.
jīn yín huā	lonicera [flower]	Lonicerae Flos	9 g.
lián qiào	forsythia [fruit]	Forsythiae Fructus	9 g.

---

* "Unsurfaced fever" describes fever obscured by exterior dampness evil where the patient's skin does not feel hot in the beginning but begins to feel hotter after some time.

MODIFICATIONS

If summerheat is prominent, the prescription is reinforced to dispel summerheat. Add:

huáng lián	coptis [root]	Coptidis Rhizoma	6 g.
qīng hāo	sweet wormwood (abbreviated decoction)	Artemisiae Apiaceae seu Annuae Herba	9 g.
lú gēn	phragmites [root]	Phragmititis Rhizoma	15 g.
hé yè	lotus [leaf]	Nelumbinis Folium	6 g.

If the body surface is obstructed by dampness, the prescription is modified to dispel superficial dampness. Add:

huò xiāng	agastache/patchouli	Agastaches seu Pogostemi Herba	9 g.
pèi lán	eupatorium	Eupatorii Herba	9 g.

If internal dampness is prominent, the prescription is modified to regulate the interior and transform dampness. Add:

cāng zhú	atractylodes [root]	Atractylodis Rhizoma	9 g.
bái dòu kòu	cardamom (abbreviated decoction)	Amomi Cardamomi Fructus	6 g.
fǎ bàn xià	processed pinellia [tuber]	Pinelliae Tuber Praeparatum	9 g.
chén pí	tangerine [peel]	Citri Exocarpium	6 g.

In cases of dark scanty urine, the prescription is modified to clear heat and disinhibit dampness through the urine. Add:

huá shí	talcum (wrapped)	Talcum	9 g.
gān cǎo	licorice [root]	Glycyrrhizae Radix	1.5 g.
fú líng	poria	Poria	9 g.

ACUPUNCTURE AND MOXIBUSTION

Main points: Needle with draining.

LU-06	*kǒng zuì*
LI-04	*hé gǔ*
CV-12	*zhōng wǎn*
ST-36	*zú sān lǐ*
TB-06	*zhī gōu*

Auxiliary points:

If heat is prominent, add:
    GV-14   *dà zhuī*
If dampness is prominent, add:
    SP-09   *yīn líng quán*
For abdominal distention and loose stools, add:
    ST-25   *tiān shū*

4. COLDS IN CASES OF QI VACUITY

Clinical Manifestations: Strong aversion to cold, fever, headache, nasal congestion, cough with white phlegm, tiredness, fatigue, shortness of breath, disinclination to speak. This is from depleted defense qi allowing external invasion of wind-cold evil.

Tongue: Pale with white coating.

Pulse: Floating, forceless.

Treatment Method: Dispel wind, dissipate cold, boost qi, resolve the exterior.

PRESCRIPTION

Ginseng and Perilla Beverage *shēn sū yǐn*

rén shēn	ginseng	Ginseng Radix	9 g.
zǐ sū yè	perilla (leaf) (abbreviated decoction)	Perillae Folium	9 g.
gé gēn	pueraria [root]	Puerariae Radix	6 g.
qián hú	peucedanum [root]	Peucedani Radix	6 g.
fǎ bàn xià	processed pinellia [tuber]	Pinelliae Tuber Praeparatum	6 g.
fú líng	poria	Poria	6 g.
jié gěng	platycodon [root]	Platycodonis Radix	3 g.
chén pí	tangerine peel	Citri Exocarpium	3 g.
zhǐ ké	bitter orange	Aurantii Fructus	3 g.
mù xiāng	saussurea [root]	Saussureae (seu Vladimiriae) Radix	3 g.
gān cǎo	licorice [root]	Glycyrrhizae Radix	3 g.
shēng jiāng	fresh ginger	Zingiberis Rhizoma Recens	3 pc.
dà zǎo	jujube	Ziziphi Fructus	3 pc.

ACUPUNCTURE AND MOXIBUSTION

Main points: In addition to those points used in the treatment of wind-cold type, add:

ST-36	*zú sān lǐ*
BL-13	*fèi shū*

5. COLDS IN CASES OF YIN VACUITY

Clinical Manifestations: Fever, slight aversion to wind or cold, headache, no perspiration or little perspiration, dizziness, vexation of the heart, heat in the palms and soles, thirst, dry throat, dry mouth, dry cough with scanty phlegm. This is from chronic yin vacuity allowing external invasion of wind-heat evil.

Tongue: Red with little coating.

Pulse: Rapid, thready.

Treatment Method: Dispel wind, clear heat, nourish yin, resolve the exterior.

PRESCRIPTION

Solomon's Seal Variant Decoction *jiā jiǎn wēi ruí tāng**

yù zhú	Solomon's seal [root]	Polygonati Yuzhu Rhizoma	9 g.
cōng bái	scallion white	Allii Fistulosi Bulbus Recens	6 g.
jié gěng	platycodon [root]	Platycodonis Radix	6 g.
bái wēi	baiwei [cynanchum root]	Cynanchi Baiwei Radix	3 g.
dàn dòu chǐ	fermented soybean (unsalted)	Glycines Semen Fermentatum Insulsum	9 g.
bò hé	mint (abbreviated decoction)	Menthae Herba	6 g.
zhì gān cǎo	(honey-fried) licorice [root]	Glycyrrhizae Radix	1.5 g.
dà zǎo	jujube	Ziziphi Fructus	2 pc.

---

*Solomon's seal is known both as *yù zhú* and *wēi ruí*.

<u>MODIFICATIONS</u>

For thirst and dry throat, add:

bĕi shā shēn	glehnia [root]	Glehniae Radix	9 g.
mài mén dōng	ophiopogon [tuber]	Ophiopogonis Tuber	9 g.

ACUPUNCTURE AND MOXIBUSTION

Main points: Needle with supplementation. In addition to those points used in the treatment of wind-heat type, add:

BL-43 (38)	*gāo huāng shū*
KI-07	*fù liū*

ALTERNATE THERAPEUTIC METHODS

1. Ear Acupuncture:

Main points: Lung, Trachea, Internal Nose, Ear Apex, Stomach, Spleen, *Sān Jiāo*.

Method: Select two to three points each session with strong stimulation. Retain needles for ten to twenty minutes.

2. Prevention

A. In spring and winter, when wind and cold are prevalent, the following decoction can prevent colds. The decoction should be taken as one dose, once daily for three consecutive days.

guàn zhòng	aspidium	Aspidii Rhizoma	9 g.
zĭ sū yè	perilla (leaf) (abbreviated decoction)	Perillae Folium	9 g.
jīng jiè	schizonepeta (abbreviated decoction)	Schizonepetae Herba et Flos	9 g.
gān căo	licorice [root]	Glycyrrhizae Radix	3 g.

B. In summer, when summerheat and dampness are prevalent, this decoction is recommended as a regular beverage:

huò xiāng	agastache/patchouli	Agastaches seu Pogostemi Herba	6 g.
pèi lán	eupatorium	Eupatorii Herba	6 g.
bò hé	mint	Menthae Herba	3 g.

C. During periods when influenza is prevalent, decoct, and take once daily:

guàn zhòng	aspidium	Aspidii Rhizoma	12 g.
băn lán gēn	isatis [root]	Isatidis Radix	6 g.
dà qīng yè	isatis [leaf]	Isatidis Folium	6 g.
gān căo	licorice [root]	Glycyrrhizae Radix	3 g.

D. A useful method in the prevention of colds is to massage M-HN-3 *(yìn táng)* and LI-04 *(hé gŭ)* with one's middle or index finger. Do this two to three times a day, for three to five minutes each time until the skin is slightly red and an aching or distended sensation is felt in the area.

E. Another method of prevention is moxibustion to ST-36 *(zú sān lĭ)* 3 to 5 moxa cones daily.

REMARKS

In the treatment of colds, herbs should be boiled gently and not decocted too long. The decoction should be taken while still warm. After taking the decoction, avoid drafts and bundle up to induce perspiration, or drink hot water to assist the medicines. After inducing perspiration, be careful to avoid drafts and keep warm to prevent catching another cold. It is recommended that the patient drink plenty of water and get sufficient rest.

The major treatment method for colds is to induce perspiration. Wind-cold patterns should be treated with warm, pungent medicines; wind-heat patterns with cool, pungent medicines; and summerheat-dampness patterns with summerheat clearing and dampness dispelling medicines.

In cases where neither heat nor cold is prevalent, a mild prescription of pungent medicines is suitable. In cases of external cold complicated by internal heat, treatment should combine relieving the exterior and clearing the interior. For epidemic cold in which patterns are severe and mainly of the wind-heat type, heat-clearing and toxin-resolving medicines should be the principal constituents.

Generally speaking, supplementing medicines are contraindicated in the treatment of colds to completely dispel evil, but in cases of poor constitution, they may be added to the prescriptions. Appropriate modifications should be made according to whether the patient is chronically qi or yin depleted.

COUGH

Ké Sòu

1. Invasion of Lung by Wind-Cold - 2. Invasion of Lung by Wind-Heat - 3. Invasion of Lung by Wind-Dryness - 4. Phlegm-Dampness Cough - 5. Liver-Fire Cough - 6. Yin Vacuity Cough

Coughing is one of the more predominant patterns presented in cases of respiratory illness. In Chinese, coughing is called *ké sòu*. *Ké* characterizes coughing with sound but without phlegm, and *sòu* characterizes coughing with phlegm but without sound. Since the majority of coughing patterns have the characteristics of both sound and phlegm, *ké* and *sòu* are usually used as a compound word.

ETIOLOGY AND PATHOGENESIS

Patterns of coughing are divided into two categories: external cough and internal cough. External coughs develop following the invasion of one or more of the six external evils. External coughs from wind-cold, wind-heat and wind-dryness are most frequently observed clinically.

Internal coughs are mainly caused by internal evils resulting from the dysfunction of the viscera and bowels. Three types of internal coughs are common. phlegm-dampness cough tends to be from repeated recurrence of coughs; this comes about when vacuity of the lung instigates vacuity of the spleen, producing dampness and phlegm. Liver-fire cough finds its major cause in emotional stress; this causes stagnation of liver qi and the production of liver fire, which rises into the lung. Yin vacuity cough results from the depletion of lung yin.

Patterns of external coughs are generally one of repletion and are marked by abrupt onset, short duration and the accompaniment of exterior symptoms such as headache, fever and aversion to cold. Patterns of internal coughs, on the other hand, are mostly vacuous and characterized by gradual onset, a protracted history of coughing and other symptoms of viscera and bowels dysfunction. In some cases, such as phlegm-dampness cough and liver-fire cough, there are often vacuity patterns complicated by repletion. Therefore, although coughing is classified as either external or internal, one can at times cause the other.

1. INVASION OF THE LUNG BY WIND-COLD

Clinical Manifestations: Choking cough, accelerated respiration, scratchy throat and expectoration of thin white phlegm, accompanied by aversion to cold, headache and stuffy runny nose.

Tongue: Thin white coating.

Pulse: Floating, taut.

Treatment Method: Dispel wind-cold, ventilate the lung, relieve coughing.

PRESCRIPTION

Choose from Rough and Ready Three Decoction *(sān ào tāng)* or Cough-Stopping Powder *(zhǐ sòu sǎn)*. Rough and Ready Three Decoction is indicated in cases of recently contracted coughs, and Cough-Stopping Powder is indicated in protracted or recurring cases of external coughs.

Rough and Ready Three Decoction *sān ào tāng*

má huáng	ephedra	Ephedrae Herba	9 g.
xìng rén	apricot kernel (abbreviated decoction)	Armeniacae Semen	9 g.
gān cǎo	licorice [root]	Glycyrrhizae Radix	6 g.

or:

Cough-Stopping Powder *zhǐ sòu sǎn*

jīng jiè	schizonepeta (abbreviated decoction)	Schizonepetae Herba et Flos	6 g.
zǐ wǎn	aster [root]	Asteris Radix et Rhizoma	9 g.
bǎi bù	stemona [root]	Stemonae Radix	9 g.
bái qián	cynanchum [root]	Cynanchi Baiqian Radix et Rhizoma	6 g.
jié gěng	platycodon [root]	Platycodonis Radix	6 g.
chén pí	tangerine [peel]	Citri Exocarpium	6 g.
gān cǎo	licorice [root]	Glycyrrhizae Radix	6 g.

MODIFICATIONS

In cases complicated by phlegm-dampness, with symptoms of coughing with sticky phlegm, oppression in the chest and slimy tongue coating, the prescription is modified to dry dampness and transform phlegm. Add:

fǎ bàn xià	processed pinellia [tuber]	Pinelliae Tuber Praeparatum	9 g.
hòu pò	magnolia [bark]	Magnoliae Cortex	9 g.
fú líng	poria	Poria	9 g.

In cases where heat is obstructed by cold, with symptoms of coughing, hoarseness, accelerated respiration, expectoration of thick sticky phlegm, irritability, thirst (in some cases) and fever, the prescription is modified to resolve the exterior and clear the interior. Add:

shí gāo	gypsum (extended decoction)	Gypsum	18 g.
huáng qín	scutellaria [root]	Scutellariae Radix	9 g.
sāng bái pí	mulberry [root bark]	Mori Radicis Cortex	9 g.

ACUPUNCTURE AND MOXIBUSTION

Main points: Needle with draining.

LU-07	*liè quē*
LI- 04	*hé gǔ*
BL-13	*fèi shū*
TB-05	*wài guān*

Auxiliary points:

For headache, add:

GB-20	*fēng chí*
GV-23	*shàng xīng*

For aching limbs, add:

BL-60	*kūn lún*
LI- 07	*wēn liū*

2. INVASION OF LUNG BY WIND-HEAT

Clinical Manifestations: Frequent coughing, heavy breathing, sore throat, dry mouth and difficult expectoration of thick sticky yellow phlegm, accompanied by fever, perspiration, aversion to wind, headache, thirst.

Tongue: Thin yellow coating.

Pulse: Rapid, floating or rapid, slippery.

Treatment Method: Dispel wind-heat, diffuse the lung, relieve coughing.

PRESCRIPTION

Mulberry Leaf and Chrysanthemum Beverage *sāng jú yǐn*

sāng yè	mulberry [leaf]	Mori Folium	9 g.
jú huā	chrysanthemum [flower]	Chrysanthemi Flos	9 g.
lián qiào	forsythia [fruit]	Forsythiae Fructus	9 g.
lú gēn	phragmites [root]	Phragmititis Rhizoma	9 g.
xìng rén	apricot kernel (abbreviated decoction)	Armeniacae Semen	9 g.
jié gěng	platycodon [root]	Platycodonis Radix	9 g.
bò hé	mint (abbreviated decoction)	Menthae Herba	6 g.
gān cǎo	licorice [root]	Glycyrrhizae Radix	6 g.

MODIFICATIONS

To increase effects of ventilating the lung and dispelling wind-heat, add:

qián hú	peucedanum [root]	Peucedani Radix	9 g.
niú bàng zǐ	arctium [fruit]	Arctii Fructus	9 g.

In cases of exuberant lung heat, the prescription is modified to clear the lung. Add:

huáng qín	scutellaria [root]	Scutellariae Radix	9 g.
zhī mǔ	anemarrhena [root]	Anemarrhenae Rhizoma	9 g.

In cases of sore throat and hoarseness, the prescription is modified to clear heat and disinhibit the throat. Add:

shè gān	belamcanda [root]	Belamcandae Rhizoma	9 g.
chì sháo yào	red peony [root]	Paeoniae Radix Rubra	9 g.

In cases where heat has injured lung yin, with symptoms of thirst, dry throat and mouth, and red tongue with little moisture, the prescription is modified to clear heat and generate liquid. Add:

běi shā shēn	glehnia [root]	Glehniae Radix	12 g.
tiān huā fěn	trichosanthes [root]	Trichosanthis Radix	12 g.

During the summer season the prescription is modified to disperse accompanying summerheat. Add:

huá shí	talcum (wrapped)	Talcum	9 g.
hé yè	lotus leaf	Nelumbinis Folium	6 g.

ACUPUNCTURE AND MOXIBUSTION

Main points: Needle with draining, or let blood.

BL-13	*fèi shū*
LU-05	*chǐ zé*
LI-11	*qū chí*
GV-14	*dà zhuī*

Auxiliary points:

For sore, dry throat, add bloodletting at:

LU-11	*shào shāng*

For excessive perspiration without relinquishment of fever, add:

ST-43	*xiàn gǔ*
KI-07	*fù liū*

3. INVASION OF LUNG BY WIND-DRYNESS

Clinical Manifestations: Dry cough without phlegm or with scanty sticky phlegm that is difficult to expectorate, or with phlegm containing streaks of blood; scratchy or sore dry throat, dry nose and mouth, exterior symptoms such as stuffy nose, headache, slight aversion to cold and fever during the early stages of some cases.

Tongue: Dry red with thin white coating or thin yellow coating.

Pulse: Floating, rapid.

Treatment Method: Course wind-dryness, moisten the lung, relieve coughing.

PRESCRIPTION

Mulberry Leaf and Apricot Kernel Decoction *sāng xìng tāng*

sāng yè	mulberry [leaf]	Mori Folium	9 g.
xìng rén	apricot [kernel] (abbreviated decoction)	Armeniacae Semen	9 g.
běi shā shēn	glehnia [root]	Gleniae Radix	9 g.
zhè bèi mǔ	Zhejiang fritillaria [bulb]	Fritillariae Verticillatae Bulbus	9 g.
dàn dòu chǐ	fermented soybean (unsalted)	Glycines Semen Fermentatum Insulsum	9 g.
shān zhī zǐ	gardenia [fruit]	Gardeniae Fructus	6 g.
lí pí	pear skin	Pyri Exocarpium	6 g.

MODIFICATIONS

In cases of severe vacuity of fluids, the prescription is modified to nourish lung yin. Add:

mài mén dōng	ophiopogon [tuber]	Ophiopogonis Tuber	9 g.
yù zhú	Solomon's seal [root]	Polygonati Yuzhu Rhizoma	9 g.

In cases of high fever, the prescription is modified to clear the lung and eliminate heat. Add:

shí gāo	gypsum (extended decoction)	Gypsum	18 g
zhī mǔ	anemarrhena [root]	Anemarrhenae Rhizoma	9 g.

In cases where phlegm is streaked with blood, the prescription is modified to clear heat and relieve bleeding. Add:

bái máo gēn	imperata [root]	Imperatae Rhizoma	15 g.

In cases where wind-dryness is accompanied by cold evil, with symptoms of dry cough with little or no phlegm, dry nose and throat, aversion to cold, fever, headache, no perspiration and thin dry white tongue coating, the prescription is changed to warm and moisten the lung and to relieve coughing. Use:

Apricot Kernel and Perilla Powder *xìng sū săn*

xìng rén	apricot kernel (abbreviated decoction)	Armeniacae Semen	6 g.
zĭ sū yè	perilla leaf (abbreviated decoction)	Perillae Folium	6 g.
zhĭ ké	bitter orange [fruit]	Aurantii Fructus	6 g.
qián hú	peucedanum [root]	Peucedani Radix	6 g.
jié gĕng	platycodon [root]	Platycodonis Radix	6 g.
zhì bàn xià	processed pinellia [tuber]	Pinelliae Tuber Praeparatum	6 g.
fú líng	poria	Poria	6 g.
chén pí	tangerine peel	Citri Exocarpium	6 g.
shēng jiāng	fresh ginger	Zingiberis Rhizoma Recens	6 g.
gān căo	licorice [root]	Glycyrrhizae Radix	6 g.
dà zăo	jujube	Ziziphi Fructus	2 pc.

Add:

zĭ wăn	aster [root]	Asteris Radix et Rhizoma	6 g.
kuăn dōng huā	tussilago [flower]	Tussilaginis Flos	6 g.
băi bù	stemona [root]	Stemonae Radix	6 g.

In cases of marked aversion to cold and no perspiration, the prescription is modified to dispel superficial cold. Add:

jīng jiè	schizonepeta (abbreviated decoction)	Schizonepetae Herba et Flos	6 g.
fáng fēng	ledebouriella [root]	Ledebouriella radix	6 g.

ACUPUNCTURE AND MOXIBUSTION

Main points: Needle with draining.

BL-13	*fèi shū*
LU-05	*chĭ zé*
LI-11	*qū chí*
LU-10	*yú jì*

Auxiliary points:

For aversion to cold without perspiration, add:

LU-07	*liè quē*
LI-04	*hé gŭ*

4. PHLEGM-DAMPNESS COUGH

Clinical Manifestations: Frequently recurring cough particularly marked on rising in the morning with expectoration of abundant dilute white phlegm, accompanied by oppression in the chest, epigastric fullness and distention, nausea, fatigue, poor appetite, loose stools.

Tongue: White slimy coating.

Pulse: Soggy or slippery.

Treatment Method: Strengthen the spleen, dry dampness, transform phlegm, relieve coughing.

PRESCRIPTION

Combine Two Matured Ingredients Decoction *(ér chén tāng)* with Three-Seed Filial Devotion Decoction *(sān zǐ yǎng qīn tāng)*.

Two Matured Ingredients Decoction *èr chén tāng*

fǎ bàn xià	processed pinellia [tuber]	Pinelliae Tuber Praeparatum	12 g.
chén pí	tangerine [peel]	Citri Exocarpium	12 g.
fú líng	poria	Poria	9 g.
gān cǎo	licorice [root]	Glycyrrhizae Radix	6 g.

with:

Three-Seed Filial Devotion Decoction *sān zǐ yǎng qīn tāng*

lái fú zǐ	radish [seed]	Raphani Semen	9 g.
zǐ sū zǐ	perilla [fruit]	Perillae Fructus	9 g.
bái jiè zǐ	white mustard [seed]	Brassicae Albae Semen	6 g.

MODIFICATIONS

To increase the effects of drying dampness and dissolving phlegm, add:

cāng zhú	atractylodes [root]	Atractylodis Rhizoma	9 g.
hòu pò	magnolia [bark]	Magnoliae Cortex	9 g.

In cases where cold phlegm is predominant, with symptoms of aversion to cold and expectoration of sticky frothy white phlegm, the prescription is modified to warm the lung and transform phlegm.
Add:

gān jiāng	dried ginger [root]	Zingiberis Rhizoma Exsiccatum	6 g.
xì xīn	asarum	Asiasari Herba cum Radice	3 g.

In cases of protracted coughing with severe symptoms of spleen vacuity, the prescription is modified to benefit spleen qi.
Add:

dǎng shēn	codonopsis [root]	Codonopsitis Radix	9 g.
bái zhú	ovate atractylodes [root]	Atractylodis Ovatae Rhizoma	9 g.

In cases where phlegm-dampness develops into phlegm-heat with symptoms of expectoration of thick purulent phlegm, slimy yellow tongue coating and rapid slippery pulse, the prescription is modified to clear heat and transform phlegm.
Use:

Phragmites Stem Decoction* *wěi jīng tāng*

lú gēn	phragmites [root]	Phragmititis Rhizoma	30 g.
yì yǐ rén	coix [seed]	Coicis Semen	30 g.
dōng guā zǐ	wax gourd [seed]	Benincasae Semen	24 g.
táo rén	peach [kernel]	Persicae Semen	9 g.

Add:

sāng bái pí	mulberry [root bark]	Mori Radicis Cortex	12 g.
guā lóu	trichosanthes [fruit]	Trichosanthis Fructus	12 g.
huáng qín	scutellaria [root]	Scutellariae Radix	9 g.
yú xīng cǎo	houttuynia	Houttuyniae Herba cum Radice	12 g.

(* Phragmites is known both as *lú gēn* and *wěi jīng*.)

After stabilizing the patient's condition, use:

Six Gentlemen Decoction *liù jūn zǐ tāng*

rén shēn	ginseng	Ginseng Radix	9 g.
bái zhú	ovate atractylodes [root]	Atractylodis Ovatae Rhizoma	9 g.
fú líng	poria	Poria	9 g.
fǎ bàn xià	processed pinellia [tuber]	Pinelliae Tuber Praeparatum	6 g.
chén pí	tangerine peel	Citri Exocarpium	6 g.
zhì gān cǎo	licorice [root] (honey-fried)	Glycyrrhizae Radix	6 g.

ACUPUNCTURE AND MOXIBUSTION

Main points: Needle with supplementation; add moxibustion.

BL-13	*fèi shū*
BL-20	*pí shū*
LU-09	*tài yuān*
SP-03	*tài bái*
ST-40	*fēng lóng*
LI-04	*hé gǔ*

Auxiliary points:

For coughing with asthma, add:

N-BW-5   *wài dìng chuǎn* (Outer Panting Stabilizer)

For oppression in the chest and epigastric fullness and distention, add:

ST-36	*zú sān lǐ*
PC-06	*nèi guān*
CV-12	*zhōng wǎn*

5. LIVER-FIRE COUGH

Clinical Manifestations: Hacking cough, scanty sticky phlegm, full distended sensation and pain throughout the chest and costal regions during coughing, flushed complexion, bitter taste in the mouth, dry scratchy throat, variation in severity of symptoms with emotional state.

Tongue: Red with thin yellow coating.

Pulse: Rapid, wiry.

Treatment Method: Clear liver fire, drain the lung, relieve coughing.

PRESCRIPTION

Combine White-Draining Powder *(xiè bái sǎn)* with Indigo and Clamshell Powder *(dài gé sǎn)*.

White-Draining Powder *xiè bái sǎn*

sāng bái pí	mulberry [root bark]	Mori Radicis Cortex	12 g.
dì gǔ pí	lycium [root bark]	Lycii Radicis Cortex	12 g.
jīng mǐ	rice	Oryzae Semen	15 g.
zhì gān cǎo	licorice [root] (honey-fried)	Glycyrrhizae Radix	6 g.

with:

Indigo and Clamshell Powder *dài gé sǎn*

qīng dài	indigo (stirred in)	Indigo Pulverata Levis	1.5 g.
hǎi gé ké	clamshell	Cyclinae Concha (seu Meretricis)	9 g.

MODIFICATIONS

To clear the liver and dispel fire, add:

shān zhī zǐ	gardenia [fruit]	Gardeniae Fructus	9 g.
huáng qín	scutellaria [root]	Scutellariae Radix	9 g.
mǔ dān pí	moutan [root bark]	Moutan Radicis Cortex	9 g.

In cases of chest pain, the prescription is modified to regulate qi and relieve pain. Add:

yù jīn	curcuma [tuber]	Curcumae Tuber	9 g.
sī guā luò	loofah	Luffae Fasciculus Vascularis	9 g.

In cases of difficult expectoration of sticky phlegm, the prescription is modified to clear heat and transform phlegm. Add:

chuān bèi mǔ	Sichuan fritillaria [bulb]	Fritillariae Cirrhosae Bulbus	9 g.
fǔ hǎi shí	pumice	Pumex	9 g.
jié gěng	platycodon [root]	Platycodonis Radix	9 g.

In cases of a persistent cough with symptoms of dry throat and mouth because of the depletion of fluids by accumulated fire, the prescription is modified to nourish lung yin and relieve coughing. Add:

běi shā shēn	glehnia [root]	Glehniae Radix	12 g.
mài mén dōng	ophiopogon [root]	Opiopogonis Radix	9 g.
tiān huā fěn	trichosanthes [root]	Trichosanthis Radix	12 g.

Also, use an astringent herb such as:

kē zǐ	chebule	Chebulae Fructus	9 g.

ACUPUNCTURE AND MOXIBUSTION

Main points: Needle with draining.

BL-13	*fèi shū*
BL-18	*gān shū*
LU-08	*jīng qú*
LR-03	*tài chōng*

Auxiliary points:

For dry scratchy throat, add:

KI-06	*zhào hǎi*

For coughing blood, add:

LU-06	*kǒng zuì*

6. YIN VACUITY COUGH

Clinical Manifestations: Dry hacking cough without phlegm, or with scanty sticky white or blood-tinged phlegm, gradual hoarseness, dry throat and mouth, afternoon tidal fever, vexing heat in the five hearts, night sweating, listlessness, emaciation.

Tongue: Red with little coating.

Pulse: Rapid, thready.

Treatment Method: Nourish yin, moisten the lung, transform phlegm, relieve coughing.

PRESCRIPTION

Adenophora/Glehnia and Ophiopogon Decoction *shā shén mài dōng tāng*

běi shā shén	glehnia [root]	Glehniae Radix	9 g.
mài mén dōng	ophiopogon	Opiopogonis	9 g.
tiān huā fěn	trichosanthes [root]	Trichosanthis Radix	12 g.
yù zhú	Solomon's seal [root]	Polygonati Yuzhu Rhizoma	9 g.
biǎn dòu	lablab [bean]	Lablab Semen	9 g.
sāng yè	mulberry [leaf]	Mori Folium	6 g.
gān cǎo	licorice [root]	Glycyrrhizae Radix	6 g.

MODIFICATIONS

To increase the effects of moistening the lung and dissolving phlegm, add:

chuān bèi mǔ	Sichuan fritillaria [bulb]	Fritillariae Cirrhosae Bulbus	9 g.
xìng rén	apricot [kernel] (abbreviated decoction)	Armeniacae Semen	6 g.

In cases of coughing with shortness of breath, the prescription is modified to preserve lung qi. Add:

wǔ wèi zǐ	schisandra [berry]	Schisandrae Fructus	6 g.
kē zǐ	chebule [fruit]	Chebulae Fructus	9 g.

In cases of afternoon tidal fever, the prescription is modified to clear vacuity-heat. Add:

dì gǔ pí	lycium [root bark]	Lycii Radicis Cortex	12 g.
yín chái hú	lanceolate stellaria [root]	Stellariae Lanceolatae Radix	6 g.
qīng hāo	sweet wormwood (abbreviated decoction)	Artemisiae Apiaceae seu Annuae Herba	6 g.
biē jiǎ	turtle shell (extended decoction)	Amydae Carapax	15 g.

In cases of night sweating, the prescription is modified to preserve yin and arrest perspiration. Add:

wū méi	mume [fruit]	Mume Fructus	9 g.
fú xiǎo mài	light wheat [grain]	Tritici Semen Leve	15 g.

In cases of phlegm containing blood, the prescription is modified to clear heat and relieve bleeding. Add:

mǔ dān pí	moutan [root bark]	Moutan Radicis Cortex	9 g.
shān zhī zǐ	gardenia [fruit]	Gardeniae Fructus	6 g.
ǒu jié	lotus [root node]	Nelumbinis Rhizomatis Nodus	9 g.

ACUPUNCTURE AND MOXIBUSTION

Main points: Needle with supplementation:

BL-13	*fèi shū*
LU-05	*chǐ zé*
LU-07	*liè quē*
KI-06	*zhào hǎi*

Auxiliary points:

For coughing blood, add:

LU-06	*kǒng zuì*
BL-17	*gé shū*

ALTERNATE THERAPEUTIC METHODS

1. Ear Acupuncture

Main points: Liver, *Shén Mén*, Lung, Trachea.

Method: Needle bilaterally to elicit a moderate sensation and retain needles ten to twenty minutes. Treat every second day, ten sessions making up one course of treatment. Vaccaria seed *(wáng bù liú xíng)* can also be fixed to auricular points with adhesive tape. [Mustard seed may also be used – Ed.]

2. Blistering Therapy

Method: With adhesive tape, fix lumps of mylabris *(bān máo)* the size of rice grains, to acupoints:

BL-13	*fèi shū*
BL-18	*gān shū*
BL-20	*pí shū*

After twelve to twenty hours, small blisters will have formed. Remove the adhesive tape and allow the blisters to be naturally reabsorbed. If signs of festering appear, apply gentian violet and cover with a sterilized gauze pad to prevent infection. This treatment method is used during the recurrence of chronic coughs.

REMARKS

In the treatment of coughs, clear distinction should first be made between external and internal types. For external coughs, the main treatment methods are to dispel evils and diffuse the lung. The early use of supplements and astringents is avoided to ensure the complete expulsion of evils. In cases of internal coughs, the emphasis of treatment is to restore to proper function to the viscera and bowels and to strengthen bodily resistance. The overuse of diaphoretics or lung-dispersing medicines should be avoided so that correct qi will not be further depleted. In cases of persistent coughing, the addition of astringents such as schisandra berry *(wǔ wèi zǐ)*, poppy husk *(mǐ ké)* and chebule *(kē zǐ)* is recommended in order to preserve lung qi and relieve coughing.

Regardless of whether patterns of coughing are external or internal, phlegm depression is common. This is from the imbalance of the ascending and descending functions of the lung. Consequently, phlegm-dissolving medicines are frequently included in prescriptions for coughs. Particularly effective in treating cough are the following herbs:

For phlegm-heat:

guā lóu	trichosanthes [fruit]	Trichosanthis Fructus	12 g.
zhè bèi mǔ	Zhejiang fritillaria [bulb]	Fritillariae Verticillatae Bulbus	9 g.
tiān zhú huáng	bamboo sugar	Bambusae Concretio Silicea	6 g.
hǎi fú shí	pumice	Pumex	9 g.
hǎi gé ké	clamshell	Cyclinae Concha (seu Meretricis)	12 g.

For phlegm-dryness:

xìng rén	apricot [kernel] (abbreviated decoction)	Armeniacae Semen	9 g.
běi shā shēn	glehnia [root]	Glehniae Radix	12 g.
zǐ wǎn	aster [root]	Asteris Radix et Rhizoma	9 g.
kuǎn dōng huā	tussilago [flower]	Tussilaginis Flos	9 g.
bǎi bù	stemona [root]	Stemonae Radix	9 g.

For phlegm-dampness:

fǎ bàn xià	processed pinellia [tuber]	Pinelliae Tuber Praeparatum	9 g.
chén pí	tangerine [peel]	Citri Exocarpium	9 g.
dǎn xīng	(bile-processed) arisaema [root]	Arisaematis Rhizoma Praeparatum	6 g.
bái jiè zǐ	white mustard [seed]	Brassicae Albae Semen	6 g.

ASTHMA

Xiào Chuăn

1. Invasion of the Lung by Wind-Cold - 2. Accumulation of Phlegm-Heat in the Lung - 3. Vacuity of the Lung - 4. Vacuity of the Kidney

Asthma, known in Chinese as *xiào chuăn*, is a frequently observed recurrent disease. *Xiào* and *chuăn* actually refer to different clinical manifestations: *xiào* patterns are characterized by short, rapid and wheezing respiration; *chuăn* patterns are characterized by labored breathing to the point that patients cannot lie flat, breathing through the mouth, raising their shoulders and flaring their nostrils during inspiration. Ancient classics state: "*Chuăn* is noted by the fashion of breathing, *xiào* is noted by the particular sound." Clinically, however, *xiào* and *chuăn* often present at the same time, and strict differentiation between the two is difficult. The two are similar in etiology, pathogenesis, differential diagnosis and treatment, and can be discussed together.

The present chapter includes the Western medical diseases of bronchial asthma, chronic asthmatic bronchitis, obstructive pulmonary emphysema and other illnesses accompanied by the symptoms of dyspnea.

ETIOLOGY AND PATHOGENESIS

Etiological factors in the pathogenesis of asthma include the six external evils, internal disruption by the seven emotions, improper diet and eating habits, stress and over-strain and extended illnesses where the physical condition is frail. Viewing *xiào* patterns separately, the main initiating factor is chronic phlegm lodged in the lung, although external evils and internal disruption are often involved in the pathogenesis.

In its initial stages, asthma is generally characterized by repletion patterns. Periodic recurrence may see its transformation into a vacuity pattern or a complex pattern of both repletion and vacuity. Pathological changes mainly appear in the lung and kidney, although the liver and spleen can also be involved.

1. INVASION OF LUNG BY WIND-COLD

Clinical Manifestations: Rapid, labored breathing, oppression in the chest, coughing and expectoration of thin white and sometimes foamy phlegm. In the early stages the accompanying symptoms often include aversion to cold, fever, headache, lack of perspiration without apparent thirst and aching joints.

Tongue: Thin white coating.

Pulse: Tight, floating.

Treatment Method: Ventilate the lung, dissipate wind-cold and calm wheezing.

PRESCRIPTION

Ephedra Decoction *má huáng tāng*

má huáng	ephedra	Ephedrae Herba	6 g.
guì zhī	cinnamon twig	Cinnamomi Ramulus	4 g.
xìng rén	apricot kernel (abbreviated decoction)	Armeniacae Semen	9 g.
zhì gān cǎo	licorice [root] (honey-fried)	Glycyrrhizae Radix	3 g.

<u>MODIFICATIONS</u>

In cases of obstruction of the lung by cold-phlegm, the prescription is modified to warm and transform cold-phlegm. Add:

fǎ bàn xià	processed pinellia [tuber]	Pinelliae Tuber Praeparatum	9 g.
chén pí	tangerine peel	Citri Exocarpium	9 g.
zǐ sū zǐ	perilla [fruit]	Perillae Fructus	9 g.
zǐ wǎn	aster [root]	Asteris Radix et Rhizoma	9 g.
bái qián	cynanchum [root]	Cynanchi Radix et Rhizoma	9 g.

In cases where perspiration has been induced without any evident relief of the asthma, the prescription is changed to regulate and harmonize construction and defense qi, diffuse the lung and calm wheezing.

Use:

Cinnamon Twig Decoction Plus Magnolia Bark and Apricot Kernel *guì zhī jiā hòu pò xìng rén tāng*

guì zhī	cinnamon twig	Cinnamomi Ramulus	9 g.
bái sháo yào	white peony [root]	Paeoniae Radix Alba	9 g.
hòu pò	magnolia bark	Magnoliae Cortex	6 g.
xìng rén	apricot kernel (abbreviated decoction)	Armeniacae Semen	6 g.
zhì gān cǎo	licorice [root] (honey-fried)	Glycyrrhizae Radix	6 g.
shēng jiāng	fresh ginger	Zingiberis Rhizoma Recens	9 g.
dà zǎo	jujube	Ziziphi Fructus	3 pc.

In cases of short rapid wheezing respiration, the prescription is changed to diffuse the the lung, transform phlegm and calm wheezing.

Use:

Belamcanda and Ephedra Decoction *shè gān má huáng tāng*

shè gān	belamcanda [root]	Belamcandae Rhizoma	6 g.
má huáng	ephedra	Ephedrae Herba	9 g.
xì xīn	asarum	Asiasari Herba cum Radice	3 g.
zǐ wǎn	aster [root]	Asteris Radix et Rhizoma	6 g.
kuǎn dōng huā	tussilago [flower]	Tussilaginis Flos	6 g.
fǎ bàn xià	pinellia [tuber] (processed)	Pinelliae Tuber Praeparatum	9 g.
wǔ wèi zǐ	schisandra [berry]	Schisandrae Fructus	3 g.
shēng jiāng	fresh ginger	Zingiberis Rhizoma Recens	9 g.
dà zǎo	jujube	Ziziphi Fructus	3 pc.

In cases of cold on the surface with internal phlegm-rheum, with expectoration of thin, clear and foamy phlegm, the prescription is changed to dispel superficial cold, transform phlegm-fluid and calm wheezing.

Use:

Minor Green-Blue Dragon Decoction *xiǎo qīng lóng tāng*

má huáng	ephedra	Ephedrae Herba	9 g.
guì zhī	cinnamon twig	Cinnamomi Ramulus	6 g.
bái sháo yào	white peony [root]	Paeoniae Radix Alba	9 g.
xì xīn	asarum	Asiasari Herba cum Radice	3 g.
gān jiāng	dried ginger [root]	Zingiberis Rhizoma Exsiccatum	6 g.
wǔ wèi zǐ	schisandra [berry]	Schisandrae Fructus	6 g.
fǎ bàn xià	pinellia [tuber] (processed)	Pinelliae Tuber Praeparatum	9 g.
zhì gān cǎo	licorice [root] (honey-fried)	Glycyrrhizae Radix	6 g.

In cases of cold on the surface complicated by internal lung heat, with symptoms of fever, aversion to cold, asthma, oppression in the chest, irritability, difficult expectoration of thick sticky phlegm, tongue coating both white and yellow in color and rapid floating pulse, the prescription is changed to dissipate cold, clear and diffuse the lung and calm wheezing. Use:

Ephedra, Apricot Kernel, Gypsum and Licorice Decoction *má xìng shí gān tāng*

má huáng	ephedra	Ephedrae Herba	6 g.
xìng rén	apricot kernel (abbreviated decoction)	Armeniacae Semen	9 g.
shí gāo	gypsum (abbreviated decoction)	Gypsum	30 g.
zhì gān cǎo	licorice [root] (honey-fried)	Glycyrrhizae Radix	6 g.

ACUPUNCTURE AND MOXIBUSTION

Main Points: Needle with draining. Moxibustion or cupping therapy may be applied to acupoints on the back.

        LU-07   *liè quē*
        LU-05   *chǐ zé*
        BL-12   *fēng mén*
        BL-13   *fèi shū*

Auxiliary points:

For stuffy nose and runny nose, add:
        ST-03   *jù liáo*
For headache and aching shoulders and back, add:
        LI-07   *wēn liū*
For fever and aversion to cold, add:
        SI-07   *zhī zhèng*
        GV-14   *dà zhuī*
        LI-04   *hé gǔ*

2. ACCUMULATION OF PHLEGM-HEAT IN THE LUNG

Clinical Manifestations: Short rapid respiration, loud husky voice, wheezing, coughing, oppression in the chest, expectoration of thick yellow phlegm, fever, perspiration, thirst with preference for cool drinks, constipation and dark urine.

Tongue: Yellow slimy coating.

Pulse: Rapid, slippery.

Treatment Method: Clear the lung, transform phlegm and calm wheezing.

PRESCRIPTION

Mulberry Root Bark Decoction *sāng bái pí tāng*

sāng bái pí	mulberry [root bark]	Mori Radicis Cortex	12 g.
fǎ bàn xià	pinellia [tuber] (processed)	Pinelliae Tuber Praeparatum	9 g.
zǐ sū zǐ	perilla [fruit]	Perillae Fructus	9 g.
xìng rén	apricot [kernel] (abbreviated decoction)	Armeniacae Semen	9 g.
zhè bèi mǔ	Zhejiang fritillaria [bulb]	Fritillariae Verticillatae Bulbus	9 g.
huáng qín	scutellaria [root]	Scutellariae Radix	9 g.
huáng lián	coptis [root]	Coptidis Rhizoma	6 g.
shān zhī zǐ	gardenia	Gardeniae Fructus	9 g.

MODIFICATIONS

In cases of fever, the prescription is modified to clear heat. Add:

shí gāo	gypsum (extended decoction)	Gypsum	30 g.
zhī mǔ	anemarrhena [root]	Anemarrhenae Rhizoma	9 g.

In cases of copious thick sticky phlegm, the prescription is modified to dispel phlegm. Add:

hǎi gé ké	clamshell	Cyclinae (seu Meretricis) Concha	12 g.
jié gěng	platycodon [root] (abbreviated decoction)	Platycodonis Radix	9 g.

In cases of thirst and dry throat, the prescription is modified to generate liquid. Add:

tiān huā fěn	trichosanthes [root]	Trichosanthis Radix	12 g.

In cases of wheezing with an inability to lie flat, copious phlegm and constipation, the prescription is modified to eliminate heat-phlegm, free the stool and calm wheezing. Add:

tíng lì zǐ	tingli [seed]	Descurainiae seu Lepidii Semen	6 g.
dà huáng	rhubarb (abbreviated decoction)	Rhei Rhizoma	6 g.
máng xiāo	mirabilite (stirred in)	Mirabilitum	9 g.

In cases where the phlegm is rust-colored and accompanied by pain in the chest, the prescription is modified to clear the lung, transform phlegm, alleviate pain and calm wheezing. Add:

yú xīng cǎo	houttuynia	Houttuyniae Herba cum Radice	15 g.
dōng guā zǐ	wax gourd [seed]	Benincasae Semen	12 g.
táo rén	peach [kernel]	Persicae Semen	6 g.
guā lóu	trichosanthes [fruit]	Trichosanthis Fructus	12 g.
yù jīn	curcuma [tuber]	Curcumae Tuber	6 g.
bái máo gēn	imperata [root]	Imperatae Rhizoma	15 g.

ACUPUNCTURE AND MOXIBUSTION

Main Points: Needle with draining.

BL-13	*fèi shū*
LU-05	*chǐ zé*
ST-40	*fēng lóng*
LI-04	*hé gǔ*
CV-22	*tiān tú*
M-BW-1b	*dìng chuǎn* (Panting Stabilizer)

3. VACUITY OF THE LUNG

Clinical Manifestations: Shortness of breath, feeble voice, weak forceless coughing and wheezing, spontaneous perspiration, sensitivity to draughts, expectoration of thin runny phlegm.

Tongue: Pale.

Pulse: Weak.

Treatment Method: Supplement the lung, boost qi and calm wheezing.

OR, THE FOLLOWING INDICATIONS:

Clinical Manifestations: Choking cough with scanty sticky phlegm, dry mouth, irritability, discomfort of the throat.

Tongue: Red with peeling coating.

Pulse: Rapid, thready.

Treatment Method: Supplement the lung, boost qi, nourish yin and calm wheezing.

PRESCRIPTION

Modified combination of Pulse-Engendering Beverage *(shēng mài yǐn)* and Lung-Supplementing Decoction *(bǔ fèi tāng)*.

Pulse-Engendering Beverage *shēng mài yǐn*

rén shēn	ginseng	Ginseng Radix	9 g.
mài mén dōng	ophiopogon [tuber]	Ophiopogonis Tuber	15 g.
wǔ wèi zǐ	schisandra [berry]	Schisandrae Fructus	6 g.

with:

Lung-Supplementing Decoction *bǔ fèi tāng*

rén shēn	ginseng	Ginseng Radix	9 g.
huáng qí	astragalus [root]	Astragali (seu Hedysari) Radix	12 g.
shú dì huáng	cooked rehmannia [root]	Rehmanniae Radix Conquita	9 g.
wǔ wèi zǐ	schisandra [berry]	Schisandrae Fructus	6 g.
zǐ wǎn	aster [root]	Asteris Radix et Rhizoma	6 g.
sāng bái pí	mulberry [root bark]	Mori Radicis Cortex	6 g.

MODIFICATIONS

In cases where vacuity of lung qi is predominant, the prescription is modified to supplement qi. Add:

shān yào	dioscorea [root]	Dioscoreae Rhizoma	30 g.
zhì gān cǎo	licorice [root] (honey-fried)	Glycyrrhizae Radix	9 g.

In cases where vacuity of lung yin is predominant, the prescription is modified to nourish yin. Add:

běi shā shēn	glehnia [root]	Glehniae Radix	12 g.
chuān bèi mǔ	Sichuan fritillaria [bulb]	Fritillariae Cirrhosae Bulbus	9 g.
huáng jīng	polygonatum [root]	Polygonati Rhizoma	12 g.

ACUPUNCTURE AND MOXIBUSTION

Main Points: Needle with supplementation and moxibustion.

M-BW-1b	*dìng chuǎn* (Panting Stabilizer)
BL-13	*fèi shū*
BL-43 (38)	*gāo huāng shū*
LU-09	*tài yuān*

Auxiliary points:
For vacuity of lung and spleen qi, add:

BL-20	*pí shū*
ST-36	*zú sān lǐ*

4. VACUITY OF THE KIDNEY

Clinical Manifestations: Persistent wheezing aggravated by physical exertion, shallow inspiration, shortness of breath, difficulty in maintaining regular rhythm of respiration, fatigue, lassitude, physical cold, cold extremities and greenish complexion.

Tongue: Pale.

Pulse: Deep, weak, thready.

Treatment Method: Supplement the kidney to and absorb qi.

PRESCRIPTION

Golden Coffer Kidney Qi Pill *jīn guì shèn qì wán*:

shú dì huáng	cooked rehmannia [root]	Rehmanniae Radix	24 g.
shān yào	dioscorea [root]	Dioscoreae Rhizoma	12 g.
shān zhū yú	cornus [fruit]	Corni Fructus	12 g.
zé xiè	alisma [tuber]	Alismatis Rhizoma	9 g.
fú líng	poria	Poria	9 g.
mǔ dān pí	moutan [root bark]	Moutan Radicis Cortex	9 g.
zhì fù zǐ	aconite [accessory tuber] (processed) (extended decoction)	Aconiti Tuber Laterale Praeparatum	3 g.
ròu guì	cinnamon bark (abbreviated decoction)	Cinnamomi Cortex	3 g.

MODIFICATIONS

In cases of swollen feet and retention of urine, the prescription is modified to disinhibit water and dampness. Add:

niú xī	achyranthes [root]	Achyranthis Bidentatae Radix	12 g.
chē qián zǐ	plantago [seed] (wrapped)	Plantaginis Semen	9 g.

In severe cases of vacuity asthma, the prescription is modified to supplement lung qi and absorb kidney qi. Add:

rén shēn	ginseng	Ginseng Radix	9 g.
wǔ wèi zǐ	schisandra [berry]	Schisandrae Fructus	6 g.
hú táo rén	walnut [kernel]	Juglandis Semen	30 g.
bǔ gǔ zhī	psoralea [seed]	Psoraleae Semen	9 g.
gé jiè	gecko	Gekko	6 g.

(or, powdered and administered separately, 1.5 g. each time)

In cases where vacuous kidney yin is predominant, with symptoms of dry mouth and throat, red complexion, red tongue and thready rapid pulse, the condition is failure of yin to check yang and failure of the kidney to govern qi. The prescription is adjusted. Delete:

zhì fù zǐ	aconite [accessory tuber] (processed)	Aconiti Tuber Laterale Praeparatum
ròu guì	cinnamon bark	Cinnamomi Cortex

Use the modified formula in conjunction with:

Pulse-Engendering Beverage *shēng mài yǐn*

rén shēn	ginseng	Ginseng Radix	9 g.
mài mén dōng	ophiopogon [tuber]	Ophiopogonis Tuber	15 g.
wǔ wèi zǐ	schisandra [berry]	Schisandrae Fructus	6 g.

In cases of congestion of the lung by phlegm-turbidity (repletion above) coupled with kidney vacuity (vacuity below), the prescription is changed to transform phlegm, downbear qi, warm the kidney and calm wheezing. Use:

Perilla Fruit Qi-Downbearing Decoction *sū zǐ jiàng qì tāng*

zǐ sū zǐ	perilla [fruit]	Perillae Fructus	9 g.
fǎ bàn xià	pinellia [tuber] (processed)	Pinelliae Tuber Praeparatum	9 g.
chén pí	tangerine peel	Citri Exocarpium	6 g.
dāng guī	tangkuei	Angelicae Sinensis Radix	6 g.
qián hú	peucedanum [root]	Peucedani Radix	6 g.
hòu pò	magnolia [bark]	Magnoliae Cortex	6 g.
ròu guì	cinnamon [bark] (abbreviated decoction)	Cinnamomi Cortex	3 g.
zhì gān cǎo	licorice [root] (honey-fried)	Glycyrrhizae Radix	6 g.

plus:

zǐ sū yè	perilla leaf (abbreviated decoction)	Perillae Folium	2 g.
shēng jiāng	fresh ginger	Zingiberis Rhizoma Recens	2 pc.
dà zǎo	jujube	Ziziphi Fructus	3 pc.

In cases of vacuous yang with phlegm depression affecting the heart and lung, with symptoms of asthma, coughing, palpitations, edema of the extremities, scanty urine, pale swollen tongue and deep thready pulse, the prescription is changed to warm the kidney, boost qi, move phlegm-rheum and calm wheezing. Use:

True Warrior Decoction *zhēn wǔ tāng*

zhì fù zǐ	aconite [accessory tuber] (processed) (extended decoction)	Aconiti Tuber Laterale Praeparatum	9 g.
fú líng	poria	Poria	9 g.
bái sháo yào	white peony [root]	Paeoniae Radix Alba	9 g.
bái zhú	ovate atractylodes [root]	Atractylodis Ovatae Rhizoma	6 g.
shēng jiāng	fresh ginger	Zingiberis Rhizoma Recens	9 g.

plus:

guì zhī	cinnamon [twig]	Cinnamomi Ramulus	9 g.
huáng qí	astragalus [root]	Astragali (seu Hedysari) Radix	15 g.
fáng jǐ	fangji [root]	Fangji Radix	9 g.
tíng lì zǐ	tingli [seed]	Descurainiae seu Lepidii Semen	6 g.

In cases of insufficiency of heart yang and static blood obstruction with symptoms of greenish-purplish lips, tongue and nails and intermittent pulse, the prescription is modified to quicken the blood and transform stasis. Add:

dān shēn	salvia [root]	Salviae Miltiorrhizae Radix	12 g.
chuān xiōng	ligusticum [root]	Ligustici Rhizoma	9 g.
chì sháo yào	red peony [root]	Paeoniae Radix Rubra	9 g.
hóng huā	carthamus [flower]	Carthami Flos	6 g.

ACUPUNCTURE AND MOXIBUSTION

Main Points: Needle with supplementation and moxibustion.

BL-23	*shèn shū*
KI-03	*tài xī*
BL-13	*fèi shū*
CV-17	*tǎn zhōng*
CV-06	*qì hǎi*
M-BW-1b	*dìng chuǎn* (Panting Stabilizer)

Auxiliary points:

For persistent asthma, add:

GV-12	*shēn zhù*
BL-43	*gāo huāng shū*

For spleen vacuity, add:

CV-12	*zhōng wǎn*
BL-20	*pí shū*

For vacuity of lung qi and heart yang, with symptoms of desertion, add:

PC-06	*nèi guān*
HT-07	*shén mén*

Apply moxibustion to:

CV-06	*qì hǎi*
CV-04	*guān yuán*
GV-04	*mìng mén*

ALTERNATE THERAPEUTIC METHODS

1. Ear Acupuncture

Main Points: Asthma point, Adrenal, Trachea, Subcortex, Sympathetic.

Method: Choose two to three points each session. Needle to elicit a strong sensation and retain needles five to ten minutes. Treat once daily, ten sessions composing one therapeutic course.

2. Plum-Blossom Needle Therapy

Location: Thenar eminence, forearm and regions along the course of the lung channel and bilaterally over the sternocleidomastoid muscles.

Method: The above regions are tapped lightly in the order given with a plum-blossom needle for fifteen minutes, until the skin is slightly red. The use of this method during asthmatic attacks can decrease their severity.

REMARKS

Differentiating between vacuity and repletion is the key factor in the treatment of asthma. Acute conditions are generally presented as repletion patterns; treatment is aimed at expelling evils from the lung and promoting respiration. In vacuity patterns, on the other hand, the conditions are generally less acute; symptoms are at times mild, at times severe and aggravated by physical exertion. During treatment, emphasis is on supplementation of the lung, spleen and kidney.

Clear differentiation between primary and secondary, acute and chronic, must be made in patterns complicated by both repletion and vacuity. During remissions from asthma, treatment should be aimed at the root of the disease to supplement and boost qi and essence. During asthmatic attacks when evils are replete, treatment should be aimed at dispelling these evils. In frail patients or those suffering from extended illnesses, both root and branch should be treated simultaneously.

STOMACH PAIN

Wèi Tòng

1. Settling of Cold Evil in the Stomach - 2. Obstruction by Food Stagnation - 3. Disruption of the Stomach by Liver Qi - 4. Accumulation of Heat in the Liver and Stomach - 5. Obstruction of the Stomach by Static Blood - 6. Depletion of Stomach Yin - 7. Vacuity-Cold of the Spleen and Stomach

Stomach pain, known in Chinese as *wèi tòng* or *wèi wǎn tòng,* manifests frequent painful sensations in the epigastrium as its major symptom. Patterns of stomach pain are often those Western medicine labels as acute and chronic gastritis, gastric and duodenal ulcers, gastric cancer and gastric neurosis.

ETIOLOGY AND PATHOGENESIS

The etiology of epigastric pain involves both repletion and vacuity. Repletion patterns include invasion of cold evil, obstruction by food stasis, stagnation of qi, accumulation of heat and blood stasis. Vacuity patterns include depletion of stomach yin and vacuity-cold of the spleen and stomach. Patterns complicated by both heat and cold, or both repletion and vacuity, are also frequently observed clinically.

Stomach pain is intimately related to the functions of the liver and spleen. Pathogenesis of stomach pain initially involves qi; as time progresses, blood becomes involved to a greater extent. Pathological changes involving qi cause relatively mild conditions, while those involving blood can cause more severe conditions. Although the etiology of stomach pain can be complex, "hindered passage gives rise to pain" (that is, stagnation of qi and/or stasis of blood) is considered the common factor. The different etiological factors influence only the characteristics and degree of pain.

1. SETTLING OF COLD EVIL IN THE STOMACH

Clinical Manifestations: Abrupt onset of epigastric pain, aggravation of pain by cold and alleviation by warmth, aversion to cold, no apparent thirst.

Tongue: White coating.

Pulse: Tight, wiry.

Treatment Method: Dissipate cold, relieve pain.

PRESCRIPTION

Lesser Galangal and Cyperus Pill *liáng fù wán*

gāo liáng jiāng	lesser galangal [root]	Alpiniae Officinarum Rhizoma	12 g.
xiāng fù zǐ	cyperus [root]	Cyperi Rhizoma	12 g.

Modifications

In cases where cold evil is severe, the prescription is modified to strengthen the cold-dispersing and qi-regulating effects.

Add:

wú zhū yú	evodia [fruit]	Evodiae Fructus	6 g.
chén pí	tangerine peel	Citri Exocarpium	9 g.

In cases manifesting chills and fever, headache, floating pulse and stomach pain caused by wind-cold, the given prescription is reinforced to rectify qi, resolve the exterior and relieve pain.

Add:

Cyperus and Perilla Powder *xiāng sū săn*

xiāng fù zĭ	cyperus [root]	Cyperi Rhizoma	9 g.
zĭ sū yè	perilla [leaf]	Perillae Folium	9 g.
chén pí	tangerine peel	Citri Exocarpium	6 g.
zhì gān căo	licorice [root] (honey-fried)	Glycyrrhizae Radix	3 g.

In cases where cold has brought about food accumulation and stagnation, with symptoms including oppression in the chest and epigastrium, loss of appetite, belching and vomiting, the prescription is modified to warm the stomach, disperse food, remove obstruction and relieve pain.

Add:

zhĭ shí	unripe bitter orange	Aurantii Fructus Immaturus	6 g.
shén qū	medicated leaven	Massa Medicata Fermentata	12 g.
jī nèi jīn	gizzard lining	Galli Gigerii Endothelium	9 g.
	(or: 3 g. powdered and stirred in)		
jiāng bàn xià	(ginger-processed) pinellia [tuber]	Pinelliae Tuber Praeparatum	9 g.
shēng jiāng	fresh ginger	Zingiberis Rhizoma Recens	9 g.

ACUPUNCTURE AND MOXIBUSTION

Main Points: Needle with draining; add moxibustion.

CV-12	*zhōng wăn*
ST-36	*zú sān lĭ*
PC-06	*nèi guān*
SP-04	*gōng sūn*

Auxiliary points:

For severe epigastric pain, add:

ST-34	*liáng qiū*

2. OBSTRUCTION BY FOOD STASIS

Clinical Manifestations: Stomach pain aggravated by the application of external pressure, eructation of foul gas, acid regurgitation, distention and fullness of the epigastrium and abdomen, decrease in pain after vomiting or expelling flatus, and, in some cases, vomiting of undigested food or difficult bowel movements.

Tongue: Thick slimy coating.

Pulse: Slippery.

Treatment Method: Disperse food, abduct stagnation, relieve pain.

PRESCRIPTION

Harmony-Preserving Pill *bǎo hé wán*

shān zhā	crataegus [fruit]	Crataegi Fructus	18 g.
shén qū	medicated leaven	Massa Medicata Fermentata	6 g.
jiāng bàn xià	(ginger-processed) pinellia [tuber]	Pinelliae Tuber Praeparatum	9 g.
fú líng	poria	Poria	9 g.
chén pí	tangerine peel	Citri Exocarpium	3 g.
lián qiào	forsythia [fruit]	Forsythiae Fructus	3 g.
lái fú zǐ	radish [seed]	Raphani Semen	3 g.

MODIFICATIONS

In cases of severe distention of the epigastrium and abdomen, the prescription is modified to move qi and abduct stagnation.

zhǐ shí	unripe bitter orange	Aurantii Fructus Immaturus	9 g.
shā rén	amomum [fruit] (abbreviated decoction)	Amomi Semen seu Fructus	6 g.
bīng láng	areca [nut]	Arecae Semen	9 g.

In cases where the preceding prescription fails to achieve therapeutic effects, and the patient shows symptoms of constipation as well as epigastric pain and distention, the given prescription is used in conjunction with Minor Qi-Infusing Decoction *(xiǎo chéng qì tāng)* to free the stool and move qi.

Minor Qi-Infusing Decoction *xiǎo chéng qì tāng*

dà huáng	rhubarb (abbreviated decoction)	Rhei Rhizoma	12 g.
zhǐ shí	unripe bitter orange	Aurantii Fructus Immaturus	9 g.
hòu pò	magnolia [bark]	Magnoliae Cortex	6 g.

Add:

mù xiāng	saussurea [root]	Saussureae (seu Vladimiriae) Radix	9 g.
xiāng fù zǐ	cyperus [root]	Cyperi Rhizoma	9 g.

In cases of severe stomach pain increased by pressure, accompanied by dry, yellow tongue coat and constipation, the pattern is food accumulation and stagnation giving rise to heat and dryness. The given prescription is used in conjunction with Major Qi-Infusing Decoction *(dà chéng qì tāng)* to drain heat, break up dryness, free the stool and abduct stagnation.

Major Qi-Infusing Decoction *dà chéng qì tāng*

dà huáng	rhubarb (abbreviated decoction)	Rhei Rhizoma	12 g.
máng xiāo	mirabilite (stirred in)	Mirabilitum	9 g.
zhǐ shí	unripe bitter orange	Aurantii Fructus Immaturus	12 g.
hòu pò	magnolia [bark]	Magnoliae Cortex	12 g.

ACUPUNCTURE AND MOXIBUSTION

Main Points: Needle with draining.

CV-11	*jiàn lǐ*
PC-06	*nèi guān*
ST-36	*zú sān lǐ*
M-LE-1	*lǐ nèi tíng* (Li Inner Court)

3. Disruption of the Stomach by Liver Qi

Clinical Manifestations: Epigastric distention and pain spreading through the costal regions, belching, acid regurgitation, difficult bowel movements. The onset of pain is associated with emotional stress.

Tongue: White coating.

Pulse: Wiry.

Treatment Method: Soothe the liver, rectify qi, harmonize the stomach, relieve pain.

PRESCRIPTION
Bupleurum Liver-Coursing Powder *chái hú shū gān sǎn*

chái hú	bupleurum [root]	Bupleuri Radix	6 g.
bái sháo yào	white peony [root]	Paeoniae Radix Alba	9 g.
xiāng fù zǐ	cyperus [root]	Cyperi Rhizoma	6 g.
chuān xiōng	ligusticum [root]	Ligustici Rhizoma	6 g.
chén pí	tangerine peel	Citri Exocarpium	6 g.
zhǐ ké	bitter orange	Aurantii Fructus	6 g.
gān cǎo	licorice [root]	Glycyrrhizae Radix	3 g.

MODIFICATIONS

In cases with severe pain, the prescription is modified to increase the qi-regulating and pain-relieving effects. Add:

chuān liàn zǐ	toosendan [fruit]	Toosendan Fructus	9 g.
yán hú suǒ	corydalis [tuber]	Corydalis Tuber	9 g.

In cases of frequent belching, the prescription is modified to redirect qi downward. Add:

chén xiāng	aquilaria [wood] (powdered and stirred in)	Aquilariae Lignum	1.5 g.
xuán fù huā	inula flower (wrapped)	Inulae Flos	6 g.

ACUPUNCTURE AND MOXIBUSTION

Main Points: Needle with draining:

LR-14	*qī mén*
CV-12	*zhōng wǎn*
PC-06	*nèi guān*
ST-36	*zú sān lǐ*
LR-03	*tài chōng*
GB-34	*yáng líng quán*

4. Accumulation of Heat in the Liver and Stomach

Clinical Manifestations: Acute, burning pain in the epigastrium, irritability, acid regurgitation, clamoring stomach, dry bitter taste in the mouth.

Tongue: Red with yellow coating.

Pulse: Wiry, rapid.

Treatment Method: Soothe the liver, clear heat, harmonize the stomach, relieve pain.

PRESCRIPTION

Liver-Transforming Brew *huà gān jiān*

mǔ dān pí	moutan [root bark]	Moutan Radicis Cortex	9 g.
shān zhī zǐ	gardenia	Gardeniae Fructus	9 g.
bái sháo yào	white peony [root]	Paeoniae Radix Alba	15 g.
qīng pí	unripe tangerine peel	Citri Exocarpium Immaturum	6 g.
chén pí	tangerine peel	Citri Exocarpium	6 g.
zé xiè	alisma [tuber]	Alismatis Rhizoma	6 g.
chuān bèi mǔ	Sichuan fritillaria [bulb]	Fritillariae Cirrhosae Bulbus	6 g.

Use in conjunction with:

Evodia and Coptis Pill (Left Metal Pill) *yú lián wán (zuǒ jīn wán)*

wú zhū yú	evodia [fruit]	Evodiae Fructus	30 g.
huáng lián	coptis [root]	Coptidis Rhizoma	180 g.

Grind the above ingredients into a powder and form pills. Take two to three gram doses twice daily with water. The two herbs may also be decocted in water, the proportion of coptis *(huáng lián)* to evodia *(wú zhū yú)* should be 6:1.

Emphasis is on the cold bitterness of *huáng lián* to clear heat. A small dose of *wú zhū yú* is used as an adjutant, having pungent dispersing properties that aid *huáng lián* in clearing heat.

Pungent drying herbal medicines can deplete yin fluids and should be used prudently in treating stomach pain of this type. If required, certain medicinals may be added to the set prescription to resolve depression and relieve pain without yin-depleting side effects. Choose from:

fó shǒu gān	Buddha's hand [fruit]	Citri Sarcodactylidis Fructus	6 g.
méi guī huā	rose	Rosae Flos	6 g.
yù jīn	curcuma [tuber]	Curcumae Tuber	9 g.

ACUPUNCTURE AND MOXIBUSTION

Main Points: Needle with draining.

CV-12	*zhōng wǎn*
ST-36	*zú sān lǐ*
PC-06	*nèi guān*
LR-02	*xíng jiān*
ST-34	*liáng qiū*
ST-44	*nèi tíng*

Auxiliary points:

In cases of acid regurgitation and clamoring stomach, add:

CV-10	*xià wǎn*
CV-11	*jiàn lǐ*

5. OBSTRUCTION OF THE STOMACH BY STATIC BLOOD

Clinical Manifestations: Stabbing stomach pain of fixed location, an increase of pain with external pressure, vomiting blood or black stools in some cases.

Tongue: Dark, purplish.

Pulse: Rough, thready.

Treatment Method: Quicken the blood, abduct stagnation, rectify qi, relieve pain.

PRESCRIPTION

Combine Sudden Smile Powder *(shī xiào sǎn)* with Salvia Beverage *(dān shēn yǐn)*.

Sudden Smile Powder *shī xiào sǎn*

wǔ líng zhī	flying squirrel droppings (wrapped)	Trogopteri seu Pteromydis Excrementum	9 g.
pú huáng	typha pollen (wrapped)	Typhae Pollen	9 g.

with:

Salvia Beverage *dān shēn yǐn*

dān shēn	salvia [root]	Salviae Miltiorrhizae Radix	30 g.
tán xiāng	sandalwood	Santali Lignum	6 g.
shā rén	amomum [fruit] (abbreviated decoction)	Amomi Semen seu Fructus	6 g.

MODIFICATIONS

In cases of vomiting blood or bloody stools, the prescription is modified to dispel stasis and relieve bleeding. Add:

sān qī	notoginseng [root] (or: 1.5 g. powder administered separately)	Notoginseng Radix	9 g.
bái jí	bletilla [tuber]	Bletillae Tuber	9 g.
dì yú	sanguisorba [root]	Sanguisorbae Radix	9 g.

In cases of vacuity-cold of the spleen and stomach with failure of the spleen to secure the blood, with symptoms of vomiting blood, black stools, sallow complexion, lack of warmth of the limbs, pale tongue and weak forceless pulse, the prescription is changed to warm the spleen and promote its ability to contain the blood.

Use:

Yellow Earth Decoction *huáng tǔ tāng*

fú lóng gān	oven earth (wrapped, extended decoction: decoct first, then discard and boil remaining herbs in its broth)	Terra Flava Usta	30 g.
shēng dì huáng	rehmannia [root] (dried)	Rehmanniae Radix	9 g.
bái zhú	ovate atractylodes [root]	Atractylodis Ovatae Rhizoma	9 g.
zhì fù zǐ	aconite [accessory tuber] (processed) (extended decoction)	Aconiti Tuber Laterale Praeparatum	9 g.
ē jiāo	ass hide glue (dissolved and stirred in)	Asini Corii Gelatinum	9 g.
huáng qín	scutellaria [root]	Scutellariae Radix	9 g.
gān cǎo	licorice [root]	Glycyrrhizae Radix	9 g.

In cases of vacuous yin with blood heat, symptoms include bleeding accompanied by dry mouth and throat, red tongue with little coating and rapid thready pulse. The prescription is modified to moisten yin, cool the blood and relieve bleeding. Add:

běi shā shēn	glehnia [root]	Glehniae Radix	12 g.
shēng dì huáng	rehmannia [root] dried/fresh	Rehmanniae Radix Exsiccata seu Recens	12 g.
mǔ dān pí	moutan [root bark]	Moutan Radicis Cortex	9 g.
ē jiāo	ass hide glue (dissolved and stirred in)	Asini Corii Gelatinum	9 g.
mài mén dōng	ophiopogon [tuber]	Ophiopogonis Tuber	12 g.

In cases of chronic bleeding giving rise to palpitations, shortness of breath, frequent dreaming, diminished sleep, fatigue, reduced food intake, pale lips and tongue and weak pulse, the prescription is changed to boost qi and nourish the blood. Use:

Spleen-Returning Decoction *guī pí tāng*

huáng qí	astragalus [root]	Astragali (seu Hedysari) Radix	9 g.
rén shēn	ginseng	Ginseng Radix	9 g.
bái zhú	ovate atractylodes [root]	Atractylodis Ovatae Rhizoma	9 g.
fú shén	root poria	Poria cum Pini Radice	9 g.
lóng yǎn ròu	longan flesh	Longanae Arillus	9 g.
suān zǎo rén	spiny jujube [kernel]	Ziziphi Spinosi Semen	9 g.
mù xiāng	saussurea [root]	Saussureae Radix (seu Vladimiriae)	6 g.
dāng guī	tangkuei	Angelicae Sinensis Radix	6 g.
yuǎn zhì	polygala [root]	Polygalae Radix	3 g.
zhì gān cǎo	licorice [root] (honey-fried)	Glycyrrhizae Radix	6 g.
shēng jiāng	fresh ginger	Zingiberis Rhizoma Recens	3 g.
dà zǎo	jujube	Ziziphi Fructus	5 pc.

ACUPUNCTURE AND MOXIBUSTION

Main Points: Needle with draining.

CV-12	*zhōng wǎn*
ST-36	*zú sān lǐ*
PC-06	*nèi guān*
SP-04	*gōng sūn*
ST-21	*liáng mén*
ST-34	*liáng qiū*

Auxiliary points:

In cases of vomiting blood or bloody stools, add:

BL-17	*gé shū*
PC-04	*xī mén*
SP-01	*yǐn bái*

6. DEPLETION OF STOMACH YIN

Clinical Manifestations: Dull indistinct epigastric pain, dry mouth and throat, hard dry stools.

Tongue: Red, lacking moisture.

Pulse: Rapid, thready.

Treatment Method: Nourish yin, boost the stomach, relieve pain.

PRESCRIPTION

Combine All-the-Way-Through Brew (*yī guàn jiān*) with Peony and Licorice Decoction (*sháo yào gān cǎo tāng*).

All-the-Way-Through Brew *yī guàn jiān*

běi shā shēn	glehnia [root]	Glehniae Radix	9 g.
mài mén dōng	ophiopogon [tuber]	Ophiopogonis Tuber	9 g.
dāng guī	tangkuei	Angelicae Sinensis Radix	9 g.
shēng dì huáng	rehmannia [root] dried/fresh	Rehmanniae Radix Exsiccata seu Recens	30 g.
gǒu qǐ zǐ	lycium [berry]	Lycii Fructus	12 g.
chuān liàn zǐ	toosendan [fruit]	Toosendan Fructus	4.5 g.

with:

Peony and Licorice Decoction *sháo yào gān cǎo tāng*

| *bái sháo yào* | white peony [root] | Paeoniae Radix Alba | 18 g. |
| *zhì gān cǎo* | licorice [root] (honey-fried) | Glycyrrhizae Radix | 6 g. |

<u>MODIFICATIONS</u>

In cases manifesting burning epigastric pain, clamoring stomach and acid regurgitation, the prescription is adjusted to clear heat and control stomach acid. Add:

Evodia and Coptis Pill (Left Metal Pill) *yú lián wán (zuǒ jīn wán)*

| *wú zhū yú* | evodia [fruit] | Evodiae Fructus | 30 g. |
| *huáng lián* | coptis [root] | Coptidis Rhizoma | 180 g. |

Grind the above ingredients into a powder and form pills. Take a two to three gram dose twice daily with water. The two herbs can also be decocted in water, with the proportion of coptis *(huáng lián)* to evodia *(wú zhū yú)*, being 6:1.

In cases of reduced food intake, the prescription is modified to strengthen spleen function.

Delete:

| *mài mén dōng* | ophiopogon [tuber] | Ophiopogonis Tuber. |

Add:

| *shān yào* | dioscorea [root] | Dioscoreae Rhizoma | 15 g. |
| *bái zhú* | ovate atractylodes [root] | Atractylodis Ovatae Rhizoma | 9 g. |

In cases of vacuous yin and blood where the stools are hard and dry, the prescription is modified to nourish the blood and moisten the intestines. Add:

hé shǒu wū	flowery knotweed [root]	Polygoni Multiflori Radix	12 g.
bǎi zǐ rén	biota [seed]	Biotae Semen	12 g.
huǒ má rén	hemp [seed]	Cannabis Semen	12 g.

ACUPUNCTURE AND MOXIBUSTION

Main Points: Needle with supplementation.

BL-20	*pí shū*
BL-21	*wèi shū*
CV-12	*zhōng wǎn*
ST-36	*zú sān lǐ*
SP-06	*sān yīn jiāo*
KI-03	*tài xī*

7. VACUITY-COLD OF THE SPLEEN AND STOMACH

Clinical Manifestations: Dull indistinct stomach pain, decrease in pain with application of external pressure or warmth, increase in pain when the stomach is empty and a decrease after food intake, regurgitation of clear fluids, reduced food intake, tiredness, fatigue, lack of warmth of the extremities (in severe cases) and loose stools.

Tongue: Pale with white coating.

Pulse: Slow, weak.

Treatment Method: Warm and supplement the spleen and stomach, relieve pain.

PRESCRIPTION

Astragalus Center-Fortifying Decoction *huáng qí jiàn zhōng tāng*

huáng qí	astragalus [root]	Astragali (seu Hedysari) Radix	9 g.
bái sháo yào	white peony [root]	Paeoniae Radix Alba	18 g.
guì zhī	cinnamon twig	Cinnamomi Ramulus	9 g.
zhì gān cǎo	licorice [root] (honey-fried)	Glycyrrhizae Radix	6 g.
shēng jiāng	fresh ginger	Zingiberis Rhizoma Recens	9 g.
dà zǎo	jujube	Ziziphi Fructus	4 pc.
yí táng	malt sugar (stirred in)	Granorum Saccharon	30 g.

MODIFICATIONS

In cases of acid regurgitation, the prescription is modified to control stomach acid. Delete or decrease the dose of:

yí táng	malt sugar	Granorum Saccharon

Add:

wú zhū yú	evodia [fruit]	Evodiae Fructus	4.5 g.
wǎ léng zǐ	ark shell	Arcae Concha Calcinatum	15 g.
	(calcined, with extended decoction; or: 3 g. powder administered separately)		

In cases of regurgitation of relatively large amounts of clear fluids, the prescription is modified to warm the stomach and transform rheum. Add:

gān jiāng	dried ginger [root]	Zingiberis Rhizoma Exsiccatum	6 g.
chén pí	tangerine peel	Citri Exocarpium	6 g.
jiāng bàn xià	(ginger-processed) pinellia [tuber]	Pinelliae Tuber Praeparatum	9 g.
fú líng	poria	Poria	12 g.

In cases accompanied by poor food intake, eructation of foul gas and thick slimy tongue coating, the prescription is modified to disperse food and dissolve obstruction. Add:

zhǐ shí	unripe bitter orange	Aurantii Fructus Immaturus	9 g.
hòu pò	magnolia bark	Magnoliae Cortex	9 g.
shén qū	medicated leaven	Massa Medicata Fermentata	12 g.
mài yá	barley sprout	Hordei Fructus Germinatus	12 g.

During attacks of epigastric pain, the given prescription may be used in conjunction with:

Lesser Galangal and Cyperus Pill *liáng fù wán*

gāo liáng jiāng	lesser galangal [root]	Alpiniae Officinarum Rhizoma	12 g.
xiāng fù zǐ	cyperus [root]	Cyperi Rhizoma	12 g.

In cases exhibiting bleeding and black stools, the prescription is changed to warm the middle burner and relieve bleeding. Use:

Yellow Earth Decoction *huáng tǔ tāng*

fú lóng gān	oven earth	Terra Flava Usta	30 g.
	(wrapped, extended decoction; decoct first and discard then boil remaining herbs in the broth)		
shú dì huáng	cooked rehmannia [root]	Rehmanniae Radix Conquita	9 g.
bái zhú	ovate atractylodes [root]	Atractylodis Ovatae Rhizoma	9 g.
zhì fù zǐ	aconite [accessory tuber]	Aconiti Tuber Laterale Praeparatum	9 g.
	(processed) (extended decoction)		

ē jiāo	ass hide glue (dissolved and stirred in)	Asini Corii Gelatinum	9 g.
huáng qín	scutellaria [root]	Scutellariae Radix	9 g.
gān cǎo	licorice [root]	Glycyrrhizae Radix	9 g.

In cases where cold is severe with acute pain and cold extremities, the prescription is changed to support yang and dissipate cold. Use:

Major Center-Fortifying Decoction *dà jiàn zhōng tāng*

huā jiāo	zanthoxylum [husk]	Zanthoxyli Pericarpium	6 g.
gān jiāng	dried ginger [root]	Zingiberis Rhizoma Exsiccatum	9 g.
rén shēn	ginseng	Ginseng Radix	9 g.
yí táng	malt sugar (stirred in)	Granorum Saccharon	50 g.

In cases with loose stools, the prescription is changed to warm and supplement the spleen. Use:

Aconite Center-Rectifying Decoction *fù zǐ lǐ zhōng tāng*

zhì fù zǐ	aconite [accessory tuber] (processed) (extended decoction)	Aconiti Tuber Laterale Praeparatum	6 g.
rén shēn	ginseng	Ginseng Radix	9 g.
bái zhú	ovate atractylodes [root]	Atractylodis Ovatae Rhizoma	9 g.
gān jiāng	dried ginger [root]	Zingiberis Rhizoma Exsiccatum	6 g.
zhì gān cǎo	licorice [root] (honey fried)	Glycyrrhizae Radix	6 g.

After alleviation of stomach pain, the following prescription may be used during recuperation:

Saussurea and Amomum Six Gentlemen Decoction *xiān shā liù jūn zǐ tāng*

rén shēn	ginseng	Ginseng Radix	9 g.
bái zhú	ovate atractylodes [root]	Atractylodis Ovatae Rhizoma	9 g.
fú líng	poria	Poria	9 g.
mù xiāng	saussurea [root]	Saussureae Radix (seu Vladimiriae)	6 g.
shā rén	amomum [fruit] (abbreviated decoction)	Amomi Semen seu Fructus	6 g.
zhì gān cǎo	licorice [root] (honey fried)	Glycyrrhizae Radix	6 g.
chén pí	tangerine peel	Citri Exocarpium	6 g.
jiāng bàn xià	(ginger-processed) pinellia [tuber]	Pinelliae Tuber Praeparatum	6 g.

ACUPUNCTURE AND MOXIBUSTION:

Main Points: Needle with supplementation; add moxibustion.

BL-20	*pí shū*
BL-21	*wèi shū*
CV-12	*zhōng wǎn*
CV-06	*qì hǎi*
ST-36	*zú sān lǐ*
PC-06	*nèi guān*
SP-04	*gōng sūn*

Auxiliary points:

For vomiting blood or bloody stools, add:

| BL-17 | *gé shū* |
| SP-03 | *tài bái* |

ALTERNATE THERAPEUTIC METHODS

1. Ear Acupuncture

Main Points: Spleen, Stomach, Liver, Sympathetic, *Shén Mén,* Subcortex.

Method: Choose two or three points per session. In cases of severe pain, needle to elicit a strong sensation, while in cases of mild pain, needle to elicit a mild sensation. Treat once daily or once every other day, ten sessions making one course of treatment.

2. Cupping Therapy

Method: Use large or medium-sized cups and apply to the upper abdomen and associated-shu points for ten to fifteen minutes.

REMARKS

Elimination of evils is the focus in treating repletion patterns of stomach pain; in treating vacuity patterns, the support of correct qi is foremost. In cases complicated by both repletion and vacuity, conjunctive methods of draining and supplementation are used.

Emphasis should be on the patient's emotional state and diet during treatment. The patient should be encouraged to avoid emotional stress, particularly during and immediately following meals. Also, it is best to eat small servings at an increased number of meals, and to avoid alcohol and spicy foods.

HICCOUGH

È Nì

1. Stomach Cold - 2. Effulgent Stomach Fire - 3. Liver Qi Stagnation - 4. Spleen and Stomach Yang Vacuity - 5. Stomach Yin Vacuity

Hiccough, known in Chinese as *è nì,* or *yuē* in certain ancient medical classics, is characterized by the counterflow of qi, resulting in the production of short spasmodic involuntary "hiccup" sounds. Hiccough may occur as an isolated dysfunction, where symptoms are mild, of short duration and cease spontaneously. Hiccough may also occur during the course of other acute and chronic disorders, and is marked by more severe symptoms that occur periodically, or persist continuously day and night without relief.

ETIOLOGY AND PATHOGENESIS

The major etiological factor causing hiccough is the stomach qi counterflow. The stomach is situated in the middle burner, connected to the diaphragm and thorax above, sending food through and downward. Pathogenic processes in which the downward passage of stomach qi is obstructed result in movement upward into the diaphragm and thorax, thereby disrupting the harmonious flow of qi and causing hiccough.

Pathogenic processes include overeating cold and raw foods, resulting in stomach cold; overeating hot spicy foods, resulting in stomach heat; emotional depression or anger, giving rise to fire and causing liver qi to disturb the stomach; chronic illness in which spleen yang is weakened, allowing obstruction of the middle burner by turbid phlegm; and febrile diseases in which stomach yin has been depleted, resulting in vacuity fire.

During the early stages, hiccoughs are usually loud, clear and forceful, and the patient's constitution basically unaffected. Patterns are generally from repletion. In chronic cases, hiccough tend to be deep and lack force, and the patients have become physically weak. These patterns are generally caused by vacuity.

1. STOMACH COLD

Clinical Manifestations: Deep, slow and forceful hiccough, milder with warmth and more severe with cold, epigastric discomfort, without apparent thirst.

Tongue: Moist white coating.

Pulse: Tardy or slow, forceful.

Treatment Method: Warm the stomach, dispel cold, relieve hiccough.

PRESCRIPTION

Clove and Persimmon Decoction *dīng xiāng shì dì tāng*

dīng xiāng	clove	Caryophylli Flos	6 g.
gāo liáng jiāng	lesser galangal [root]	Alpiniae Officinarum Rhizoma	9 g.
shì dì	persimmon [calyx]	Kaki Calyx	9 g.
zhì gān cǎo	licorice [root] (honey fried)	Glycyrrhizae Radix	3 g.

MODIFICATIONS

The prescription is often reinforced to increase its effectiveness in arresting hiccough. Add:

| *dāo dòu* | sword bean | Canavaliae Semen | 9 g. |

In cases with severe cold, the prescription is modified to dissipate cold and redirect qi downward. Add:

| *wú zhū yú* | evodia [fruit] | Evodiae Fructus | 4.5 g. |
| *ròu guì* | cinnamon [bark] (abbreviated decoction) | Cinnamomi Cortex | 4.5 g. |

In cases accompanied by phlegm and food stasis, the prescription is modified to transform phlegm and disperse food. Add:

hòu pò	magnolia [bark]	Magnoliae Cortex	6 g.
chén pí	tangerine peel	Citri Exocarpium	6 g.
fǎ bàn xià	pinellia [tuber] (processed)	Pinelliae Tuber Praeparatum	9 g.
fú líng	poria	Poria	9 g.

ACUPUNCTURE AND MOXIBUSTION

Main Points: Needle with draining; add moxibustion.

CV-12	*zhōng wǎn*
LI-04	*hé gǔ*
PC-06	*nèi guān*
ST-36	*zú sān lǐ*
BL-17	*gé shū*

Auxiliary points:

In cases with severe cold, add moxibustion to:

| CV-13 | *shàng wǎn* |
| ST-21 | *liáng mén* |

In cases of obstruction of food matter, add:

| CV-11 | *jiàn lǐ* |
| M-LE-1 | *lǐ nèi tíng* (Li Inner Court) |

2. EFFULGENT STOMACH FIRE

Clinical Manifestations: Loud clear hiccough, halitosis, irritability, thirst with preference for cold fluids, dark scanty urine, constipation.

Tongue: Yellow coating.

Pulse: Rapid, slippery.

Treatment Method: Drain heat, downbear stomach qi, relieve hiccough.

PRESCRIPTION

Bamboo Leaf and Gypsum Decoction *zhú-yè shí-gāo tāng*

zhú yè	black bamboo [leaf]	Bambusae Folium	15 g.
mài mén dōng	ophiopogon [tuber]	Ophiopogonis Tuber	15 g.
shí gāo	gypsum (extended decoction)	Gypsum	30 g.
rén shēn	ginseng	Ginseng Radix	6 g.
fǎ bàn xià	pinellia [tuber] (processed)	Pinelliae Tuber Praeparatum	9 g.
gān cǎo	licorice [root]	Glycyrrhizae Radix	3 g.
jīng mǐ	rice	Oryzae Semen	15 g.

MODIFICATIONS

The prescription is often modified to avoid fostering heat.

Delete:

rén shēn	ginseng	Ginseng Radix

Add:

běi shā shēn	glehnia [root]	Glehniae Radix	9 g.

The prescription is often reinforced to clear the stomach and move qi downward.
Add:

shì dì	persimmon [calyx]	Kaki Calyx	9 g.
zhú rú	bamboo shavings	Bambusae Caulis in Taeniam	9 g.

In cases of constipation with fullness of the abdomen, the given prescription is reinforced to free the stool and eliminate heat.
Add:

Minor Qi-Infusing Decoction *xiǎo chéng qì tāng*

dà huáng	rhubarb (abbreviated decoction)	Rhei Rhizoma	12 g.
zhǐ shí	unripe bitter orange	Aurantii Fructus Immaturus	9 g.
hòu pò	magnolia [bark]	Magnoliae Cortex	6 g.

ACUPUNCTURE AND MOXIBUSTION

Main Points: Needle with draining.

BL-17	*gé shū*
CV-12	*zhōng wǎn*
ST-36	*zú sān lǐ*
PC-06	*nèi guān*
ST-44	*nèi tíng*

3. LIVER QI STAGNATION

Clinical Manifestations: Hiccough brought on or worsened by emotional stress, with distention and pain in the chest and hypochondrium, reduced food intake, borborygmus and flatulence.

Tongue: Thin coating.

Pulse: Wiry, forceful.

Treatment Method: Soothe the liver, calm the stomach, relieve hiccough.

PRESCRIPTION
Five Milled Ingredients Drink *wǔ mò yǐn zǐ*

mù xiāng	saussurea [root]	Saussureae Radix seu Vladimiriae	9 g.
bīng láng	areca [nut]	Arecae Semen	9 g.
zhǐ shí	unripe bitter orange	Aurantii Fructus Immaturus	9 g.
wū yào	lindera [root]	Linderae Radix	9 g.
chén xiāng	aquilaria [wood] (powdered and stirred in)	Aquilariae Lignum	6 g.

MODIFICATIONS

The prescription is often reinforced to soothe the liver and relieve stagnation. Add:

chuān liàn zǐ	toosendan [fruit]	Toosendan Fructus	9 g.
yán hú suǒ	corydalis [tuber]	Corydalis Tuber	9 g.

The prescription is often reinforced to move qi downward and relieve hiccough. Add:

dīng xiāng	clove	Caryophylli Flos	4.5 g.
dài zhě shí	hematite (extended decoction)	Haematitum	15 g.

In cases of stagnation of liver qi giving rise to fire, with symptoms of irritability, constipation, bitter taste in the mouth, red tongue and rapid wiry pulse, the prescription is modified to drain the liver and harmonize the stomach. Add:

huáng lián	coptis [root]	Coptidis Rhizoma	6 g.
zhǐ shí	unripe bitter orange	Aurantii Fructus Immaturus	9 g.
dà huáng	rhubarb (abbreviated decoction)	Rhei Rhizoma	6 g.

In cases of counterflow ascent of stomach qi with obstruction by phlegm, symptoms will include dizziness, occasional nausea, thin slimy tongue coating and slippery wiry pulse. The given prescription is reinforced to transform phlegm, downbear qi, harmonize the stomach and relieve hiccough. Add:

Inula and Hematite Decoction *xuán fù huā dài zhě shí tāng*

xuán fù huā	inula flower (wrapped)	Inulae Flos	9 g.
dài zhě shí	hematite (extended decoction)	Haematitum	9 g.
rén shēn	ginseng	Ginseng Radix	6 g.
shēng jiāng	fresh ginger	Zingiberis Rhizoma Recens	9 g.
fǎ bàn xià	pinellia [tuber] (processed)	Pinelliae Tuber Praeparatum	9 g.
zhì gān cǎo	licorice [root] (honey fried)	Glycyrrhizae Radix	6 g.
dà zǎo	jujube	Ziziphi Fructus	4 pc.
plus:			
fú líng	poria	Poria	9 g.
chén pí	tangerine peel	Citri Exocarpium	9 g.

ACUPUNCTURE AND MOXIBUSTION

Main Points: Needle with draining.

CV-12	*zhōng wǎn*
BL-17	*gé shū*
PC-06	*nèi guān*
ST-36	*zú sān lǐ*
CV-17	*tǎn zhōng*
LR-03	*tài chōng*
LR-14	*qī mén*

4. SPLEEN AND STOMACH YANG VACUITY

Clinical Manifestations: Low, weak hiccough that interferes with respiration, pale complexion, lack of warmth of the limbs, heaviness and fatigue, low food intake.

Tongue: Pale with white coating.

Pulse: Deep, thready, weak.

Treatment Method: Warm and supplement the spleen and stomach, harmonize the middle burner, downbear qi, relieve hiccough.

PRESCRIPTION

Center-Rectifying Decoction *lǐ zhōng tāng*

rén shēn	ginseng	Ginseng Radix	12 g.
bái zhú	ovate atractylodes [root]	Atractylodis Ovatae Rhizoma	9 g.
gān jiāng	dried ginger [root]	Zingiberis Rhizoma Exsiccatum	9 g.
zhì gān cǎo	licorice [root] (honey-fried)	Glycyrrhizae Radix	6 g.

MODIFICATIONS

The prescription is often reinforced to warm the middle burner and relieve hiccough. Add:

dāo dòu	sword bean	Canavaliae Semen	9 g.
wú zhū yú	evodia [fruit]	Evodiae Fructus	4.5 g.
dīng xiāng	clove	Caryophylli Flos	6 g.

In cases of prolonged hiccough with hardness in the epigastrium, the given prescription may be used with Inula and Hematite Decoction *(xuán fù huā dài zhě-shí tāng)* to consolidate the effects of harmonizing the middle burner and moving qi downward.

Inula and Hematite Decoction *xuán fù huā dài zhě shí tāng*

xuán fù huā	inula flower (wrapped)	Inulae Flos	9 g.
dài zhě shí	hematite (extended decoction)	Haematitum	9 g.
rén shēn	ginseng	Ginseng Radix	6 g.
shēng jiāng	fresh ginger	Zingiberis Rhizoma Recens	9 g.
fǎ bàn xià	pinellia [tuber] (processed)	Pinelliae Tuber Praeparatum	9 g.
zhì gān cǎo	licorice [root] (honey-fried)	Glycyrrhizae Radix	6 g.
dà zǎo	jujube	Ziziphi Fructus	4 pc.

In cases where kidney yang is also vacuous, with physical cold, cold extremities, weak aching knees and lower back, pale tongue and slow deep pulse, the prescription is modified to warm the kidney and assist yang. Add:

zhì fù zǐ	aconite [accessory tuber] (processed) (extended decoction)	Aconiti Tuber Laterale Praeparatum	6 g.
ròu guì	cinnamon bark (abbreviated decoction)	Cinnamomi Cortex	6 g.

In cases accompanied by food stasis, the prescription is modified to disperse food and remove food stagnation. Add:

chén pí	tangerine peel	Citri Exocarpium	6 g.
mài yá	barley sprout	Hordei Fructus Germinatus	9 g.

In cases where spleen qi has been greatly depleted, with low weak intermittent hiccough and loose stools, the prescription is changed to supplement spleen qi and relieve hiccough. Use:

Center-Supplementing Qi-Boosting Decoction *bǔ zhōng yì qì tāng*

huáng qí	astragalus [root]	Astragali (seu Hedysari) Radix	15 g.
rén shēn	ginseng	Ginseng Radix	9 g.
bái zhú	ovate atractylodes [root]	Atractylodis Ovatae Rhizoma	9 g.
dāng guī	tangkuei	Angelicae Sinensis Radix	9 g.
chén pí	tangerine peel	Citri Exocarpium	6 g.
shēng mā	cimicifuga [root]	Cimicifugae Rhizoma	3 g.
chái hú	bupleurum [root]	Bupleuri Radix	3 g.
zhì gān cǎo	licorice [root] (honey-fried)	Glycyrrhizae Radix	6 g.

plus:

dāo dòu	sword bean	Canavaliae Semen	9 g.
wú zhū yú	evodia [fruit]	Evodiae Fructus	4.5 g.
dīng xiāng	clove	Caryophylli Flos	6 g.

ACUPUNCTURE AND MOXIBUSTION

Main Points: Needle with supplementation; add moxibustion.

CV-12	*zhōng wǎn*
PC-06	*nèi guān*
ST-36	*zú sān lǐ*
BL-17	*gé shū*
CV-06	*qì hǎi*

5. STOMACH YIN VACUITY

Clinical Manifestations: Fast and abrupt hiccough, irritability, uneasiness, dry mouth.

Tongue: Dry, red with cracked surface in some cases.

Pulse: Rapid, thready.

Treatment Method: Nourish stomach yin, generate liquid, relieve hiccough.

PRESCRIPTION

Stomach-Boosting Decoction *yì wèi tāng*

běi shā shēn	glehnia [root]	Glehniae Radix	9 g.
shēng dì huáng	rehmannia [root] (dried)	Rehmanniae Radix	12 g.
mài mén dōng	ophiopogon [tuber]	Ophiopogonis Tuber	9 g.
yù zhú	Solomon's seal [root]	Polygonati Yuzhu Rhizoma	9 g.
bīng táng	rock candy	Saccharon Crystallinum	3 g.

MODIFICATIONS

To reinforce the effects of the prescription to relieve hiccough, add:

pí pá yè	loquat [leaf]	Eriobotryae Folium	9 g.
shì dì	persimmon [calyx]	Kaki Calyx	9 g.
shí hú	dendrobium [stem] (extended decoction)	Dendrobii Caulis	12 g.

In cases of weakened stomach qi without desire for food, the prescription is reinforced to boost qi and harmonize the middle burner.

Add:

Tangerine Peel and Bamboo Shavings Decoction *jú pí zhú rú tāng*

chén pí	tangerine [peel]	Citri Exocarpium	12 g.
zhú yè	black bamboo [leaf]	Bambusae Folium	12 g.
shēng jiāng	fresh ginger	Zingiberis Rhizoma Recens	9 g.
rén shēn	ginseng	Ginseng Radix	3 g.
gān cǎo	licorice [root]	Glycyrrhizae Radix	6 g.
dà zǎo	jujube	Ziziphi Fructus	5 pc.

ACUPUNCTURE AND MOXIBUSTION

Main Points: Needle with supplementation.

CV-12	*zhōng wǎn*
PC-06	*nèi guān*
ST-36	*zú sān lǐ*
BL-17	*gé shū*
KI-03	*tài xī*
SP-06	*sān yīn jiāo*

ALTERNATE THERAPEUTIC METHODS

1. Ear Acupuncture

Main Points: Diaphragm, Sympathetic, Stomach, Liver, Spleen.

Method: In the proximity of the above points, locate painful pressure-points. Needle to elicit strong stimulation and retain for thirty minutes. In stubborn cases of hiccough, implanted needle therapy may be used.

2. Cupping Therapy

Main Points:

BL-17	*gé shū*
BL-46 (41)	*gé guān*
BL-18	*gān shū*
CV-12	*zhōng wǎn*
ST-18	*rǔ gēn*

Method: Cup at each point for ten to fifteen minutes.

REMARKS

During differential diagnosis it is primarily important to determine whether these patterns are from vacuity or repletion, heat or cold. During treatment, methods to downbear stomach qi and relieve hiccough are mainly used. Acumoxa therapy is very effective in cases of recent onset from repletion, and less effective in chronic cases that are from vacuity.

Hiccough without relief during the later stages of severe illnesses is an indication that stomach qi is extremely weak. Prognosis is unfavorable and comprehensive treatment including Western medicines should be used.

VOMITING

Ǒu Tù

**1. Exterior Evil Invading the Stomach - 2. Food Accumulation and
Stagnation - 3. Obstruction and Stagnation of Phlegm-Dampness -
4. Liver Qi Invading the Stomach - 5. Spleen and Stomach Vacuity Cold
- 6. Stomach Yin Vacuity**

Vomiting is a frequently observed clinical manifestation that is presented in
a wide variety of illnesses. In Chinese, vomiting is called *ǒu tù, ǒu* referring to the
condition in which there is vomit with sound, and *tù* referring to the condition in
which there is vomit without sound. The condition in which there is sound but no
vomit is known as dry retching *(gān ǒu)*. Since *ǒu* and *tù* often manifest simultaneously and are not obviously distinguishable, the compound term *ǒu tù* is generally used. Although *ǒu tù* and *gān ǒu* are in fact different phenomena, they are
basically equivalent in differential diagnosis and treatment, and both are therefore included in this discussion of vomiting.

Biomedically labeled diseases addressed in this chapter include vomiting
because of acute and chronic gastritis, gastrectasis (dilation of the stomach), car-
diospasm and esophageal spasm. For cases of vomiting secondary to other acute
and chronic conditions, reference should be made to the appropriate chapter. (Also
see the Remarks section at the end of this chapter.)

ETIOLOGY AND PATHOGENESIS

The stomach functions to store and decompose food; stomach qi controls
descent and facilitates the downward passage of food. Vomiting is the result of
the counterflow of stomach qi upward; it may be brought about by the six extenal
evils, internal disruption by the seven affects, improper diet and eating habits or
taxation.

On the basis of different etiological factors and different physical conditions,
vomiting cases are clinically divided into vacuity and repletion patterns. Cases due
to repletion, usually caused by evils, are generally acute and of short duration.
Cases from vacuity are caused by weakening of the stomach resulting in an inability to control descent. In these cases, the condition is often chronic and long lasting.

1. EXTERIOR EVIL INVADING THE STOMACH

Clinical Manifestations: Sudden onset of vomiting accompanied by aversion to
cold, fever, headache, general aches and pains, oppression in the chest, epigastric
fullness.

Tongue: White slimy coating.

Pulse: Floating, wiry.

Treatment Method: Dispel evils, transform turbidity with aromatic herbs, relieve vomiting.

PRESCRIPTION

Agastache/Patchouli Qi-Righting Powder *huò xiāng zhèng qì sǎn*

huò xiāng	agastache/patchouli	Agastaches seu Pogostemi Herba	6 g.
zǐ sū yè	perilla leaf (abbreviated decoction)	Perillae Folium	4.5 g.
bái zhǐ	angelica [root]	Angelicae Dahuricae Radix	3 g.
dà fù pí	areca [husk]	Arecae Pericarpium	3 g.
fú líng	poria	Poria	9 g.
bái zhú	ovate atractylodes [root]	Atractylodis Ovatae Rhizoma	6 g.
chén pí	tangerine peel	Citri Exocarpium	6 g.
jiāng bàn xià	(ginger-processed) pinellia [tuber]	Pinelliae Tuber Praeparatum	6 g.
hòu pò	magnolia bark	Magnoliae Cortex	3 g.
jié gěng	platycodon [root]	Platycodonis Radix	4.5 g.
zhì gān cǎo	licorice [root] (honey-fried)	Glycyrrhizae Radix	3 g.
shēng jiāng	fresh ginger	Zingiberis Rhizoma Recens	3 g.
dà zǎo	jujube	Ziziphi Fructus	2 pc.

MODIFICATIONS

In cases of food collection and stagnation with symptoms of oppression in the chest and abdominal distention, the prescription is modified to abduct stagnation.

Delete:

bái zhú	ovate atractylodes [root]	Atractylodis Ovatae Rhizoma
zhì gān cǎo	licorice [root] (honey-fried)	Glycyrrhizae Radix
dà zǎo	jujube	Ziziphi Fructus

Add:

shén qū	medicated leaven	Massa Medicata Fermentata	9 g.
jī nèi jīn	gizzard lining	Galli Gigerii Endothelium	9 g.

In cases of strong wind-cold evil, with aversion to cold and fever without perspiration, the prescription is modified to dispel wind-cold evil and relieve exterior symptoms. Add:

fáng fēng	ledebouriella [root]	Ledebouriellae Radix	6 g.
jīng jiè	schizonepeta (abbreviated decoction)	Schizonepetae Herba et Flos	6 g.

In cases of attack by summerheat-dampness, showing symptoms of vomiting, irritability and thirst, the prescription is modified to dispel summerheat-dampness and to relieve vomiting.

Delete:

bái zhǐ	angelica [root]	Angelicae Dahuricae Radix
bái zhú	ovate atractylodes [root]	Atractylodis Ovatae Rhizoma
zhì gān cǎo	licorice [root] (honey-fried)	Glycyrrhizae Radix
dà zǎo	jujube	Ziziphi Fructus

Add:

huáng lián	coptis [root]	Coptidis Rhizoma	6 g.
pèi lán	eupatorium	Eupatorii Herba	9 g.
hé yè	lotus leaf	Nelumbinis Folium	6 g.

ACUPUNCTURE AND MOXIBUSTION

Main points: Needle with draining.

LI-04	*hé gŭ*
BL-11	*dà zhù*
CV-12	*zhōng wăn*
PC-06	*nèi guān*
ST-36	*zú sān lĭ*
GB-20	*fēng chí*

Auxiliary points:

For retention of food, add:

CV-11	*jiàn lĭ*

For accumulation of internal phlegm, add:

ST-40	*fēng lóng*

2. FOOD ACCUMULATION AND STAGNATION

Clinical Manifestations: Vomiting of acidic fluid or the undigested contents of the stomach, distention and fullness of the epigastrium and abdomen, eructation, loss of appetite, foul stools that may be either loose or hard.

Tongue: Thick slimy coating.

Pulse: Replete, slippery.

Treatment Method: Disperse food, abduct stagnation, relieve vomiting.

PRESCRIPTION

Harmony-Preserving Pill *băo hé wán*

shān zhā	crataegus [fruit]	Crataegi Fructus	18 g.
shén qū	medicated leaven	Massa Medicata Fermentata	9 g.
jiāng bàn xià	(ginger-processed) pinellia [tuber]	Pinelliae Tuber Praeparatum	9 g.
fú líng	poria	Poria	9 g.
chén pí	tangerine peel	Citri Exocarpium	6 g.
lián qiào	forsythia [fruit]	Forsythiae Fructus	6 g.
lái fú zĭ	radish [seed]	Raphani Semen	6 g.

MODIFICATIONS

In cases of accumulation of a great amount of food, manifested by abdominal fullness and constipation, the prescription is modified to move stagnation.

Minor Qi-Infusing Decoction *xiăo chéng qì tāng*

dà huáng	rhubarb (abbreviated decoction)	Rhei Rhizoma	12 g.
zhĭ shí	unripe bitter orange	Aurantii Fructus Immaturus	9 g.
hòu pò	magnolia [bark]	Magnoliae Cortex	6 g.

ACUPUNCTURE AND MOXIBUSTION

Main points: Needle with draining.

CV-12	*zhōng wăn*
ST-36	*zú sān lĭ*
PC-06	*nèi guān*
CV-11	*jiàn lĭ*
CV-21	*xuán jī*
SP-14	*fù jié*

Auxiliary points:

For abdominal distention, add:

CV-06   *qì hǎi*

3. OBSTRUCTION AND STAGNATION OF PHLEGM-DAMPNESS

Clinical Manifestations: Vomiting of clear liquid and mucus, epigastric full-ness, loss of appetite, dizziness, palpitation.

Tongue: White slimy coating.

Pulse: Slippery.

Treatment Method: Warm and dispel phlegm-rheum, calm the stomach, relieve vomiting.

PRESCRIPTION

Use Minor Pinellia Decoction *(xiǎo bàn xià tāng)* with Poria (Hoelen), Cinnamon Twig, Ovate Atractylodes and Licorice Decoction *(líng guì zhú gān tāng)*.

Minor Pinellia Decoction *xiǎo bàn xià tāng*

zhì bàn xià	pinellia [tuber] (processed)	Pinelliae Tuber Praeparatum	9 g.
shēng jiāng	fresh ginger	Zingiberis Rhizoma Recens	9 g.

with:

Poria (Hoelen), Cinnamon Twig, Ovate Atractylodes and Licorice Decoction *líng guì zhú gān tāng*

fú líng	poria	Poria	12 g.
guì zhī	cinnamon [twig]	Cinnamomi Ramulus	9 g.
bái zhú	ovate atractylodes [root]	Atractylodis Ovatae Rhizoma	6 g.
zhì gān cǎo	licorice [root] (honey-fried)	Glycyrrhizae Radix	6 g.

MODIFICATIONS

In cases where the phlegm stagnation has given rise to heat, with symptoms of dizziness, vertigo, irritability, insomnia, nausea and vomiting, the prescription is changed so as to transform phlegm, clear heat and relieve vomiting. Use:

Gallbladder-Warming Decoction *wēn dǎn tāng*

zhì bàn xià	pinellia [tuber] (processed)	Pinelliae Tuber Praeparatum	9 g.
zhú rú	bamboo shavings	Bambusae Caulis in Taeniam	6 g.
zhǐ shí	unripe bitter orange	Aurantii Fructus Immaturus	6 g.
chén pí	tangerine peel	Citri Exocarpium	6 g.
zhì gān cǎo	licorice [root] (honey-fried)	Glycyrrhizae Radix	6 g.
fú líng	poria	Poria	9 g.
shēng jiāng	fresh ginger	Zingiberis Rhizoma Recens	2 pc.
dà zǎo	jujube	Ziziphi Fructus	3 pc.

ACUPUNCTURE AND MOXIBUSTION

Main points: Needle with even supplementation, even draining; add moxibustion.

SP-09   *yīn líng quán*
SP-04   *gōng sūn*
CV-12   *zhōng wǎn*
ST-40   *fēng lóng*
ST-36   *zú sān lǐ*
PC-06   *nèi guān*

Auxiliary points:

With borborygmus, add:
      ST-25   *tiān shū*

4. LIVER QI INVADING THE STOMACH

Clinical Manifestations: Vomiting, acid regurgitation, frequent eructation, oppression in the chest, hypochondriac pain.

Tongue: Thin white or thin slimy coating.

Pulse: Wiry.

Treatment Method: Soothe the liver, calm the stomach, downbear qi, relieve vomiting.

PRESCRIPTION

Combine Pinellia and Magnolia Bark Decoction *(bàn-xià hòu-pò tāng)* with Evodia and Coptis Pill (Left Metal Pill) *(yú lián wán [zuǒ jīn wán])*

Pinellia and Magnolia Bark Decoction *bàn xià hòu pò tāng*

jiāng bàn xià	(ginger-processed) pinellia [tuber]	Pinelliae Tuber Praeparatum	12 g.
hòu pò	magnolia [bark]	Magnoliae Cortex	9 g.
fú líng	poria	Poria	12 g.
shēng jiāng	fresh ginger	Zingiberis Rhizoma Recens	9 g.
zǐ sū yè	perilla [leaf] (abbreviated decoction)	Perillae Folium	6 g.

Evodia and Coptis Pill (Left Metal Pill) *yú lián wán (zuǒ jīn wán)*

wú zhū yú	evodia [fruit]	Evodiae Fructus	30 g.
huáng lián	coptis [root]	Coptidis Rhizoma	180 g.

Grind the above ingredients into a powder and form pills. Take two to three gram dose twice daily with water. The two herbs can also be decocted in water, with the proportion of coptis *(huáng lián)* to evodia *(wú zhū yú)* being 6:1.

MODIFICATIONS

In cases manifesting bitter taste in the mouth, clamoring stomach and constipation, the prescription is modified to clear heat and free the stool. Add:

dà huáng	rhubarb (abbreviated decoction)	Rhei Rhizoma	6 g.
zhǐ shí	unripe bitter orange	Aurantii Fructus Immaturus	9 g.

In cases with severe heat, the prescription is modified to clear the liver and drain fire. Add:

zhú rú	bamboo shavings	Bambusae Caulis in Taeniam	9 g.
shān zhī zǐ	gardenia	Gardeniae Fructus	9 g.

ACUPUNCTURE AND MOXIBUSTION

Main points: Needle with even supplementation, even draining.
      CV-12   *zhōng wǎn*
      GB-34   *yáng líng quán*
      LR-03   *tài chōng*
      ST-36   *zú sān lǐ*
      PC-06   *nèi guān*

5. SPLEEN AND STOMACH VACUITY COLD

Clinical Manifestations: Vomiting brought on by a slight increase in food intake, sallow or pale complexion, fatigue, general weakness, cold extremities, loose stools.

Tongue: Pale with white coating.

Pulse: Weak, thready.

Treatment Method: Warm the middle burner, strengthen the spleen, calm the stomach, downbear qi.

PRESCRIPTION

Center-Rectifying Decoction *lǐ zhōng tāng*

rén shēn	ginseng	Ginseng Radix	12 g.
bái zhú	ovate atractylodes [root]	Atractylodis Ovatae Rhizoma	9 g.
gān jiāng	dried ginger [root]	Zingiberis Rhizoma Exsiccatum	9 g.
zhì gān cǎo	licorice [root] (honey-fried)	mix-fried Glyccerhiza Radix	6 g.

MODIFICATIONS

To reinforce the effect against vomiting, the prescription is modified to rectify and downbear qi. Add:

jiāng bàn xià	(ginger-processed) pinellia [tuber]	Pinelliae Tuber Praeparatum	9 g.
chén pí	tangerine peel	Citri Exocarpium	6 g.
shā rén	amomum [fruit] (abbreviated decoction)	Amomi Semen seu Fructus	6 g.

In cases of prolonged vomiting of clear fluid, the prescription is modified to warm the stomach and relieve vomiting. Add:

wú zhū yú	evodia [fruit]	Evodiae Fructus	4.5 g.

ACUPUNCTURE AND MOXIBUSTION

Main points: Needle with supplementation; add moxibustion.

BL-20	*pí shū*
BL-21	*wèi shū*
CV-12	*zhōng wǎn*
ST-36	*zú sān lǐ*
PC-06	*nèi guān*
SP-04	*gōng sūn*

6. STOMACH YIN VACUITY

Clinical Manifestations: Repeated vomiting with spells of retching, thirst, dry throat, hunger without desire for food.

Tongue: Red with little coating.

Pulse: Rapid, thready.

Treatment Method: Nourish stomach yin, downbear qi, relieve vomiting.

PRESCRIPTION

Ophiopogon Decoction *mài mén dōng tāng*

mài mén dōng	ophiopogon [tuber]	Ophiopogonis Tuber	15 g.
rén shēn	ginseng	Ginseng Radix	6 g.
jiāng bàn xià	(ginger-processed) pinellia [tuber]	Pinelliae Tuber Praeparatum	6 g.
gān cǎo	licorice [root])	Glycyrrhizae Radix	3 g.
jīng mǐ	rice	Oryzae Semen	15 g.
dà zǎo	jujube	Ziziphi Fructus	3 pc.

MODIFICATIONS

Ginseng *(rén shēn)* is often replaced by:

běi shā shēn	glehnia [root]	Glehniae Radix	12 g.

In cases of severe fluid depletion, the prescription is modified to generate liquid. Reduce:

jiāng bàn xià	(ginger-processed) pinellia [tuber]	Pinelliae Tuber Praeparatum

Add:

shí hú	dendrobium [stem] (extended decoction)	Dendrobii Caulis	12 g.
tiān huā fěn	trichosanthes [root]	Trichosanthis Radix	12 g.
zhī mǔ	anemarrhena [root]	Anemarrhenae Rhizoma	9 g.
zhú rú	bamboo shavings	Bambusae Caulis in Taeniam	6 g.

In cases of dry stools and constipation, the prescription is modified to moisten the intestines and promote elimination. Add:

huǒ má rén	hemp [seed]	Cannabis Semen	15 g.
fēng mì	honey (stirred in)	Mel	20 g.

ACUPUNCTURE AND MOXIBUSTION

Main points: Needle with supplementation.

CV-12	*zhōng wǎn*
ST-36	*zú sān lǐ*
PC-06	*nèi guān*
SP-04	*gōng sūn*
SP-06	*sān yīn jiāo*
KI-03	*tài xī*

ALTERNATE THERAPEUTIC METHODS

1. Ear Acupuncture

Main points: Stomach, Liver, Sympathetic, Subcortex, *Shén Mén.*

Method: Select two to three acupoints each session and retain needles for twenty to thirty minutes. Needle once daily.

REMARKS

Because vomiting is a symptom in many illnesses, several other conditions recognized by Western medicine may give rise to vomiting. These can include acute contagious diseases, intestinal obstruction, gastrointestinal tumors, morning sickness, uremia and certain craniocerebral conditions. Treatment should always be focused on the primary illness. During differential diagnosis and treatment of vomiting it may be useful to refer to the chapters on Esophageal Constriction and Dribbling Urinary Block.

ESOPHAGEAL CONSTRICTION

Yē Gé

1. Congestion of Qi and Phlegm - 2. Depletion of Fluids with Accumulation of Heat - 3. Accumulation of Blood Stasis - 4. Vacuity of Qi and Devitalization of Yang

SUPPLEMENT: STOMACH REFLUX

(Fǎn Wèi)

1. Spleen Vacuity Cold with Counterflow Ascent of Stomach Qi

In Chinese, esophageal constriction is known as *yē gé*. The word *yē* refers to difficulty in swallowing food; *gé* refers to an involuntary resistance to swallowing food or drink, or vomiting immediately after the intake of food or drink. *Yē* patterns may occur in isolation, or they may indicate the development of *gé* patterns, hence the compound word, *yē gé*.

Esophageal constriction includes disorders Western medicine labels spasms of the cardiac sphincter, hiatal hernia, esophagitis, esophageal diverticulosis, esophageal cancer and other functional disorders of the esophagus. In patients who are middle-aged or older the possibility of cancer should be considered during diagnosis.

ETIOLOGY AND PATHOGENESIS

Two etiological factors influence the development of esophageal constriction. The first is internal disruption of the liver and spleen from anxiety, depression, worry or anger, resulting in phlegm stagnation, stagnation of qi and blood stasis. The second is indulgence in smoking, alcohol, rich and sweet foods or hot and spicy foods. These habits can foster the transformation of dampness into heat and injure yin, resulting in a depletion of fluids and blood. In both cases, the stomach, liver, spleen and kidney may be damaged along with the pathological changes occurring in the esophagus.

Generally speaking, mild cases of esophageal constriction are caused by the stagnation of liver and spleen qi leading to the binding depression of qi and phlegm, or by the depletion of stomach yin, causing sluggish activity of the esophagus. Both result in difficulty in swallowing. More severe cases develop when the binding depression of qi and phlegm causes stagnant blood. The resulting phlegm stagnation and static blood block stomach qi. If stomach yin is severely depleted, kidney yin will be injured. Such morbid developments present with pain on swallowing, vomiting directly following ingestion or difficulty swallowing liquids. With continued development of these pathological changes, injury to yin leads to injury of yang, thus dysfunction of both the spleen and kidney. Such cases are critical with a poor prognosis.

1. CONGESTION OF QI AND PHLEGM

Clinical Manifestations: Sensation of obstruction in the throat when swallowing, fullness and oppression in the chest and diaphragm, minor relief of symptoms when in a favorable emotional state.

Tongue: Thin slimy coating.

Pulse: Wiry, slippery.

Treatment Method: Rectify qi, transform phlegm, resolve depression.

PRESCRIPTION
Diaphragm-Arousing Powder *qǐ gé sǎn*

běi shā shēn	glehnia [root]	Glehniae Radix	12 g.
dān shēn	salvia [root]	Salviae Miltiorrhizae Radix	12 g.
fú líng	poria	Poria	9 g.
yù jīn	curcuma [tuber]	Curcumae Tuber	9 g.
chuān bèi mǔ	Sichuan fritillaria [bulb]	Fritillariae Cirrhosae Bulbus	9 g.
shā rén ké	amomum [husk]	Amomi Pericarpium	6 g.
hé yè dì	lotus leaf base	Nelumbinis Basis Folii	6 g.
mǐ pí kāng	rice bran	Oryza sativa	6 g.

MODIFICATIONS

To reinforce the transformation of phlegm and resolution of depression, add:

guā lóu	trichosanthes [fruit]	Trichosanthis Fructus	9 g.
chén pí	tangerine peel	Citri Exocarpium	6 g.
dǎn xīng	bile (processed) arisaema [root]	Arisaematis Rhizoma cum Felle Bovis	4.5 g.
xuán fù huā	inula flower (wrapped)	Inulae Flos	6 g.
dài zhě shí	hematite (extended decoction)	Haematitum	9 g.

In cases of injury to fluids with dry mouth, dry throat and constipation, the prescription is modified to generate liquid and moisten dryness. Add:

Humor-Increasing Decoction *zēng yè tāng*

xuán shēn	scrophularia [root]	Scrophulariae Radix	30 g.
mài mén dōng	ophiopogon [tuber]	Ophiopogonis Tuber	24 g.
shēng dì huáng	rehmannia [root] (dried/fresh)	Rehmanniae Radix Exsiccata seu Recens	24 g.

plus:

fēng mì	honey (stirred in)	Mel	30 g.

ACUPUNCTURE AND MOXIBUSTION

Main points: Needle with even supplemention, even draining; add moxibustion.

CV-22	*tiān tú*
CV-17	*tǎn zhōng*
CV-13	*shàng wǎn*
ST-36	*zú sān lǐ*
PC-06	*nèi guān*
BL-21	*wèi shū*

2. Depletion of Fluids with Accumulation of Heat

Clinical Manifestations: Difficulty swallowing accompanied by sensations of obstruction and pain, liquids ingest easily but solids with difficulty, emaciation, dry mouth and throat, constipation, vexing heat in the five hearts.

Tongue: Dry, red, sometimes presenting a cracked surface.

Pulse: Thready, rapid.

Treatment Method: Nourish yin, generate liquid, clear heat.

PRESCRIPTION

Adenophora-Glehnia and Ophiopogon Decoction *shā-shēn mài-dōng tāng*

běi shā shēn	glehnia [root]	Glehniae Radix	9 g.
mài mén dōng	ophiopogon [tuber]	Ophiopogonis Tuber	9 g.
tiān huā fěn	trichosanthes root	Trichosanthis Radix	12 g.
yù zhú	Solomon's seal [root]	Polygonati Yuzhu Rhizoma	9 g.
bái biǎn dòu	lablab [bean]	Lablab Semen	12 g.
sāng yè	mulberry leaf	Mori Folium	6 g.
gān cǎo	licorice [root]	Glycyrrhizae Radix	6 g.

MODIFICATIONS

To reinforce nourishing yin and clearing heat, add:

xuán shēn	scrophularia [root]	Scrophulariae Radix	9 g.
dān shēn	salvia [root]	Salviae Miltiorrhizae Radix	9 g.
shēng dì huáng	rehmannia [root] (dried) (dried/fresh)	Rehmanniae Radix Exsiccata seu Recens	12 g.
shí hú	dendrobium [stem] (extended decoction)	Dendrobii Caulis	9 g.
jīn yín huā	lonicera [flower]	Lonicerae Flos	9 g.
shān dòu gēn	bushy sophora [root]	Sophorae Subprostratae Radix	6 g.
yín chái hú	lanceolate stellaria [root]	Stellariae Lanceolatae Radix	6 g.
lù fēng fáng	hornet's nest	Vespae Nidus	6 g.

In cases of hard stools or constipation, the prescription is modified to clear heat and free the stool. Add:

dà huáng	rhubarb (abbreviated decoction)	Rhei Rhizoma	6 g.

Discontinue rhubarb *(dà huáng)* after the bowels begin to move, to avoid depletion of fluids.

ACUPUNCTURE AND MOXIBUSTION

Main points: Needle with supplementation.

CV-22	*tiān tú*
CV-17	*tǎn zhōng*
CV-13	*shàng wǎn*
ST-36	*zú sān lǐ*
PC-06	*nèi guān*
SP-06	*sān yīn jiāo*

Auxiliary points:

For constipation, add:

KI-06	*zhào hǎi*

3. ACCUMULATION OF BLOOD STASIS

Clinical Manifestations: Spasmodic pain of fixed location in the chest, inability to swallow solid foods and difficulty in swallowing liquids, hard stools in the form of small balls, vomiting of dark red liquids in some cases, dull, grayish complexion, emaciation, dry skin.

Tongue: Dry, dark purplish.

Pulse: Rough, thready.

Treatment Method: Nourish yin, moisten dryness, move static blood, break masses.

PRESCRIPTION

Combine Diaphragm-Arousing Powder *(qǐ gé sǎn)* with Peach Kernel and Carthamus Beverage *(táo hóng yǐn)*.

Diaphragm-Arousing Powder *qǐ gé sǎn*

běi shā shēn	glehnia [root]	Glehniae Radix	12 g.
dān shēn	salvia [root]	Salviae Miltiorrhizae Radix	12 g.
fú líng	poria	Poria	9 g.
yù jīn	curcuma [tuber]	Curcumae Tuber	9 g.
chuān bèi mǔ	Sichuan fritillaria [bulb]	Fritillariae Cirrhosae Bulbus	9 g.
shā rén ké	amomum [husk]	Amomi Pericarpium	6 g.
hé yè dì	lotus leaf base (calyx of leaf)	Nelumbinis Basis Folii	6 g.
mǐ pí kāng	rice [husk]	Oryza Testa	6 g.

Peach Kernel and Carthamus Beverage *táo hóng yǐn*

táo rén	peach [kernel]	Persicae Semen	9 g.
hóng huā	carthamus [flower]	Carthami Flosa	6 g.
chuān xiōng	ligusticum [root]	Ligustici Rhizoma	6 g.
dāng guī wěi	tangkuei tail	Angelicae Sinensis Radicis Extremitas	9 g.
wēi líng xiān	clematis [root]	Clematidis Radix	9 g.

MODIFICATIONS

In severe cases, the prescription is modified to dispel static blood, free the connections, soften tumors and transform phlegm. Add:

sān qī	notoginseng [root]	Notoginseng Radix	9 g.
	(or: 1.5 g. powdered and administered separately)		
chì sháo yào	red peony [root]	Paeoniae Radix Rubra	9 g.
hǎi zǎo	sargassum	Sargassi Herba	12 g.
kūn bù	kelp	Algae Thallus	12 g.
guā lóu	trichosanthes [fruit]	Trichosanthis Fructus	9 g.

ACUPUNCTURE AND MOXIBUSTION

Main points: Needle with even supplementation, even draining; add moxibustion.

BL-17	*gé shū*
CV-22	*tiān tú*
CV-17	*tǎn zhōng*
PC-06	*nèi guān*
CV-13	*shàng wǎn*
ST-36	*zú sān lǐ*

4. VACUITY OF QI AND DEVITALIZATION OF YANG

Clinical Manifestations: Prolonged cases of inability to swallow food or liquids, with emaciation, pale complexion, listlessness, physical cold, shortness of breath, regurgitation of clear fluids, edema of the face and limbs.

Tongue: Pale with white coating.

Pulse: Weak, thready.

Treatment Method: Supplement spleen qi, warm kidney yang.

PRESCRIPTION

Combine Qi-Supplementing Spleen-Moving Decoction *(bǔ qì yùn pí tāng)* with Right-Restoring [Kidney Yang] Pill *(yòu guī wán).*

Qi-Supplementing Spleen-Moving Decoction *bǔ qì yùn pí tāng*

rén shēn	ginseng	Ginseng Radix	9 g.
bái zhú	ovate atractylodes [root]	Atractylodis Ovatae Rhizoma	9 g.
fú líng	poria	Poria	9 g.
huáng qí	astragalus [root]	Astragali (seu Hedysari) Radix	12 g.
jiāng bàn xià	(ginger-processed) pinellia [tuber]	Pinelliae Tuber Praeparatum	6 g.
chén pí	tangerine peel	Citri Exocarpium	6 g.
shā rén	amomum [fruit] (abbreviated decoction)	Amomi Semen seu Fructus	3 g.
gān cǎo	licorice [root]	Glycyrrhizae Radix	6 g.
shēng jiāng	fresh ginger	Zingiberis Rhizoma Recens	3 g.
dà zǎo	jujube	Ziziphi Fructus	3 pc.

Right-Restoring [Kidney Yang] Pill *yòu guī wán*

shú dì huáng	cooked rehmannia [root]	Rehmanniae Radix Conquita	24 g.
shān yào	dioscorea [root]	Dioscoreae Rhizoma	12 g.
shān zhū yú	cornus [fruit]	Corni Fructus	9 g.
gǒu qǐ zǐ	lycium [berry]	Lycii Fructus	12 g.
lù jiǎo jiāo	deerhorn glue (dissolved and stirred in)	Cervi Gelatinum Cornu	12 g.
tù sī zǐ	cuscuta [seed]	Cuscutae Semen	12 g.
dù zhòng	eucommia [bark]	Eucommiae Cortex	12 g.
dāng guī	tangkuei	Angelicae Sinensis Radix	9 g.
ròu guì	cinnamon bark (abbreviated decoction)	Cinnamomi Cortex	6 g.
zhì fù zǐ	aconite [accessory tuber] (processed) (extended decoction)	Aconiti Tuber Laterale Praeparatum	6 g.

MODIFICATIONS

Clinically, Qi-Supplementing Spleen-Moving Decoction *(bǔ qì yùn pí tāng)* is administered first until the patient is able to ingest small amounts of food, after which Qi-Supplementing Spleen-Moving Decoction *(bǔ qì yùn pí tāng)* and Right-Restoring [Kidney Yang] Pill *(yòu guī wán)* are alternated.

ACUPUNCTURE AND MOXIBUSTION

Main points: Needle with supplementation; add moxibustion.

BL-23	*shèn shū*
BL-20	*pí shū*
BL-21	*wèi shū*

BL-17	*gé shū*
CV-22	*tiān tú*
CV-17	*tǎn zhōng*
PC-06	*nèi guān*
CV-13	*shàng wǎn*
ST-36	*zú sān lǐ*

Auxiliary points:

For shortness of breath, add moxibustion to:

| CV-06 | *qì hǎi* |

For cold limbs and feeble pulse, add moxibustion to:

| GV-04 | *mìng mén* |

ALTERNATE THERAPEUTIC METHODS

1. Ear Acupuncture

Main Points: *Shén Mén*, Stomach, Esophagus, Diaphragm.

Method: Needle bilaterally to elicit a moderate sensation. Treat once daily, ten sessions per therapeutic course.

SUPPLEMENT:

STOMACH REFLUX

Fǎn Wèi

1. SPLEEN AND STOMACH VACUITY COLD WITH STOMACH QI COUNTERFLOW

Clinical Manifestations: Distention and fullness of the epigastrium and abdomen after eating, vomiting in the evening of food eaten in the morning and vomiting in the morning of food eaten in the evening, vomit containing undigested food, accompanied by symptoms of tiredness, fatigue and lusterless complexion.

Tongue: Pale with thin white coating.

Pulse: Thready, tardy, forceless.

Treatment Method: Warm and strengthen the spleen and stomach, downbear qi.

PRESCRIPTION

Clove and Aquilaria Diaphragm-Freeing Powder *dīng chén tòu gé sǎn*

rén shēn	ginseng	Ginseng Radix	12 g.
bái zhú	ovate atractylodes [root]	Atractylodis Ovatae Rhizoma	9 g.
mù xiāng	saussurea [root]	Saussureae Radix (seu Vladimiriae)	9 g.
jiāng bàn xià	(ginger-processed) pinellia [tuber]	processed Pinelliae Tuber	9 g.
shā rén	amomum [fruit] (abbreviated decoction)	Amomi Semen seu Fructus	6 g.
chén pí	tangerine peel	Citri Exocarpium	6 g.
huò xiāng	agastache/patchouli	Agastaches seu Pogostemi Herba	9 g.

hòu pò	magnolia [bark]	Magnoliae Cortex	9 g.
xiāng fù zǐ	cyperus [root]	Cyperi Rhizoma	6 g.
qīng pí	unripe tangerine peel	Citri Exocarpium Immaturum	6 g.
dīng xiāng	clove	Caryophylli Flos	4.5 g.
chén xiāng	aquilaria [wood] (powdered and stirred in)	Aquilariae Lignum	1.5 g.
ròu dòu kòu	nutmeg	Myristicae Semen	6 g.
cǎo guǒ	tsaoko [fruit]	Amomi Tsao-Ko Fructus	4.5 g.
shén qū	medicated leaven	Massa Medicata Fermentata	15 g.
mài yá	barley sprout	Hordei Fructus Germinatus	15 g.
zhì gān cǎo	licorice [root] (honey-fried)	Glycyrrhizae Radix	3 g.

MODIFICATIONS

In cases of severe vomiting, the prescription is modified to suppress the counterflow ascent of stomach qi and relieve vomiting.
Add:

| *xuán fù huā* | inula flower (wrapped) | Inulae Flos | 6 g. |
| *dài zhě shí* | hematite (extended decoction) | Haematitum | 9 g. |

In cases of pale complexion, cold extremities, pale tongue and deep thready pulse, the pattern is one of chronic vomiting leading to vacuity of kidney yang. The prescription is changed to warm and supplement spleen and kidney yang.
Use:

Aconite Center-Rectifying Decoction *fù zǐ lǐ zhōng tāng*

zhì fù zǐ	aconite [accessory tuber] (processed) (extended decoction)	Aconiti Tuber Laterale Praeparatum	6 g.
rén shēn	ginseng	Ginseng Radix	9 g.
bái zhú	ovate atractylodes [root]	Atractylodis Ovatae Rhizoma	9 g.
gān jiāng	dried ginger [root]	Zingiberis Rhizoma Exsiccatum	6 g.
zhì gān cǎo	licorice [root] (honey-fried)	Glycyrrhizae Radix	6 g.

plus:

wú zhū yú	evodia [fruit]	Evodiae Fructus	4.5 g.
dīng xiāng	clove	Caryophylli Flos	4.5 g.
ròu guì	cinnamon bark (abbreviated decoction)	Cinnamomi Cortex	6 g.

In cases of chronic vomiting leading to vacuity of qi and yin, with symptoms of dry mouth and lips, constipation, red tongue with little coating and a thready pulse, the prescription is altered to supplement qi and yin, harmonize the stomach and downbear qi.
Use:

Major Pinellia Decoction *dà bàn xià tāng*

jiāng bàn xià	(ginger-processed) pinellia [tuber]	Pinelliae Tuber Praeparatum	9 g.
rén shēn	ginseng	Ginseng Radix	9 g.
fēng mì	honey (stirred in)	Mel	50 g.

plus:

běi shā shēn	glehnia [root]	Glehniae Radix	12 g.
hòu pò	magnolia bark	Magnoliae Cortex	6 g.
mài mén dōng	ophiopogon [tuber]	Ophiopogonis Tuber	12 g.

American ginseng *(xī yáng shēn)* may be substituted for ginseng *(rén shēn)*.

ACUPUNCTURE AND MOXIBUSTION

Main points: Needle with supplementation; add moxibustion.

BL-21	*wèi shū*
BL-20	*pí shū*
CV-12	*zhōng wǎn*
LR-13	*zhāng mén*
ST-36	*zú sān lǐ*
PC-06	*nèi guān*
CV-06	*qì hǎi*

Auxiliary points:

For severe vomiting, add:

BL-17	*gé shū*
M-UE-16	*zhōng kuí* (Central Eminence)

For vacuity of kidney yang, add:

BL-23	*shèn shū*

For vacuity of both qi and yin, add:

CV-04	*guān yuán*
SP-06	*sān yīn jiāo*

REMARKS

Esophageal constriction patterns are classified as vacuity at the root and repletion at the branch. Superficially, patterns show qi stagnation, obstruction by phlegm and blood stasis. The root vacuity progresses through stages of depletion of fluids, consumption of blood and injury to yin causing injury to yang. During the early stages of esophageal constriction, repletion is predominant, with the root vacuity becoming predominant during the later stages.

Since the development of esophageal constriction usually involves improper dietary habits as well as emotional factors, it is important that the diet be regulated and emotional disruption be kept to a minimum during treatment. Decoctions should be taken slowly in small amounts and at frequent intervals.

During clinical examination, esophageal constriction needs to be clearly distinguished from stomach reflux and plum-pit qi. Stomach reflux is characterized by stagnation of food matter in the stomach, with symptoms of food eaten in the morning being vomited in the evening and food eaten in the evening being vomited in the morning. Stomach reflux is generally the result of vacuity cold of the spleen and stomach with stomach qi counterflow, accompanied by cold. It resembles the pyloric obstruction and pyloric spasms of Western medicine. Esophageal constriction, on the other hand, is characterized by the inability to swallow food and drink, or vomiting upon ingestion, and is most often caused by yin vacuity accompanied by fire.

Compared to plum-pit qi, esophageal constriction presents an involuntary resistance to swallowing food and drink, whereas plum-pit qi patterns present a sensation of throat discomfort and obstruction but no actual difficulty ingesting foods.

ABDOMINAL PAIN

Fù Tòng

1. Obstruction by Cold Evil - **2. Obstruction by Damp-Heat** -
3. Vacuity of Spleen Yang - **4. Obstruction by Food Stagnation** -
5. Qi Stagnation and Blood Stasis - **5A. Predominant Qi Stagnation** -
5B. Predominant Blood Stasis

Abdominal pain refers to pain in the region around the umbilicus to the pubic bone, and is distinguished from epigastric pain. This symptom is frequently encountered clinically and is presented in a wide variety of illnesses. This chapter discusses treatment of conditions known in Western medicine as acute and chronic gastroenteritis, enterospasm, psychosomatic gastrointestinal conditions and dyspepsia. For the treatment of abdominal pain from gynecological disorders, or disorders usually requiring surgery, refer to the appropriate chapters.

ETIOLOGY AND PATHOGENESIS

Patterns of abdominal pain are caused by the external evils of cold, dampness or heat, or by internal disruption because of improper diet and poor eating habits, emotional stress or constitutional yang vacuity. These factors cause stagnation and obstruction of the flow of qi, leading to blockage of the connecting vessels, or to reduced nourishment of the channels, resulting in abdominal pain.

The pathogenesis of abdominal pain includes cold, heat, repletion and vacuity. Clinically, one may give rise to another, one may transform into another or two or more may manifest.

1. OBSTRUCTION BY COLD EVIL

Clinical Manifestations: Acute and sudden abdominal pain that is decreased by the external application of heat and increased by cold, no apparent thirst, copious clear urine, loose stools.

Tongue: White slimy coating.

Pulse: Deep, tight.

Treatment Method: Warm the middle burner, dissipate cold, regulate qi, relieve pain.

PRESCRIPTION

Combine Lesser Galangal and Cyperus Pill *(liáng fù wán)* with Qi-Righting Lindera and Cyperus Powder *(zhèng qì tiān xiāng sǎn)*.

Lesser Galangal and Cyperus Pill *liáng fù wán*

gāo liáng jiāng	lesser galangal [root]	Alpiniae Officinarum Rhizoma	12 g.
xiāng fù zǐ	cyperus [root]	Cyperi Rhizoma	12 g.

with:

Qi-Righting Lindera and Cyperus Powder *zhèng qì tiān xiāng sǎn*

wū yào	lindera [root]	Linderae Radix	9 g.
gān jiāng	dried ginger [root]	Zingiberis Rhizoma Exsiccatum	9 g.
xiāng fù zǐ	cyperus [root]	Cyperi Rhizoma	9 g.
zǐ sū zǐ	perilla [fruit]	Perillae Fructus	9 g.
chén pí	tangerine peel	Citri Exocarpium	6 g.

MODIFICATIONS

In cases of excruciating pain in the umbilical region relieved by heat or pressure, vacuous kidney yang with invasion of cold evil is indicated. The prescription is thus changed to warm and invigorate kidney yang. Use:

Vessel-Freeing Counterflow Cold Decoction *tōng mài sì nì tāng*

zhì fù zǐ	aconite [accessory tuber] (processed) (extended decoction)	Aconiti Tuber Laterale Praeparatum	15 g.
gān jiāng	dried ginger [root]	Zingiberis Rhizoma Exsiccatum	9 g.
zhì gān cǎo	licorice [root] (honey-fried)	Glycyrrhizae Radix	6 g.

ACUPUNCTURE AND MOXIBUSTION

Main points: Needle with draining; add moxibustion.

CV-12	*zhōng wǎn*
ST-36	*zú sān lǐ*
SP-04	*gōng sūn*
SP-15	*dà hèng*
LI-04	*hé gǔ*

Auxiliary points:
For severe abdominal pain accompanied by diarrhea and cold limbs, add salt moxibustion to:

CV-08	*shén què*

2. OBSTRUCTION BY DAMP-HEAT

Clinical Manifestations: Abdominal pain that is increased by external pressure, abdominal fullness and distention, constipation or difficult elimination of loose stools, irritability, thirst, scanty dark urine.

Tongue: Yellow slimy coating.

Pulse: Slippery, rapid.

Treatment Method: Free the stool, dispel damp-heat.

PRESCRIPTION

Major Qi-Infusing Decoction *dà chéng qì tāng*

dà huáng	rhubarb (abbreviated decoction)	Rhei Rhizoma	12 g.
máng xiāo	mirabilite (stirred in)	Mirabilitum	9 g.
zhǐ shí	unripe bitter orange	Aurantii Fructus Immaturus	12 g.
hòu pò	magnolia [bark]	Magnoliae Cortex	15 g.

<u>MODIFICATIONS</u>

In cases of difficult elimination of loose stools, the prescription is modified to clear heat and disinhibit dampness.

Delete:

máng xiāo	mirabilite	Mirabilitum	

Add:

huáng qín	scutellaria [root]	Scutellariae Radix	9 g.
shān zhī zǐ	gardenia	Gardeniae Fructus	9 g.

In cases where abdominal pain extends through the costal regions, the prescription is modified to soothe the liver, regulate qi and relieve pain.

Add:

chái hú	bupleurum [root]	Bupleuri Radix	9 g.
yù jīn	curcuma [tuber]	Curcumae Tuber	9 g.

ACUPUNCTURE AND MOXIBUSTION

Main points: Needle with draining.

CV-10	*xià wǎn*
ST-21	*liáng mén*
LI-11	*qū chí*
ST-25	*tiān shū*
SP-09	*yīn líng quán*

Auxiliary points:

For thirst, add:

ST-44	*nèi tíng*

3. VACUITY OF SPLEEN YANG

Clinical Manifestations: Dull periodic abdominal pain relieved by heat or external pressure that increases when hungry or fatigued, loose stools, tiredness, physical cold.

Tongue: Pale with white coating.

Pulse: Deep, thready.

Treatment Method: Warm and supplement spleen yang, relieve pain.

PRESCRIPTION

Minor Center-Fortifying Decoction *xiǎo jiàn zhōng tāng*

bái sháo yào	white peony [root]	Paeoniae Radix Alba	18 g.
guì zhī	cinnamon [twig]	Cinnamomi Ramulus	9 g.
zhì gān cǎo	licorice [root] (honey-fried)	Glycyrrhizae Radix	6 g.
shēng jiāng	fresh ginger	Zingiberis Rhizoma Recens	9 g.
yí táng	malt sugar (stirred in)	Granorum Saccharon	30 g.
dà zǎo	jujube	Ziziphi Fructus	4 pc.

<u>MODIFICATIONS</u>

In cases of shortness of breath and poor spirits, the prescription is modified to supplement qi. Add:

huáng qí	astragalus [root]	Astragali (seu Hedysari) Radix	12 g.

In cases of severe abdominal pain accompanied by vomiting, cold limbs and a tight thready pulse, the prescription is changed to warm the middle burner and dissipate cold. Use:

Major Center-Fortifying Decoction *dà jiàn zhōng tāng*

huā jiāo	zanthoxylum [husk]	Zanthoxyli Pericarpium	6 g.
gān jiāng	dried ginger [root]	Zingiberis Rhizoma Exsiccatum	9 g.
rén shēn	ginseng	Ginseng Radix	9 g.
yí táng	malt sugar (stirred in)	Granorum Saccharon	50 g.

In cases of abdominal pain accompanied by diarrhea, cold limbs and a slow deep pulse, the prescription is changed to warm and supplement the spleen and kidney yang. Use:

Aconite Center-Rectifying Decoction *fù zǐ lǐ zhōng tāng*

zhì fù zǐ	aconite [accessory tuber] (processed) (extended decoction)	Aconiti Tuber Laterale Praeparatum	6 g.
rén shēn	ginseng	Ginseng Radix	9 g.
bái zhú	ovate atractylodes [root]	Atractylodis Ovatae Rhizoma	9 g.
gān jiāng	dried ginger [root]	Zingiberis Rhizoma Exsiccatum	6 g.
zhì gān cǎo	licorice [root] (honey-fried)	Glycyrrhizae Radix	6 g.

ACUPUNCTURE AND MOXIBUSTION

Main points: Needle with supplementation; add moxibustion.

ST-36	*zú sān lǐ*
SP-06	*sān yīn jiāo*

Auxiliary points:

For loose stools and diarrhea, add:

BL-20	*pí shū*
BL-23	*shèn shū*
CV-04	*guān yuán*
LR-13	*zhāng mén*

4. OBSTRUCTION BY FOOD STASIS

Clinical Manifestations: Abdominal fullness, distention and pain increased by external pressure, refusal of food, belching of foul gas, acid regurgitation; sometimes constipation or, in some cases, abdominal pain that occurs just prior to a bout of diarrhea and that disappear with the emptying of the bowels.

Tongue: Slimy coating.

Pulse: Replete, slippery.

Treatment Method: Disperse food, abduct stagnation, relieve pain.

PRESCRIPTION

For mild cases:

Harmony-Preserving Pill *bǎo hé wán*

shān zhā	crataegus [fruit]	Crataegi Fructus	18 g.
shén qū	medicated leaven	Massa Medicata Fermentata	9 g.
zhì bàn xià	pinellia [tuber] (processed)	Pinelliae Tuber Praeparatum	9 g.
fú líng	poria	Poria	9 g.
chén pí	tangerine peel	Citri Exocarpium	6 g.

| *lián qiào* | forsythia [fruit] | Forsythiae Fructus | 6 g. |
| *lái fú zǐ* | radish [seed] | Raphani Semen | 6 g. |

For severe cases:

Unripe Bitter Orange Stagnation-Abducting Pill *zhǐ-shí dǎo zhì wán*

zhǐ shí	unripe bitter orange	Aurantii Fructus Immaturus	12 g.
shén qū	medicated leaven	Massa Medicata Fermentata	9 g.
bái zhú	ovate atractylodes [root]	Atractylodis Ovatae Rhizoma	9 g.
huáng lián	coptis [root]	Coptidis Rhizoma	6 g.
huáng qín	scutellaria [root]	Scutellariae Radix	6 g.
fú líng	poria	Poria	9 g.
zé xiè	alisma [tuber]	Alismatis Rhizoma	6 g.
dà huáng	rhubarb (abbreviated decoction)	Rhei Rhizoma	9 g.

ACUPUNCTURE AND MOXIBUSTION

Main points: Needle with draining.

CV-12	*zhōng wǎn*
ST-25	*tiān shū*
ST-21	*liáng mén*
ST-36	*zú sān lǐ*
M-LE-1	*lǐ nèi tíng* (Li Inner Court)

Auxiliary points:

For acid regurgitation, add:

| GB-34 | *yáng líng quán* |

5A. QI STAGNATION AND BLOOD STASIS – PREDOMINANT QI STAGNATION

Clinical Manifestations: Distention, fullness and pain in the epigastrium and abdomen increasing with anger, indeterminate moving location of pain, relief following belching or expulsion of gas.

Tongue: Thin coating.

Pulse: Wiry.

Treatment Method: Soothe the liver, regulate qi.

PRESCRIPTION

Bupleurum Liver-Coursing Powder *chái hú shū gān sǎn*

chái hú	bupleurum [root]	Bupleuri Radix	6 g.
bái sháo yào	white peony [root]	Paeoniae Radix Alba	9 g.
xiāng fù zǐ	cyperus [root]	Cyperi Rhizoma	6 g.
chuān xiōng	ligusticum [root]	Ligustici Rhizoma	6 g.
chén pí	tangerine peel	Citri Exocarpium	6 g.
zhǐ ké	bitter orange	Aurantii Fructus	6 g.
zhì gān cǎo	licorice [root] (honey-fried)	Glycyrrhizae Radix	3 g.

ACUPUNCTURE AND MOXIBUSTION

Main points: Needle with even supplementation, even draining.

CV-17	*tăn zhōng*
LR-03	*tài chōng*
PC-06	*nèi guān*
GB-34	*yáng líng quán*

Auxiliary points:

For costal pain, add:

LR-14	*qī mén*

For upper abdominal pain, add:

CV-12	*zhōng wǎn*

For pain in the umbilical region, add:

CV-06	*qì hǎi*
CV-10	*xià wǎn*

5B. Qi Stagnation and Blood Stasis – Predominant Blood Stasis

Clinical Manifestations: Predominance of blood stasis, pain is severe and the location of the pain is definite and stationary.

Tongue: Purplish.

Pulse: Wiry or rough.

Treatment Method: Quicken the blood and dissolve stasis, warm the channels, relieve pain.

PRESCRIPTION

Lesser Abdomen Stasis-Expelling Decoction *shào fù zhú yū tāng*

dāng guī	tangkuei	Angelicae Sinensis Radix	9 g.
chì sháo yào	red peony [root]	Paeoniae Radix Rubra	6 g.
pú huáng	typha pollen (wrapped)	Typhae Pollen	9 g.
mò yào	myrrh	Myrrha	6 g.
chuān xiōng	ligusticum [root]	Ligustici Rhizoma	3 g.
wŭ líng zhī	flying squirrel's droppings (wrapped)	Trogopteri seu Pteromipcis Excrementum	6 g.
yán hú suŏ	corydalis [tuber]	Corydalis Tuber	3 g.
gān jiāng	dried ginger [root]	Zingiberis Rhizoma Exsiccatum	3 g.
ròu guì	cinnamon [bark] (abbreviated decoction)	Cinnamomi Cortex	3 g.
xiǎo huí xiāng	fennel	Foeniculi Fructus	3 g.

MODIFICATIONS

In cases of post-operative pain following abdominal surgery, the prescription is modified to dispel stasis and relieve pain. Add:

zé lán	lycopus	Lycopi Herba	9 g.
hóng huā	carthamus [flower]	Carthami Flosa	6 g.

In cases of pain following traumatic injury, the prescription is modified to dispel blood stasis and promote regeneration. Add:

wáng bù liú xíng	vaccaria [seed]	Vaccariae Semen	6 g.
sān qī	notoginseng [root]	Notoginseng Radix	9 g.
	(or powdered and administered separately, each time 1.5 g.)		

ACUPUNCTURE AND MOXIBUSTION

Main points: Needle with even supplementation, even draining.

CV-17	*tăn zhōng*
LR-03	*tài chōng*
BL-17	*gé shū*
SP-06	*sān yīn jiāo*

Auxiliary points:

See: 5A. Predominant Qi Stagnation

ALTERNATE THERAPEUTIC METHODS

1. Ear Acupuncture:

Main points: Large Intestine, Small Intestine, Stomach, Spleen, *Shén Mén,* Sympathetic.

Method: Select two to three points each session. Needle to elicit a moderate sensation and retain the needles for ten to twenty minutes. One session each day or every second day, ten sessions constituting one therapeutic course.

2. Cupping Therapy

Method: Apply large-sized cups to the given acupoints on the abdomen and back. Choose three to four acupoints per session, one or two sessions each day. This method is suitable in cases of abdominal pain caused by cold or obstruction by food stasis.

REMARKS

In the clinical manifestations of abdominal pain, etiological factors, location of pain and characteristics of pain serve as the basis for differentiation of cold and heat, repletion and vacuity, qi and blood, viscera and bowels. In general, pain from repletion is aggravated by pressure while pain from vacuity is somewhat relieved by pressure; pain after eating is from repletion while pain when hungry is from vacuity; pain from cold is relieved by heat while pain from heat is relieved by cold compresses; and pain from stagnation of qi manifests as abdominal distention and pain with indeterminate moving location, whereas pain from blood stasis manifests as a stabbing pain with a definite fixed location.

Differential diagnosis may also be made according to the location of abdominal pain. Pain in the inguinal region, sometimes extending into the costal region, is often found in illnesses of the liver and gallbladder. Pain in the lower abdomen and umbilical region often involves the spleen, small intestine, kidney or bladder. Conscientious differential diagnosis made on the basis of the characteristic functions of each of the viscera and bowels, as well as the accompanying symptoms and signs of abdominal pain, will enable administration of an effective treatment.

DIARRHEA

Xiè Xiè

1. Attack by External Cold and Dampness - 2. Attack by External Damp-Heat - 3. Retention of Food in the Stomach and Intestines - 4. Disharmony of the Liver and Spleen - 5. Vacuity of the Spleen and Stomach - 6. Vacuity of Kidney Yang

Diarrhea refers to conditions in which the frequency of bowel movements is increased, stools are soft and runny or, in severe cases, the stools are like water. In Chinese, diarrhea is *xiè xiè,* the first *xiè* having the meaning of loose unformed stools with rather mild sensations at elimination, while the second *xiè* refers to runny watery stools with acute sensations during elimination. Diarrhea may occur in any of the four seasons, although it is most commonly seen in summer and autumn.

Diarrhea patterns include acute and chronic enteritis, indigestion, intestinal parasitic diseases, disorders of the pancreas, liver or gallbladder, endocrinic and metabolic disorders and emotional stress.

ETIOLOGY AND PATHOGENESIS

The etiology of diarrhea is often complex. A constant factor in its pathogenesis, however, is disruption of the normal functioning of the spleen and stomach. Clinically, diarrhea is divided into acute or chronic conditions based on etiological factors and the duration of the illness.

Acute diarrhea is often brought on by internal injury because of improper diet, external evils such as cold, heat, dampness and summerheat or emotional stress leading to disharmony between the liver and spleen. Chronic diarrhea is most often caused by vacuity of the spleen and kidney leading to disruption of the transporting and transforming functions of the spleen.

1. ATTACK BY EXTERNAL COLD AND DAMPNESS

Clinical Manifestations: Diarrhea with watery stools, borborygmus, abdominal pain, congestion in the epigastrium and loss of appetite. Accompanying symptoms may include fever, aversion to cold, stuffy nose, headache, no apparent thirst, general aches and pains.

Tongue: Thin white slimy coating.

Pulse: Soft, tardy.

Treatment Method: Dispel cold, transform dampness and relieve diarrhea.

PRESCRIPTION

Agastache/Patchouli Qi-Righting Powder *huò xiāng zhèng qì sǎn*

huò xiāng	agastache/patchouli	Agastaches seu Pogostemi Herba	6 g.
zǐ sū yè	perilla leaf (abbreviated decoction)	Perillae Folium	4.5 g.
bái zhǐ	angelica [root]	Angelicae Dahuricae Radix	3 g.
dà fù pí	areca husk	Arecae Pericarpium	3 g.
fú líng	poria	Poria	9 g.
bái zhú	ovate atractylodes [root]	Atractylodis Ovatae Rhizoma	6 g.
chén pí	tangerine peel	Citri Exocarpium	6 g.
zhì bàn xià	pinellia [tuber] (processed)	Pinelliae Tuber Praeparatum	6 g.
hòu pò	magnolia bark	Magnoliae Cortex	3 g.
jié gěng	platycodon [root]	Platycodonis Radix	4.5 g.
zhì gān cǎo	licorice [root] (honey-fried)	Glycyrrhizae Radix	3 g.
shēng jiāng	fresh ginger	Zingiberis Rhizoma Recens	3 g.
dà zǎo	jujube	Ziziphi Fructus	2 pc.

MODIFICATIONS

Where wind cold exterior symptoms are severe, the prescription is modified to increase the action of dispelling wind and cold. Add:

jīng jiè	schizonepeta (abbreviated decoction)	Schizonepetae Herba et Flos	6 g.
fáng fēng	ledebouriella [root]	Ledebouriellae Radix	6 g.

Where dampness is prevalent, with symptoms of oppression in the chest, abdominal distention, scanty urine, general fatigue, and white slimy tongue coating, the prescription is modified to fortify the spleen, dry dampness and promote diuresis. Add:

Stomach-Calming Poria (Hoelen) Five Decoction *wèi líng tāng*

cāng zhú	atractylodes [root]	Atractylodis Rhizoma	9 g.
bái zhú	ovate atractylodes [root]	Atractylodis Ovatae Rhizoma	9 g.
fú líng	poria	Poria	12 g.
zhū líng	polyporus	Polyporus	9 g.
hòu pò	magnolia [bark]	Magnoliae Cortex	6 g.
chén pí	tangerine [peel]	Citri Exocarpium	6 g.
zé xiè	alisma [tuber]	Alismatis Rhizoma	9 g.
guì zhī	cinnamon [twig]	Cinnamomi Ramulus	9 g.
zhì gān cǎo	licorice [root] (honey-fried)	Glycyrrhizae Radix	6 g.

ACUPUNCTURE AND MOXIBUSTION

Main points: Needle with supplementation; add moxibustion.

ST-25	*tiān shū*
CV-12	*zhōng wǎn*
ST-36	*zú sān lǐ*
LI-04	*hé gǔ*
SP-09	*yīn líng quán*

2. ATTACK BY EXTERNAL DAMP-HEAT

Clinical Manifestations: Diarrhea, abdominal pain, urgent bowel movements or diarrhea with difficulty in defecation, yellow pasty foul stools, burning sensation in the anal region, irritability, thirst, dark scanty urine.

Tongue: Yellow slimy coating.

Pulse: Rapid, slippery.

Treatment Method: Clear heat, eliminate dampness and relieve diarrhea.

PRESCRIPTION

Pueraria, Scutellaria and Coptis Decoction
gé gēn huáng qín huáng lián tāng

gé gēn	pueraria [root]	Puerariae Radix	15 g.
huáng qín	scutellaria [root]	Scutellariae Radix	9 g.
huáng lián	coptis [root]	Coptidis Rhizoma	6 g.
zhì gān cǎo	licorice [root] (honey-fried)	Glycyrrhizae Radix	6 g.

MODIFICATIONS

To increase heat-clearing, add:

jīn yín huā	lonicera [flower]	Lonicerae Flos	12 g.

To strengthen damp-draining, add:

fú líng	poria	Poria	12 g.
mù tōng	mutong [stem]	Mutong Caulis	6 g.
chē qián zǐ	plantago [seed]	Plantaginis Semen	9 g.

Where dampness is prevalent, with symptoms of fullness of the chest and abdomen, no apparent thirst or thirst without the desire to drink, slightly yellow thick slimy tongue coating, and soft tardy pulse, the prescription is modified to dry dampness and relieve the middle burner. Add:

Stomach-Calming Powder *píng wèi sǎn*

cāng zhú	atractylodes [root]	Atractylodis Rhizoma	15 g.
hòu pò	magnolia [bark]	Magnoliae Cortex	9 g.
chén pí	tangerine [peel]	Citri Exocarpium	9 g.
zhì gān cǎo	licorice [root] (honey-fried)	Glycyrrhizae Radix	3 g.

plus:

shēng jiāng	fresh ginger	Zingiberis Rhizoma Recens	3 g.
dà zǎo	jujube	Ziziphi Fructus	2 pc.

With indigestion from food stasis, the prescription is modified to disperse food and abduct stagnation. Add:

shén qū	medicated leaven	Massa Medicata Fermentata	9 g.
mài yá	barley sprout	Hordei Fructus Germinatus	12 g.
shān zhā	crataegus [fruit]	Crataegi Fructus	12 g.

With diarrhea from summerheat-dampness, with symptoms including watery stools, spontaneous perspiration, grainy complexion, irritability, thirst, and dark urine, the prescription is modified to clear summerheat and dispel dampness. Add:

huò xiāng	agastache/patchouli	Agastaches seu Pogostemi Herba	9 g.
xiāng fú mǐ	cyperus [root]	Cyperi Rhizoma	6 g.
biǎn dòu	lablab [bean]	Lablab Semen	12 g.
hé yè	lotus leaf	Nelumbinis Folium	6 g.

ACUPUNCTURE AND MOXIBUSTION

Main points: Needle with draining.

ST-25	*tiān shū*
ST-36	*zú sān lǐ*
ST-44	*nèi tíng*
SP-09	*yīn líng quán*
LI-11	*qū chí*

3. RETENTION OF FOOD IN THE STOMACH AND INTESTINES

Clinical Manifestations: Abdominal pain, borborygmus, stools foul with rotten egg odor, abdominal pain relieved after bowel movement, fullness of the epigastrium and abdomen, belching of foul gas, acid regurgitation, loss of appetite.

Tongue: Thick, slimy or filthy coating.

Pulse: Slippery.

Treatment Method: Disperse food, abduct stagnation and relieve diarrhea.

PRESCRIPTION

Harmony-Preserving Pill *bǎo hé wán*

shān zhā	crataegus [fruit]	Crataegi Fructus	18 g.
shén qū	medicated leaven	Massa Medicata Fermentata	9 g.
zhì bàn xià	processed pinellia [tuber]	Pinelliae Tuber Praeparatum	9 g.
fú líng	poria	Poria	9 g.
chén pí	tangerine peel	Citri Exocarpium	6 g.
lián qiào	forsythia [fruit]	Forsythiae Fructus	6 g.
lái fú zǐ	radish seed	Raphani Semen	6 g.

MODIFICATIONS

For accumulation of food that has given rise to heat, with yellow slimy tongue coating and rapid slippery pulse, the prescription is modified to clear heat, disperse food and abduct stagnation. Use:

Unripe Bitter Orange Stagnation-Abducting Pill *zhǐ shí dǎo zhì wán*

zhǐ shí	unripe bitter orange	Aurantii Fructus Immaturus	12 g.
shén qū	medicated leaven	Massa Medicata Fermentata	9 g.
bái zhú	ovate atractylodes [root]	Atractylodis Ovatae Rhizoma	9 g.
huáng lián	coptis [root]	Coptidis Rhizoma	6 g.
huáng qín	scutellaria [root]	Scutellariae Radix	6 g.
fú líng	poria	Poria	9 g.
zé xiè	alisma [tuber]	Alismatis Rhizoma	6 g.
dà huáng	rhubarb (abbreviated decoction)	Rhei Rhizoma	9 g.

ACUPUNCTURE AND MOXIBUSTION

Main points: Needle with draining.

ST-25	*tiān shū*
CV-12	*zhōng wǎn*
ST-36	*zú sān lǐ*
M-LE-1	*lǐ nèi tíng* (Li Inner Court)

4. DISHARMONY OF LIVER AND SPLEEN

Clinical Manifestations: Distention and congestion in the chest and hypochondrium, belching, poor appetite, abdominal pain and diarrhea brought on by depression, anger or anxiety, no relief of pain with bowel movements.

Tongue: Thin white coating.

Pulse: Wiry.

Treatment Method: Repress the liver, support the spleen and relieve diarrhea.

PRESCRIPTION

Pain and Diarrhea Formula *tòng xiè yào fāng*

bái zhú	ovate atractylodes [root]	Atractylodis Ovatae Rhizoma	9 g.
bái sháo yào	white peony [root]	Paeoniae Radix Alba	6 g.
chén pí	tangerine peel	Citri Exocarpium	4.5 g.
fáng fēng	ledebouriella [root]	Ledebouriellae Radix	6 g.

MODIFICATIONS

In cases of persistent diarrhea, the prescription is modified to raise spleen qi. Add:

shēng má	cimicifuga [root] (honey-fried)	Cimicifugae Rhizoma	3 g.

ACUPUNCTURE AND MOXIBUSTION

Main points: Needle with draining.

ST-25	*tiān shū*
CV-12	*zhōng wǎn*
ST-36	*zú sān lǐ*
BL-18	*gān shū*
GB-34	*yáng líng quán*
LR-03	*tài chōng*

5. VACUITY OF THE SPLEEN AND STOMACH

Clinical Symptoms: Loose stools, increased frequency of bowel movements with consumption of oily or greasy foods, loss of appetite, epigastric fullness and discomfort after eating, sallow complexion, lack of vitality, fatigue.

Tongue: Pale with white coating.

Pulse: Weak, thready.

Treatment Method: Strengthen the spleen, benefit the stomach, relieve diarrhea.

PRESCRIPTION

Ginseng, Poria and Ovate Atractylodes Powder *shēn líng bái zhú sǎn*

rén shēn	ginseng	Ginseng Radix	12 g.
fú líng	poria	Poria	12 g.
bái zhú	ovate atractylodes [root]	Atractylodis Ovatae Rhizoma	12 g.
shān yào	dioscorea [root]	Dioscoreae Rhizoma	12 g.
bái biǎn dòu	lablab [bean]	Lablab Semen	9 g.

lián zǐ	lotus [fruit-seed]	Nelumbinis Fructus seu Semen	6 g.
yì yǐ rén	coix [seed]	Coicis Semen	6 g.
shā rén	amomum [fruit] (abbreviated decoction)	Amomi Semen seu Fructus	6 g.
jié gěng	platycodon [root] (abbreviated decoction)	Platycodonis Radix	6 g.
zhì gān cǎo	licorice [root] (honey-fried)	Glycyrrhizae Radix	12 g.

MODIFICATIONS

In cases of vacuity of spleen yang with prevalence of internal cold where symptoms include abdominal cold and pain and cold extremities, the prescription is modified to warm the spleen and dispel cold. Employ:

Aconite Center-Rectifying Decoction *fù-zǐ lǐ zhōng tāng*

zhì fù zǐ	aconite [accessory tuber] (processed) (extended decoction)	Aconiti Tuber Laterale Praeparatum	6 g.
rén shēn	ginseng	Ginseng Radix	9 g.
bái zhú	ovate atractylodes [root]	Atractylodis Ovatae Rhizoma	9 g.
gān jiāng	dried ginger [root]	Zingiberis Rhizoma Exsiccatum	6 g.
zhì gān cǎo	licorice [root] (honey-fried)	Glycyrrhizae Radix	6 g.

plus:

| *wú zhū yú* | evodia [fruit] | Evodiae Fructus | 6 g. |
| *ròu guì* | cinnamon [bark] (abbreviated decoction) | Cinnamomi Cortex | 6 g. |

In extended cases of diarrhea with weakened spleen qi leading to anal prolapse, use:

Center-Supplementing Qi-Boosting Decoction *bǔ zhōng yì qì tāng*

huáng qí	astragalus [root]	Astragali (seu Hedysari) Radix	15 g.
rén shēn	ginseng	Ginseng Radix	9 g.
bái zhú	ovate atractylodes [root]	Atractylodis Ovatae Rhizoma	9 g.
dāng guī	tangkuei	Angelicae Sinensis Radix	9 g.
chén pí	tangerine peel	Citri Exocarpium	6 g.
shēn má	cimicifuga [root]	Cimicifugae Rhizoma	3 g.
chái hú	bupleurum [root]	Bupleuri Radix	3 g.
zhì gān cǎo	licorice [root] (honey-fried)	Glycyrrhizae Radix	6 g.

ACUPUNCTURE AND MOXIBUSTION

Main points: Needle with supplementation; add moxibustion.

BL-20	*pí shū*
BL-26	*guān yuán shū*
CV-12	*zhōng wǎn*
ST-25	*tiān shū*
ST-36	*zú sān lǐ*
SP-03	*tài bái*

6. VACUITY OF KIDNEY AND SPLEEN YANG

Clinical Manifestations: Diarrhea usually occurring just before dawn; abdominal coldness and pain and borborygmus prior to bowel movements; physical cold, cold extremities, sore weak lower back and knees.

Tongue: Pale with white coating.

Pulse: Deep, thready, weak.

Treatment Method: Warm and supplement spleen and kidney yang and relieve diarrhea.

PRESCRIPTION

Four Spirits Pill *sì shén wán*

bǔ gǔ zhī	psoralea [seed]	Psoraleae Semen	12 g.
ròu dòu kòu	nutmeg	Myristicae Semen	6 g.
wǔ wèi zǐ	schisandra [berry]	Schisandrae Fructus	6 g.
wú zhū yú	evodia [fruit]	Evodiae Fructus	3 g.

MODIFICATIONS

To increase the kidney and spleen warming effect, add:

zhì fù zǐ	aconite [accessory tuber] (processed) (extended decoction)	Aconiti Tuber Laterale Praeparatum	6 g.
pào jiāng	blast-fried ginger (charred)	Zingiberis Rhizoma Tostum	6 g.

In cases where the patient is of advanced age and poor constitution and shows signs of prolapse and chronic diarrhea, the prescription is modified to boost qi and fortify the spleen. Add:

huáng qí	astragalus [root]	Astragali (seu Hedysari) Radix	12 g.
dǎng shēn	codonopsis [root]	Codonopsitis Radix	9 g.
bái zhú	ovate atractylodes [root]	Atractylodis Ovatae Rhizoma	9 g.

To reinforce the basic prescription to relieve diarrhea with astringent herbs, add:

Peach Blossom Decoction *táo huā tāng*

chì shí zhī	halloysite (wrapped)	Halloysitum Rubrum	12 g.
gān jiāng	dried ginger [root]	Zingiberis Rhizoma Exsiccatum	4.5 g.
gēng mǐ	non-glutinous rice	Oryzae Semen	15 g.

ACUPUNCTURE AND MOXIBUSTION

Main points: Needle with supplementation; add moxibustion.

BL-23	*shèn shū*
BL-20	*pí shū*
GV-04	*mìng mén*
CV-04	*guān yuán*
KI-03	*tài xī*
ST-36	*zú sān lǐ*

ALTERNATE THERAPEUTIC METHODS

1. Ear Acupuncture

Main points: Small Intestine, Large Intestine, Stomach, Spleen, Liver, Kidney, Sympathetic, *Shén Mén*.

Method: Select three to five acupoints each treatment session. In cases of acute diarrhea, retain needles for five to ten minutes; treat once or twice daily. In cases of chronic diarrhea, retain needles for ten to twenty minutes, treat once daily. Ten treatments make up one therapeutic course.

REMARKS

During the initial stages of diarrhea from external invasion, tonics and astringents should be avoided to prevent evils from fixating deeply. In cases of persistent diarrhea, care should be taken not to overuse diuretics, so as to avoid injury to yin fluids. During treatment, attention should be paid to the patient's diet, restricting raw and cold foods and prohibiting meat, fish and oily greasy foods.

DYSENTERY

Lì Jí

1. Damp-Heat Dysentery - 2. Epidemic Toxic Dysentery - 3. Cold-Dampness Dysentery - 4. Yin Vacuity Dysentery - 5. Vacuity-Cold Dysentery - 6. Chronic Intermittent Dysentery

Dysentery is a contagious intestinal infection that commonly occurs in summer and autumn. Its characteristic features include an increased frequency of bowel movements, tenesmus (straining to free the stool), abdominal pain and stool mixed with mucus, pus and blood. Refer to this chapter for differential diagnosis and treatment of all cases of bacterial and amoebic dysentery.

ETIOLOGY AND PATHOGENESIS:

The etiology of dysentery usually involves attack by epidemic heat and dampness, or the intake of raw, cold or contaminated foods. When the intestinal tract is obstructed by external evils and food matter, the large intestine fails to pass fecal material, leading to stagnation of qi and blood. Eventually the connecting vessels are injured, and the feces become mixed with pus and blood. In cases where evils have mainly injured qi, stools contain more pus than blood, while in cases where evils have mainly injured blood, stools contain more blood than pus. In cases where both qi and blood have been injured, stools are mixed with equal proportions of pus and blood.

On the basis of differing etiological factors, clinical manifestations and duration of illness, dysentery may be divided into the following six types:

1. *Damp-heat dysentery,* resulting from the accumulation of damp-heat in the intestinal tract.

2. *Epidemic toxiin dysentery,* a critical condition caused by heat-toxin and characterized by high fever and coma.

3. *Cold-dampness dysentery,* caused by accumulation of damp-cold in the spleen and stomach blocking the passage of qi to the large intestine.

4. *Yin vacuity dysentery,* presented in cases of yin vacuous constitutions.

5. *Vacuity-cold dysentery,* in cases of extended dysentery leading to vacuity of spleen and kidney yang.

6. *Chronic intermittent dysentery,* presented in cases of extended recurring dysentery where evils linger and correct qi is insufficient.

In addition, there exists an advanced condition known as "fasting dysentery." In this type of dysentery, patients cannot ingest food or vomit upon eating. It is generally a development of damp-heat or epidemic toxic dysentery.

1. DAMP-HEAT DYSENTERY

Clinical Symptoms: Abdominal pain, tenesmus, stools mixed with both pus and blood, burning sensation in the anus, dark scanty urine, irritability, thirst, fever and, in some cases, aversion to cold in the early stages.

Tongue: Yellow slimy coating.

Pulse: Rapid, slippery.

Treatment Method: Clear heat, transform dampness, rectify qi and blood.

PRESCRIPTION
Peony Decoction *sháo yào tāng*

bái sháo yào	white peony [root]	Paeoniae Radix Alba Yao	15 g.
huáng lián	coptis [root]	Coptidis Rhizoma	9 g.
huáng qín	scutellaria [root]	Scutellariae Radix	9 g.
dāng guī	tangkuei	Angelicae Sinensis Radix	9 g.
dà huáng	rhubarb (abbreviated decoction)	Rhei Rhizoma	9 g.
bīng láng	areca [nut]	Arecae Semen	5 g.
mù xiāng	saussurea [root]	Saussureae (seu Vladimiriae) Radix	5 g.
gān cǎo	licorice [root]	Glycyrrhizae Radix	5 g.
ròu guì	cinnamon [bark]	Cinnamomi Cortex	3 g.

MODIFICATIONS

In cases accompanied by fever, perspiration and headache, the prescription is modified to alleviate exterior symptoms and to relieve dysentery.
Use:
Pueraria, Scutellaria and Coptis Decoction
gé gēn huáng qín huáng lián tāng

gé gēn	pueraria [root]	Puerariae Radix	15 g.
huáng qín	scutellaria [root]	Scutellariae Radix	9 g.
huáng lián	coptis [root]	Coptidis Rhizoma	6 g.
zhì gān cǎo	licorice [root] (honey-fried)	Glycyrrhizae Radix	6 g.

plus:

jīn yín huā	lonicera [flower]	Lonicerae Flos	12 g.

In cases where heat is predominant and the stools contain more blood and less pus, the prescription is modified to clear heat and disperse toxins.
Use:
Pulsatilla Decoction *bái tóu wēng tāng*

bái tóu wēng	pulsatilla [root]	Pulsatillae Radix	15 g.
huáng bǎi	phellodendron [bark]	Phellodendri Cortex	12 g.
qín pí	ash [bark]	Fraxini Cortex	12 g.
huáng lián	coptis [root]	Coptidis Rhizoma	6 g.

In cases accompanied by food accumulation and stagnation, the prescription is modified to clear food matter and promote evacuation.
Add:

zhǐ shí	unripe bitter orange	Aurantii Fructus Immaturus	9 g.
shān zhā	crataegus [fruit]	Crataegi Fructus	12 g.
shén qū	medicated leaven	Massa Medicata Fermentata	9 g.

In cases where the blood is obstructed by heat with severe abdominal pain, the prescription is modified to cool the blood and clear stasis.

Add:

dì yú	sanguisorba [root]	Sanguisorbae Radix	9 g.
táo rén	peach [kernel]	Persicae Semen	9 g.
chì sháo yào	red peony [root]	Paeoniae Radix Rubra	9 g.
mǔ dān pí	moutan [root bark]	Moutan Radicis Cortex	9 g.

ACUPUNCTURE AND MOXIBUSTION

Main points: Needle with draining.

LI-04	*hé gǔ*
ST-25	*tiān shū*
ST-37	*shàng jù xū*
LI-11	*qū chí*
SP-09	*yīn líng quán*

Auxiliary points:

For fever, add:

GV-14	*dà zhuī*

For tenesmus, add:

BL-29	*zhōng lǚ shū*
GV-01	*cháng qiáng*

For inability to take food or drink, add:

CV-12	*zhōng wǎn*
PC-06	*nèi guān*

2. EPIDEMIC TOXIC DYSENTERY

Clinical Symptoms: Sudden onset of illness, high fever, thirst, headache, irritability, loss of consciousness with convulsions in severe cases, acute abdominal pain, tenesmus, stools mixed with pus and blood.

Tongue: Dark red with dry yellow coating

Pulse: Rapid, slippery

Treatment Method: Clear heat, cool the blood, disperse toxins.

PRESCRIPTION

Pulsatilla Decoction *bái tóu wēng tāng*

bái tóu wēng	pulsatilla [root]	Pulsatillae Radix	15 g.
huáng bǎi	phellodendron [bark]	Phellodendri Cortex	12 g.
qín pí	ash [bark]	Fraxini Cortex	12 g.
huáng lián	coptis [root]	Coptidis Rhizoma	6 g.

MODIFICATIONS

To strengthen heat clearing and toxin dispersing add:

jīn yín huā	lonicera [flower]	Lonicerae Flos	9 g.
huáng qín	scutellaria [root]	Scutellariae Radix	9 g.
chì sháo yào	red peony [root]	Paeoniae Radix Rubra	9 g.
mǔ dān pí	moutan [root bark]	Moutan Radicis Cortex	9 g.
dì yú	sanguisorba [root]	Sanguisorbae Radix	9 g.

In cases where heat-toxin has invaded the construction aspect (*yíng fèn*) with provoked internal wind, there will be symptoms of high fever, loss of consciousness, convulsions and delirium. The patient's condition is critical and certain patent medicines should be added to clear construction, open the orifices and stop convulsions. Use one of the following prepared medicines:

PEACEFUL PALACE BOVINE BEZOAR PILL (*ān gōng niú huáng wán*)

PURPLE SNOW ELIXIR (*zǐ xuě dān*)

SUPREME JEWEL ELIXIR (*zhì bǎo dān*).

In cases of extreme weakness of correct qi with severe exuberant heat-toxin, there will be symptoms of pale complexion, cold extremities, perspiration, heavy breathing and a weak faint pulse. The following prescription should be given immediately to restore yang and prevent collapse.
Use:

Ginseng and Aconite Decoction *shēn fù tāng*

| *rén shēn* | ginseng | Ginseng Radix | 30 g. |
| *zhì fù zǐ* | aconite [accessory tuber] (processed) | Aconiti Tuber Laterale Conquitum | 15 g. |

If oral administration is not possible, nasal feeding may be used. Acupuncture and moxibustion may also prove effective during this state. After alleviating prostration, continue treatment of the original pattern.

ACUPUNCTURE AND MOXIBUSTION

Main points: Needle with draining.

LI-04	*hé gǔ*
ST-25	*tiān shū*
ST-37	*shàng jù xū*
GV-14	*dà zhuī*
M-UE-1-5	*shí xuān* (Ten Diffusing Points) (Bleed)

Auxiliary points:

For loss of consciousness with convulsions, to open the orifices and return consciousness, needle:

GV-26	*shuǐ gōu*
KI-01	*yǒng quán*

To drain heat and extinguish wind:

LR-03	*tài chōng*
BL-40 (54)	*wěi zhōng*

3. COLD-DAMPNESS DYSENTERY

Clinical Symptoms: Sticky stools mixed with pus and blood (pus being more predominant), abdominal pain, tenesmus, oppression in the chest and fullness of the epigastrium, aversion to cold and preference for warmth, loss of appetite, no apparent thirst, heaviness of the head and limbs.

Tongue: Pale with white slimy coating.

Pulse: Soft, tardy.

Treatment Method: Warm and dissipate cold dampness, rectify qi, dissolve stasis.

PRESCRIPTION

Stomach-Calming Poria Five Decoction *wèi líng tāng*

cāng zhú	atractylodes [root]	Atractylodis Rhizoma	9 g.
bái zhú	ovate atractylodes [root]	Atractylodis Ovatae Rhizoma	9 g.
fú líng	poria	Poria	9 g.
zhū líng	polyporus	Polyporus	9 g.
hòu pò	magnolia [bark]	Magnoliae Cortex	9 g.
chén pí	tangerine [peel]	Citri Exocarpium	9 g.
zé xiè	alisma [tuber]	Alismatis Rhizoma	12 g.
guì zhī	cinnamon [twig]	Cinnamomi Ramulus	6 g.
zhì gān cǎo	licorice [root] (honey-fried)	Glycyrrhizae Radix	3 g.

MODIFICATIONS

Since diuresis is contraindicated in the treatment of dysentery, the prescription is modified to invigorate the blood.

Delete:

zé xiè	alisma [tuber]	Alismatis Rhizoma
fú líng	poria	Poria

Add:

bái sháo yào	white peony [root]	Paeoniae Radix Alba	12 g.
dāng guī	tangkuei	Angelicae Sinensis Radix	9 g.

In all of the above cases, reinforce the prescription to rectify qi and dissipate cold.
Add:

bīng láng	areca [nut]	Arecae Semen	9 g.
mù xiāng	saussurea [root]	Saussureae (seu Vladimiriae) Radix	9 g.
pào jiāng	blast-fried ginger (charred)	Zingiberis Rhizoma Tostum	6 g.

ACUPUNCTURE AND MOXIBUSTION

Main points: Needle with supplementation; add moxibustion.

LI-04	*hé gǔ*
ST-25	*tiān shū*
ST-37	*shàng jù xū*
SP-09	*yīn líng quán*
CV-12	*zhōng wǎn*

4. YIN VACUITY DYSENTERY

Clinical Symptoms: Stools mixed with pus and blood, elimination of fresh blood and thick mucus (in some cases), burning pain in the abdomen, loss of appetite, irritability, thirst.

Tongue: Dark red with little coating.

Pulse: Rapid, thready.

Treatment Method: Clear heat, nourish yin, relieve dysentery.

PRESCRIPTION
Carriage-Halting Pill *zhù chē wán*

huáng lián	coptis [root]	Coptidis Rhizoma	9 g.
dāng guī	tangkuei	Angelicae Sinensis Radix	6 g.
ē jiāo	ass hide glue (dissolved and stirred in)	Asini Corii Gelatinum	9 g.
pào jiāng	blast-fried ginger (charred)	Zingiberis Rhizoma Tostum	1.5 g.

MODIFICATIONS

The prescription may be reinforced to relieve pain. Add:

| *bái sháo yào* | white peony [root] | Paeoniae Radix Alba | 12 g. |
| *gān cǎo* | licorice [root] | Glycyrrhizae Radix | 6 g. |

In cases where vacuity fire has depleted fluids giving rise to symptoms of severe thirst, scanty urine and dry tongue, the prescription is modified to nourish yin and generate liquid.

Add:

| *běi shā shēn* | glehnia [root] | Glehniae Radix | 12 g. |
| *shí hú* | dendrobium [stem] (extended decoction) | Dendrobii Caulis | 12 g. |

In cases where large amounts of blood are present in the stool, the prescription is modified to cool the blood and relieve bleeding.

Add:

mǔ dān pí	moutan [root bark]	Moutan Radicis Cortex	9 g.
hàn lián cǎo	eclipta	Ecliptae Herba	12 g.
dì yú	sanguisorba [root]	Sanguisorbae Radix	9 g.

In cases where damp-heat has not been completely dispersed, with symptoms of bitter taste in the mouth and burning sensation of the anus, the prescription is modified to clear heat and disinhibit dampness.

Add:

| *huáng bǎi* | phellodendron [bark] | Phellodendri Cortex | 9 g. |
| *qín pí* | ash [bark] | Fraxini Cortex | 9 g. |

ACUPUNCTURE AND MOXIBUSTION

Main points: Needle with supplementation.

LI-04	*hé gǔ*
ST-25	*tiān shū*
ST-37	*shàng jù xū*
KI-06	*zhào hǎi*
SP-06	*sān yīn jiāo*

5. VACUITY-COLD DYSENTERY

Clinical Symptoms: Liquid stools mixed with pus, incontinence of stools (in severe cases), dull cold abdominal pain, loss of appetite, fatigue, physical cold, cold extremities, lower back ache.

Tongue: Pale with white coating.

Pulse: Deep, thready.

Treatment Method: Warm and supplement the spleen and kidney, relieve dysentery with astringent herbs.

PRESCRIPTION
True Man Viscus-Nourishing Decoction *zhēn rén yǎng zàng tāng*

rén shēn	ginseng	Ginseng Radix	9 g.
bái zhú	ovate atractylodes [root]	Atractylodis Ovatae Rhizoma	12 g.
bái sháo yào	white peony [root]	Paeoniae Radix Alba	15 g.
dāng guī	tangkuei	Angelicae Sinensis Radix	9 g.
mù xiāng	saussurea [root]	Saussureae Radix (seu Vladimiriae)	9 g.
hē zǐ	chebule	Chebulae Fructus	9 g.
ròu guì	cinnamon bark (abbreviated decoction)	Cinnamomi Cortex	6 g.
yīng sù ké	poppy [husk]	Papaveris Pericarpium	12 g.
ròu dòu kòu	nutmeg	Myristicae Semen	9 g.
zhì gān cǎo	licorice [root] (honey-fried)	Glycyrrhizae Radix	6 g.

MODIFICATIONS

In cases where the above prescription does not achieve significant therapeutic effects, the prescription is modified to consolidate the yang restoring action.

Add:

zhì fù zǐ	aconite [accessory tuber] (processed) (extended decoction)	Aconiti Tuber Laterale Praeparatum	6 g.
pào jiāng	blast-fried ginger (charred)	Zingiberis Rhizoma Tostum	6 g.

In cases of prolonged dysentery, with vacuous spleen qi leading to anal prolapse, the prescription is modified to benefit spleen qi and rectify prolapse. Use:

Center-Supplementing Qi-Boosting Decoction *bǔ zhōng yì qì tāng*

huáng qí	astragalus [root]	Astragali seu Hedysari Radix	15 g.
rén shēn	ginseng	Ginseng Radix	9 g.
bái zhú	ovate atractylodes [root]	Atractylodis Ovatae Rhizoma	9 g.
dāng guī	tangkuei	Angelicae Sinensis Radix	9 g.
chén pí	tangerine [peel]	Citri Exocarpium	6 g.
shēng má	cimicifuga [root]	Cimicifugae Rhizoma	3 g.
chái hú	bupleurum [root]	Bupleuri Radix	3 g.
zhì gān cǎo	licorice [root] (honey-fried)	Glycyrrhizae Radix	6 g.

ACUPUNCTURE AND MOXIBUSTION

Main points: Needle with supplementation; add moxibustion.

LI-04	*hé gǔ*
ST-25	*tiān shū*
ST-37	*shàng jù xū*
BL-20	*pí shū*
BL-23	*shèn shū*

Auxiliary points:

For anal prolapse, add:

GV-01	*cháng qiáng*
GV-20	*bǎi huì* (moxibustion)

6. CHRONIC INTERMITTENT DYSENTERY

Clinical Symptoms: Recurring dysentery showing no improvement over an extended time, abdominal pain, tenesmus, stools mixed with both pus and blood duirng attacks of dysentery, tiredness, fatigue, lethargy and loss of appetite.

Tongue: Pale with slimy coating.

Pulse: Thready.

Treatment Method: Warm and strengthen the spleen, clear heat, rectify qi, dissolve stasis.

PRESCRIPTION
Coptis Rectifying Decoction *lián lǐ tāng*

rén shēn	ginseng	Ginseng Radix	12 g.
bái zhú	ovate atractylodes [root]	Atractylodis Ovatae Rhizoma	9 g.
huáng lián	coptis [root]	Coptidis Rhizoma	9 g.
fú líng	poria	Poria	9 g.
zhì gān cǎo	licorice [root] (honey-fried)	Glycyrrhizae Radix	6 g.

MODIFICATIONS

To rectify qi and remove stasis, delete:

fú líng	poria	Poria

Add:

bīng láng	areca [nut]	Arecae Semen	9 g.
mù xiāng	saussurea [root]	Saussureae seu Vladimiriae Radix	9 g.
zhǐ shí	unripe bitter orange	Aurantii Fructus Immaturus	9 g.

In cases of extreme vacuity of spleen yang, with symptoms of cold abdomen with pain, cold extremities and stools mixed with pus, the prescription is modified to warm the spleen and dissipate cold.

Delete:

huáng lián	coptis [root]	Coptidis Rhizoma

and add:

zhì fù zǐ	aconite, accessory tuber (processed) (extended decoction)	Processed Aconiti Tuber Laterale	6 g.
ròu guì	cinnamon bark (abbreviated decoction)	Cinnamomi Cortex	6 g.

In cases of persistent dysentery, with patterns complicated by both heat and cold, the prescription is modified to warm the organs and clear the intestines.

Use:

Mume Pill *wū méi wán*

wū méi	mume [fruit]	Mume Fructus	12 g.
zhì fù zǐ	aconite [accessory tuber] (processed) (extended decoction)	Aconiti Tuber Laterale Praeparatum	6 g.
gān jiāng	dried ginger [root]	Zingiberis Rhizoma Exsiccatum	6 g.
huā jiāo	zanthoxylum	Zanthoxyli Pericarpium	1.5 g.
guì zhī	cinnamon twig	Cinnamomi Ramulus	6 g.
xì xīn	asarum	Asiasari Herba cum Radice	1.5 g.
rén shēn	ginseng	Ginseng Radix	9 g.
dāng guī	tangkuei	Angelicae Sinensis Radix	6 g.
huáng lián	coptis [root]	Coptidis Rhizoma	6 g.
huáng bǎi	phellodendron [bark]	Phellodendri Cortex	9 g.

In treating cases between recurrences of dysentery, the prescription is modified to prevent recurrence.

Use:

Saussurea and Amomum Six Gentlemen Decoction *xiāng shā liù jūn zǐ tāng*

rén shēn	ginseng	Ginseng Radix	9 g.
bái zhú	ovate atractylodes [root]	Atractylodis Ovatae Rhizoma	9 g.
fú líng	poria	Poria	9 g.
mù xiāng	saussurea [root]	Saussureae seu Vladimiriae Radix	6 g.
shā rén	amomum [fruit] (abbreviated decoction)	Amomi Semen seu Fructus	6 g.
zhì gān cǎo	licorice [root] (honey-fried)	Glycyrrhizae Radix	6 g.

In cases of extended illnesses with symptoms of dark red stools resembling fruit preserves, abdominal pain and relatively mild tenesmus, brucea *(yā dàn zǐ)* may be used to treat dysentery.* The method of administration is to remove the shells of the seeds and package the inner kernels in capsules. The adult dosage is fifteen capsules each time, three times daily over seven to ten days. Since brucea *(yā dàn zǐ)* is a gastrointestinal irritant, it should be taken after meals.

ACUPUNCTURE AND MOXIBUSTION

Main points: Needle with even supplementation, even draining.

LI-04	*hé gǔ*
ST-25	*tiān shū*
ST-37	*shàng jù xū*
CV-04	*guān yuán*
ST-36	*zú sān lǐ*

ALTERNATE THERAPEUTIC METHODS

1. Ear Acupuncture

Main Points: Large Intestine, Small Intestine, Stomach, Lower portion of Rectum, *Shén Mén*, Spleen, Kidney

Method: Select three to five points each session. In cases of acute dysentery needle to elicit a strong sensation and retain the needles twenty to thirty minutes once daily. In cases of chronic dysentery, elicit a mild sensation and retain needles for five to ten minutes every second day.

REMARKS

In the differential diagnosis of dysentery, it is necessary to clearly distinguish cold from heat and vacuity from repletion. Generally speaking, repletion patterns are observed at the onset of illness, while vacuity patterns manifest as cases become prolonged. Cases of chronic intermittent dysentery generally show as pattern of root vacuity and branch repletion.

Concerning treatment, use the clearing method when dysentery is caused by heat, use the warming method when it is due to cold, promote elimination when it is of short duration and supplement when of extended duration. Use the clear and warm methods together when patterns are complicated by both heat and cold. Drain and supplement when patterns are complicated by both repletion and vacuity.

Though symptoms such as stool mixed with blood and pus, abdominal pain and tenesmus may be alleviated after several days of treatment, continue treatment for an additional five to seven days to ensure thorough clearing of evils, so as to prevent recurrence of the illness.

---

*Brucea *(yā dàn zǐ)* has proven clinically effective against amoebas in their cyst stage. — (Ed.)

CONSTIPATION

Biàn Bì

1. Heat Constipation - 2. Qi Stagnation Constipation - 3. Qi Vacuity Constipation - 4. Blood Vacuity Constipation - 5. Cold Constipation

Fecal block *(biàn bì)* refers to conditions in which the bowels have difficulty evacuating stools. This includes conditions where the feces are too hard to pass, where too much time is spent moving the bowels, or where evacuation is difficult even though the sensation of needing to move the bowels is present. The major factor causing constipation is dysfunction of the large intestine.

Constipation patterns are present in what is known as habitual constipation in Western medicine, in certain cases of neurosis, during the recovery stages of enteritis, postpartum, after surgery or illnesses that weaken peristalsis or during certain pathological conditions of the rectum or anus. For cases of high fever accompanied by constipation, refer either to this chapter, or to the differentiation and treatment of febrile diseases.

ETIOLOGY AND PATHOGENESIS

Although the pathogenesis of constipation usually involves the inability of the large intestine to move feces, it is also intimately connected with the functioning of the spleen, stomach and kidney. The pathogenesis of constipation includes the stagnation of internal heat and dryness resulting in lack of fluids, stagnation of the flow of qi from emotional upset and vacuity of qi or blood from internal injury from strain, stress or a lack of physical exercise. Constipation is classified as five categories according to its etiology, pathogenesis and clinical manifestations: heat constipation, qi stagnation constipation, qi vacuity constipation, blood vacuity constipation and cold constipation.

1. HEAT CONSTIPATION

Clinical Manifestations: Constipation, elimination at several day intervals, dark scanty urine, flushed complexion, fever, thirst, halitosis and abdominal distention with pain in some cases.

Tongue: Red with dry yellow coating.

Pulse: Rapid, slippery.

Treatment Method: Clear heat, moisten the intestines.

PRESCRIPTION

Hemp Seed Pill *má zǐ rén wán*

huǒ má rén	hemp [seed]	Cannabis Semen	15 g.
bái sháo yào	white peony [root]	Paeoniae Radix Alba	9 g.
zhǐ shí	unripe bitter orange	Aurantii Fructus Immaturus	9 g.
hòu pò	magnolia [bark]	Magnoliae Cortex	9 g.
dà huáng	rhubarb (abbreviated decoction)	Rhei Rhizoma	9 g.
xìng rén	apricot [kernel]	Armeniacae Semen	9 g.

MODIFICATIONS

In cases where there is injury to fluids, the prescription is modified to nourish yin and generate liquid.

Add:

shēng dì huáng	rehmannia [root] dried/fresh	Rehmanniae Radix Exsiccata seu Recens	9 g.
xuán shēn	scrophularia [root]	Scrophulariae Radix	9 g.
mài mén dōng	ophiopogon [tuber]	Ophiopogonis Tuber	9 g.

In cases accompanied by injury to the liver by depression or anger, with symptoms of irritability, red eyes and wiry pulse, the prescription can be reinforced to clear the liver and move the bowels. Use the prepared medicine, TOILETTE PILL *(gēng yī wán)*.

ACUPUNCTURE AND MOXIBUSTION

Main points: Needle with draining.

ST-25	*tiān shū*
BL-25	*dà cháng shū*
TB-06	*zhī gōu*
KI-06	*zhào hǎi*
LI-04	*hé gǔ*
LI-11	*qū chí*

Auxiliary points:

For irritability, fever and thirst, add:

HT-08	*shào fǔ*
CV-23	*lián quán*

For headache, add:

M-HN-3	*yìn táng* (Hall of Impression)

For halitosis, add:

CV-24	*chéng jiāng*

2. QI STAGNATION CONSTIPATION

Clinical Manifestations: Constipation, frequent belching, sensation of stuffiness and blockage in the chest and hypochondrium, reduced food intake and abdominal distention and pain in severe cases.

Tongue: Thin slimy coating.

Pulse: Wiry.

Treatment Method: Normalize qi, move stagnation.

PRESCRIPTION

Six Milled Ingredients Beverage *liù mò yǐn*

chén xiāng	aquilaria [wood] (powdered and stirred in)	Aquilariae Lignum	3 g.
bīng láng	areca [nut]	Arecae Semen	9 g.
mù xiāng	saussurea [root]	Saussureae seu Vladimiriae Radix	9 g.
wū yào	lindera [root]	Linderae Radix	9 g.
zhǐ shí	unripe bitter orange	Aurantii Fructus Immaturus	9 g.
dà huáng	rhubarb (abbreviated decoction)	Rhei Rhizoma	9 g.

MODIFICATIONS

In cases of prolonged stagnation of qi giving rise to fire, with symptoms of bitter tasting mouth, dry throat, yellow tongue coating and rapid wiry pulse, the prescription is modified to clear heat and drain fire. Add:

huáng qín	scutellaria [root]	Scutellariae Radix	9 g.
shān zhī zǐ	gardenia	Gardeniae Fructus	9 g.

ACUPUNCTURE AND MOXIBUSTION

Main points: Needle with draining.

ST-25	*tiān shū*
BL-25	*dà cháng shū*
TB-06	*zhī gōu*
CV-06	*qì hǎi*
CV-12	*zhōng wǎn*
LR-03	*tài chōng*

Auxiliary points:

For severe costal pain, add:

LR-14	*qī mén*
GB-24	*rì yuè*

3. QI VACUITY CONSTIPATION

Clinical Manifestations: Difficult elimination despite the need to move the bowels, the stools are neither too hard nor dry and there is neither abdominal pain nor distention. These symptoms may be accompanied by shortness of breath, spontaneous perspiration, fatigue or tiredness.

Tongue: Pale, delicate.

Pulse: Weak.

Treatment Method: Boost qi, free the stool.

PRESCRIPTION

Astragalus Decoction *huáng-qí tāng*

huáng qí	astragalus [root]	Astragali (seu Hedysari) Radix	30 g.
chén pí	tangerine [peel]	Citri Exocarpium	9 g.
huǒ má rén	hemp [seed]	Cannabis Semen	15 g.
fēng mì	honey (stirred in)	Mel	15 g.

MODIFICATIONS

In severe cases of qi vacuity, the prescription is modified to increase the supplementation of qi. Add:

rén shēn	ginseng	Ginseng Radix	9 g.
bái zhú	ovate atractylodes [root]	Atractylodis Ovatae Rhizoma	9 g.

ACUPUNCTURE AND MOXIBUSTION

Main points: Needle with supplementation; add moxibustion.

ST-25	*tiān shū*
BL-25	*dà cháng shū*
SP-06	*sān yīn jiāo*
BL-20	*pí shū*
ST-36	*zú sān lǐ*
CV-04	*guān yuán*

4. BLOOD VACUITY CONSTIPATION

Clinical Manifestations: Dry hard stools, pale complexion, dizziness and vertigo, palpitations, pale lips.

Tongue: Pale.

Pulse: Rough, thready.

Treatment Method: Nourish the blood, moisten the intestines.

PRESCRIPTION

Intestine-Moistening Pill *rùn cháng wán*

shēng dì huáng	rehmannia [root] dried/fresh	Rehmanniae Radix Exsiccata seu Recens	12 g.
dāng guī	tangkuei	Angelicae Sinensis Radix	12 g.
huǒ má rén	hemp [seed]	Cannabis Semen	15 g.
táo rén	peach [kernel]	Persicae Semen	9 g.
zhǐ ké	bitter orange	Aurantii Fructus	9 g.

MODIFICATIONS

For aged patients or postpartum difficulty moving the bowels, the prescription is modified to boost qi, promote production of blood and moisten the intestines. Add:

huáng qí	astragalus [root]	Astragali (seu Hedysari) Radix	12 g.
hé shǒu wū	flowery knotweed [root]	Polygoni Multiflori Radix	12 g.
ròu cōng róng	cistanche [stem]	Cistanches Caulis	12 g.

In cases compounded by yin vacuity and subsequent internal heat with symptoms of constipation accompanied by thirst, irritability, red tongue with little coating and a rapid thready pulse, the prescription is modified to replenish yin and clear heat.

Add:

xuán shēn	scrophularia [root]	Scrophulariae Radix	9 g.
zhī mǔ	anemarrhena [root]	Anemarrhenae Rhizoma	9 g.

ACUPUNCTURE AND MOXIBUSTION

Main points: Needle with supplementation; add moxibustion.

ST-25	*tiān shū*
BL-25	*dà cháng shū*
ST-36	*zú sān lǐ*
SP-14	*fù jié*
CV-04	*guān yuán*
SP-06	*sān yīn jiāo*

Auxiliary points:

For yin vacuity with internal heat, add:

KI-06	*zhào hǎi*

For palpitations, add:

PC-06	*nèi guān*

5. COLD CONSTIPATION

Clinical Manifestations: Difficult elimination with clear copious urine, pale complexion, dizziness and vertigo, cold extremities, a preference for heat and an aversion to cold, abdominal coldness and pain, coldness and aching of the lower back and knees.

Tongue: Pale with white coating.

Pulse: Slow, deep.

Treatment Method: Warm kidney yang, replenish kidney essence, moisten bowels, promote elimination.

PRESCRIPTION

Ferry Brew *jì chuān jiān*

dāng guī	tangkuei	Angelicae Sinensis Radix	12 g.
ròu cōng róng	cistanche [stem]	Cistanches Caulis	12 g.
niú xī	achyranthes [root]	Achyranthis Bidentatae Radix	6 g.
zé xiè	alisma [tuber]	Alismatis Rhizoma	4.5 g.
shēng má	cimicifuga [root]	Cimicifugae Rhizoma	3 g.
zhǐ ké	bitter orange	Aurantii Fructus	3 g.

MODIFICATIONS

To warm yang and supplement the kidney, add:

ròu guì	cinnamon bark (abbreviated decoction)	Cinnamomi Cortex	6 g.
shú dì huáng	cooked rehmannia [root]	Rehmanniae Radix Conquita	12 g.

ACUPUNCTURE AND MOXIBUSTION

Main points: Needle with supplementation; add moxibustion.

ST-25	*tiān shū*
BL-25	*dà cháng shū*
CV-06	*qì hǎi*
BL-23	*shèn shū*
CV-04	*guān yuán shu*
KI-06	*zhào hǎi*

Auxiliary points:

For severe yang vacuity, add moxibustion of:

      CV-08   *shén què*

For lower back pain, add:

      BL-40 (54) *wěi zhōng*

For anal prolapse, add:

      GV-01   *cháng qiáng*
      GV-20   *bǎi huì*

ALTERNATE THERAPEUTIC METHODS

1. Ear Acupuncture

Main points: Large Intestine, lower portion of Rectum, Brain.

Method: Elicit a moderate to strong sensation. Retain needles for twenty to thirty minutes. Needle once daily.

REMARKS

Patients suffering from constipation should add more fruits and vegetables to the diet, participate in physical exercise and foster the habit of moving the bowels at a fixed time each day.

LATERAL COSTAL PAIN

Xié Tòng

1. Stagnation of Liver Qi - 2. Stasis of Liver Blood - 3. Liver and Gallbladder Damp-Heat - 4. Vacuity of Liver Yin

SUPPLEMENT: GALLBLADDER INFLAMMATION; GALLSTONES

Dǎn Náng Yán; Dǎn Shí Zhèng

1. Stagnation of Liver and Gallbladder Qi - 2. Obstruction by Damp-Heat - 3. Heat-Toxins of the Liver and Gallbladder

Lateral costal pain, a commonly observed clinical symptom, may involve one or both sides of the costal region. The degree of pain differs from case to case. Chronic illnesses generally exhibit dull or indistinct pain in the costal region, while acute or severe conditions can exhibit excruciating pain.

Costal pain may be present in acute and chronic disorders of the liver, gallbladder and pleura, including the Western medical conditions of hepatitis, hepatomegaly, cholecystitis and cholelithiasis. Cases of traumatic injury to the costal region, costal chondritis, and intercostal neuralgia are also included. Please refer to the chapter on Parasitic Worms *(chóng zhèng)* for the treatment of costal pain because of biliary roundworm.

ETIOLOGY AND PATHOGENESIS

The pathogenesis of costal pain mainly involves the liver and gallbladder. It is classified as either repletion or vacuity, although repletion patterns are most often observed. Repletion patterns usually involve qi stagnation, from which blood stasis or the accumulation of damp-heat are a secondary event. Vacuity patterns involve a depletion of yin and blood leading to malnourishment of the liver.

Vacuity and repletion are not absolute or invariable and may present simultaneously or in mutual transformation. Repletion patterns can in time produce heat and deplete yin, while cases of liver and kidney yin vacuity can lead to, or be accompanied by, qi stagnation and blood stasis.

1. STAGNATION OF LIVER QI

Clinical Symptoms: Distending pain of indeterminate location in the costal region and oppression in the chest, sometimes accompanied by frequent sighing, irritability or mental depression, bitter taste in the mouth or acid regurgitation. These symptoms are often affected by the emotional state of the patient.

Tongue: Thin white coating.

Pulse: Wiry.

Treatment Method: Soothe the liver, rectify qi, relieve pain.

PRESCRIPTION
Bupleurum Liver-Coursing Powder *chái hú shū gān sǎn*

chái hú	bupleurum [root]	Bupleuri Radix	6 g.
bái sháo yào	white peony [root]	Paeoniae Radix Alba	9 g.
xiāng fù zǐ	cyperus [root]	Cyperi Rhizoma	6 g.
chuān xiōng	ligusticum [root]	Ligustici Rhizoma	6 g.
chén pí	tangerine [peel]	Citri Exocarpium	6 g.
zhǐ ké	bitter orange	Aurantii Fructus	6 g.
zhì gān cǎo	licorice [root] (honey-fried)	Glycyrrhizae Radix	3 g.

MODIFICATIONS

In cases of severe costal pain, the prescription is reinforced to increase the effects of regulating qi and relieving pain. Add:

qīng pí	unripe tangerine [peel]	Citri Exocarpium Immaturum	6 g.
chuān liàn zǐ	toosendan [fruit]	Toosendan Fructus	6 g.
yù jīn	curcuma [tuber]	Curcumae Tuber	6 g.

In cases where the stagnation of qi gives rise to heat, with symptoms of pulling pain in the costal regions, dryness and bitterness in the mouth, dark urine, constipation, red tongue with yellow coating and rapid wiry pulse, the prescription is modified to clear the liver, rectify qi and relieve pain.

Delete:

chuān xiōng	ligusticum [root]	Ligustici Rhizoma

Select from and add:

mǔ dān pí	moutan [root bark]	Moutan Radicis Cortex	9 g.
shān zhī zǐ	gardenia	Gardeniae Fructus	9 g.
huáng lián	coptis [root]	Coptidis Rhizoma	6 g.
chuān liàn zǐ	toosendan [fruit]	Toosendan Fructus	9 g.
yán hú suǒ	corydalis [tuber]	Corydalis Tuber	9 g.

In cases where the qi stagnation gives rise to heat that injures liver yin, with dull pain in the the costal region aggravated by overwork, dizziness and vertigo, insomnia, a red tongue with thin dry coating and a thready wiry pulse, the prescription is modified to nourish yin and clear heat.

Delete:

chuān xiōng	ligusticum [root]	Ligustici Rhizoma

Add:

dāng guī	tangkuei	Angelicae Sinensis Radix	9 g.
hé shǒu wū	flowery knotweed [root]	Polygoni Multiflori Radix	9 g.
gǒu qǐ zǐ	lycium [berry]	Lycii Fructus	9 g.
shān zhī zǐ	gardenia [fruit]	Gardeniae Fructus	6 g.
jú huā	chrysanthemum [flower]	Chrysanthemi Flos	6 g.

In cases where liver qi adversely affects the transporting function of the spleen, with costal pain accompanied by borborygmus, abdominal pain or diarrhea, the prescription is modified to fortify the spleen, inhibit the liver and relieve diarrhea. Add:

bái zhú	ovate atractylodes [root]	Atractylodis Ovatae Rhizoma	9 g.
fáng fēng	ledebouriella [root]	Ledebouriellae Radix	4.5 g.
fú líng	poria	Poria	9 g.
yì yǐ rén	coix [seed]	Coicis Semen	15 g.

In cases accompanied by disturbance of the stomach's descending function, with symptoms of nausea and vomiting, the prescription is modified to harmonize the stomach, downbear qi and relieve vomiting. Add:

xuán fù huā	inula flower (wrapped)	Inulae Flos	9 g.
dài zhě shí	hematite (extended decoction)	Haematitum	12 g.
jiāng bàn xià	(ginger-processed) pinellia [tuber]	Pinelliae Tuber Praeparatum	9 g.
shēng jiāng	fresh ginger	Zingiberis Rhizoma Recens	6 g.

In cases accompanied by poor appetite and abdominal distention after eating, the prescription is modified to revitalize the spleen and stomach and disperse food. Add:

jī nèi jīn	gizzard lining	Galli Gigerii Endothelium	9 g.
shén qū	medicated leaven	Massa Medicata Fermentata	12 g.
shān zhā	crataegus [fruit]	Crataegi Fructus	9 g.
shā rén	amomum [fruit] (abbreviated decoction)	Amomi Semen seu Fructus	6 g.

In cases of acid regurgitation, the prescription is modified to restrain acid. Add:

wǎ léng zǐ	ark shell (extended decoction)	Arcae Concha	15 g.
huáng lián	coptis [root]	Coptidis Rhizoma	9 g.
wú zhū yú	evodia [fruit]	Evodiae Fructus	1.5 g.

ACUPUNCTURE AND MOXIBUSTION

Main points: Needle with draining.

BL-18	*gān shū*
LR-14	*qī mén*
LR-03	*tài chōng*
TB-06	*zhī gōu*
GB-34	*yáng líng quán*

Auxiliary points:

For acid regurgitation, add:

BL-21	*wèi shū*

For insomnia, add:

HT-07	*shén mén*

2. STASIS OF LIVER BLOOD

Clinical Symptoms: Stabbing pain of definite location in the costal region which increases with external pressure and intensifies at night, sometimes accompanied by a mass under the ribs.

Tongue: Dark, purplish, sometimes with stasis macules on the tongue.

Pulse: Deep, wiry or deep, rough.

Treatment Method: Rectify qi, dispel blood stasis, relieve pain.

PRESCRIPTION

Infradiaphragmatic Stasis-Expelling Decoction *gé xià zhú yū tāng*

wǔ líng zhī	flying squirrel droppings (wrapped)	Trogopteri seu Pteromydis Excrementum	9 g.
dāng guī	tangkuei	Angelicae Sinensis Radix	9 g.
táo rén	peach [kernel]	Persicae Semen	9 g.
hóng huā	carthamus [flower]	Carthami Flosa	9 g.
chuān xiōng	ligusticum [root]	Ligustici Rhizoma	6 g.
mǔ dān pí	moutan [root bark]	Moutan Radicis Cortex	6 g.
wū yào	lindera [root]	Linderae Radix	6 g.
xiāng fù zǐ	cyperus [root]	Cyperi Rhizoma	4.5 g.
chì sháo yào	red peony [root]	Paeoniae Radix Rubra	6 g.
zhǐ ké	bitter orange	Aurantii Fructus	4.5 g.
yán hú suǒ	corydalis [tuber]	Corydalis Tuber	3 g.
gān cǎo	licorice [root]	Glycyrrhizae Radix	9 g.

MODIFICATIONS

In cases of rather severe costal pain caused by traumatic injury, the treatment principle is to quicken the blood, dispel stasis and relieve pain. Use:

Origin-Restorative Blood-Quickening Decoction *fù yuán huó xuè tāng*

táo rén	peach [kernel]	Persica Semen	9 g.
chái hú	bupleurum [root]	Bupleuri Radix	9 g.
dà huáng tàn	rhubarb (charred)	Rhei Rhizoma Carbonistatum	30 g.
dāng guī	tangkuei	Angelicae Sinensis Radix	9 g.
tiān huā fěn	trichosanthes [root]	Trichosanthis Radix	12 g.
hóng huā	carthamus [flower]	Carthami Flosa	6 g.
chuān shān jiǎ	pangolin scales	Manitis Squama	6 g.
gān cǎo	licorice [root]	Glycyrrhizae Radix	6 g.
huáng jiǔ	yellow wine	Vinum Aureum	20 cc.

In cases where a mass is present under the ribs and correct qi is still strong, the prescription is modified to dispel stasis and dissipate binds.

Add to the above:

sān léng	sparganium [root]	Sparganii Rhizoma	9 g.
é zhú	zedoary	Zedoariae Rhizoma	9 g.
zhè chóng	wingless cockroach	Eupolyphaga seu Opisthoplatia	9 g.

ACUPUNCTURE AND MOXIBUSTION

Main points: Needle with draining.

BL-17	*gé shū*
LR-03	*tài chōng*
LI-04	*hé gǔ*
SP-06	*sān yīn jiāo*
GB-25	*jǐng mén*
SP-21	*dà bāo*
LR-14	*qī mén*

Auxiliary points:

For traumatic costal injury, add:

A-Shi Points	*ā shì xué* (Ouch Points)

3. LIVER AND GALLBLADDER DAMP-HEAT

Clinical Symptoms: Severe costal pain, bitter taste in the mouth, oppression in the chest, loss of appetite, nausea, vomiting, jaundice (in some cases), dark urine.

Tongue: Yellow slimy coating.

Pulse: Slippery, rapid or wiry, rapid.

Treatment Method: Clear heat, disinhibit dampness, relieve pain.

PRESCRIPTION

Gentian Liver-Draining Decoction *lóng dǎn xiè gān tāng*

lóng dǎn cǎo	gentian [root]	Gentianae Radix	6 g.
huáng qín	scutellaria [root]	Scutellariae Radix	9 g.
shān zhī zǐ	gardenia [fruit]	Gardeniae Fructus	9 g.
zé xiè	alisma [tuber]	Alismatis Rhizoma	12 g.
mù tōng	mutong [stem]	Mutong Caulis	9 g.
dāng guī	tangkuei	Angelicae Sinensis Radix	3 g.
chē qián zǐ	plantago seed (wrapped)	Plantaginis Semen	9 g.
shēng dì huáng	rehmannia [root] dried/fresh	Rehmanniae Radix Exsiccata seu Recens	9 g.
chái hú	bupleurum [root]	Bupleuri Radix	6 g.
gān cǎo	licorice [root]	Glycyrrhizae Radix	6 g.

MODIFICATIONS

To reinforce the effects of the prescription, and to course the liver, harmonize the stomach, rectify qi and relieve pain, add:

chuān liàn zǐ	toosendan [fruit]	Toosendan Fructus	9 g.
qīng pí	unripe tangerine [peel]	Citri Exocarpium Immaturum	6 g.
yù jīn	curcuma [tuber]	Curcumae Tuber	9 g.
jiāng bàn xià	(ginger-processed) pinellia [tuber]	Pinelliae Tuber Praeparatum	6 g.

In cases of fever and jaundice, the prescription is modified to clear heat, disinhibit dampness and dispel jaundice.
Add:

yīn chén hāo	capillaris	Artemisiae Capillaris Herba	30 g.
huáng bǎi	phellodendron [bark]	Phellodendri Cortex	9 g.

In cases where the accumulation of damp-heat has led to the formation of stones that obstruct the gallbladder and give rise to a severe costal pain that radiates through the back and shoulder, the prescription is modified to dredge the gallbladder and expel stones.
Add:

jīn qián cǎo	moneywort	Jinqiancao Herba	30 g.
yù jīn	curcuma [tuber]	Curcumae Tuber	12 g.
hǎi jīn shā	lygodium spore (wrapped)	Lygodii Spora	12 g.

In cases where heat has depleted fluids, with abdominal distention, fullness and constipation, the prescription is modified to drain heat and promote elimination.
Add:

dà huáng	rhubarb (abbreviated decoction)	Rhei Rhizoma	9 g.
máng xiāo	mirabilite (stirred in)	Mirabilitum	9 g.

ACUPUNCTURE AND MOXIBUSTION

Main points: Needle with draining.

LR-14	*qī mén*
GB-24	*rì yuè*
TB-06	*zhī gōu*
GB-34	*yáng líng quán*
LR-03	*tài chōng*
SP-09	*yīn líng quán*

Auxiliary points:

For severe heat, add:

   GV-14   *dà zhuī*

For nausea and abdominal distention, add:

   ST-36   *zú sān lǐ*
   CV-12   *zhōng wǎn*

For irritability, add:

   PC-04   *xī mén*

For jaundice, add:

   GV-09   *zhì yáng*

4. VACUITY OF LIVER YIN

Clinical Symptoms: Dull or indistinct costal pain aggravated by overwork, with irritability, dry mouth and throat, dizziness and vertigo.

Tongue: Red with little coating.

Pulse: Thready, wiry, rapid.

Treatment Method: Nourish yin, soothe the liver, relieve pain.

PRESCRIPTION

All-the-Way-Through* Brew *yī guàn jiān*

běi shā shēn	glehnia [root]	Glehniae Radix	9 g.
mài mén dōng	ophiopogon [tuber]	Ophiopogonis Tuber	9 g.
dāng guī	tangkuei	Angelicae Sinensis Radix	9 g.
shēng dì huáng	rehmannia [root] (dried/fresh)	Rehmanniae Radix Exsiccata seu Recens	30 g.
gǒu qǐ zǐ	lycium [berry]	Lycii Fructus	12 g.
chuān liàn zǐ	toosendan [fruit]	Toosendan Fructus	4.5 g.

(* Linking liver and kidney yin dysfunction)

MODIFICATIONS

To increase the pain-relieving effects of this prescription, add:

yán hú suǒ	corydalis [tuber]	Corydalis Tuber	9 g.

In cases of irritability, palpitations and insomnia, the prescription is modified to clear heat and quiet the spirit. Add:

shān zhī zǐ	gardenia [fruit]	Gardeniae Fructus	6 g.
suān zǎo rén	spiny jujube [kernel]	Ziziphi Spinosi Semen	12 g.

In cases where dizziness and vertigo are marked, the prescription is modified to supplement the liver and kidney. Add:

nǚ zhēn zǐ	ligustrum [fruit]	Ligustri Fructus	9 g.
hàn lián cǎo	eclipta	Ecliptae Herba	9 g.
huáng jīng	polygonatum [root]	Polygonati Huangjing Rhizoma	12 g.

In cases of distending costal pain, the prescription is modified to rectify qi and relieve pain. Add:

xiāng fù zǐ	cyperus [root]	Cyperi Rhizoma	6 g.
yù jīn	curcuma [tuber]	Curcumae Tuber	6 g.

In cases of bitter taste in the mouth and dry throat, occasionally accompanied by nosebleeding, the prescription is modified to clear heat and relieve bleeding. Add:

huáng qín	scutellaria [root]	Scutellariae Radix	9 g.
bái máo gēn	imperata [root]	Imperatae Rhizoma	30 g.
pú huáng	typha pollen (wrapped)	Typhae Pollen	9 g.

ACUPUNCTURE AND MOXIBUSTION

Main points: Needle with supplementation.

LR-14	*qī mén*
BL-18	*gān shū*
BL-23	*shèn shū*
SP-10	*xuè hǎi*
SP-06	*sān yīn jiāo*
KI-03	*tài xī*

Auxiliary points:

For tidal fever, add:

> BL-43 (38) *gāo huāng shū*

ALTERNATE THERAPEUTIC METHODS

1. Ear Acupuncture

Main points: Liver, Gall bladder, *Shén Mén,* Thorax.

Method: Select points on the affected side. For repletion patterns, needle to elicit a strong sensation. For vacuity patterns needle to elicit a mild sensation. Retain needles for 30 minutes or use the needle embedding method.

2. Plum-Blossom Needle Therapy

Method: Lightly tap the site of pain in the costal region and the back-shu points. Tap above, below and on the same level as the site of pain. This can be accompanied by cupping therapy.

REMARKS

The differential diagnosis of costal pain should be centered on qi and blood. In cases of qi stagnation, a distending pain that is mobile and has no definite location will manifest. In cases of blood stasis, there is a stabbing pain of fixed location, often with swelling. Costal pain because of damp-heat can be quite severe and can be accompanied by bitter taste in the mouth and yellow slimy tongue coating. Costal pain because of yin vacuity is generally vague but constant.

In the treatment of repletion patterns, the methods most often used involve regulating qi, dispelling stasis, clearing heat and draining dampness. For vacuity patterns, treatment involves nourishing yin and soothing the liver, with the prescriptions typically including qi regulating medicinals. It is important that the medicinals chosen do not have drying properties that further damage yin.

In the treatment of costal pain, the therapeutic effects are greatly improved when acupuncture is combined with herbal medicines.

SUPPLEMENT:

GALLBLADDER INFLAMMATION; GALLSTONES

Dăn Náng Yán, Dăn Shí Zhèng

1. Stagnation of Liver and Gallbladder Qi - 2. Obstruction by Damp-Heat - 3. Heat-Toxins of the Liver and Gallbladder

Gallbladder inflammation, or cholecystitis, includes both acute and chronic conditions It is most often the result of blockage of the bile ducts, retention of bile and subsequent infection by intestinal bacteria. Cholelithiasis includes the formation of gallstones in the gallbladder, common bile duct or bile ducts within the liver. In general, gallstones result from stasis of the bile followed by infection of the bile ducts and poor regulation of the cholesterol metabolism. Gallbladder inflammation and gallstones have several clinical manifestations in common, such as costal pain or tenderness in the upper right quadrant, nausea and vomiting, fever, poor digestion and jaundice in some cases. Symptoms are often aggravated following a fatty or greasy meal. The two often mutually give rise to each other or are concomitant and their differential diagnosis and treatment according to traditional Chinese medicine are basically the same, being gallbladder repletion patterns. For these reasons, gallbladder inflammation and gallstone will be discussed as a single unit.

Although traditional Chinese medicine has no equivalent terms for gallbladder inflammation or gallstone, similar sets of symptoms are recorded under the classifications of costal pain and jaundice. Further discussion is addressed in the relevant chapters. In modern clinical practice, x-rays, cholecystography or ultrasound are often used to confirm a diagnosis of gallstones.

ETIOLOGY AND PATHOGENESIS

In traditional Chinese medicine, the gallbladder, known as the "clear-centered bowel," is the storage place of bile and requires unrestricted passage for proper function. The gallbladder is coupled with the liver and is considered exterior to it. The etiology of gallbladder inflammation and gallstones includes a variety of factors such as emotional upset, excessive exposure to heat or cold, improper diet and eating habits, excessive consumption of rich greasy foods and, on occasion, intestinal or liver parasites. These factors cause stagnation of liver and gallbladder qi, blockage by accumulated damp-heat, disruption of bile secretion and, ultimately, pain because of impairment of free flow. When bile deviates from its normal course of flow, jaundice can result. Also, stagnation of liver and gallbladder qi over an extended period can transform into fire and give rise to toxins. Prolonged accumulation of damp-heat can further stagnate qi as well as blood, and lead to the formation of stones and gravel.

1. STAGNATION OF LIVER AND GALLBLADDER QI

Clinical Manifestations: Dull upper right abdominal pain or tenderness that spreads to the right shoulder and back, increase in pain following a fatty meal, congestion and fullness of the epigastrium and abdomen, oppression of the chest, belching, loss of appetite, no apparent fever or jaundice, frequent recurrence of symptoms.

Tongue: Thin coating.

Pulse: Wiry.

Treatment Method: Disperse the liver, disinhibit the gallbladder, rectify qi and relieve pain.

PRESCRIPTION

Liver-Clearing Qi-Moving Decoction *qīng gān xíng qī tāng*

chái hú	bupleurum [root]	Bupleuri Radix	9 g.
zhì bàn xià	pinellia [tuber] (processed)	Pinelliae Tuber Praeparatum	9 g.
yù jīn	curcuma [tuber]	Curcumae Tuber	9 g.
yán hú suǒ	corydalis [tuber]	Corydalis Tuber	9 g.
mù xiāng	saussurea [root]	Saussureae Radix (seu Vladimiriae)	9 g.
chuān liàn zǐ	toosendan [fruit]	Toosendan Fructus	9 g.
huáng qín	scutellaria [root]	Scutellariae Radix	9 g.
bái sháo yào	white peony [root]	Paeoniae Radix Alba	9 g.
xiāng fù zǐ	cyperus [root]	Cyperi Rhizoma	9 g.
zhǐ ké	bitter orange	Aurantii Fructus	9 g.
gān cǎo	licorice [root]	Glycyrrhizae Radix	6 g.

MODIFICATIONS

In cases accompanied by gallstones, the prescription is modified to expel stones. Add:

jīn qián cǎo	moneywort	Jinqiancao Herba	30 g.
hǎi jīn shā	lygodium spore (wrapped)	Lygodii Spora	9 g.
jī nèi jīn	gizzard lining	Galli Gigerii Endothelium	9 g.
dà huáng	rhubarb (abbreviated decoction)	Rhei Rhizoma	9 g.

In cases of weakened spleen with dampness, with symptoms of lack of strength and white slimy tongue coating, the prescription is modified to strengthen the spleen and dispel dampness. Add:

dǎng shēn	codonopsis [root]	Codonopsitis Radix	9 g.
cāng zhú	atractylodes [root]	Atractylodis Rhizoma	9 g.
bái zhú	ovate atractylodes [root]	Atractylodis Ovatae Rhizoma	9 g.
fú líng	poria	Poria	12 g.

In cases of extended illness where yin is depleted, with symptoms of dry mouth and throat, irritability, heat in the chest, red tongue with little coating, and thready wiry pulse, the prescription is modified to nourish yin and cool heat. Add:

shēng dì huáng	rehmannia [root] (fresh/dried)	Rehmanniae Radix Excicata seu Recens	12 g.
mài mén dōng	ophiopogon [tuber]	Ophiopogonis Tuber	9 g.
shí hú	dendrobium [stem] (extended decoction)	Dendrobii Caulis	9 g.

In cases of extended illness with repeatedly recurring stabbing upper right abdominal pain, the prescription is modified to quicken the blood and relieve pain. Add:

dān shēn	salvia [root]	Salviae Miltiorrhizae Radix	12 g.
chì sháo yào	red peony [root]	Paeoniae Radix Rubra	9 g.

ACUPUNCTURE AND MOXIBUSTION

Main points: Needle with draining.

GB-34	*yáng líng quán*
GB-24	*rì yuè*
BL-19	*dǎn shū*
M-LE-23	*dǎn náng xué* (Gallbladder Point)
BL-18	*gān shū*
LR-03	*tài chōng*

Auxiliary points:

For nausea and vomiting, add:

PC-06	*nèi guān*
CV-13	*shàng wǎn*

For conglomeration and fullness of the epigastrium and abdomen, add:

ST-25	*tiān shū*

For vacuity of spleen qi with dampness, add:

ST-36	*zú sān lǐ*
SP-09	*yīn líng quán*

For stagnation of qi with yin vacuity, add:

SP-06	*sān yīn jiāo*

2. OBSTRUCTION BY DAMP-HEAT

Clinical Manifestations: Distending pain or twisting pain of the right upper abdomen aggravated by external pressure, radiation of pain to the right shoulder and back, periodic increase in severity of pain, accompanied by bitter taste in the mouth, poor appetite, nausea and vomiting, constipation, yellow urine, chills and fever or fever with no chills and, in some cases, jaundice.

Tongue: Red with yellow slimy coating.

Pulse: Rapid, wiry, slippery.

Treatment Method: Disperse the liver, disinhibit the gallbladder, clear heat and drain dampness.

PRESCRIPTION

Gallbladder-Clearing Dampness-Disinhibiting Decoction
qīng dǎn lì shī tāng

chái hú	bupleurum [root]	Bupleuri Radix	9 g.
zhì bàn xià	pinellia [tuber] (processed)	Pinelliae Tuber Praeparatum	9 g.
shān zhī zǐ	gardenia [fruit]	Gardeniae Fructus	9 g.
chē qián zǐ	plantago seed (wrapped)	Plantaginis Semen	12 g.
mù tōng	mutong [stem]	Mutong Caulis	9 g.
huáng qín	scutellaria [root]	Scutellariae Radix	9 g.
yù jīn	curcuma [tuber]	Curcumae Tuber	12 g.
yīn chén hāo	capillaris	Artemisiae Capillaris Herba	30 g.
dà huáng	rhubarb (abbreviated decoction)	Rhei Rhizoma	9 g.

MODIFICATIONS

In cases of gallstones, add:

jīn qián cǎo	moneywort	Jinqiancao Herba	30 g.
hǔ zhàng	bushy knotweed [root]	Polygoni Cuspidati Rhizoma	30 g.

In cases of severe pain, add:

yán hú suǒ	corydalis [tuber]	Corydalis Tuber	9 g.
chuān liàn zǐ	toosendan [fruit]	Toosendan Fructus	9 g.

ACUPUNCTURE AND MOXIBUSTION

Main points: Needle with draining.

GB-34	*yáng líng quán*
M-LE-23	*dǎn náng xué* (Gallbladder Point)
BL-19	*dǎn shū*
GB-24	*rì yuè*
SP-09	*yīn líng quán*
ST-36	*zú sān lǐ*

Auxiliary points:

For fever, add:

LR-02	*xíng jiān*
GB-43	*xiá xī*

For jaundice, add:

GV-09	*zhì yáng*
SI-04	*wàn gǔ*

For severe pain, add:

GB-40	*qiū xū*
M-BW-35	*huá tuó jiā jí* (Hua Tuo's Paravertebrals)

3. HEAT-TOXINS OF THE LIVER AND GALLBLADDER

Clinical Manifestations: Constant severe pain in the right upper abdomen, radiation of pain into the right shoulder and back, aggravation of pain with external pressure, accompanied by high fever, aversion to cold, bitter taste in the mouth, thirst, constipation, dark scanty urine and, in severe cases, loss of consciousness and delirium.

Tongue: Red or deep red with dry yellow coating.

Pulse: Rapid, wiry or rapid, surging.

Treatment Method: Disperse the liver, disinhibit the gallbladder, clear heat and resolve toxins.

PRESCRIPTION

Gallbladder-Clearing Fire-Draining Decoction *qīng dǎn xiè huǒ tāng*

chái hú	bupleurum [root]	Bupleuri Radix	9 g.
zhì bàn xià	processed pinellia	Processed Pinelliae Tuber	9 g.
yīn chén hāo	capillaris	Artemisiae Capillaris Herba	30 g.
yù jīn	curcuma [tuber]	Curcumae Tuber	9 g.
bǎn lán gēn	isatis root	Isatidis Radix	12 g.
lián qiáo	forsythia [fruit]	Forsythiae Fructus	12 g.
máng xiāo	mirabilite (powdered and stir in)	Mirabilitum	9 g.
huáng qín	scutellaria [root]	Scutellariae Radix	9 g.
lóng dǎn cǎo	gentian [root]	Gentianae Radix	9 g.
shān zhī zǐ	gardenia [fruit]	Gardeniae Fructus	9 g.
mù xiāng	saussurea [root]	Saussureae Radix (seu Vladimiriae)	9 g.
jīn yín huā	lonicera [flower]	Lonicerae Flos	12 g.
dà huáng	rhubarb (abbreviated decoction)	Rhei Rhizoma	9 g.

<u>Modifications</u>

For loss of consciousness and delirium, add the prepared medicine, Peaceful Palace Bovine Bezoar Pill *(ān gōng niú huáng wán)*.

ACUPUNCTURE AND MOXIBUSTION

Main points: Needle with draining.

GB-34	*yáng líng quán*
M-LE-23	*dǎn náng xué* (Gallbladder Point)
GV-14-	*dà zhuī*
GB-24	*rì yuè*
BL-19	*dǎn shū*
LI-11	*qū chí*

Auxiliary points:

For jaundice, add:

LR-03	*tài chōng*
GV-09	*zhì yáng*
SI-04	*wàn gǔ*

For constipation, add:

ST-25	*tiān shū*
TB-06	*zhī gōu*

For loss of consciousness and delirium, add:

PC-06	*nèi guān*
GV-26	*shuǐ gōu*

ALTERNATE THERAPEUTIC METHODS

1. Ear Acupuncture

Auricular Points: Liver, Sympathetic, *Shén Mén*, Gallbladder, Endocrine, Triple Burner.

Method: Select three to four points each session, needling to elicit a strong sensation and retain needles for thirty minutes, manipulating at intervals. Treat once every one to two days, ten sessions per therapeutic course. Auricular seed plaster therapy may also be used.

2. Auricular Seed Plaster Therapy

Mature seeds from vaccaria *(wáng bù liú xíng)* are placed in the centers of 0.5 cm square pieces of adhesive plaster.* These plasters are adhered to selected auricular points, after which they are pressed with the fingertip for several minutes. Patients are instructed to press the plasters themselves for five to ten minutes, three to four times throughout the day. When symptoms are active, the number of times and length of time of pressure may be increased. Plasters are changed every five days, alternating left and right ears. One course of treatment is generally one month in length, with a break of seven days between courses. Evaluation of therapeutic results should be done after one to two courses of treatment.

3. Electro-Acupuncture

Treatment Method: Select a closely packed wave or an intermittent wave with a strong amplitude, as high as the patient can tolerate. Treat once daily for thirty minutes each session, five to ten sessions per therapeutic course. Allow five days rest between two consecutive sessions.

---

*Editor's note: If *wáng bù liú xíng* cannot be obtained, mustard seeds may be used.

Main points:

GB-24	*rì yuè*
LR-14	*qī mén*
M-LE-23	*dǎn náng xué* (Gallbladder Point)

Auxiliary points:

ST-36	*zú sān lǐ*
CV-12	*zhōng wǎn*

4. Folk Remedies

A. ***Corn silk (yù mǐ xū)*** Steep 60 g. of corn silk in boiling water or decoct in water. Administer two cups daily. Indicated for cases of gravel-like gallstones or gallbladder inflammation.

B. ***Moneywort (jīn qián cǎo)*** Decoct 60-120 g. in water. Administer two cups daily. Indicated in cases of gravel-like gallstones or gallbladder inflammation.

REMARKS

Chinese herbal medicine and acumoxa therapy are relatively effective in relieving pain and regulating the gallbladder in cases of inflammation and gallstone. During treatment, patients should maintain a worry-free state of mind, avoid overeating, abstain from hot spicy and greasy foods and maintain regular bowel movements. In cases where the gallstones are large (a diameter over one centimeter), surgery should be considered. In cases of severe obstruction and infection accompanied by shock and other serious complications, emergency treatment should be undertaken immediately.

JAUNDICE

Huáng Dăn

1A. Heat-Predominant Yang Jaundice - 1B. Dampness-Predominant Yang Jaundice - 1C. Acute Yang Jaundice - 2. Yin Jaundice

Jaundice presents with yellow discoloration of the eyes and skin as well as dark yellow urine as its main symptoms. Jaundice may occur in a variety of bio-medically-described illnesses including acute and chronic hepatitis, pancreatitis, cholecystitis, cholelithiasis and hepatic cirrhosis.

ETIOLOGY AND PATHOGENESIS

The major etiological factor in the development of jaundice is dampness, with the pathological changes occurring mainly in the spleen, stomach, liver and gallbladder. The spleen, which regulates digestion and transportation of food and water, functions most efficiently when free of dampness. Obstruction of the middle burner by dampness may result from factors such as improper diet, over-consumption of liquor or rich sweet foods or attack by exterior damp-heat. Such obstruction may further affect the smoothing and dispersing functions of the liver and gallbladder, resulting in circulation of bile outside its regular channels, causing jaundice.

On the basis of etiological factors and physical constitution, jaundice is divided into yang and yin types. In patients with yang jaundice, heat is severe; there is often a pre-existing physical constitution characterized by a profusion of stomach fire and dampness transforming into damp-heat. Since heat and dampness tend to be present in differing degrees, the pathogenesis of yang jaundice is further classified as heat-predominant or damp-predominant. Acute jaundice is an extreme repletion of heat-toxins that enters the construction and gathers in the pericardium. In these cases, the onset of jaundice is abrupt and the patterns are severe.

In yin jaundice, yin is replete and coldness predominates. These patients generally exhibit spleen yang vacuity. In such cases dampness has transformed to cold-damp causing vacuity and creating yin jaundice.

Clinically, yang jaundice and yin jaundice may, under certain conditions, undergo mutual transformation, giving rise to complicated patterns involving both heat and cold, repletion and vacuity.

1A. HEAT-PREDOMINANT YANG JAUNDICE

Clinical Manifestations: Bright yellow discoloration of the eyes and skin, fever, thirst, oppression in the chest, nausea, vomiting, distention and fullness of the epigastrium and abdomen, dark yellow scanty urine, constipation.

Tongue: Yellow slimy coating.

Pulse: Rapid, wiry.

Treatment Method: Clear heat, disinhibit dampness, free the stool, dispel jaundice.

PRESCRIPTION

Capillaris Decoction *yīn chén hāo tāng*

yīn chén hāo	capillaris	Artemisiae Capillaris Herba	30 g.
shān zhī zǐ	gardenia [fruit]	Gardeniae Fructus	15 g.
dà huáng	rhubarb	Rhei Rhizoma	9 g.

MODIFICATIONS

The prescription is often reinforced to dispel jaundice by adding diuretics. Use:

zhū líng	polyporus	Polyporus	9 g.
zé xiè	alisma [tuber]	Alismatis Rhizoma	9 g.
chē qián zǐ	plantago seed (wrapped)	Plantaginis Semen	9 g.
huá shí	talcum (wrapped)	Talcum	12 g.

The prescription is often reinforced to dispel jaundice by adding heat-clearing detoxifying herbs. Use:

| *bǎn lán gēn* | isatis [root] | Isatidis Radix | 12 g. |
| *chuí pén cǎo* | hanging stonecrop | Sedi Sarmentosi Herba | 15 g. |

In cases of severe costal pain, the prescription is modified to clear the liver, rectify qi and relieve pain. Add:

chái hú	bupleurum [root]	Bupleuri Radix	9 g.
yù jīn	curcuma [tuber]	Curcumae Tuber	9 g.
chuān liàn zǐ	toosendan [fruit]	Toosendan Fructus	9 g.

In cases of vexation and nausea, the prescription is modified to clear the heart, eliminate vexation, move qi downward and relieve nausea. Add:

| *huáng lián* | coptis [root] | Coptidis Rhizoma | 6 g. |
| *zhú rú* | bamboo shavings | Bambusae Caulis in Taeniam | 9 g. |

In cases of distention and fullness of the epigastrium and abdomen, the prescription is modified to move qi and disperse distention. Add:

| *zhǐ shí* | unripe bitter orange | Aurantii Fructus Immaturus | 9 g. |
| *hòu pò* | magnolia [bark] | Magnoliae Cortex | 9 g. |

In cases where constipation has been relieved and yet the tongue coating is still slimy, the prescription is modified to prevent injury to spleen yang. Add spleen-reinforcing, dampness-dispelling medicines such as:

| *bái zhú* | ovate atractylodes [root] | Atractylodis Ovatae Rhizoma | 9 g. |
| *fú líng* | poria | Poria | 12 g. |

Delete bitter heat-clearing medicinals such as:

| *dà huáng* | rhubarb | Rhei Rhizoma | |

In cases where the bile duct has been obstructed by gallstones, with symptoms of yellow discoloration of the skin and eyes and pain in the right hypochondrium spreading to the back and shoulder, aversion to cold, fever and (in some cases) light grayish stools, the prescription is changed to clear the liver, drain the gallbladder, remove stones and dispel jaundice. Use:

Major Bupleurum Decoction *dà chái hú tāng*

chái hú	bupleurum [root]	Bupleuri Radix	12 g.
bái sháo yào	white peony [root]	Paeoniae Radix Alba	9 g.
huáng qín	scutellaria [root]	Scutellariae Radix	9 g.
zhì bàn xià	pinellia [tuber] (processed)	Pinelliae Tuber Praeparatum	9 g.
zhǐ shí	unripe bitter orange	Aurantii Fructus Immaturus	9 g.
dà huáng	rhubarb (abbreviated decoction)	Rhei Rhizoma	9 g.
shēng jiāng	fresh ginger	Zingiberis Rhizoma Recens	12 g.
dà zǎo	jujube	Ziziphi Fructus	4 pc.

Add:

yīn chén hāo	capillaris	Artemisiae Capillaris Herba	15 g.
jīn qián cǎo	moneywort	Jinqiancao Herba	30 g.
yù jīn	curcuma [tuber]	Curcumae Tuber	9 g.

In cases of obstruction of the bile duct by parasitic worms, with sudden onset of jaundice and periodic piercing pain in the hypochondrium, the prescription is changed to quiet worms, relieve pain, drain the gallbladder and dispel jaundice. Use:

Mume Pill *wū méi wán*

wū méi	mume [fruit]	Mume Fructus	12 g.
zhì fù zǐ	aconite [accessory tuber] (processed) (extended decoction)	Aconiti Tuber Laterale Praeparatum	6 g.
gān jiāng	dried ginger [root]	Zingiberis Rhizoma Exsiccatum	6 g.
huā jiāo	zanthoxylum [husk]	Zanthoxyli Pericarpium	1.5 g.
guì zhī	cinnamon [twig]	Cinnamomi Ramulus	6 g.
xì xīn	asarum	Asiasari Herba cum Radice	1.5 g.
rén shēn	ginseng	Ginseng Radix	9 g.
dāng guī	tangkuei	Angelicae Sinensis Radix	6 g.
huáng lián	coptis [root]	Coptidis Rhizoma	6 g.
huáng bǎi	phellodendron [bark]	Phellodendri Cortex	9 g.

Add:

yīn chén hāo	capillaris	Artemisiae Capillaris Herba	15 g.
shān zhī zǐ	gardenia [fruit]	Gardeniae Fructus	9 g.
chuān liàn zǐ	toosendan [fruit]	Toosendan Fructus	9 g.
bīng láng	areca [nut]	Arecae Semen	12 g.

ACUPUNCTURE AND MOXIBUSTION

Main points: Needle with draining.

GV-09	*zhì yáng*
GB-34	*yáng líng quán*
LR-03	*tài chōng*
BL-18	*gān shū*
BL-19	*dǎn shū*
GV-14	*dà zhuī*

Auxiliary points:

For abdominal distention and constipation, add:

ST-25	*tiān shū*
BL-25	*dà cháng shū*

For costal pain, add:

LR-14	*qī mén*
TB-06	*zhī gōu*

1B. DAMPNESS-PREDOMINANT YANG JAUNDICE

Clinical Manifestations: Yellow discoloration of the skin and eyes (although less bright than that of heat-predominant yang jaundice), unsurfaced fever, feeling of body heaviness, fullness and discomfort of the chest and epigastrium, loss of appetite, nausea, vomiting, thirst with little liquid intake, abdominal distention, loose stools with difficult elimination, dark scanty urine.

Tongue: Slightly yellow thick slimy coating.

Pulse: Wiry and slippery or soft and tardy.

Treatment Method: Disinhibit dampness, clear heat, dispel jaundice.

PRESCRIPTION

Capillaris and Poria Five Powder *yīn chén wǔ líng sǎn*

yīn chén hāo	capillaris	Artemisiae Capillaris Herba	15 g.
zé xiè	alisma [tuber]	Alismatis Rhizoma	15 g.
fú líng	poria	Poria	9 g.
zhū líng	polyporus	Polyporus	9 g.
bái zhú	ovate atractylodes [root]	Atractylodis Ovatae Rhizoma	9 g.
guì zhī	cinnamon [twig]	Cinnamomi Ramulus	3 g.

MODIFICATIONS

To reinforce transformation of dampness and dispel jaundice, add:

huò xiāng	agastache/patchouli	Agastaches seu Pogostemi Herba	9 g.
bái dòu kòu	cardamom (abbreviated decoction)	Amomi Cardamomi Fructus	6 g.

In cases accompanied by nausea and vomiting, the prescription is modified to downbear qi and stop nausea and vomiting. Add:

jiāng bàn xià	(ginger-processed) pinellia [tuber]	Pinelliae Tuber Praeparatum	9 g.
chén pí	tangerine peel	Citri Exocarpium	9 g.

In cases of marked abdominal distention, the prescription is modified to move qi and disperse distention. Add:

dà fù pí	areca [husk]	Arecae Pericarpium	9 g.
zhǐ shí	unripe bitter orange	Aurantii Fructus Immaturus	9 g.

In cases of yang jaundice where heat evil and dampness are equal in degree, the prescription is changed to eliminate damp-heat and dispel jaundice. Use:

Sweet Dew Toxin-Dispersing Elixir *gān lù xiāo dú dān*

huá shí	talcum (wrapped)	Talcum	15 g.
yīn chén hāo	capillaris	Artemisiae Capillaris Herba	12 g.
huáng qín	scutellaria [root]	Scutellariae Radix	9 g.
shí chāng pú	acorus [root]	Acori Rhizoma	6 g.
chuān bèi mǔ	Sichuan fritillaria [bulb]	Fritillariae Cirrhosae Bulbus	6 g.
mù tōng	mutong [stem]	Mutong Caulis	6 g.
huò xiāng	agastache/patchouli	Agastaches seu Pogostemi Herba	6 g.
shè gān	belamcanda [root]	Belamcandae Rhizoma	6 g.
lián qiào	forsythia [fruit]	Forsythiae Fructus	6 g.
bò hé	mint (abbreviated decoction)	Menthae Herba	3 g.
bái dòu kòu	cardamom (abbreviated decoction)	Amomi Cardamomi Fructus	4.5 g.

ACUPUNCTURE AND MOXIBUSTION

Main points: Needle with draining.

GV-09	*zhì yáng*
BL-18	*gān shū*
BL-19	*dǎn shū*
GB-34	*yáng líng quán*
SP-09	*yīn líng quán*
LR-03	*tài chōng*

Auxiliary points:

For fever, add:

LI-04	*hé gǔ*

For nausea and oppression in the chest, add:

PC-06	*nèi guān*
SP-04	*gōng sūn*

For fullness of the epigastrium and loose stools, add:

ST-36	*zú sān lǐ*

1C. ACUTE YANG JAUNDICE

Clinical Manifestations: Jaundice of sudden onset and rapid development, high fever, vexing thirst, costal pain, abdominal fullness, loss of consciousness, delirium, epistaxis, hemafecia or (in some cases) dermal stasis macules.

Tongue: Dark red with dry yellow coating.

Pulse: Wiry, rapid, slippery or rapid, thready.

Treatment Method: Clear heat, resolve toxins, cool the blood, open the orifices, dispel jaundice.

PRESCRIPTION

Rhinoceros Horn Powder *xī jiǎo sǎn*

xī jiǎo	rhinoceros horn* (powdered and stirred in)	Rhinocerotis Cornu	6 g.
huáng lián	coptis [root]	Coptidis Rhizoma	9 g.
shēng má	cimicifuga [root]	Cimicifugae Rhizoma	9 g.
shān zhī zǐ	gardenia [fruit]	Gardeniae Fructus	9 g.
yīn chén hāo	capillaris	Artemisiae Capillaris Herba	30 g.

*Use of *xī jiǎo* (rhinoceros horn) is prohibited in North America by the endangered species laws. Water Buffalo Horn *(shuǐ niú jiǎo)* may be substituted. Increase the dose to 15 g., extended decoction.)

MODIFICATIONS

To increase the effects of clearing heat, resolving toxins and cooling the blood, add:

dà qīng yè	isatis [leaf]	Isatidis Folium	15 g.
pú gōng yīng	dandelion	Taraxaci Herba cum Radice	15 g.
shēng dì huáng	rehmannia [root] dried/fresh	Rehmanniae Radix Exsiccata seu Recens	15 g.
mǔ dān pí	moutan [root bark]	Moutan Radicis Cortex	9 g.
shí hú	dendrobium [stem] (extended decoction)	Dendrobii Caulis	12 g.

In cases of loss of consciousness and delirium, a prepared medicine may be added to clear heat, resolve toxins, relieve convulsions and open the orifices. Choose from

Peaceful Palace Bovine Bezoar Pill *(ān gōng niú huáng wán)* or Supreme Jewel Elixir *(zhì bǎo dān)*.

In cases manifesting severe epistaxis, hemafecia or dermal stasis macules, the prescription is modified to cool the blood and relieve bleeding. Add:

dì yú	sanguisorba [root] (charred)	Sanguisorbae Radix	12 g.
cè bǎi yè	biota leaf (charred)	Biotae Folium	12 g.

In cases of dark scanty urine with urine retention, or in cases of drum distention (ascites), the prescription is modified to clear heat and free and disinhibit the urine. Add:

mù tōng	mutong [stem]	Mutong Caulis	6 g.
bái máo gēn	imperata [root]	Imperatae Rhizoma	15 g.
dà fù pí	areca [husk]	Arecae Pericarpium	9 g.
chē qián cǎo	plantago (wrapped)	Plantaginis Herba	12 g.

ACUPUNCTURE AND MOXIBUSTION

Main points: Needle with draining.

GV-09	*zhì yáng*
BL-18	*gān shū*
BL-19	*dǎn shū*
GV-14	*dà zhuī*
GB-34	*yáng líng quán*
LR-03	*tài chōng*

Auxiliary points:

For loss of consciousness, let blood at:

GV-26	*shuǐ gōu*
PC-09	*zhōng chōng*
HT-09	*shào chōng*

For epistaxis and hemafecia, add:

BL-40 (54)	*wěi zhōng*
KI-01	*yǒng quán*

2. Yin Jaundice

Clinical Manifestations: Dull yellow discoloration of the eyes and skin, feelings of heaviness and fatigue, oppression of the epigastrium, reduced food intake, abdominal distention, loose stools, lassitude, physical cold, no apparent thirst.

Tongue: Pale with white slimy coating.

Pulse: Soft, tardy or slow, deep.

Treatment Method: Supplement the spleen, harmonize the stomach, warm and transform cold-dampness.

PRESCRIPTION

Capillaris, Atractylodes and Aconite Decoction *yīn-chén zhú fù tāng*

yīn chén hāo	capillaris	Artemisiae Capillaris Herba	12 g.
gān jiāng	dried ginger [root]	Zingiberis Rhizoma Exsiccatum	9 g.
zhì fù zǐ	aconite [accessory tuber] (processed) (extended decoction)	Aconiti Tuber Laterale Praeparatum	6 g.
ròu guì	cinnamon bark (extended decoction)	Cinnamomi Cortex	3 g
zhì gān cǎo	licorice [root] (honey-fried)	Glycyrrhizae Radix	6 g.

MODIFICATIONS

To move qi and disinhibit dampness, add:

yù jīn	curcuma [tuber]	Curcumae Tuber	9 g.
fú líng	poria	Poria	12 g.
zé xiè	alisma [tuber]	Alismatis Rhizoma	9 g.

In cases of marked abdominal distention and thick slimy tongue coating, the prescription is modified to dry dampness and disperse distention.

Delete:

zhì gān cǎo	licorice [root] (honey-fried)	Glycyrrhizae Radix	6 g.

Add:

cāng zhú	atractylodes [root]	Atractylodis Rhizoma	9 g.
hòu pò	magnolia [bark]	Magnoliae Cortex	9 g.

In cases of distention of the epigastrium and abdomen, dull costal pain, no desire for food, heaviness and fatigue of the four limbs, irregular alternation of constipation and diarrhea and thready wiry pulse, the pattern is one of liver depression and spleen vacuity; the prescription is changed to soothe the liver and support the spleen. Use:

Free Wanderer Pill *xiāo yáo wán*

chái hú	bupleurum [root]	Bupleuri Radix	9 g.
bái sháo yào	white peony [root]	Paeoniae Radix Alba	12 g.
dāng guī	tangkuei	Angelicae Sinensis Radix	9 g.
bái zhú	ovate atractylodes [root]	Atractylodis Ovatae Rhizoma	9 g.
fú líng	poria	Poria	9 g.
zhì gān cǎo	licorice [root] (honey-fried)	Glycyrrhizae Radix	6 g.
bò hé	mint (abbreviated decoction)	Menthae Herba	3 g.
shēng jiāng	fresh ginger	Zingiberis Rhizoma Recens	3 g.

ACUPUNCTURE AND MOXIBUSTION

Main points: Needle with even supplementation, even draining; add moxibustion.

BL-20	*pí shū*
ST-36	*zú sān lǐ*
BL-19	*dǎn shū*
SP-09	*yīn líng quán*
SP-06	*sān yīn jiāo*
CV-12	*zhōng wǎn*

Auxiliary points:

For lassitude and chills, add:

GV-04	*mìng mén*
CV-06	*qì hǎi*

For loose stools, add:

CV-04	*guān yuán*
ST-25	*tiān shū*

ALTERNATE THERAPEUTIC METHODS

1. Ear Acupuncture

Main points: Gallbladder, Liver, Spleen, Stomach, Diaphragm, Root of Auricular Vagus.

Method: Select two to three points each session. Needle once daily to elicit a moderate sensation. Ten sessions constitute one therapeutic course.

REMARKS

Pattern recognition is based on the differentiation of yang and yin jaundice. Clinically, the course of yang jaundice is relatively short, while the course of yin jaundice is long.

In addition to herbal medicines and acupuncture-moxibustion, modification of the patient's diet is an important part of treatment. The diet should include foods that are fresh, light and neutral in taste. Rich, oily or sweet foods, which can obstruct the spleen and give rise to dampness, should be avoided. Liquor and hot spicy foods should also be eliminated from the diet. In addition, jaundice patients should get plenty of bed-rest, avoid overwork and maintain an optimistic outlook to facilitate a quick and complete recovery.

DRUM DISTENTION

Gŭ Zhàng

1. Stagnation of Qi and Obstruction by Dampness - 2. Burdening of the Spleen by Cold-Dampness - 3. Accumulation of Damp-Heat - 4. Stagnation of Spleen Qi and Liver Blood - 5. Vacuity of Spleen and Kidney Yang - 6. Vacuity of Liver and Kidney Yin

Drum distention, named because of the resemblance of a swollen and distended abdomen to a skin stretched over a drum, presents enlargement and distention of the abdomen, greenish-yellow discoloration of the skin and a protrusion of superficial abdominal blood vessels as its distinguishing features. Drum distention patterns are observed in the later stages of various ascites conditions, including hepatic cirrhosis, tuberculosis, peritonitis, kala-azar (a protozoan disease), schistosomiasis (from liver flukes), malnutrition and malignant abdominal tumors.

ETIOLOGY AND PATHOGENESIS

The etiology of drum distention includes the following: emotional stress and consequent stagnation of liver qi; habitual consumption of alcohol or improper diet and eating habits, which injure the spleen and stomach; infection by schistosomes (liver flukes); and prolonged cases of jaundice or abdominal tumors. All of these factors may lead to dysfunction of the liver, spleen and kidney, causing stagnation and accumulation of qi, blood and water; the result is progressive abdominal swelling and drum distention.

In the past, on the basis of etiology, pathogenesis and clinical manifestations, drum distention was categorized as either "qi drum," "blood drum," or "water drum." Such division, however, can only distinguish primary from secondary pathogenesis, since qi stagnation, static blood and stationary water often exist together, none being the sole cause of the illness. Patterns of drum distention are now seen to be characterized by root vacuity with branch repletion, or complication by both vacuity and repletion.

1. STAGNATION OF QI AND OBSTRUCTION BY DAMPNESS

Clinical Manifestations: Distention and enlargement of the abdomen, which is not hard when pressed, sensation of distention and fullness or pain of the hypochondrium, reduced food intake, an increase in distention after meals, belching, scanty urine.

Tongue: Thin slimy coating.

Pulse: Wiry.

Treatment Method: Soothe the liver, rectify qi, move dampness, reduce distention.

PRESCRIPTION

Combine Bupleurum Liver-Coursing Powder *(chái hú shū gān sǎn)* with Stomach-Calming Poria (Hoelen) Five Decoction *(wèi líng tāng)*.

Bupleurum Liver-Coursing Powder *chái hú shū gān sǎn*

chái hú	bupleurum [root]	Bupleuri Radix	6 g.
bái sháo yào	white peony [root]	Paeoniae Radix Alba	9 g.
xiāng fù zǐ	cyperus [root]	Cyperi Rhizoma	6 g.
chuān xiōng	ligusticum [root]	Ligustici Rhizoma	6 g.
chén pí	tangerine [peel]	Citri Exocarpium	6 g.
zhǐ ké	bitter orange	Aurantii Fructus	6 g.
gān cǎo	licorice [root]	Glycyrrhizae Radix	3 g.

with:

Stomach-Calming Poria (Hoelen) Five Decoction *wèi líng tāng*

cāng zhú	atractylodes [root]	Atractylodis Rhizoma	9 g.
bái zhú	ovate atractylodes [root]	Atractylodis Ovatae Rhizoma	9 g.
fú líng	poria	Poria	9 g.
hòu pò	magnolia [bark]	Magnoliae Cortex	9 g.
chén pí	tangerine [peel]	Citri Exocarpium	9 g.
zé xiè	alisma [tuber]	Alismatis Rhizoma	12 g.
guì zhī	cinnamon [twig]	Cinnamomi Ramulus	6 g.
gān cǎo	licorice [root]	Glycyrrhizae Radix	3 g.

MODIFICATIONS

In cases of severe abdominal distention, the prescription is modified to break qi and remove obstruction. Add:

mù xiāng	saussurea [root]	Saussureae seu Vladimiriae Radix	9 g.
bīng láng	areca [nut]	Arecae Semen	9 g.

In cases of regurgitation of clear fluids, the prescription is modified to harmonize the stomach and move qi downward. Add:

zhì bàn xià	(ginger-processed) pinellia [tuber]	Pinelliae Tuber Praeparatum	9 g.
gān jiāng	dried ginger [root]	Zingiberis Rhizoma Exsiccatum	6 g.

ACUPUNCTURE AND MOXIBUSTION

Main points: Needle with draining.

CV-06	*qì hǎi*
LR-03	*tài chōng*
CV-09	*shuǐ fēn*
CV-12	*zhōng wǎn*
ST-25	*tiān shū*
SP-09	*yīn líng quán*

Auxiliary points:

For costal pain, add:

GB-34	*yáng líng quán*
TB-06	*zhī gōu*

For constipation, add:

SP-14	*fù jié*

2. BURDENING OF THE SPLEEN BY COLD-DAMPNESS

Clinical Manifestations: Distention, enlargement and fullness of the abdomen (similar to a large bladder of water when pressed), epigastric fullness and oppression, some decrease in symptoms with the external application of heat, edema of the lower limbs, tiredness, fatigue, heaviness of the limbs, scanty urine, loose stools.

Tongue: White slimy coating.

Pulse: Tardy.

Treatment Method: Strengthen the spleen, dissipate cold, move qi, drain dampness.

PRESCRIPTION

Spleen-Firming Beverage *shí pí yǐn*

hòu pò	magnolia bark	Magnoliae Cortex	6 g.
bái zhú	ovate atractylodes [root]	Atractylodis Ovatae Rhizoma	6 g.
mù guā	chaenomeles [fruit]	Chaenomelis Fructus	6 g.
mù xiāng	saussurea [root]	Saussureae Radix (seu Vladimiriae)	6 g.
cǎo guǒ	tsaoko [fruit]	Amomi Tsao-Ko Fructus	6 g.
bīng láng	areca [nut]	Arecae Semen	6 g.
zhì fù zǐ	aconite [accessory tuber] (processed) (extended decoction)	Aconiti Tuber Laterale Praeparatum	6 g.
pào jiāng	dried ginger (charred)	Zingiberis Rhizoma Tostum	6 g.
fú líng	poria	Poria	6 g.
zhì gān cǎo	licorice [root] (honey-fried)	Glycyrrhizae Radix	3 g.
shēng jiāng	fresh ginger	Zingiberis Rhizoma Recens	3 g.
dà zǎo	jujube	Ziziphi Fructus	3 pc.

MODIFICATIONS

In cases where water and dampness are extreme the prescription is reinforced to free and disinhibit the urine. Add:

ròu guì	cinnamon bark (abbreviated decoction)	Cinnamomi Cortex	6 g.
zhū líng	polyporus	Polyporus	9 g.
zé xiè	alisma [tuber]	Alismatis Rhizoma	9 g.

In cases of qi vacuity presenting shortness of breath and pale complexion, the prescription is modified to supplement lung and spleen qi. Add:

huáng qí	astragalus [root]	Astragali (seu Hedysari) Radix	12 g.
rén shēn	ginseng	Ginseng Radix	9 g.

In cases of marked costal pain and abdominal distention, the prescription is modified to rectify qi and relieve the middle burner. Add:

yù jīn	curcuma [tuber]	Curcumae Tuber	9 g.
qīng pí	unripe tangerine [peel]	Citri Exocarpium Immaturum	6 g.
shā rén	amomum [fruit] (abbreviated decoction)	Amomi Semen seu Fructus	6 g.

ACUPUNCTURE AND MOXIBUSTION

Main points: Needle with draining; add moxibustion.

BL-20	*pí shū* (moxibustion)
SP-04	*gōng sūn*

CV-09   *shuǐ fēn* (moxibustion)
LR-13   *zhāng mén*
SP-09   *yīn líng quán*
CV-12   *zhōng wǎn*

Auxiliary points:

For loose stools, add:

ST-36   *zú sān lǐ*

3. ACCUMULATION OF DAMP-HEAT

Clinical Manifestations: Enlargement, fullness, hardness and pain of the abdomen; irritability, fever, bitter taste in the mouth, thirst without desire for drink, dark urine excreted with difficulty, constipation or loose sticky stools, jaundice in some cases.

Tongue: Redness of the sides and tip of the tongue, yellow slimy sometimes grayish-black coating.

Pulse: Rapid, wiry.

Treatment Method: Clear heat, transform dampness, free the stool, dispel water.

PRESCRIPTION

Combine Center Fullness Separating and Dispersing Decoction *(zhōng mǎn fēn xiāo tāng)* with Capillaris Decoction *(yīn-chén-hāo tāng)*.

Center Fullness Separating and Dispersing Decoction
zhōng mǎn fēn xiāo tāng

hòu pò	magnolia [bark]	Magnoliae Cortex	12 g.
zhǐ shí	unripe bitter orange	Aurantii Fructus Immaturus	9 g.
huáng lián	coptis [root]	Coptidis Rhizoma	9 g.
huáng qín	scutellaria [root]	Scutellariae Radix	9 g.
zhī mǔ	anemarrhena [root]	Anemarrhenae Rhizoma	9 g.
zhì bàn xià	pinellia [tuber] (processed)	Pinelliae Tuber Praeparatum	9 g.
chén pí	tangerine peel	Citri Exocarpium	9 g.
fú líng	poria	Poria	12 g.
zhū líng	polyporus	Polyporus	12 g.
zé xiè	alisma [tuber]	Alismatis Rhizoma	12 g.
shā rén	amomum [fruit] (abbreviated decoction)	Amomi Semen seu Fructus	4.5 g.
gān jiāng	dried ginger [root]	Zingiberis Rhizoma Exsiccatum	3 g.
jiāng huáng	turmeric	Curcumae Longae Rhizoma	3 g.
bái zhú	ovate atractylodes [root]	Atractylodis Ovatae Rhizoma	3 g.
zhì gān cǎo	licorice [root] (honey-fried)	Glycyrrhizae Radix	3 g.
rén shēn	ginseng	Ginseng Radix	3 g.

with:

Capillaris Decoction *yīn chén hāo tāng*

yīn chén hāo	capillaris	Artemisiae Capillaris Herba	18 g.
shān zhī zǐ	gardenia	Gardeniae Fructus	12 g.
dà huáng	rhubarb (abbreviated decoction)	Rhei Rhizoma	6 g.

MODIFICATIONS

In cases of severe heat with jaundice, the prescription is modified to clear heat and dispel jaundice.

Delete:

rén shēn	ginseng	Ginseng Radix
gān jiāng	dried ginger [root]	Zingiberis Rhizoma Exsiccatum

Increase doses of:

yīn chén hāo	capillaris	Artemisiae Capillaris Herba	to 30 g.
shān zhī zǐ	gardenia	Gardeniae Fructus	to 15 g.
dà huáng	rhubarb (abbreviated decoction)	Rhei Rhizoma	to 9 g.

In cases of dark urine excreted with difficulty, the prescription is modified to move water and disinhibit the orifices. Add:

huá shí	talcum (wrapped)	Talcum	12 g.
hú lú	bottle gourd	Lagenariae Depressae Fructus	15 g.

In very severe cases, an alternate prescription is temporarily used until the bowels have been emptied. Use:

Boats and Carts Pill *zhōu chē (jū) wán*

qiān niú zǐ	morning glory [seed]	Pharbitidis Semen	120 g.
gān suì	kansui [root]	Kansui Radix	30 g.
yuán huā	genkwa [flower]	Daphnes Genkwa Flos	30 g.
dà jǐ	euphorbia root	Euphorbiae Radix	30 g.
dà huáng	rhubarb	Rhei Rhizoma	60 g.
qīng pí	unripe tangerine peel	Citri Exocarpium Immaturum	15 g.
chén pí	tangerine peel	Citri Exocarpium	15 g.
mù xiāng	saussurea [root]	Saussureae Radix (seu Vladimiriae)	15 g.
bīng láng	areca [nut]	Arecae Semen	15 g.
qīng fěn	calomel	Calomelas	3 g.

Powder the above ingredients and make into small pills. Take a 3-6 g. dosage with water before breakfast each day. Careful attention should be paid to the protection of spleen and stomach qi, avoiding overuse of the drastic purgatives and diuretics found in Boats and Carts Pill.

ACUPUNCTURE AND MOXIBUSTION

Main points: Needle with draining.

CV-09	*shuǐ fēn*
GB-34	*yáng líng quán*
LR-02	*xíng jiān*
ST-44	*nèi tíng*
ST-25	*tiān shū*
ST-37	*shàng jù xū*

Auxiliary points:

For severe heat, add:

GV-14	*dà zhuī*

For severe dampness, add:

SP-09	*yīn líng quán*

For jaundice, add:

      BL-48 (43)   *yáng gāng*
      SI-04   *wàn gǔ*

4. STAGNATION OF SPLEEN QI AND LIVER BLOOD

Clinical Manifestations: Enlargement, hardness, distention and fullness of the abdomen, protrusion of distended blood vessels from the abdominal surface, stabbing pain in the abdomen and hypochondrium, dull blackish complexion, spider webbing on the face, neck and chest, red spots on the palms, purplish discoloration of the lips, thirst without desire for drink, black stools.

Tongue: Purple, sometimes with stasis macules on the tongue.

Pulse: Rough, thready.

PRESCRIPTION

Construction-Regulating Beverage *tiáo yíng yǐn*

é zhú	zedoary	Zedoariae Rhizoma	9 g.
chuān xiōng	ligusticum [root]	Ligustici Rhizoma	9 g.
dāng guī	tangkuei	Angelicae Sinensis Radix	12 g.
yán hú suǒ	corydalis [tuber]	Corydalis Tuber	9 g.
chì sháo yào	red peony [root]	Paeoniae Radix Rubra	9 g.
qū mài	dianthus	Dianthi Herba	9 g.
dà huáng	rhubarb (abbreviated decoction)	Rhei Rhizoma	6 g.
bīng láng	areca [nut]	Arecae Semen	9 g.
chén pí	tangerine peel	Citri Exocarpium	9 g.
dà fù pí	areca [husk]	Arecae Pericarpium	9 g.
tíng lì zǐ	tingli [seed]	Descurainiae seu Lepidii Semen	9 g.
chì fú líng	red poria	Poria Rubra	12 g.
sāng bái pí	mulberry [root bark]	Mori Radicis Cortex	9 g.
xì xīn	asarum	Asiasari Herba cum Radice	1.5 g.
bái zhǐ	angelica [root]	Angelicae Dahuricae Radix	3 g.
ròu guì	cinnamon [bark] (abbreviated decoction)	Cinnamomi Cortex	3 g.
zhì gān cǎo	licorice [root] (honey-fried)	Glycyrrhizae Radix	3 g.
shēng jiāng	fresh ginger	Zingiberis Rhizoma Recens	3 g.
dà zǎo	jujube	Ziziphi Fructus	3 pc.

MODIFICATIONS

In cases where stools are black, the prescription is modified to dispel stasis and relieve bleeding. Add:

sān qī	notoginseng [root]	Notoginseng Radix	9 g.
cè bǎi yè	biota [leaf]	Biotae Folium	12 g.

In cases of extreme abdominal distention where the pulse is rapid, wiry and forceful and the physical condition still strong, Boats and Carts Pill *(zhōu chē [jū] wán)* (above) may be temporarily administered to initially purge the bowels and disinhibit water. Once the edema has been alleviated, treatment of blood stasis may be undertaken. Careful attention should be paid to protection of spleen and stomach qi, avoiding overuse of the drastic purgatives and diuretics in Boats and Carts Pill.

ACUPUNCTURE AND MOXIBUSTION

Main points: Needle with draining.

LR-14	*qī mén*
LR-13	*zhāng mén*
CV-05	*shí mén*
SP-06	*sān yīn jiāo*
CV-09	*shuǐ fēn*
ST-36	*zú sān lǐ*

5. VACUITY OF SPLEEN AND KIDNEY YANG

Clinical Manifestations: Enlargement, fullness and distention of the abdomen, symptoms milder in the morning and more severe at night, greenish-yellow complexion, epigastric fullness, poor food intake, tiredness, physical cold, cold extremities, edema of the lower limbs and in some cases, difficult urination.

Tongue: Pale or light purple, enlarged.

Pulse: Deep, thready, wiry.

Treatment Method: Warm and supplement spleen and kidney yang, move qi downward, disinhibit water.

PRESCRIPTION

In cases predominantly vacuous of spleen yang, combine Aconite Center-Rectifying Decoction *(fù zǐ lǐ zhōng tāng)* with Poria Five Powder *(wǔ líng sǎn)*.

Aconite Center-Rectifying Decoction *fù zǐ lǐ zhōng tāng*

zhì fù zǐ	aconite [accessory tuber] (processed) (extended decoction)	Aconiti Tuber Laterale Praeparatum	6 g.
rén shēn	ginseng	Ginseng Radix	9 g.
bái zhú	ovate atractylodes [root]	Atractylodis Ovatae Rhizoma	9 g.
gān jiāng	dried ginger [root]	Zingiberis Rhizoma Exsiccatum	6 g.
zhì gān cǎo	licorice [root] (honey-fried)	Glycyrrhizae Radix	6 g.

with:

Poria (Hoelen) Five Powder *wǔ líng sǎn*

fú líng	poria	Poria	9 g.
zhū líng	polyporus	Polyporus	9 g.
zé xiè	alisma [tuber]	Alismatis Rhizoma	15 g.
bái zhú	ovate atractylodes [root]	Atractylodis Ovatae Rhizoma	9 g.
guì zhī	cinnamon [twig]	Cinnamomi Ramulus	6 g.

In cases with predominance of kidney yang vacuity, use:

Life Saver Kidney Qi Pill *jì shēng shèn qì wán*

shú dì huáng	cooked rehmannia [root]	Rehmanniae Radix Conquita	6 g.
shān yào	dioscorea [root]	Dioscoreae Rhizoma	12 g.
shān zhū yú	cornus [fruit]	Corni Fructus	12 g.
zé xiè	alisma [tuber]	Alismatis Rhizoma	12 g.
fú líng	poria	Poria	12 g.
mǔ dān pí	moutan [root bark]	Moutan Radicis Cortex	12 g.
zhì fù zǐ	aconite [accessory tuber] (processed) (extended decoction)	Aconiti Tuber Laterale Praeparatum	6 g.
ròu guì	cinnamon bark (abbreviated decoction)	Cinnamomi Cortex	6 g.
chuān niú xī	cyathula [root]	Cyathulae Radix	6 g.
chē qián zǐ	plantago seed (wrapped)	Plantaginis Semen	12 g.

ACUPUNCTURE AND MOXIBUSTION

Main points: Needle with even supplementation, even draining; add moxibustion.

BL-20	*pí shū*
BL-23	*shèn shū*
CV-09	*shuǐ fēn*
KI-07	*fù liū*
CV-04	*guān yuán*
ST-36	*zú sān lǐ*

Auxiliary points:

For severe physical cold, add moxibustion of:

GV-04	*mìng mén*
BL-24	*qì hǎi shū*

6. VACUITY OF LIVER AND KIDNEY YIN

Clinical Manifestations: Enlargement, distention and fullness of the abdomen, protrusion of the superficial abdominal blood vessels in severe cases, dull complexion, purplish lips, dry mouth, irritability, bleeding of the nose and gums (in some cases), dark scanty urine.

Tongue: Dark red with little dry coating.

Pulse: Rapid, thready, wiry.

Treatment Method: Nourish liver and kidney yin, rectify qi, quicken the blood, dispel stasis.

PRESCRIPTION

Combine Six-Ingredient Rehmannia Pill *(liù wèi dì huáng wán)* with Infradiaphragmatic Stasis-Expelling Decoction *(gé xià zhú yū tāng)*.

Six-Ingredient Rehmannia Pill *liù wèi dì huáng wán*

shú dì huáng	cooked rehmannia [root]	Rehmanniae Radix Conquita	24 g.
shān zhū yú	cornus [fruit]	Corni Fructus	12 g.
shān yào	dioscorea [root]	Dioscoreae Rhizoma	12 g.
zé xiè	alisma [tuber]	Alismatis Rhizoma	9 g.
fú líng	poria	Poria	9 g.
mǔ dān pí	moutan [root bark]	Moutan Radicis Cortex	9 g.

with:

Infradiaphragmatic Stasis-Expelling Decoction *gé xià zhú yū tāng*

wǔ líng zhī	flying squirrel droppings (wrapped)	Trogopteri seu Pteromydis Excrementum	9 g.
dāng guī	tangkuei	Angelicae Sinensis Radix	9 g.
táo rén	peach [kernel]	Persicae Semen	9 g.
hóng huā	carthamus [flower]	Carthami Flosa	9 g.
chuān xiōng	ligusticum [root]	Ligustici Rhizoma	6 g.
mǔ dān pí	moutan [root bark]	Moutan Radicis Cortex	6 g.
wū yào	lindera [root]	Linderae Radix	6 g.
xiāng fù zǐ	cyperus [root]	Cyperi Rhizoma	4.5 g.
chì sháo yào	red peony [root]	Paeoniae Radix Rubra	6 g.
zhǐ ké	bitter orange	Aurantii Fructus	4.5 g.
yán hú suǒ	corydalis [tuber]	Corydalis Tuber	3 g.
gān cǎo	licorice [root]	Glycyrrhizae Radix	9 g.

MODIFICATIONS

In severe cases of yin vacuity, the prescription is reinforced to nourish yin and generate liquid. Add:

xuán shēn	scrophularia [root]	Scrophulariae Radix	9 g.
shí hú	dendrobium [stem] (extended decoction)	Dendrobii Caulis	9 g.
mài mén dōng	ophiopogon [tuber]	Ophiopogonis Tuber	12 g.

In cases of extreme abdominal distention, the prescription is modified to move qi and relieve distention. Add:

lái fú zǐ	radish [seed]	Raphani Semen	9 g.
dà fù pí	areca [husk]	Arecae Pericarpium	9 g.

In cases accompanied by tidal fever and irritability, the prescription is modified to clear vacuity heat and eliminate vexation. Add:

yín chái hú	lanceolate stellaria [root]	Stellariae Lanceolatae Radix	9 g.
dì gǔ pí	lycium [root bark]	Lycii Radicis Cortex	9 g.
biē jiǎ	turtle shell (extended decoction)	Amydae Carapax	30 g.
zhú yè	black bamboo [leaf]	Bambusae Folium	9 g.

In cases of bleeding nose and gums, the prescription is modified to cool the blood and relieve bleeding. Add:

bái máo gēn	imperata [root]	Imperatae Rhizoma	30 g.
xiān hè cǎo	agrimony	Agrimoniae Herba	12 g.

In cases of scanty urine, the prescription is modified to remove water. Add:

zhū líng	polyporus	Polyporus	9 g.
huá shí	talcum (wrapped)	Talcum	9 g.

To free yang in cases of scanty urine, add a small dose of:

ròu guì	cinnamon [bark] (abbreviated decoction)	Cinnamomi Cortex	1.5 g.

ACUPUNCTURE AND MOXIBUSTION

Main points: Needle with even supplementation, even draining.

BL-18	gān shū
BL-23	shèn shū
CV-05	shí mén
CV-09	shuǐ fēn
SP-06	sān yīn jiāo
KI-07	fù liū

Auxiliary points:

For tidal fever, add:

KI-03	tài xī
BL-43 (38)	gāo huāng shū

ALTERNATE THERAPEUTIC METHODS

1. Ear Acupuncture

Auricular points: Liver, Kidney, Pancreas, Large Intestine.

Method: Select two or three points per session, needle to elicit a moderate sensation and retain the needles for ten to twenty minutes. Treat once every two days, ten sessions per therapeutic course.

REMARKS

Drum distention is a severe pattern; in the early stages of illness, it is generally the result of spleen and liver dysfunction, with stagnation of qi and obstruction by dampness. Clear distinction must be made as to the predominance of qi stagnation, static blood, damp-heat, or cold-dampness before the appropriate therapeutic methods can be administered. In cases of extended illness or when the patient's physical condition is frail, pathogenesis may involve vacuity of spleen and kidney yang or vacuity of liver and kidney yin. Since drum distention patterns are a root vacuity with branch repletion, or are complicated by both repletion and vacuity, treatment should couple draining and supplementation; draining, however, should not be too harsh.

During the treatment of drum distention, strict attention should be paid to the regulation of the patient's dietary habits, emotional state and exposure to the elements. Low salt diets, or in cases of severe urine retention, salt-free diets, are generally recommended. Patients should be advised to free themselves from worry and anxiety during treatment, as well as to avoid chills and draughts to prevent invasion of evils thereby introducing further pathological changes.

EDEMA

Shuǐ Zhǒng

1. Attack by Wind-Heat - 2. Inundation by Water-Dampness - 3. Accumulation of Damp-Heat - 4. Decline of Spleen Yang - 5. Vacuity of Kidney Yang

Edema is the accumulation of fluid in the body. It permeates the tissues and results in the swelling of the eyelids, face, limbs, trunk or the entire body. Edema can be divided into yang edema and yin edema on the basis of etiology, pathogenesis and clinical manifestations. Yang edema is relatively acute, generally beginning with the head and face, and swelling is most severe above the waist. Yin edema develops slowly, usually beginning with the feet, and swelling is most severe below the waist.

Edema is a common symptom of many diseases recognized by Western medicine. These include congestive heart failure, acute and chronic nephritis, endocrine disease and nutritional imbalance, all of which can be treated with the information in this chapter.

ETIOLOGY AND PATHOGENESIS

Patterns of edema can be caused either by external evil attack or internal disruption. In either case, pathological changes occur mainly in the lung, spleen and kidney, with the kidney playing the fundamental role. Etiological factors which result in the dysfunction of the lung and spleen, such as attack by external wind-heat or invasion of water-dampness or damp-heat, generally cause the repletion patterns of yang edema.

Factors that can bring about spleen and kidney vacuity, such as internal disruption from improper diet and eating habits, taxation or overindulgence in sexual activity, are generally patterns of root vacuity with branch repletion. These are classified as yin edema.

Mutual transformation between yin edema and yang edema is possible. In cases of prolonged yang edema with a constant decline in correct qi, for example, there is a danger of transformation to yin edema. Conversely, in cases of yin edema compounded by external evil attack, the severity of swelling can increase and give rise to symptoms of yang edema.

In addition, obstruction of the water passages of the triple burner by static blood can cause very persistent cases of edema.

1. ATTACK BY WIND-HEAT

Clinical Manifestations: Abrupt onset of edema beginning with the eyelids and face, and gradually spreading to the limbs and entire body; sensitivity to drafts, fever, heavy aching limbs, difficult urination and sore red swollen throat.

Tongue: Red.

Pulse: Rapid, slippery, floating. Cases of relatively severe edema may also present deep pulse.

Treatment Method: Course wind, clear heat, diffuse the lung, remove water.

PRESCRIPTION

Spleen-Effusing Decoction Plus Ovate Atractylodes *yuè bì jiā zhú tāng*

má huáng	ephedra	Ephedrae Herba	9 g.
shí gāo	gypsum (extended decoction)	Gypsum	18 g.
shēng jiāng	fresh ginger	Zingiberis Rhizoma Recens	9 g.
gān cǎo	licorice [root]	Glycyrrhizae Radix	6 g.
dà zǎo	jujube	Ziziphi Fructus	5 pc.
bái zhú	ovate atractylodes [root]	Atractylodis Ovatae Rhizoma	9 g.

<u>MODIFICATIONS</u>

To reinforce the prescription's diuretic effects, add:

chē qián zǐ	plantago seed (wrapped)	Plantaginis Semen	12 g
zé xiè	alisma [tuber]	Alismatis Rhizoma	9 g.
shí wéi	pyrrosia [leaf]	Pyrrosiae Folium	9 g.
bái máo gēn	imperata [root]	Imperatae Rhizoma	30 g.

In cases with sore red swollen throat, the prescription is modified to clear heat and disinhibit the pharynx.

Delete:

shēng jiāng	fresh ginger	Zingiberis Rhizoma Recens
dà zǎo	jujube	Ziziphi Fructus

Add:

bǎn lán gēn	isatis [root]	Isatidis Radix	12 g.
pú gōng yīng	dandelion	Taraxaci Herba cum Radice	9 g.
jié gěng	platycodon [root]	Platycodonis Radix	9 g.
lián qiáo	forsythia [fruit]	Forsythiae Fructus	9 g.

In cases accompanied by coughing and difficult breathing, the prescription is modified.

Add:

qián hú	peucedanum [root]	Peucedani Radix	9 g.
xìng rén	apricot [kernel] (abbreviated decoction)	Armeniacae Semen	9 g.
sāng bái pí	mulberry [root bark]	Mori Radicis Cortex	12 g.
tíng lì zǐ	tingli [seed]	Descurainiae seu Lepidii Semen	6 g.

In cases of hematuria, the prescription is modified to clear heat and relieve bleeding.

Add:

xiǎo jì	cephalanoplos	Cephalanoploris Herba seu Radix	12 g.
bái máo gēn	imperata [root]	Imperatae Rhizoma	30 g.

In cases tending toward wind cold manifesting difficult breathing, aversion to cold, coughing, thin white tongue coating and slippery, floating or tight pulse, the prescription is modified to course wind and dispel cold.

Delete:

| *shí gāo* | gypsum | Gypsum | |

Add:

zǐ sū yè	perilla leaf (abbreviated decoction)	Perillae Folium	9 g.
fáng fēng	ledebouriella [root]	Ledebouriellae Radix	9 g.
guì zhī	cinnamon [twig]	Cinnamomi Ramulus	6 g.

ACUPUNCTURE AND MOXIBUSTION

Main points: Needle with draining.

BL-13	*fèi shū*
BL-12	*fēng mén*
LU-07	*liè quē*
LI-04	*hé gǔ*
LI-06	*piān lì*
TB-05	*wài guān*

Auxiliary points:

For severe edema of the face, add:

GV-26   *shuǐ gōu*

For sore throat, add bloodletting at:

LU-11   *shào shāng*

2. INUNDATION BY WATER-DAMPNESS

Clinical Manifestations: Generalized pitting edema, scanty urine, sensation of heaviness and fatigue, oppression in the chest, loss of appetite, nausea. Exterior patterns are generally not present; onset of illness is relatively slow.

Tongue: White slimy coating.

Pulse: Deep, tardy.

Treatment Method: Fortify the spleen, transform dampness, invigorate yang, drain water.

PRESCRIPTION

Modified combination of Five-Peel Powder (Beverage) *(wǔ pí sǎn [yǐn])* and Stomach-Calming Poria (Hoelen) Five Decoction *(wèi líng tāng)*.

Five-Peel Powder (Beverage) *wǔ pí sǎn (yǐn)*

sāng bái pí	mulberry root bark	Mori Radicis Cortex	12 g.
fú líng pí	poria skin	Poriae Cortex	15 g.
jiāng pí	ginger skin	Zingiberis Rhizomatis Cortex	9 g.
chén pí	tangerine peel	Citri Exocarpium	9 g.
dà fù pí	areca husk	Arecae Pericarpium	9 g.

with:

Stomach-Calming Poria (Hoelen) Five Decoction *wèi líng tāng*

cāng zhú	atractylodes [root]	Atractylodis Rhizoma	9 g.
bái zhú	ovate atractylodes [root]	Atractylodis Ovatae Rhizoma	9 g.
fú líng	poria	Poria	9 g.
zhū líng	polyporus	Polyporus	9 g.

hòu pò	magnolia [bark]	Magnoliae Cortex	9 g.
chén pí	tangerine [peel]	Citri Exocarpium	9 g.
zé xiè	alisma [tuber]	Alismatis Rhizoma	12 g.
guì zhī	cinnamon [twig]	Cinnamomi Ramulus	6 g.
zhì gān cǎo	licorice [root] (honey-fried)	Glycyrrhizae Radix	6 g.

MODIFICATIONS

In cases of severe edema accompanied by difficult breathing, the prescription is modified to diffuse the lung, calm panting and dispel water. Add:

má huáng	ephedra	Ephedrae Herba	9 g.
xìng rén	apricot kernel (abbreviated decoction)	Armeniacae Semen	9 g.
tíng lì zǐ	tingli [seed]	Descurainiae seu Lepidii Semen	9 g.

ACUPUNCTURE AND MOXIBUSTION

Main points: Needle with draining.

BL-20	*pí shū*
SP-09	*yīn líng quán*
CV-12	*zhōng wǎn*
CV-09	*shuǐ fēn*
ST-36	*zú sān lǐ*
BL-22	*sān jiāo shū*

Auxiliary points:

For severe edema accompanied by difficult breathing, add:

| BL-13 | *fèi shū* |
| LU-07 | *liè quē* |

3. ACCUMULATION OF DAMP-HEAT

Clinical Manifestations: General edema, moist shiny skin, oppression in the chest, fullness and discomfort of the epigastrium, irritability, thirst, dark scanty urine, constipation.

Tongue: Yellow slimy coating.

Pulse: Soft, rapid or deep, rapid.

Treatment Method: Dispel damp, clear heat, disinhibit water and disperse swelling.

PRESCRIPTION

Coursing and Piercing Drink *shū záo yǐn zǐ*

zé xiè	alisma [tuber]	Alismatis Rhizoma	12 g.
chì xiǎo dòu	rice bean	Phaseoli Calcarati Semen	15 g.
shāng lù	phytolacca [root]	Phytolaccae Radix	6 g.
qiāng huó	notopterygium [root]	Notopterygii Rhizoma	9 g.
dà fù pí	areca [husk]	Arecae Pericarpium	9 g.
jiāo mù	zanthoxylum [seed]	Zanthoxyli Semen	3 g.
mù tōng	mutong [stem]	Mutong Caulis	9 g.
qín jiāo	large gentian [root]	Gentianae Macrophyllae Radix	9 g.
bīng láng	areca [nut]	Arecae Semen	9 g.
fú líng pí	poria skin	Poriae Cortex	15 g.
shēng jiāng	fresh ginger	Zingiberis Rhizoma Recens	3 g.

MODIFICATIONS

In cases of abdominal fullness and constipation, the prescription is modified to assist draining.
Add:

Fangji, Zanthoxylum, Tingli and Rhubarb Pill *jǐ jiāo lì huáng wán*

fáng jǐ	fangji [root]	Fangji Radix	12 g.
jiāo mù	zanthoxylum [seed]	Zanthoxyli Semen	4.5 g.
tíng lì zǐ	tingli [seed]	Descurainiae seu Lepidii Semen	9 g.
dà huáng	rhubarb (abbreviated decoction)	Rhei Rhizoma	9 g.

In cases of heavy breathing, asthma, inability to lie flat, fullness of the chest and rapid wiry pulse, the prescription is modified to drain the lung and calm panting. Combine with the given prescription:

Tingli and Jujube Lung-Draining Decoction *tíng lì dà zǎo xiè fèi tāng*

tíng lì zǐ	tingli [seed]	Descurainiae seu Lepidii Semen	9 g.
dà zǎo	jujube	Ziziphi Fructus	10 pc.

In cases where damp-heat has injured the blood vessels causing painful urination and hematuria, the prescription is modified to cool the blood and relieve bleeding.
Add:

dà jì	cirsium	Cirsii Herba seu Radix	12 g.
xiǎo jì	cephalanoplos	Cephalanoploris Herba seu Radix	12 g.
bái máo gēn	imperata [root]	Imperatae Rhizoma	30 g.

ACUPUNCTURE AND MOXIBUSTION

Main points: Needle with draining.

SP-09	*yīn líng quán*
CV-09	*shuǐ fēn*
BL-39 (53)	*wěi yáng*
LI-04	*hé gǔ*
LI-11	*qū chí*
BL-22	*sān jiāo shū*

Auxiliary points:
For hematuria, add:

SP-10	*xuè hǎi*
SP-06	*sān yīn jiāo*

4. DECLINE OF SPLEEN YANG

Clinical Manifestations: Generalized pitting edema that is more severe in the legs, distention and fullness of the epigastrium and abdomen, loss of appetite, loose stools, sallow complexion, tiredness, lack of warmth in the limbs, scanty urine.

Tongue: Pale with a white glossy coating.

Pulse: Deep, tardy or deep, weak.

Treatment Method: Warm and invigorate spleen yang, transform dampness, disinhibit water.

PRESCRIPTION

Spleen-Firming Beverage *shí pí yǐn*

hòu pò	magnolia [bark]	Magnoliae Cortex	6 g.
bái zhú	ovate atractylodes [root]	Atractylodis Ovatae Rhizoma	6 g.
mù guā	chaenomeles [fruit]	Chaenomelis Fructus	6 g.
mù xiāng	saussurea [root]	Saussureae Radix (seu Vladimiriae)	6 g.
cǎo guǒ	tsaoko [fruit]	Amomi Tsao-Ko Fructus	6 g.
bīng láng	areca [nut]	Arecae Semen	6 g.
zhì fù zǐ	aconite [accessory tuber] (processed) (extended decoction)	Aconiti Tuber Laterale Praeparatum	6 g.
pào jiāng	dried ginger (charred)	Zingiberis Rhizoma Tostum	6 g.
fú líng	poria	Poria	6 g.
zhì gān cǎo	licorice [root] (honey-fried)	Glycyrrhizae Radix	3 g.
shēng jiāng	fresh ginger	Zingiberis Rhizoma Recens	3 g.
dà zǎo	jujube	Ziziphi Fructus	3 pc.

MODIFICATIONS

In cases of severe qi vacuity with shortness of breath and weak voice, the prescription is modified to fortify the spleen and benefit qi.
Add:

huáng qí	astragalus [root]	Astragali (seu Hedysari) Radix	12 g.
rén shēn	ginseng	Ginseng Radix	9 g.

In cases where water dampness is severe with greatly diminished urine secretion, the prescription is modified to aid the function of the urinary bladder and free and disinhibit the urine.
Add:

guì zhī	cinnamon [twig]	Cinnamomi Ramulus	9 g.
zhū líng	polyporus	Polyporus	9 g.
zé xiè	alisma [tuber]	Alismatis Rhizoma	9 g.

ACUPUNCTURE AND MOXIBUSTION

Main points: Needle with even supplementation, even draining; add moxibustion.

BL-20	*pí shū*
ST-36	*zú sān lǐ*
CV-06	*qì hǎi*
CV-09	*shuǐ fēn*
SP-09	*yīn líng quán*
SP-06	*sān yīn jiāo*

Auxiliary points:

For epigastric fullness and discomfort, add:

CV-12	*zhōng wǎn*

For loose stools, add:

ST-25	*tiān shū*

5. VACUITY OF KIDNEY YANG

Clinical Manifestations: Generalized pitting edema more severe below the waist, palpitations, shortness of breath, aching, cold and heaviness of the lower back, diminished secretion of urine, cold limbs, lassitude, physical cold, pale or grayish dull complexion.

Tongue: Pale, swollen with white coating.

Pulse: Deep, thready, or slow, deep, forceless.

Treatment Method: Warm and invigorate kidney yang, disinhibit water and disperse swelling.

PRESCRIPTION

True Warrior Decoction *zhēn wǔ tāng*

zhì fù zǐ	aconite [accessory tuber] (processed) (extended decoction)	Aconiti Tuber Laterale Praeparatum	9 g.
fú líng	poria	Poria	9 g.
bái sháo yào	white peony [root]	Paeoniae Radix Alba	9 g.
bái zhú	ovate atractylodes [root]	Atractylodis Ovatae Rhizoma	6 g.
shēng jiāng	fresh ginger	Zingiberis Rhizoma Recens	9 g.

MODIFICATIONS

The prescription is often reinforced to warm and supplement kidney yang.
Add:

hú lú bā	fenugreek [seed]	Foeni-Graeci Semen	9 g.
bā jǐ tiān	morinda [root]	Morindae Radix	9 g.
ròu guì	cinnamon [bark] (abbreviated decoction)	Cinnamomi Cortex	6 g.

In cases where water evil has flooded into the lung causing difficult breathing, the prescription is modified to drain the lung and calm panting.
Add:

tíng lì zǐ	tingli [seed]	Descurainiae seu Lepidii Semen	9 g.

In cases with palpitations, purplish-black lips and weak rapid pulse, water qi has intimidated the heart, obstructed heart yang and led to obstruction by static blood. The prescription is modified to warm yang and dispel stasis.

Increase the dosage of:

zhì fù zǐ	aconite [accessory tuber] (processed) (extended decoction)	Aconiti Tuber Laterale Praeparatum	12 g.

Add:

guì zhī	cinnamon [twig]	Cinnamomi Ramulus	9 g.
dān shēn	salvia [root]	Salviae Miltiorrhizae Radix	12 g.
yì mǔ cǎo	leonurus	Leonuri Herba	12 g.
hóng huā	carthamus [flower]	Carthami Flos	9 g.
zhì gān cǎo	licorice [root] (honey-fried)	Glycyrrhizae Radix	9 g.

In acute cases, there will be tiredness, drowsiness, nausea and, when severe, the taste of urine in the mouth. The prescription is modified to resolve toxins and transform turbidity. Add:

dà huáng	rhubarb	Rhei Rhizoma	6 g.
zhì bàn xià	pinellia [tuber] (processed)	Pinelliae Tuber Praeparatum	9 g.
huáng lián	coptis [root]	Coptidis Rhizoma	6 g.

In cases compounded with attack by external cold, with symptoms of increased edema, aversion to cold and no perspiration, the prescription is modified to dissipate cold evil.

Delete:

bái sháo yào	white peony [root]	Paeoniae Radix Alba

Add:

má huáng	ephedra	Ephedrae Herba	9 g.
xì xīn	asarum	Asiasari Herba cum Radice	3 g.
gān cǎo	licorice [root]	Glycyrrhizae Radix	6 g.

In cases of prolonged yang vacuity resulting in injury to yin, with symptoms including recurrent edema, aching lower back, seminal emission, dry mouth and throat, vexing heat in the five hearts, bleeding gums, red tongue and weak thready pulse, the prescription is changed to nourish kidney yin and disinhibit water.

Use:

Left-Restoring [Kidney Yin] Pill *zuǒ guī wán*

shú dì huáng	cooked rehmannia [root]	Rehmanniae Radix Conquita	24 g.
shān yào	dioscorea [root]	Dioscoreae Rhizoma	12 g.
shān zhū yú	cornus [fruit]	Corni Fructus	12 g.
gǒu qǐ zǐ	lycium [berry]	Lycii Fructus	12 g.
chuān niú xī	cyathula [root]	Cyathulae Radix	9 g.
tù sī zǐ	cuscuta [seed]	Cuscutae Semen	12 g.
lù jiǎo jiāo	deerhorn glue (dissolved)	Cervi Gelatinum Cornu	12 g.
guī bǎn jiāo	tortoise plastron (dissolved)	Testudinis Plastrum	12 g.

Add:

zé xiè	alisma [tuber]	Alismatis Rhizoma	9 g.
fú líng	poria	Poria	9 g
dōng kuí zǐ	mallow [seed]	Malvae Verticillatae Semen	9 g.

ACUPUNCTURE AND MOXIBUSTION

Main points: Needle with even supplementation, even draining; add moxibustion.

BL-23	*shèn shū*
BL-20	*pí shū*
CV-04	*guān yuán*
CV-09	*shuǐ fēn*
KI-07	*fù liū*
CV-06	*qì hǎi*

Auxiliary points:

For swelling of the feet, add:

GB-41	*zú lín qì*
SP-05	*shāng qiū*

ALTERNATE THERAPEUTIC METHODS

1. Ear Acupuncture

Main points: Liver, Spleen, Kidney, Subcortex, Urinary Bladder, Abdomen.

Method: Select two or three points per session. Needle bilaterally to elicit a moderate sensation. Treat once every two days.

REMARKS

In the treatment of edema, blood-invigorating stasis-dissolving medicinals are often added to promote diuresis, disinhibit water and disperse swelling. The rationale is that with the movement of blood, water also moves. These would include:

yì mǔ cǎo	leonurus	Leonuri Herba	12 g.
zé lán	lycopus	Lycopus Herba	12 g.
táo rén	peach [kernel]	Persica Semen	9 g.
hóng huā	carthamus [flower]	Carthami Flos	9 g.

During the initial stages of edema, patients should follow a salt-free diet; this may be gradually changed to a low-salt diet after the edema has been brought under control and the swelling has begun to subside. Return to a normal diet should proceed only after there is complete drainage of the excessive fluids. Also, hot, spicy foods should be restricted and patients should abstain from alcohol, cigarettes and other stimulants. Patients should also pay attention to recuperation, prevention of colds and not overworking themselves or overindulging in sexual activity. This is to avoid further injury to qi and essence.

THORACIC BI

Xiōng Bì

1. Heart Static Blood Obstruction - 2. Congestion by Phlegm-Turbidity - 3. Congealed Yin Cold - 4. Heart and Kidney Yin Vacuity - 5. Qi and Yin Vacuity - 6. Yang Qi Vacuity and Debilitation

Thoracic bi refers to patterns characterized by oppression in the chest with chest pain. In some cases the pain will radiate through to the back, with shortness of breath or difficult respiration preventing patients from lying flat. Mild cases manifest simple congestion and discomfort in the chest, while severe cases manifest twisting pain in the chest accompanied by shortness of breath and difficult respiration. With continued development, thoracic bi may result in the condition known as *zhēn xīn tòng* (true cardiac pain), with critical symptoms of intense prolonged chest pain accompanied by perspiration, cold extremities, pale complexion, faint thready or intermittent pulse and cyanotic lips, hands and feet.

Thoracic bi is observed in coronary arteriosclerotic heart disease as well as other heart diseases as diagnosed by Western medicine.

ETIOLOGY AND PATHOGENESIS

The etiology of thoracic bi may include invasion by cold evil, improper diet and eating habits, emotional stress and frail constitution with old age. The site of pathological change is generally the heart, although the spleen and kidney may also be affected. Pathogenesis in all cases involves root vacuity and branch repletion. Vacuity patterns include depleted yin, yang, qi and blood, while repletion patterns include yin cold, phlegm-turbidity and blood stasis. Since the majority of clinically observed thoracic bi patterns are complicated by both repletion and vacuity, simultaneous treatment of both repletion and vacuity is undertaken according to the predominance and severity of symptoms.

1. HEART STATIC BLOOD OBSTRUCTION

Clinical Manifestations: Stabbing chest pain of fixed location, pain more severe at night, periodic spells of palpitation.

Tongue: Dark, purple.

Pulse: Deep, rough.

Treatment Method: Quicken the blood, dissolve stasis, relieve pain.

PRESCRIPTION

House of Blood Stasis-Expelling Decoction *xuè fǔ zhú yū tāng*

táo rén	peach [kernel]	Persicae Semen	12 g.
hóng huā	carthamus [flower]	Carthami Flos	9 g.
dāng guī	tangkuei	Angelicae Sinensis Radix	9 g.
shēng dì huáng	rehmannia [root] dried/fresh	Rehmanniae Radix Exsiccata seu Recens	9 g.
chuān xiōng	ligusticum [root]	Ligustici Rhizoma	4.5 g.
chì sháo yào	red peony [root]	Paeoniae Radix Rubra	6 g.
niú xī	achyranthes [root]	Achyranthis Bidentatae Radix	9 g.
jié gěng	platycodon [root]	Platycodonis Radix	4.5 g.
chái hú	bupleurum [root]	Bupleuri Radix	3 g.
zhǐ ké	bitter orange	Aurantii Fructus	6 g.
gān cǎo	licorice [root]	Glycyrrhizae Radix	3 g.

MODIFICATIONS

In cases of severe chest pain, the prescription is modified to quicken the blood, rectify qi and relieve pain.
Add:

jiàng xiāng	dalbergia [wood]	Dalbergiae Lignum	6 g.
yù jīn	curcuma [tuber]	Curcumae Tuber	9 g.
yán hú suǒ	corydalis [tuber]	Corydalis Tuber	9 g.

ACUPUNCTURE AND MOXIBUSTION

Main points: Needle with draining.

CV-17	*tǎn zhōng*
CV-14	*jù què*
BL-15	*xīn shū*
BL-17	*gé shū*
HT-06	*yīn xī*

Auxiliary points:

For purple tongue and cyanotic lips, bleed:

LU-11	*shào shāng*
HT-09	*shào chōng*
PC-09	*zhōng chōng*

2. CONGESTION BY PHLEGM-TURBIDITY

Clinical Manifestations: Sensations of congestion and pain in the chest, pain radiating through to the back and shoulders (in some cases), shortness of breath, rapid respiration, heaviness of the limbs, overweight, excessive phlegm.

Tongue: White slimy coating.

Pulse: Slippery.

Treatment Method: Free yang, dispel phlegm-turbidity.

PRESCRIPTION

Trichosanthes, Chinese Chive and Pinellia Decoction
guā lóu xiè bái bàn xià tāng

guā lóu	trichosanthes [fruit]	Trichosanthis Fructus	12 g.
xiè bái	Chinese chive [bulb]	Allii Bulbus	9 g.
fǎ bàn xià	pinellia [tuber] (processed)	Pinelliae Tuber Praeparatum	12 g.
bái jiǔ	white liquor	Granorum Spiritus Incolor	50 cc.

MODIFICATIONS

To reinforce invigorating yang and dispelling phlegm-turbidity, add:

gān jiāng	dried ginger [root]	Zingiberis Rhizoma Exsiccatum	6 g.
chén pí	tangerine [peel]	Citri Exocarpium	9 g.
bái dòu kòu	cardamom (abbreviated decoction)	Amomi Cardamomi Fructus	6 g.

ACUPUNCTURE AND MOXIBUSTION

Main points: Needle with draining.

CV-14	*jù què*
CV-17	*tǎn zhōng*
PC-04	*xī mén*
LU-09	*tài yuān*
ST-40	*fēng lóng*

Auxiliary points:

For pain radiating through to the back, add cupping to the following points:

BL-13	*fèi shū*
BL-15	*xīn shū*

3. CONGEALED YIN COLD

Clinical Manifestations: Chest pain radiating through to the back and aggravated by exposure to cold, with oppression in the chest, shortness of breath, palpitations, difficult respiration, inability to lie flat, pale complexion, cold extremities.

Tongue: White coating.

Pulse: Deep, thready.

Treatment Method: Free yang, dissipate cold, relieve pain.

PRESCRIPTION

Trichosanthes, Chinese Chive and White Liquor Decoction
guā lóu xiè bái bái jiǔ tāng

guā lóu	trichosanthes [fruit]	Trichosanthis Fructus	12 g.
xiè bái	Chinese chive [bulb]	Allii Bulbus	12 g.
bái jiǔ	white liquor	Granorum Spiritus Incolor	50 cc.

MODIFICATIONS

To reinforce the therapeutic effects of the prescription, add:

zhì fù zǐ	aconite [accessory tuber] (processed) (extended decoction)	Aconiti Tuber Laterale Praeparatum	9 g.
guì zhī	cinnamon [twig]	Cinnamomi Ramulus	9 g.
zhǐ shí	unripe bitter orange	Aurantii Fructus Immaturus	9 g.
dān shēn	salvia [root]	Salviae Miltiorrhizae Radix	12 g.
tán xiāng	sandalwood	Santali Lignum	3 g.

In cases of profuse phlegm-dampness, presenting chest pain with coughing and expectoration of phlegm and mucus, the prescription is modified to promote movement of qi and transform phlegm. Add:

shēng jiāng	fresh ginger	Zingiberis Rhizoma Recens	9 g.
chén pí	tangerine [peel]	Citri Exocarpium	9 g.
fú líng	poria	Poria	12 g.
xìng rén	apricot [kernel] (abbreviated decoction)	Armeniacae Semen	9 g.

ACUPUNCTURE AND MOXIBUSTION

Main points: Needle with draining; add moxibustion.

BL-15	xīn shū
BL-14	jué yīn shū
PC-06	nèi guān
HT-05	tōng lǐ

Auxiliary points:

For cold extremities, add moxibustion to:

| CV-06 | qì hǎi |
| CV-04 | guān yuán |

4. HEART AND KIDNEY YIN VACUITY

Clinical Manifestations: Congestion and pain in the chest, palpitations, night sweating, irritability, insomnia, weak aching lower back and legs, tinnitus, dizziness and vertigo.

Tongue: Red with little coating.

Pulse: Rapid, thready.

Treatment Method: Nourish heart and kidney yin, quiet the spirit, relieve pain.

PRESCRIPTION

Left-Restoring [Kidney Yin] Beverage *zuǒ guī yǐn*

shú dì huáng	cooked rehmannia [root]	Rehmanniae Radix Conquita	24 g.
shān yào	dioscorea [root]	Dioscoreae Rhizoma	12 g.
gǒu qǐ zǐ	lycium [berry]	Lycii Fructus	12 g.
shān zhū yú	cornus [fruit]	Corni Fructus	12 g.
fú líng	poria	Poria	9 g.
zhì gān cǎo	licorice [root] (honey-fried)	Glycyrrhizae Radix	6 g.

MODIFICATIONS

To reinforce the effects of nourishing heart yin and calming the spirit, add:

mài mén dōng	ophiopogon [tuber]	Ophiopogonis Tuber	12 g.
wǔ wèi zǐ	schisandra [berry]	Schisandrae Fructus	6 g.
bǎi zǐ rén	biota [seed]	Biotae Semen	12 g.
suān zǎo rén	spiny jujube [kernel]	Ziziphi Spinosi Semen	12 g.

In cases of severe chest pain, the prescription is modified to nourish the blood, free the connections and relieve pain. Add:

dāng guī	tangkuei	Angelicae Sinensis Radix	9 g.
dān shēn	salvia [root]	Salvia Radix	12 g.
chuān xiōng	ligusticum [root]	Ligustici Rhizoma	6 g.
yù jīn	curcuma [tuber]	Curcumae Tuber	9 g.

In cases of yin vacuity with hyperactive yang, presenting dizziness and vertigo, with numbness of the tongue and extremities, the prescription is modified to nourish yin and subdue yang. Add:

hé shǒu wū	flowery knotweed [root] (processed)	Polygoni Multiflori Radix Praeparatum	12 g.
nǔ zhēn zǐ	ligustrum [fruit]	Ligustri Fructus	12 g.
gōu téng	uncaria [stem and thorn] (abbreviated decoction)	Uncariae Ramulus cum Unco	9 g.
shí jué míng	abalone shell (extended decoction)	Haliotidis Concha	15 g.
mǔ lì	oyster shell (extended decoction)	Ostreae Concha	15 g.
biē jiǎ	turtle shell (extended decoction)	Amydae Carapax	18 g.

ACUPUNCTURE AND MOXIBUSTION

Main points: Needle with even supplementation, even draining.

BL-15	*xīn shū*
BL-23	*shèn shū*
HT-06	*yīn xī*
KI-03	*tài xī*
CV-17	*tǎn zhōng*
BL-17	*gé shū*

Auxiliary points:

For insomnia, add:

HT-07	*shén mén*

5. QI AND YIN VACUITY

Clinical Manifestations: Periodic congestion and dull pain in the chest, palpitations, shortness of breath, fatigue, sluggish speech, lusterless complexion, dizziness and vertigo, increase in severity of symptoms with physical exertion.

Tongue: Reddish, sometimes with tooth marks.

Pulse: Weak, thready or intermittent.

Treatment Method: Supplement qi, nourish yin, relieve pain.

PRESCRIPTION

Combine Pulse-Engendering Beverage *(shēng mài yǐn)* with Ginseng Construction-Nourishing Decoction (Pill) *(rén shēn yǎng róng tāng [wán])*

Pulse-Engendering Beverage *shēng mài yǐn*

rén shēn	ginseng	Ginseng Radix	9 g.
mài mén dōng	ophiopogon [tuber]	Ophiopogonis Tuber	15 g.
wǔ wèi zǐ	schisandra [berry]	Schisandrae Fructus	6 g.

with:

Ginseng Construction-Nourishing Decoction (Pill)
rén shēn yǎng róng tāng (wán)

rén shēn	ginseng	Ginseng Radix	9 g.
bái zhú	ovate atractylodes [root]	Atractylodis Ovatae Rhizoma	9 g.
fú líng	poria	Poria	9 g.
huáng qí	astragalus [root]	Astragali (seu Hedysari) Radix	12 g.
shú dì huáng	cooked rehmannia [root]	Rehmanniae Radix Conquita	9 g.
dāng guī	tangkuei	Angelicae Sinensis Radix	9 g.
bái sháo yào	white peony [root]	Paeoniae Radix Alba	12 g.
chén pí	tangerine [peel]	Citri Exocarpium	9 g.
ròu guì	cinnamon [bark]	Cinnamomi Cortex	3 g.
	(abbreviated decoction)		
wǔ wèi zǐ	schisandra [berry]	Schisandrae Fructus	6 g.
yuǎn zhì	polygala [root]	Polygalae Radix	6 g.
zhì gān cǎo	licorice [root] (honey-fried)	Glycyrrhizae Radix	6 g.
shēng jiāng	fresh ginger	Zingiberis Rhizoma Recens	3 g.
dà zǎo	jujube	Ziziphi Fructus	3 pc.

MODIFICATIONS

In cases of severe chest pain, the prescription is modified to invigorate the blood, free the connections and relieve pain. Add:

dān shēn	salvia [root]	Salviae Miltiorrhizae Radix	12 g.
yì mǔ cǎo	leonurus	Leonuri Herba	15 g.
yù jīn	curcuma [tuber]	Curcumae Tuber	9 g.
sān qī	notoginseng [root]	Notoginseng Radix	9 g.
	(or, powdered and administered separately, 1.5 g. each time)		

In cases of intermittent pulse, the prescription is modified to boost qi, nourish the blood and restore the pulse. Combine with:

Honey-Fried Licorice Decoction *zhì gān cǎo tāng*

zhì gān cǎo	licorice [root] (honey-fried)	Glycyrrhizae Radix	12 g.
rén shēn	ginseng	Ginseng Radix	6 g.
shēng dì huáng	rehmannia [root] dried/fresh	Rehmanniae Radix Exsiccata seu Recens	30 g
guì zhī	cinnamon [twig]	Cinnamomi Ramulus	9 g.
ē jiāo	ass hide glue (dissolved and stirred in)	Asini Corii Gelatinum	6 g.
mài mén dōng	ophiopogon [tuber]	Ophiopogonis Tuber	9 g.
huǒ má rén	hemp [seed]	Cannabis Semen	9 g.
shēng jiāng	fresh ginger	Zingiberis Rhizoma Recens	9 g.
dà zǎo	jujube	Ziziphi Fructus	6 pc.
bái jiǔ	white liquor (stirred in)	Granorum Spiritus Incolor	10 cc.

ACUPUNCTURE AND MOXIBUSTION

Main points: Needle with supplementation; add moxibustion.

BL-15	xīn shū
PC-06	nèi guān
CV-17	tǎn zhōng
ST-36	zú sān lǐ
BL-17	gé shū

Auxiliary points:

For shortness of breath, add moxibustion to:

BL-24	qì hǎi shū
BL-23	shèn shū

6. YANG QI VACUITY

Clinical Manifestations: Oppression in the chest, shortness of breath, pain radiating through to the back (in severe cases), palpitations, perspiration, aching lower back, pale complexion, pale or purplish lips and nails.

Tongue: Pale or dark purple.

Pulse: Deep, thready or deep, faint.

Treatment Method: Warm yang, boost qi, relieve pain.

PRESCRIPTION

Combine Ginseng and Aconite Decoction *(shēn fù tāng)* with Right-Restoring [Kidney Yang] Beverage *(yòu guī yǐn)*.

Ginseng and Aconite Decoction *shēn fù tāng*

rén shēn	ginseng	Ginseng Radix	30 g.
zhì fù zǐ	aconite [accessory tuber] (processed) (extended decoction)	Aconiti Tuber Laterale Praeparatum	15 g.

with:

Right-Restoring (Kidney Yang) Beverage *yòu guī yǐn*

shú dì huáng	cooked rehmannia [root]	Rehmanniae Radix Conquita	24 g.
shān yào	dioscorea [root]	Dioscoreae Rhizoma	12 g.
gǒu qǐ zǐ	lycium [berry]	Lycii Fructus	12 g.
shān zhū yú	cornus [fruit]	Corni Fructus	12 g.
dù zhòng	eucommia [bark]	Eucommiae Cortex	9 g.
zhì gān cǎo	licorice [root] (honey-fried)	Glycyrrhizae Radix	6 g.
zhì fù zǐ	aconite [accessory tuber] (processed) (extended decoction)	Aconiti Tuber Laterale Praeparatum	9 g.
ròu guì	cinnamon [bark] (abbreviated decoction)	Cinnamomi Cortex	6 g.

MODIFICATIONS

In cases presenting excessive perspiration and deep faint barely perceptible pulse, the prescriptions are modified to secure yang qi desertion.

Add:

duàn lóng gǔ	calcined dragon bone (extended decoction)	Mastodi Ossis Fossilia Calcinatum	30 g.
duàn mǔ lì	calcined oyster shell (extended decoction)	Ostreae Concha Calcinatum	30 g.

In cases where yang vacuity has led to yin vacuity, the prescription is modified to warm yang and nourish yin.

Add:

mài mén dōng	ophiopogon [tuber]	Ophiopogonis Tuber	9 g.
wǔ wèi zǐ	schisandra [berry]	Schisandrae Fructus	6 g.

In kidney yang vacuity that can no longer control water, leading to water qi intimidating the heart, there will be symptoms of palpitations, short rapid respiration, inability to lie flat, diminished secretion of urine and edema of the limbs. The prescription is changed to warm kidney yang and to free and disinhibit the urine.

Use:

True Warrior Decoction *zhēn wǔ tāng*

zhì fù zǐ	aconite [accessory tuber] (processed) (extended decoction)	Aconiti Tuber Laterale Praeparatum	9 g.
fú líng	poria	Poria	9 g.
bái sháo yào	white peony [root]	Paeoniae Radix Alba	9 g.
bái zhú	ovate atractylodes [root]	Atractylodis Ovatae Rhizoma	6 g.
shēng jiāng	fresh ginger	Zingiberis Rhizoma Recens	9 g.
Add:			
fáng jǐ	fangji [root]	Fangji Radix	6 g.
zhū líng	polyporus	Polyporus	9 g.
chē qián zǐ	plantago seed (wrapped)	Plantaginis Semen	9 g.

ACUPUNCTURE AND MOXIBUSTION

Main points: Needle with supplementation; add moxibustion.

BL-23	*shèn shū*
CV-04	*guān yuán*
CV-17	*tǎn zhōng*
PC-06	*nèi guān*
HT-05	*tōng lǐ*
BL-15	*xīn shū*

Auxiliary points:

For cold extremities, add moxibustion to:

CV-06	*qì hǎi*

ALTERNATE THERAPEUTIC METHODS

1. Ear Acupuncture

Main Points: Heart, Small Intestine, Sympathetic, Subcortex, Thorax, Lower Blood Pressure Groove, Liver, Lung, Brain, Occiput.

Method: Select two or three points each session, needle to elicit a strong sensation and retain needles for sixty minutes. Treat every other day, two weeks making one therapeutic course.

REMARKS

More severe thoracic bi patterns present true cardiac pain and are associated with the critical heart diseases described by Western medicine such as acute myocardial infarction. In such cases, emergency measures must be taken and comprehensive treatment with Western medicine should be begun. Apart from this, congestion and pain in the chest may also manifest during the early stages of diaphragmatic or esophageal tumors; therefore, careful distinction between these conditions should be made during diagnosis.

PALPITATION

Xīn Jì

1. Heart and Gallbladder Qi Vacuity - 2. Heart Blood Vacuity - 3. Yin Vacuity with Effulgent Fire - 4. Heart Yang Vacuity - 5. Oppression of the Heart by Water and Phlegm-Fluid - 6. Obstruction of the Heart by Blood Stasis

In traditional Chinese medicine, palpitation refers to patterns in which the heart rate becomes so irregular or accelerated that patients become aware of it, experiencing sensations of nervousness, anxiety or terror. Mild cases of palpitation, known in Chinese as *jīng jì* (fright palpitation) manifest as periodic temporary heart palpitation brought on by sudden fright or exertion. The condition of these patients is generally good. Racing of the heart, known as *zhēng chōng* (fearful throbbing), manifests as an irregular or accelerated heart rate that occurs without the initiating stimulus of fright or exertion. These spells of palpitation continue without relief and the condition of these patients is relatively poor.

Palpitations are brought on or increased in severity by emotional stress and overwork, and may be accompanied by symptoms of insomnia, poor memory, dizziness and tinnitus. They are frequently observed in neurosis, tachycardia and various arrhythmias described by Western medicine.

ETIOLOGY AND PATHOGENESIS

Etiological factors include heart and gallbladder qi vacuity, heart blood vacuity, depleted yin with yin vacuity fire effulgence, heart yang vacuity, water qi intimidating the heart and blood stasis obstructing the channels. In general, mild palpitations manifest as repletion patterns, while severe palpitations are vacuity patterns in the majority of cases. Repletion patterns may also exist in the midst of vacuity. Therefore, thorough differentiation must be undertaken during clinical examination.

1. HEART AND GALLBLADDER QI VACUITY

Clinical Manifestations: Easily frightened, fearfulness, insomnia, profuse dreaming.

Tongue: Thin white coating.

Pulse: Slightly rapid; weak in heart position.

Treatment Method: Supplement heart and gallbladder qi, suppress fright, quiet the spirit.

PRESCRIPTION

Spirit-Quieting Mind-Stabilizing Pill *ān shén dìng zhì wán*

fú líng	poria	Poria	9 g.
fú shén	root poria	Poria cum Pini Radice	9 g.
yuǎn zhì	polygala [root]	Polygalae Radix	6 g.
rén shēn	ginseng	Ginseng Radix	9 g.
shí chāng pú	acorus [root]	Acori Rhizoma	6 g.
lóng chǐ	dragon bone (extended decoction)	Mastodi Dentis Fossilia	30 g.

MODIFICATIONS

To suppress fright and quiet the spirit, the prescription is reinforced. Add:

hǔ pò	amber (powdered and stirred in)	Succinum	3 g.
zhū shā	cinnabar* (powdered and stirred in)	Cinnabaris	0.5 g.
cí shí	loadstone (extended decoction)	Magnetitum	30 g.
zhì gān cǎo	licorice [root] (honey-fried)	Glycyrrhizae Radix	9 g.

*Overuse of cinnabar *(zhū shā)* should be avoided. It should be given with caution to those with abnormal liver or kidney function.

In cases of heart yin vacuity, the prescription is modified to nourish the heart and quiet the spirit. Add:

bǎi zǐ rén	biota [seed]	Biotae Semen	12 g.
wǔ wèi zǐ	schisandra [berry]	Schisandrae Fructus	6 g.
suān zǎo rén	spiny jujube [kernel]	Ziziphi Spinosi Semen	15 g.

In cases of palpitations with irritability, susceptibility to fright, copious phlegm, poor appetite, nausea, yellow slimy tongue coating and rapid slippery pulse, the prescription is changed to clear phlegm-heat and calm the heart.
Use:

Coptis Gallbladder-Warming Decoction *huáng lián wēn dǎn tāng*

huáng lián	coptis [root]	Coptidis Rhizoma	6 g.
fǎ bàn xià	pinellia [tuber] (processed)	Pinelliae Tuber Praeparatum	6 g.
chén pí	tangerine peel	Citri Exocarpium	9 g.
fú líng	poria	Poria	9 g.
zhǐ shí	unripe bitter orange	Aurantii Fructus Immaturus	9 g.
zhú rú	bamboo shavings	Bambusae Caulis in Taeniam	6 g.
zhì gān cǎo	licorice [root] (honey-fried)	Glycyrrhizae Radix	3 g.
dà zǎo	jujube	Ziziphi Fructus	2 pc.

plus:

suān zǎo rén	spiny jujube [kernel]	Ziziphi Spinosi Semen	12 g.
yuǎn zhì	polygala [root]	Polygalae Radix	9 g.

ACUPUNCTURE AND MOXIBUSTION

Main Points: Needle with supplementation.

BL-15	*xīn shū*
CV-14	*jù què*
HT-07	*shén mén*
PC-06	*nèi guān*
HT-05	*tōng lǐ*
GB-40	*qiū xū*

Auxiliary points:
For susceptibility to fright, add:
   PC-07 *dà líng*
For phlegm-heat, add:
   ST-40 *fēng lóng*
   BL-19 *dǎn shū*

2. HEART BLOOD VACUITY

Clinical Manifestations: Palpitations, dizziness, vertigo, lusterless complexion, fatigue.

Tongue: Pale.

Pulse: Weak, thready.

Treatment Method: Boost qi, supplement blood, nourish the heart, quiet the spirit.

PRESCRIPTION

Spleen-Returning Decoction *guī pí tāng*

huáng qí	astragalus [root]	Astragali (seu Hedysari) Radix	9 g.
rén shēn	ginseng	Ginseng Radix	9 g.
bái zhú	ovate atractylodes [root]	Atractylodis Ovatae Rhizoma	9 g.
fú shén	root poria	Poria cum Pini Radice	9 g.
lóng yǎn ròu	longan [flesh]	Longanae Arillus	9 g.
suān zǎo rén	spiny jujube [kernel]	Ziziphi Spinosi Semen	9 g.
mù xiāng	saussurea [root]	Saussureae Radix (seu Vladimiriae)	6 g.
dāng guī	tangkuei	Angelicae Sinensis Radix	6 g.
yuǎn zhì	polygala [root]	Polygalae Radix	3 g.
zhì gān cǎo	licorice [root] (honey-fried)	Glycyrrhizae Radix	6 g.
shēng jiāng	fresh ginger	Zingiberis Rhizoma Recens	3 g.
dà zǎo	jujube	Ziziphi Fructus	5 pc.

MODIFICATIONS

In cases of palpitations with intermittent or irregular pulse, the prescription is changed to boost qi, nourish the blood and restore the pulse. Use:

Honey-Fried Licorice Decoction *zhì gān cǎo tāng*

zhì gān cǎo	licorice [root] (honey-fried)	Glycyrrhizae Radix	12 g.
rén shēn	ginseng	Ginseng Radix	6 g.
shēng dì huáng	rehmannia [root] dried/fresh	Rehmanniae Radix Exsiccata seu Recens	30 g.
guì zhī	cinnamon [twig]	Cinnamomi Ramulus	9 g.
ē jiāo	ass hide glue (dissolved and stirred in)	Asini Corii Gelatinum	6 g.
mài mén dōng	ophiopogon [tuber]	Ophiopogonis Tuber	9 g.
huǒ má rén	hemp [seed]	Cannabis Semen	9 g.
shēng jiāng	fresh ginger	Zingiberis Rhizoma Recens	9 g.
dà zǎo	jujube	Ziziphi Fructus	10 pc.
bái jiǔ	white liquor	Granorum Spiritus Incolor	10 cc.

In cases of palpitations caused by depletion of heart yin during the latter stages of febrile disease, the prescription is changed to boost qi, nourish yin and relieve palpitations. Use:

Pulse-Engendering Beverage *shēng mài yǐn*

rén shēn	ginseng	Ginseng Radix	9 g.
mài mén dōng	ophiopogon [tuber]	Ophiopogonis Tuber	15 g.
wǔ wèi zǐ	schisandra [berry]	Schisandrae Fructus	6 g.

ACUPUNCTURE AND MOXIBUSTION

Main Points: Needle with supplementation; add moxibustion.

BL-15	*xīn shū*
CV-14	*jù què*
HT-07	*shén mén*
PC-06	*nèi guān*
BL-20	*pí shū*
ST-36	*zú sān lǐ*
BL-17	*gé shū*

Auxiliary points:
For loss of appetite, add:

| BL-21 | *wèi shū* |

3. YIN VACUITY WITH EFFULGENT FIRE

Clinical Manifestations: Palpitations, irritability, insomnia, dizziness, vertigo, vexing heat in the five hearts, lower backache, tinnitus.

Tongue: Red with little or no coating.

Pulse: Rapid, thready.

Treatment Method: Nourish yin, downbear fire, supplement the heart, quiet the spirit.

PRESCRIPTION

Celestial Emperor Heart-Supplementing Elixir *tiān wáng bǔ xīn dān*

shēng dì huáng	rehmannia [root] dried/fresh	Rehmanniae Radix Exsiccata seu Recens	30 g
tiān mén dōng	asparagus [tuber]	Asparagi Tuber	12 g.
mài mén dōng	ophiopogon [tuber]	Ophiopogonis Tuber	12 g.
suān zǎo rén	spiny jujube [kernel]	Ziziphi Spinosi Semen	12 g.
dāng guī	tangkuei	Angelicae Sinensis Radix	9 g.
dān shēn	salvia [root]	Salviae Miltiorrhizae Radix	9 g.
xuán shēn	scrophularia [root]	Scrophulariae Radix	9 g.
rén shēn	ginseng	Ginseng Radix	6 g.
fú líng	poria	Poria	6 g.
wǔ wèi zǐ	schisandra [berry]	Schisandrae Fructus	6 g.
yuǎn zhì	polygala [root]	Polygalae Radix	6 g.
jié gěng	platycodon [root]	Platycodonis Radix	6 g.
bǎi zǐ rén	biota [seed]	Biotae Semen	12 g.
zhū shā	cinnabar (powdered and stirred in	Cinnabaris	0.5 g.

MODIFICATIONS

In cases of dry throat and bitter taste in the mouth, the prescription is modified to clear heat. Add:

| *huáng lián* | coptis [root] | Coptidis Rhizoma | 6 g. |

In cases presenting vexing heat in the five hearts, nocturnal seminal emission and lower backache, the prescription is changed to nourish yin and downbear fire. Use:

Anemarrhena, Phellodendron and Rehmannia Decoction
zhī bǎi dì huáng tāng

shú dì huáng	cooked rehmannia [root]	Rehmanniae Radix Conquita	24 g.
shān zhū yú	cornus [fruit]	Corni Fructus	12 g.
shān yào	dioscorea [root]	Dioscoreae Rhizoma	12 g.
zé xiè	alisma [tuber]	Alismatis Rhizoma	9 g.
fú líng	poria	Poria	9 g.
mǔ dān pí	moutan [root bark]	Moutan Radicis Cortex	9 g.
zhī mǔ	anemarrhena [root]	Anemarrhenae Rhizoma	9 g.
huáng bǎi	phellodendron [bark]	Phellodendri Cortex	9 g.

ACUPUNCTURE AND MOXIBUSTION

Main Points: Needle with even supplementation, even draining.

BL-15	*xīn shū*
CV-14	*jù què*
BL-14	*jué yīn shū*
BL-23	*shèn shū*
KI-03	*tài xī*
HT-07	*shén mén*
PC-06	*nèi guān*

Auxiliary points:

For tinnitus, add:

TB-03	*zhōng zhù*

For irritability, add:

PC-08	*láo gōng*

4. HEART YANG VACUITY

Clinical Manifestations: Palpitations, chest pain or oppression, shortness of breath, pale complexion, cold extremities, physical cold.

Tongue: Pale.

Pulse: Weak or deep, rapid, thready.

Treatment Method: Warm and supplement heart yang, quiet the spirit, alleviate palpitations.

PRESCRIPTION

Cinnamon Twig, Licorice, Dragon Bone and Oyster Shell Decoction
guì zhī gān cǎo lóng gǔ mǔ lì tāng

guì zhī	cinnamon [twig]	Cinnamomi Ramulus	9 g.
zhì gān cǎo	licorice [root] (honey-fried)	Glycyrrhizae Radix	9 g.
lóng gǔ	dragon bone (extended decoction)	Mastodi Ossis Fossilia	30 g.
mǔ lì	oyster shell (extended decoction)	Ostreae Concha	30 g.

MODIFICATIONS

To boost qi and warm yang, add:

rén shēn	ginseng	Ginseng Radix	9 g.
zhì fù zǐ	aconite [accessory tuber] (processed)	Aconiti Tuber Laterale Praeparatum	9 g.

ACUPUNCTURE AND MOXIBUSTION

Main Points: Needle with supplementation; add moxibustion.

BL-15	*xīn shū*
CV-14	*jù què*
HT-07	*shén mén*
PC-06	*nèi guān*
CV-06	*qì hǎi*
CV-04	*guān yuán*

Auxiliary points:

For severe physical cold and cold extremities, apply moxibustion to:

BL-23	*shèn shū*

5. OPPRESSION OF THE HEART BY WATER AND PHLEGM-FLUID

Clinical Manifestations: Palpitations, dizziness, vertigo, expectoration of phlegm and mucus, fullness and discomfort of the chest and epigastrium, cold extremities, physical cold, scanty urine, thirst without desire for drink and edema of the lower limbs (in some cases).

Tongue: White glossy coating.

Pulse: Deep wiry or wiry slippery.

Treatment Method: Warm yang, transform phlegm-rheum, quiet the spirit, alleviate palpitations.

PRESCRIPTION

Poria (Hoelen), Cinnamon Twig, Ovate Atractylodes and Licorice Decoction
líng guì zhú gān tāng

fú líng	poria	Poria	12 g.
guì zhī	cinnamon [twig]	Cinnamomi Ramulus	9 g.
bái zhú	ovate atractylodes [root]	Atractylodis Ovatae Rhizoma	6 g.
zhì gān cǎo	licorice [root] (honey-fried)	Glycyrrhizae Radix	6 g.

MODIFICATIONS

In cases of upward flow of water and phlegm-rheum causing nausea and vomiting, the prescription is modified to harmonize the stomach and downbear qi. Add:

zhì bàn xià	(processed) pinellia [root]	Pinelliae Tuber Praeparatum	9 g.
chén pí	tangerine peel	Citri Exocarpium	6 g.
shēng jiāng	fresh ginger	Zingiberis Rhizoma Recens	6 g.

In cases where kidney yang is depleted, there may be an inability to control water, causing intimidation of the heart by water qi. Symptoms include palpitations, coughing, asthma, inability to lie flat, retention of urine and severe edema. The prescription is changed to warm yang and remove water. Use:

True Warrior Decoction *zhēn wǔ tāng*

zhì fù zǐ	aconite [accessory tuber] (processed) (extended decoction)	Aconiti Tuber Laterale Praeparatum	9 g.
fú líng	poria	Poria	9 g.
bái sháo yào	white peony [root]	Paeoniae Radix Alba	9 g.
bái zhú	ovate atractylodes [root]	Atractylodis Ovatae Rhizoma	6 g.
shēng jiāng	fresh ginger	Zingiberis Rhizoma Recens	9 g.

plus:

guì zhī	cinnamon [twig]	Cinnamomi Ramulus	6 g.
huáng qí	astragalus [root]	Astragali (seu Hedysari) Radix	9 g.
fáng jǐ	fangji [root]	Fangji Radix	6 g.
tíng lì zǐ	tingli [seed]	Descurainiae seu Lepidii Semen	6 g.

ACUPUNCTURE AND MOXIBUSTION

Main Points: Needle with even supplementation, even draining.

BL-15	*xīn shū*
CV-14	*jù què*
HT-07	*shén mén*
CV-09	*shuǐ fēn*
PC-06	*nèi guān*
SP-09	*yīn líng quán*
CV-04	*guān yuán*

Auxiliary points:

For epigastric fullness and discomfort, add:

CV-12	*zhōng wǎn*

For loose stools, add:

ST-25	*tiān shū*
BL-20	*pí shū*

6. Obstruction of the Heart by Blood Stasis

Clinical Manifestations: Palpitations, oppression in the chest, periodic chest pain, purplish discoloration of the lips and nails.

Tongue: Dark purple, sometimes with stasis macules on the tongue.

Pulse: Rough, thready or intermittent.

Treatment Method: Quicken the blood, dissolve stasis, rectify qi, clear connections.

PRESCRIPTION

Peach Kernel and Carthamus Brew *táo rén hóng huā jiān*

táo rén	peach [kernel]	Persicae Semen	9 g.
hóng huā	carthamus [flower]	Carthami Flos	9 g.
dān shēn	salvia [root]	Salviae Miltiorrhizae Radix	12 g.
chì sháo yào	red peony [root]	Paeoniae Radix Rubra	9 g.
xiāng fù zǐ	cyperus [root]	Cyperi Rhizoma	6 g.
yán hú suǒ	corydalis [tuber]	Corydalis Tuber	9 g.
dāng guī	tangkuei	Angelicae Sinensis Radix	9 g.
shēng dì huáng	rehmannia [root] dried/fresh	Rehmanniae Radix Exsiccata seu Recens	9 g.
qīng pí	unripe tangerine [peel]	Citri Exocarpium Immaturum	6 g.
chuān xiōng	ligusticum [root]	Ligustici Rhizoma	6 g.

Modifications

This prescription may be reinforced to warm and invigorate heart yang, quiet the spirit and alleviate palpitations.

Add:

Cinnamon Twig, Licorice, Dragon Bone and Oyster Shell Decoction
guì zhī gān cǎo lóng gǔ mǔ lì tāng

guì zhī	cinnamon [twig]	Cinnamomi Ramulus	9 g.
zhì gān cǎo	licorice [root] (honey-fried)	Glycyrrhizae Radix	9 g.
lóng gǔ	dragon bone (extended decoction)	Mastodi Ossis Fossilia	30 g.
mǔ lì	oyster shell (extended decoction)	Ostreae Concha	30 g.

ACUPUNCTURE AND MOXIBUSTION

Main Points: Needle with even supplementation, even draining; add moxibustion.

BL-15	*xīn shū*
CV-14	*jù què*
HT-07	*shén mén*
CV-17	*tǎn zhōng*
SP-10	*xuè hǎi*
CV-06	*qì hǎi*
SP-06	*sān yīn jiāo*

Auxiliary points:

For faint pulse, add:

PC-06	*nèi guān*
LU-09	*tài yuān*

ALTERNATE THERAPEUTIC METHODS

1. Ear Acupuncture

Main points: Heart, Sympathetic, *Shén Mén*, Subcortex, Small Intestine.

Method: Needle to elicit a mild sensation, manipulating two to three times during the needle retention period. Treat once daily, ten sessions per therapeutic course.

REMARKS

During the treatment of palpitations, patients are advised to avoid emotional stress as much as possible. Relaxation in a tranquil environment, plenty of rest, a regular schedule and abstinence from hot spicy foods are recommended in all cases.

INSOMNIA

Bú Mèi

1. Liver Depression Transforming into Fire - 2. Phlegm-Fire Harassing the Interior - 3. Yin Vacuity with Effulgent Fire - 4. Heart and Spleen Vacuity - 5. Heart and Gallbladder Qi Vacuity

Insomnia refers to a class of patterns characterized by the inability to remain asleep long enough for adequate rest. The condition can vary greatly in severity. In mild cases, patients experience difficulty falling asleep, are easily awakened once asleep, find it difficult to fall back to sleep once awakened or experience fitful sleep. In severe cases, patients are unable to fall asleep throughout the entire night.

Headache, dizziness, vertigo, palpitations and forgetfulness often occur with insomnia. These symptoms are frequently observed in diseases Western medicine labels as anxiety, neurasthenia and neurosis. In cases where the insomnia is caused by fever, asthma, coughing or pain, emphasis should be placed on the root illness.

ETIOLOGY AND PATHOGENESIS

Insomnia's numerous etiological factors include emotional disruption or stress, improper diet and eating habits, excessive sexual activity and frail constitution following an extended illness. All these lead to dysfunction of the interchange of yin and yang, where yang fails to enter yin, causing insomnia. Insomnia patterns may be from repletion or vacuity but vacuity patterns are more common.

Repletion patterns may be caused by stagnation of liver qi and liver depression transforming into fire that rises to disturb the spirit, or by obstruction of the stomach by food matter giving rise to phlegm-heat and insomnia. Vacuity patterns are from yin vacuity of qi and blood, affecting the heart, spleen, liver or kidney. Prolonged repletion patterns with depletion of qi and blood may develop into vacuity patterns.

1. LIVER DEPRESSION TRANSFORMING INTO FIRE

Clinical Manifestations: Insomnia, irritability, headache, distending pain of the hypochondrium, bloodshot eyes, bitter taste in the mouth, thirst, dark urine, constipation.

Tongue: Red with yellow coating

Pulse: Rapid, wiry

Treatment Method: Soothe the liver, clear heat, quiet the spirit.

PRESCRIPTION

Gentian Liver-Draining Decoction *lóng dǎn xiè gān tāng*

lóng dǎn cǎo	gentian [root]	Gentianae Radix	6 g.
huáng qín	scutellaria [root]	Scutellariae Radix	9 g.
shān zhī zǐ	gardenia	Gardeniae Fructus	9 g.
zé xiè	alisma [tuber]	Alismatis Rhizoma	12 g.
mù tōng	mutong [stem]	Mutong Caulis	9 g.
dāng guī	tangkuei	Angelicae Sinensis Radix	3 g.
chē qián zǐ	plantago seed (wrapped)	Plantaginis Semen	9 g.
shēng dì huáng	rehmannia [root] dried/fresh	Rehmanniae Radix Exsiccata seu Recens	9 g.
chái hú	bupleurum [root]	Bupleuri Radix	6 g.
gān cǎo	licorice [root]	Glycyrrhizae Radix	6 g.

MODIFICATIONS

To settle the heart and quiet the spirit, add:

fú shén	root poria	Poria cum Pini Radice	9 g.
lóng gǔ	dragon bone (extended decoction)	Mastodi Ossis Fossilia	15 g.
mǔ lì	oyster shell (extended decoction)	Ostreae Concha	15 g.

In cases of oppression of the chest, distention of the hypochondrium and frequent heavy sighing, the prescription is modified to soothe the liver and resolve stagnation. Add:

yù jīn	curcuma [tuber]	Curcumae Tuber	9 g.
xiāng fù zǐ	cyperus [root]	Cyperi Rhizoma	9 g.

ACUPUNCTURE AND MOXIBUSTION

Main Points: Needle with draining.

HT-07	*shén mén*
SP-06	*sān yīn jiāo*
LR-03	*tài chōng*
BL-18	*gān shū*
PC-05	*jiān shǐ*
N-HN-54	*ān mián* (Quiet Sleep)

Auxiliary points:

For headache and vertigo, add:

GB-20	*fēng chí*

For bloodshot eyes, add:

M-HN-9	*tài yáng* (Greater Yang)
LI-15	*jiān yú*

For tinnitus, add:

TB-17	*yì fēng*
TB-03	*zhōng zhǔ*

2. PHLEGM-FIRE HARASSING THE INTERIOR

Clinical Manifestations: Insomnia, heaviness of the head, copious phlegm, discomfort, pain and distention of the epigastrium; aversion to eating, belching, acid regurgitation, nausea, irritability, bitter taste in the mouth.

Tongue: Yellow slimy coating.

Pulse: Rapid, slippery.

Treatment Method: Clear heat, transform phlegm, harmonize the stomach, quiet the spirit.

PRESCRIPTION

Gallbladder-Warming Decoction *wēn dǎn tāng*

fǎ bàn xià	pinellia [tuber] (processed)	Pinelliae Tuber Praeparatum	6 g.
zhú rú	bamboo shavings	Bambusae Caulis in Taeniam	6 g.
zhǐ shí	unripe bitter orange	Aurantii Fructus Immaturus	6 g.
chén pí	tangerine peel	Citri Exocarpium	6 g.
zhì gān cǎo	licorice [root] (honey-fried)	Glycyrrhizae Radix	6 g.
fú líng	poria	Poria	9 g.
shēng jiāng	fresh ginger	Zingiberis Rhizoma Recens	2 pc.
dà zǎo	jujube	Ziziphi Fructus	3 pc.

MODIFICATIONS

To reinforce the effects of clearing heat and reducing fire, add:

huáng lián	coptis [root]	Coptidis Rhizoma	6 g.
shān zhī zǐ	gardenia	Gardeniae Fructus	9 g.

In cases of palpitations and easy fright, the prescription is modified to suppress fright, quiet the spirit and stabilize the mind. Add:

zhēn zhū mǔ	mother-of-pearl (extended decoction)	Concha Margaritifera	30 g.
zhū shā	cinnabar (powdered and stirred in)	Cinnabaris	0.5 g.

In cases of obstruction by phlegm and food matter with disruption of the stomach, the prescription is modified to disperse food, disperse stagnation and harmonize the stomach. Add:

fǎ bàn xià	pinellia [tuber] (processed)	Pinelliae Tuber Praeparatum	9 g.
shén qū	medicated leaven	Massa Medicata Fermentata	12 g.
shān zhā	crataegus [fruit]	Crataegi Fructus	12 g.
lái fú zǐ	radish [seed]	Raphani Semen	9 g.

ACUPUNCTURE AND MOXIBUSTION

Main Points: Needle with draining.

CV-12	*zhōng wǎn*
ST-40	*fēng lóng*
BL-21	*wèi shū*
ST-36	*zú sān lǐ*
HT-07	*shén mén*
SP-06	*sān yīn jiāo*

Auxiliary points:

For irritability, nausea and vomiting, add:

PC-06	*nèi guān*

For dizziness and vertigo, add:

M-HN-3	*yìn táng* (Hall of Impression)
LI-04	*hé gǔ*

3. YIN VACUITY WITH EFFULGENT FIRE

Clinical Manifestations: Insomnia, irritability, dizziness and vertigo, tinnitus, aching lower back, palpitations, dry mouth, vexing heat in the five hearts, forgetfulness, nocturnal emission in some cases.

Tongue: Red with little coating.

Pulse: Rapid, thready.

Treatment Method: Nourish kidney yin, downbear heart fire and quiet the spirit.

PRESCRIPTION

Coptis and Ass Hide Glue Decoction *huáng lián ē jiāo tāng*

huáng lián	coptis [root]	Coptidis Rhizoma	4.5 g.
ē jiāo	ass hide glue (dissolved and stirred in)	Asini Corii Gelatinum	12 g.
huáng qín	scutellaria [root]	Scutellariae Radix	9 g.
bái sháo yào	white peony [root]	Paeoniae Radix Alba	9 g.
jī zǐ huáng	egg yolk (stirred in during cooling)	Galli Vitellus	2 pc.

MODIFICATIONS

To increase yin supplementation, add:

nǚ zhēn zǐ	ligustrum [fruit]	Ligustri Fructus	12 g.
hàn lián cǎo	eclipta	Ecliptae Herba	12 g.

In extreme yin vacuity with dry parched throat, the prescription is modified to nourish yin and moisten the throat. Add:

xuán shēn	scrophularia [root]	Scrophulariae Radix	9 g.
mài mén dōng	ophiopogon [tuber]	Ophiopogonis Tuber	9 g.
shí hú	dendrobium [stem] (extended decoction)	Dendrobii Caulis	12 g.

In cases of marked exuberant fire and irritability, the prescription is modified to clear fire and relieve irritability. Add:

shān zhī zǐ	gardenia	Gardeniae Fructus	9 g.
zhú yè	black bamboo [leaf]	Bambusae Folium	12 g.

In cases of dizziness, vertigo and tinnitus, the prescription is modified to nourish yin and subdue yang. Add:

guī bǎn	tortoise plastron (extended decoction)	Testudinis Plastrum	30 g.
mǔ lì	oyster shell (extended decoction)	Ostreae Concha	15 g.
cí shí	loadstone (extended decoction)	Magnetitum	15 g.

ACUPUNCTURE AND MOXIBUSTION

Main Points: Needle with even supplementation, even draining.

HT-07	*shén mén*
SP-06	*sān yīn jiāo*
BL-15	*xīn shū*
BL-23	*shèn shū*
KI-03	*tài xī*
PC-06	*nèi guān*

Auxiliary points:

For tinnitus, add:

SI-19	*tīng gōng*

For seminal emission, add:

BL-52 (47)	*zhì shì*

4. HEART AND SPLEEN VACUITY

Clinical Manifestations: Frequent dreaming, light sleep, palpitations, forgetfulness, dizzy spells, vertigo, fatigue, tiredness, listlessness, loss of appetite, lusterless complexion.

Tongue: Pale with thin coating.

Pulse: Weak, thready.

Treatment Method: Supplement the heart and spleen to promote the production of qi and blood.

PRESCRIPTION

Spleen-Returning Decoction *guī pí tāng*

huáng qí	astragalus [root]	Astragali (seu Hedysari) Radix	9 g.
rén shēn	ginseng	Ginseng Radix	9 g.
bái zhú	ovate atractylodes [root]	Atractylodis Ovatae Rhizoma	9 g.
fú shén	root poria	Poria cum Pini Radice	9 g.
lóng yǎn ròu	longan [flesh]	Longanae Arillus	9 g.
suān zǎo rén	spiny jujube [kernel]	Ziziphi Spinosi Semen	9 g.
mù xiāng	saussurea [root]	Saussureae Radix (seu Vladimiriae)	6 g.
dāng guī	tangkuei	Angelicae Sinensis Radix	6 g.
yuǎn zhì	polygala [root]	Polygalae Radix	3 g.
zhì gān cǎo	licorice [root] (honey-fried)	Glycyrrhizae Radix	6 g.
shēng jiāng	fresh ginger	Zingiberis Rhizoma Recens	3 g.
dà zǎo	jujube	Ziziphi Fructus	5 pc.

MODIFICATIONS

To enhance nourishing heart blood, add:

shú dì huáng	cooked rehmannia [root]	Rehmanniae Radix Conquita	12 g.
bái sháo yào	white peony [root]	Paeoniae Radix Alba	9 g.
ē jiāo	ass hide glue (dissolved and stirred in)	Asini Corii Gelatinum	9 g.

In cases of more severe insomnia, the prescription is modified to nourish the heart and quiet the spirit.

Add:

wǔ wèi zǐ	schisandra [berry]	Schisandrae Fructus	6 g.
yè jiāo téng	flowery knotweed [stem]	Polygoni Multiflori Caulis	15 g.
bǎi zǐ rén	biota [seed]	Biotae Semen	12 g.
lóng gǔ	dragon bone (extended decoction)	Mastodi Ossis Fossilia	15 g.
mǔ lì	oyster shell (extended decoction)	Ostreae Concha	15 g.

ACUPUNCTURE AND MOXIBUSTION

Main Points: Needle with supplementation; add moxibustion.

HT-07	*shén mén*
SP-06	*sān yīn jiāo*
BL-20	*pí shū*
BL-15	*xīn shū*
ST-36	*zú sān lǐ*

Auxiliary points:
For forgetfulness, add:

BL-52 (47)	*zhì shì*	
M-HN-1	*sì shén cōng* (Alert Spirit Quartet)	
GV-20	*bǎi huì*	

5. HEART AND GALLBLADDER QI VACUITY

Clinical Manifestations: Insomnia, frequent dreaming, tendency to wake with a start, timidity, palpitations, proneness to fright, shortness of breath, fatigue, copious clear urine.

Tongue: Pale.

Pulse: Thready, wiry.

Treatment Method: Supplement qi, suppress fright, quiet the spirit, stabilize the mind.

PRESCRIPTION

Spirit-Quieting Mind-Stabilizing Pill *ān shén dìng zhì wán*

fú líng	poria	Poria	9 g.
fú shén	root poria	Poria cum Pini Radice	9 g.
yuǎn zhì	polygala [root]	Polygalae Radix	6 g.
rén shēn	ginseng	Ginseng Radix	9 g.
shí chāng pú	acorus [root]	Acori Rhizoma	6 g.
lóng chǐ	dragon bone (extended decoction)	Mastodi Dentis Fossilia	30 g.

MODIFICATIONS

In cases accompanied by yin vacuity and blood vacuity, with agitation and insomnia, the prescription is modified to nourish yin and blood, quiet the spirit and eliminate vexation. Add:

suān zǎo rén	spiny jujube [kernel]	Ziziphi Spinosi Semen	18 g.
chuān xiōng	ligusticum [root]	Ligustici Rhizoma	3 g.
zhī mǔ	anemarrhena [root]	Anemarrhenae Rhizoma	6 g.

ACUPUNCTURE AND MOXIBUSTION

Main Points: Needle with supplementation; add moxibustion.

HT-07	*shén mén*
SP-06	*sān yīn jiāo*
BL-15	*xīn shū*
BL-19	*dǎn shū*
PC-07	*dà líng*
GB-40	*qiū xū*

ALTERNATE THERAPEUTIC METHODS

1. Ear Acupuncture

Main Points: Subcortex, Brain, Sympathetic, Heart, Spleen, Endocrine, *Shén Mén*.

Method: Select two to three points per session. Needle to elicit a mild sensation and retain needles for thirty minutes. Treat once daily, ten sessions per therapeutic course.

2. Plum Blossom Needle Therapy

Main Points:

M-HN-1	*sì shén cōng* (Alert Spirit Quartet)

with either:

Back transport points	*bèi shū xué*
M-BW-35	*huá tuó jiā jí* (Hua Tuo's Paravertebrals)

Method: Use a plum blossom needle to lightly tap over the above points. Move from the top to the bottom of the back and repeat two or three times. Treat once daily, ten sessions per therapeutic course.

REMARKS

In the treatment of insomnia, attention must be paid to the patient's psychological state. Patients should be advised to rid themselves of all worry and anxiety, avoid emotional stress and refrain from smoking or drinking alcohol, tea or coffee before retiring. Patients should also participate in appropriate forms of physical exercise. Treatment coordinated with qigong therapy exercises is also very effective.

HEADACHE

Tóu Tòng

1. Wind-Cold Headache - 2. Wind-Heat Headache - 3. Wind-Dampness Headache - 4. Liver Yang Headache - 5. Kidney Yin Vacuity Headache - 6. Kidney Yang Vacuity Headache - 7. Qi Vacuity Headache - 8. Blood Vacuity Headache - 9. Phlegm-Turbidity Headache - 10. Blood Stasis Headache

Headache, one of the most commonly encountered clinical complaints, occurs both as an isolated phenomenon and as a symptom of a wide variety of acute and chronic conditions. The present chapter centers on conditions in which headache is the major symptom. Headaches that are symptomatic to a specific disease, for example, a fever, generally disappear with effective treatment of that disease. Thus, these have not been included.

In Western medicine, headaches are part of the diseases and conditions of herbal medicine, neurology, psychology, ophthalmology and otorhinolaryngology. Refer to this chapter for the various presentations of headache, including those caused by neurosis, hypertension, migraine and traumatic injury.

ETIOLOGY AND PATHOGENESIS

Although many factors can be involved, all headaches may be classified as caused by either the invasion of external evils or to internal disruption. The head is the meeting place of the three hand yang channels, the three foot yang channels and the liver channel of foot jueyin. Also, the qi and blood of the five viscera and six bowels all ascend to the head.

Generally speaking, headaches are caused by stagnation of qi and blood. This may result from invasion by external evils or internal disruption of the viscera and bowels. Headaches from external attack are of the repletion type: they are short in duration and are caused by wind evil, cold, dampness or heat, with wind evil being the most prevalent external factor.

Headaches from internal disruption are generally persistent and involve the liver, spleen and kidney. The rise of liver yang, vacuity of qi and blood or depletion of kidney yang, yin or essence are involved. Patterns are generally vacuity types, but they can be observed as repletion in the midst of vacuity, such as with phlegm-turbidity and blood stasis headaches.

1. WIND-COLD HEADACHE

Clinical Manifestations: Headache extending through the neck and back aggravated by draughts with aversion to cold and no apparent thirst.

Tongue: Thin white coating.

Pulse: Tight, floating.

Treatment Method: Course wind, dissipate cold and relieve pain.

PRESCRIPTION
Tea-Blended Ligusticum Powder *chuān xiōng chá tiáo sǎn*

chuān xiōng	ligusticum [root]	Ligustici Rhizoma	9 g.
jīng jiè	schizonepeta	Schizonepetae Herba et Flos	9 g.
bái zhǐ	angelica [root]	Angelicae Dahuricae Radix	6 g.
qiāng huó	notopterygium [root]	Notopterygii Rhizoma	6 g.
xì xīn	asarum	Asiasari Herba cum Radice	3 g.
fáng fēng	ledebouriella [root]	Ledebouriellae Radix	6 g.
gān cǎo	licorice [root]	Glycyrrhizae Radix	6 g.
bò hé	mint (abbreviated decoction)	Menthae Herba	9 g.

Take with hot green or black tea to enhance the diaphoretic effect.

<u>MODIFICATIONS</u>

In cases where cold evil has invaded the liver channel giving rise to headaches at the apex, dry retching or vomiting of clear frothy fluid and, in severe cases, cold extremities with white tongue coating and wiry pulse, the prescription is changed to relieve jueyin headache.

Use:

Evodia Decoction *wú zhū yú tāng*

wú zhū yú	evodia [fruit]	Evodiae Fructus	6 g.
rén shēn	ginseng	Ginseng Radix	9 g.
shēng jiāng	fresh ginger	Zingiberis Rhizoma Recens	18 g.
dà zǎo	jujube	Ziziphi Fructus	4 pc.

The prescription is often modified to strengthen pain relief.

Add:

zhì bàn xià	pinellia [tuber] (processed)	Pinelliae Tuber Praeparatum	9 g.
gǎo běn	Chinese lovage [root]	Ligustici Sinensis Rhizoma et Radix	6 g.
chuān xiōng	ligusticum [root]	Ligustici Rhizoma	6 g.

ACUPUNCTURE AND MOXIBUSTION

Main Points: Needle with draining.

GB-20	*fēng chí*
BL-12	*fēng mén*
LI-04	*hé gǔ*
LU-7	*liè quē*

Auxiliary Points:

Acupuncture points may be selected according to the routes of the channels over the head:

For occipital headache, add:

BL-60	*kūn lún*
SI-03	*hòu xī*
BL-10	*tiān zhù*
GV-19	*hòu dǐng*

For frontal headache, add:

ST-08	*tóu wéi*
GV-23	*shàng xīng*
ST-44	*nèi tíng*
GB-14	*yáng bái*
M-HN-3	*yìn táng* (Hall of Impression)

For lateral headache, add:

M-HN-9	*tài yáng* (Greater Yang)
GB-08	*shuài gǔ*
TB-05	*wài guān*
GB-41	*zú lín qì*

For headache at the apex, add:

GV-20	*bǎi huì*
SI-03	*hòu xī*
BL-67	*zhì yīn*
LR-03	*tài chōng*
BL-07	*tōng tiān*

2. WIND-HEAT HEADACHE

Clinical Manifestations: Distending headache, or splitting headache in severe cases, fever, sensitivity to draughts, flushed complexion, bloodshot eyes, thirst, constipation, dark urine.

Tongue: Red with yellow coating.

Pulse: Rapid, floating.

Treatment Method: course wind, clear heat and relieve pain.

PRESCRIPTION

Ligusticum, Dahurican Angelica and Gypsum Decoction
xiōng zhǐ shí-gāo tāng

chuān xiōng	ligusticum [root]	Ligustici Rhizoma	9 g.
bái zhǐ	angelica [root]	Angelicae Dahuricae Radix	9 g.
shí gāo	gypsum (extended decoction)	Gypsum	30 g.
jú huā	chrysanthemum [flower]	Chrysanthemi Flos	9 g.
gǎo běn	Chinese lovage [root]	Ligustici Sinensis Rhizoma et Radix	6 g.
qiāng huó	notopterygium [root]	Notopterygii Rhizoma	6 g.

MODIFICATIONS

In many cases, this prescription is modified to reinforce wind-dispersing and heat-clearing. Delete:

gǎo běn	Chinese lovage [root]	Ligustici Sinensis Rhizoma et Radix
qiāng huó	notopterygium [root]	Notopterygii Rhizoma

Add:

huáng qín	scutellaria [root]	Scutellariae Radix	9 g.
bài jiàng cǎo	baijiang	Baijiang Herba cum Radice	9 g.
shān zhī zǐ	gardenia [fruit]	Gardeniae Fructus	9 g.
bò hé	mint (abbreviated decoction)	Menthae Herba	9 g.

In cases of severe heat and depletion of fluids with symptoms of red dry tongue and marked thirst, the prescription is modified to generate liquid and relieve thirst.

Add:

shí hú	dendrobium [stem] (extended decoction)	Dendrobii Caulis	12 g.
tiān huā fěn	trichosanthes [root]	Trichosanthis Radix	12 g.
lú gēn	phragmites [root]	Phragmititis Rhizoma	15 g.

In cases of constipation, sores on the mouth or nose and fever, a prepared medicine may be additionally prescribed to downbear fire and free the stool. Use the prepared medicine, COPTIS UPPER-BODY-CLEARING PILL *(huáng lián shàng qīng wán)*.

In cases accompanied by stuffy nose with turbid yellow mucus and severe frontal headache, the prescription is modified to course wind and open the orifices.

Add:

cāng ěr zǐ	xanthium [fruit]	Xanthii Fructus	9 g.
xīn yí	magnolia [flower] (wrapped)	Magnoliae Flos	9 g.
bò hé	mint (abbreviated decoction)	Menthae Herba	9 g.

ACUPUNCTURE AND MOXIBUSTION

Main points: Needle with draining.

LI-04	*hé gǔ*
GB-20	*fēng chí*
LI-11	*qū chí*
GB-14	*yáng bái*

Auxiliary points:

May be accompanied with acupuncture points selected on the basis of the routes of the channels over the head. See 1. Wind-Cold Headache.

3. WIND-DAMPNESS HEADACHE

Clinical Manifestations: Headache as if head is tightly bound, heaviness of the limbs, loss of appetite, oppression in the chest, scanty urine and, in some cases, loose stools.

Tongue: White slimy coating.

Pulse: Soft.

Treatment Method: course wind, dispel dampness and relieve pain.

PRESCRIPTION

Notopterygium Dampness-Overcoming Decoction
qiāng huó shèng shī tāng

qiāng huó	notopterygium [root]	Notopterygii Rhizoma	6 g.
dú huó	tuhuo [angelica root]	Angelicae Duhuo Radix	6 g.
gǎo běn	Chinese lovage [root]	Ligustici Sinensis Rhizoma et Radix	6 g.
fáng fēng	ledebouriella [root]	Ledebouriellae Radix	6 g.
màn jīng zǐ	vitex [fruit]	Viticis Fructus	6 g.
chuān xiōng	ligusticum [root]	Ligustici Rhizoma	6 g.
zhì gān cǎo	licorice [root] (honey-fried)	Glycyrrhizae Radix	3 g.

MODIFICATIONS

In cases of congestion of the epigastrium, loss of appetite and loose stools, the prescription is modified to dry dampness and disperse food.

Add:

cāng zhú	atractylodes [root]	Atractylodis Rhizoma	9 g.
hòu pò	magnolia [bark]	Magnoliae Cortex	9 g.
chén pí	tangerine [peel]	Citri Exocarpium	6 g.
zhǐ ké	bitter orange	Aurantii Fructus	6 g.

In cases of nausea and vomiting, the prescription is modified to redirect stomach qi downward and relieve vomiting.

Add:

jiāng bàn xià	(ginger-processed) pinellia [tuber]	Pinelliae Tuber Praeparatum	9 g.
shēng jiāng	fresh ginger	Zingiberis Rhizoma Recens	9 g.

In cases of headache occurring during the summer where summerheat and dampness have invaded the body causing symptoms of fever, difficult perspiration, oppression in the chest, thirst, nausea, vomiting and loss of appetite, the prescription is changed to clear summerheat and transform dampness.

Use:

Coptis and Elsholtzia Beverage *huáng lián xiāng rú yǐn*

huáng lián	coptis [root]	Coptidis Rhizoma	6 g.
xiāng rú	elsholtzia	Elsholtziae Herba	6 g.
biǎn dòu	lablab [bean]	Lablab Semen	9 g.
hòu pò	magnolia [bark]	Magnoliae Cortex	6 g.

plus:

huò xiāng	agastache/patchouli	Agastaches seu Pogostemi Herba	9 g.
pèi lán	eupatorium	Eupatorii Herba	9 g.
hé yè	lotus [leaf]	Nelumbinis Folium	6 g.

ACUPUNCTURE AND MOXIBUSTION

Main points: Needle with draining and moxibustion.

LU-07	*liè quē*
GB-20	*fēng chí*
TB-08	*sān yáng luò*
LI-04	*hé gǔ*

Auxiliary points:

May be accompanied with acupuncture points selected on the basis of the routes of the channels over the head. See 1. Wind-Cold Headache.

4. LIVER YANG HEADACHE

Clinical Manifestations: Headache accompanied by dizziness and vertigo, irritability, restless sleep; in some cases costal pain, flushed complexion, bitter taste in the mouth.

Tongue: Thin yellow coating.

Pulse: Wiry, forceful.

Treatment Method: Settle the liver, subdue yang and relieve pain.

PRESCRIPTION

Gastrodia and Uncaria Beverage *tiān má gōu téng yǐn*

tiān má	gastrodia [root]	Gastrodiae Rhizoma	9 g.
gōu téng	uncaria [stem and thorn] (abbreviated decoction)	Uncariae Ramulus cum Unco	12 g.
shí jué míng	abalone shell (extended decoction)	Haliotidis Concha	18 g.
shān zhī zǐ	gardenia [fruit]	Gardeniae Fructus	9 g.
huáng qín	scutellaria [root]	Scutellariae Radix	9 g.
chuān niú xī	cyathula [root]	Cyathulae Radix	12 g.
dù zhòng	eucommia [bark]	Eucommiae Cortex	9 g.
yì mǔ cǎo	leonurus	Leonuri Herba	9 g.
sāng jì shēng	mistletoe	Loranthi seu Visci Ramus	9 g.
yè jiāo téng	flowery knotweed [stem]	Polygoni Multiflori Caulis	9 g.
fú shén	root poria	Poria cum Pini Radice	9 g.

MODIFICATIONS

To increase the sedative and yang quelling effects, add:

mǔ lì	oyster shell (extended decoction)	Ostreae Concha	15 g.
lóng gǔ	dragon bone (extended decoction)	Mastodi Ossis Fossilia	15 g.

In cases of vacuity of liver and kidney yin with symptoms of headache that is mild in the morning, severe in the evening, sometimes aggravated by overwork, with red tongue with little coating and thready wiry pulse, the prescription is modified to nourish the liver and kidney.
Add:

shēng dì huáng	rehmannia [root] dried/fresh	Rehmanniae Radix Exsiccata seu Recens	9 g.
hé shǒu wū	flowery knotweed [root]	Polygoni Multiflori Radix	9 g.
nǚ zhēn zǐ	ligustrum [fruit]	Ligustri Fructus	9 g.
gǒu qǐ zǐ	lycium [berry]	Lycii Fructus	9 g.
hàn lián cǎo	eclipta	Ecliptae Herba	9 g.
shí hú	dendrobium [stem] (extended decoction)	Dendrobii Caulis	9 g.

In cases with severe headache, costal pain, bitter taste in the mouth, flushed complexion, constipation, dark urine, yellow tongue coating and rapid wiry pulse, the differentiation should include exuberance of liver fire. The prescription is modified to clear the liver and drain fire.
Add:

lóng dǎn cǎo	gentian [root]	Gentianae Radix	6 g.
yù jīn	curcuma [tuber]	Curcumae Tuber	9 g.
xià kū cǎo	prunella [spike]	Prunellae Spica	12 g.

ACUPUNCTURE AND MOXIBUSTION

Main points: Needle with even supplementation, even draining.

GB-05	*xuán lú*
GB-04	*hàn yàn*
LR-03	*tài chōng*
KI-03	*tài xī*
GB-20	*fēng chí*
GB-43	*xiá xī*

Auxiliary points:

For bloodshot eyes, add:

TB-01 *guān chōng* (bleed)

For sensation of scorching heat in the face, add:

ST-44 *nèi tíng*

5. KIDNEY YIN VACUITY HEADACHE

Clinical Manifestations: Headache and sensation of emptiness of the head accompanied by dizziness and vertigo, weak, aching lower back, lassitude, fatigue, seminal emission, tinnitus and insomnia.

Tongue: Red with little coating.

Pulse: Thready, forceless.

Treatment Method: Supplement kidney yin, relieve pain.

PRESCRIPTION

Major Origin-Supplementing Brew *dà bǔ yuán jiān*

shú dì huáng	cooked rehmannia [root]	Rehmanniae Radix Conquita	24 g.
shān zhū yú	cornus [fruit]	Corni Fructus	12 g.
shān yào	dioscorea [root]	Dioscoreae Rhizoma	12 g.
gǒu qǐ zǐ	lycium [berry]	Lycii Fructus	12 g.
rén shēn	ginseng	Ginseng Radix	9 g.
dāng guī	tangkuei	Angelicae Sinensis Radix	9 g.
zhì gān cǎo	licorice [root] (honey-fried)	Glycyrrhizae Radix	6 g.

ACUPUNCTURE AND MOXIBUSTION

Main points: Needle with supplementation.

GV-20 *bǎi huì*

BL-23 *shèn shū*

BL-18 *gān shū*

KI-03 *tài xī*

SP-06 *sān yīn jiāo*

GV-23 *shàng xīng*

Auxiliary points:

For insomnia, add:

HT-07 *shén mén*

For tinnitus, add:

SI-19 *tīng gōng*

6. KIDNEY YANG VACUITY HEADACHE

Clinical Manifestations: Headache, accompanied by physical cold, pale complexion, cold extremities, aching lower back, tiredness and fatigue.

Tongue: Pale.

Pulse: Deep, slow, thready.

Treatment Method: Warm and supplement kidney yang, relieve pain.

PRESCRIPTION

Right-Restoring [Kidney Yang] Pill *yòu guī wán*

shú dì huáng	cooked rehmannia [root]	Rehmanniae Radix Conquita	24 g.
shān yào	dioscorea [root]	Dioscoreae Rhizoma	12 g.
shān zhū yú	cornus [fruit]	Corni Fructus	9 g.
gǒu qǐ zǐ	lycium [berry]	Lycii Fructus	12 g.
lù jiǎo jiāo	deerhorn glue (dissolved and stirred in)	Cervi Gelatinum Cornu	12 g.
tù sī zǐ	cuscuta [seed]	Cuscutae Semen	12 g.
dù zhòng	eucommia [bark]	Eucommiae Cortex	12 g.
dāng guī	tangkuei	Angelicae Sinensis Radix	9 g.
ròu guì	cinnamon [bark] (abbreviated decoction)	Cinnamomi Cortex	6 g.
zhì fù zǐ	aconite [accessory tuber] (processed) (extended decoction)	Processed Aconiti Tuber Laterale	6 g.

MODIFICATIONS

In cases accompanied by invasion of the kidney channel of foot-shaoyin by internal cold evil, the prescription is changed to assist yang and dissipate cold. Use:

Ephedra, Aconite and Asarum Decoction *má huáng fù zǐ xì xīn tāng*

má huáng	ephedra	Ephedrae Herba	6 g.
zhì fù zǐ	aconite [accessory tuber] (processed) (extended decoction)	Aconiti Tuber Laterale Praeparatum	3 g.
xì xīn	asarum	Asiasari Herba cum Radice	3 g.

ACUPUNCTURE AND MOXIBUSTION

Main points: Needle with supplementation.

GV-20	*bǎi huì*
BL-23	*shèn shū* (add moxibustion)
CV-04	*guān yuán* (add moxibustion)
KI-03	*tài xī*
GV-04	*mìng mén* (add moxibustion)
GV-23	*shàng xīng*

7. QI VACUITY HEADACHE

Clinical Manifestations: Constant dull headache aggravated by overwork; lack of strength, fatigue, loss of appetite.

Tongue: Pale with thin white coating.

Pulse: Weak.

Treatment Method: Supplement qi and relieve pain.

PRESCRIPTION

Center-Supplementing Qi-Boosting Decoction *bǔ zhōng yì qì tāng*

huáng qí	astragalus [root]	Astragali (seu Hedysari) Radix	15 g.
rén shēn	ginseng	Ginseng Radix	9 g.
bái zhú	ovate atractylodes [root]	Atractylodis Ovatae Rhizoma	9 g.
dāng guī	tangkuei	Angelicae Sinensis Radix	9 g.
chén pí	tangerine [peel]	Citri Exocarpium	6 g.
shēng má	cimicifuga [root]	Cimicifugae Rhizoma	3 g.
chái hú	bupleurum [root]	Bupleuri Radix	3 g.
zhì gān cǎo	licorice [root] (honey-fried)	Glycyrrhizae Radix	6 g.

MODIFICATIONS

To assist in relieving headache, add:

chuān xiōng	ligusticum [root]	Ligustici Rhizoma	6 g.
xì xīn	asarum	Asiasari Herba cum Radice	3 g.
màn jīng zǐ	vitex [fruit]	Viticis Fructus	9 g.

ACUPUNCTURE AND MOXIBUSTION

Main points: Needle with supplementation.

GV-20	*bǎi huì*
CV-06	*qì hǎi* (add moxibustion)
BL-20	*pí shū* (add moxibustion)
ST-36	*zú sān lǐ* (add moxibustion)
LI-04	*hé gǔ*
GV-23	*shàng xīng*

Auxiliary points:

For frontal headache, add:

M-HN-3	*yìn táng* (Hall of Impression)

8. BLOOD VACUITY HEADACHE

Clinical Manifestations: Headache accompanied by dizziness, vertigo, luster-less complexion, blurred vision, palpitations, difficulty falling asleep, tiredness, fatigue, aggravation of symptoms with overwork and in some cases, a history of bleeding.

Tongue: Pale.

Pulse: Weak, thready.

Treatment Method: Nourish the blood and relieve pain.

PRESCRIPTION

Supplemented Four Agents Decoction *jiā wèi sì wù tāng*

dāng guī	tangkuei	Angelicae Sinensis Radix	12 g.
bái sháo yào	white peony [root]	Paeoniae Radix Alba	12 g.
shú dì huáng	cooked rehmannia [root]	Rehmanniae Radix Conquita	12 g.
chuān xiōng	ligusticum [root]	Ligustici Rhizoma	9 g.
jú huā	chrysanthemum [flower]	Chrysanthemi Flos	9 g.
màn jīng zǐ	vitex [fruit]	Viticis Fructus	9 g.
huáng qín	scutellaria [root]	Scutellariae Radix	3 g.
gān cǎo	licorice [root]	Glycyrrhizae Radix	6 g.

MODIFICATIONS

In cases with marked tinnitus, insomnia, dizziness and vertigo, the prescription is modified to nourish liver yin and blood. Add:

hé shǒu wū	flowery knotweed [root]	Polygoni Multiflori Radix	12 g.
gǒu qǐ zǐ	lycium [berry]	Lycii Fructus	9 g.
huáng jīng	polygonatum [root]	Polygonati Huangjing Rhizoma	12 g.
suān zǎo rén	spiny jujube [kernel]	Ziziphi Spinosi Semen	15 g.

ACUPUNCTURE AND MOXIBUSTION

Main points: Needle with supplementation; add moxibustion.

BL-18	*gān shū*
BL-17	*gé shū*
BL-20	*pí shū* (add moxibustion)
SP-06	*sān yīn jiāo*
GV-23	*shàng xīng*
ST-36	*zú sān lǐ* (add moxibustion)

Auxiliary points:

For insomnia and palpitations, add:

HT-07	*shén mén*
PC-06	*nèi guān*

9. PHLEGM-TURBIDITY HEADACHE

Clinical Manifestations: Headache and dizziness as if under the crushing weight of a heavy object, congestion and fullness of the chest and epigastrium, nausea, vomiting of phlegm and mucus.

Tongue: White slimy coating.

Pulse: Slippery.

Treatment Method: Transform phlegm-turbidity and relieve pain.

PRESCRIPTION

Pinellia, Ovate Atractylodes and Gastrodia Decoction
bàn xià bái zhú tiān má tāng

fǎ bàn xià	pinellia [tuber] (processed)	Pinelliae Tuber Praeparatum	9 g.
tiān má	gastrodia [root]	Gastrodiae Rhizoma	6 g.
fú líng	poria	Poria	6 g.
jú hóng	red tangerine [peel]	Citri Exocarpium Rubrum	6 g.
bái zhú	ovate atractylodes [root]	Atractylodis Ovatae Rhizoma	15 g.
gān cǎo	licorice [root]	Glycyrrhizae Radix	3 g.
shēng jiāng	fresh ginger	Zingiberis Rhizoma Recens	3 g.
dà zǎo	jujube	Ziziphi Fructus	2 pc.

MODIFICATIONS

To reinforce the effects of dissolving phlegm-turbidity and relieving pain, add:

hòu pò	magnolia [bark]	Magnoliae Cortex	6 g.
bái jí lí	tribulus [fruit]	Tribuli Fructus	6 g.
màn jīng zǐ	vitex [fruit]	Viticis Fructus	9 g.

In cases of accumulated phlegm-turbidity giving rise to heat, with symptoms of bitter taste in the mouth, difficult bowel movements, slimy yellow tongue coating and rapid slippery pulse, the prescription is modified to move qi, clear heat and transform phlegm-turbidity.

Delete:

bái zhú	ovate atractylodes [root]	Atractylodis Ovatae Rhizoma

Add:

huáng qín	scutellaria [root]	Scutellariae Radix	9 g.
zhú rú	bamboo shavings	Bambusae Caulis in Taeniam	9 g.
zhǐ shí	unripe bitter orange	Aurantii Fructus Immaturus	9 g.

ACUPUNCTURE AND MOXIBUSTION

Main points: Needle with draining.

GV-20	*bǎi huì*
LI-04	*hé gǔ*
ST-36	*zú sān lǐ*
M-HN-3	*yìn táng* (Hall of Impression)
CV-12	*zhōng wǎn*
ST-40	*fēng lóng*

Auxiliary points:
For vomiting, add:

PC-06	*nèi guān*

For loose stools, add:

ST-25	*tiān shū*

10. BLOOD STASIS HEADACHE

Clinical Manifestations: Persistent stabbing headache with fixed location of pain, with a possible history of traumatic injury to the head.

Tongue: Dark, purplish.

Pulse: Rough, thready.

Treatment Method: quicken the blood, dissolve stasis, relieve pain.

PRESCRIPTION

Orifice-Freeing Blood-Quickening Decoction *tōng qiào huó xuè tāng*

chì sháo yào	red peony [root]	Paeoniae Radix Rubra	3 g.
chuān xiōng	ligusticum [root]	Ligustici Rhizoma	3 g.
táo rén	peach [kernel]	Persicae Semen	9 g.
hóng huā	carthamus [flower]	Carthami Flosa	9 g.
cōng bái	scallion white	Allii Fistulosi Bulbus Recens	3 g.
dà zǎo	jujube	Ziziphi Fructus	5 pc.
shè xiāng	musk (stirred in)	Moschus	0.1 g.
huáng jiǔ	yellow wine	Vinum Aureum	50 cc.

MODIFICATIONS

The prescription may be modified to rectify qi, open the orifices and relieve pain. Add:

yù jīn	curcuma [tuber]	Curcumae Tuber	9 g.
shí chāng pú	acorus [root]	Acori Rhizoma	6 g.
xì xīn	asarum	Asiasari Herba cum Radice	3 g.
bái zhǐ	angelica [root]	Angelicae Dahuricae Radix	9 g.

In cases of severe headache, entymological medicines may be used to quicken the blood, free the connections and relieve pain. Use:

quán xiē	scorpion	Buthus	3 g.
wú gōng	centipede	Scolopendra	3 g.
zhè chóng	wingless cockroach	Eupolyphaga seu Opisthoplatia	6 g.

In cases of extended illness with vacuity of both qi and blood, the prescription is modified to supplement qi and blood.

Add:

huáng qí	astragalus [root]	Astragali (seu Hedysari) Radix	12 g.
dāng guī	tangkuei	Angelicae Sinensis Radix	9 g.

In cases where headache has been relieved but dizziness, vertigo, forgetfulness, insomnia and dream-troubled sleep persist, the prescription is modified to nourish the heart, supplement the kidney and quiet the spirit.

Delete:

shè xiāng	musk	Moschus

Add:

hé shǒu wū	flowery knotweed [root]	Polygoni Multiflori Radix	12 g.
gǒu qí zhǐ	lycium [berry	Lycii Fructus	9 g.
shí chāng pú	acorus [root]	Acori Rhizoma	6 g.
suān zǎo rén	spiny jujube [kernel]	Ziziphi Spinosi Semen	12 g.
tiān má	gastrodia [root]	Gastrodiae Rhizoma	9 g.

ACUPUNCTURE AND MOXIBUSTION

Main points: Needle with draining.

LI-04	*hé gǔ*
LR-03	*tài chōng*
ST-36	*zú sān lǐ*
SP-10	*xuè hǎi*
SP-06	*sān yīn jiāo*
A-Shi Points	*ā shì xué* (Ouch Points)

Auxiliary points:

For pain of the supraorbital ridge, add:

      BL-02   *zǎn zhú*

For lateral headache, add:

      M-HN-9   *tài yáng* (Greater Yang)

For occipital headache, add:

      TB-18   *zī mài*

For headache at the apex, add:

      M-HN-1   *sì shén cōng* (Alert Spirit Quartet)

ALTERNATE THERAPEUTIC METHODS

1. Ear Acupuncture

Main Points: Occipital, Frontal, Subcortex, *Shén Mén*.

Method: Needle unilaterally or bilaterally to elicit a strong sensation. Retain needles for twenty to thirty minutes, applying manipulation at five minute intervals. Alternately, needles may be implanted at the above points for three to seven days. In cases of persistent headache, let blood from the veins on the posterior surface of the ear.

2. Plum-Blossom Needle Therapy

Method: Use a plum-blossom needle to tap over the head, temples, back of the neck and the *huá tuó jiā jí* points. In cases of repletion patterns with extreme pain, tap more forcefully. Treat once daily, ten sessions per therapeutic course.

REMARKS

During the differential diagnosis and treatment of headache, attention must be paid to the duration of illness, as well as to the characteristics and specific location of pain. In cases of headaches because of the invasion of external evils, for example, onset is generally abrupt; pain is continuous and relatively severe, with characteristics of twitching, burning, distending or heaviness. Patterns are mainly replete and dominated by the presence of external wind. Treatment, however, must also take into account evils such as cold, heat and dampness, all of which may coexist with wind in headache.

The onset of headaches from internal disruption is generally slower, with intermittent mild pain aggravated by work. They may be qualified as dull, empty or dizzying. These patterns are mainly vacuous and treatment should emphasize supplementation. Repletion patterns or patterns of repletion in the midst of vacuity, such as headache caused by phlegm-turbidity or blood stasis, are also possible. Blood stasis headaches are characterized by stabbing pain at a distinct, fixed location. Patients often have histories of traumatic injury to the head or persistent headaches over an extended period. Phlegm-turbidity headaches are usually accompanied by nausea and vomiting of phlegm and mucus.

The specific location of pain is very significant in the differential diagnosis of headaches. Generally speaking, taiyang channel headache occurs in the occipital region of the head and extends down the back of the neck. Yangming channel headache occurs in the forehead and along the supraorbital ridge. Shaoyang channel headache occurs over the lateral regions of the head and often involves the ears. Jueyin channel headache occurs at the crown of the skull and sometimes involves the eyes.

On the basis of the location of pain in relation to the paths of the channels over the head, prescriptions for headaches may include "homing medicines" which direct treatment into their specific channels and ultimately to the site of pathological change.

For taiyang channel headache along the occiput or neck, use:

qiāng huó	notopterygium [root]	Notopterygii Rhizoma	9 g.
màn jīng zǐ	vitex [fruit]	Viticis Fructus	9 g.
gǎo běn	Chinese lovage [root]	Ligustici Sinensis Rhizoma et Radix	9 g.

For yangming channel headache along the forehead, use:

gé gēn	pueraria [root]	Puerariae Radix	9 g.
bái zhǐ	angelica [root]	Angelicae Dahuricae Radix	9 g.

For shaoyang channel headache along the lateral side of the head above the ears, use:

chái hú	bupleurum [root]	Bupleuri Radix	6 g.
chuān xiōng	ligusticum [root]	Ligustici Rhizoma	6 g.

For jueyin channel headache along the apex, use:

wú zhū yú	evodia [fruit]	Evodiae Fructus	6 g.

Effective results may be achieved by combining acupuncture and moxibustion with herbal treatment. Tuina massage is also useful. In the differential diagnosis of headache, care must be taken to rule out headache from pathological or carcinogenic changes in the cranium and brain, requiring treatment of the original disease.

DIZZINESS AND VERTIGO

Xuàn Yūn

1. Ascendant Hyperactivity of Liver Yang - 2. Vacuity of Qi and Blood - 3. Vacuity of Kidney Essence and Yin - 4. Vacuity of Kidney Essence and Yang - 5. Obstruction of the Middle Burner by Phlegm-Dampness - 6. Obstruction of the Middle Burner by Phlegm-Fire

SUPPLEMENT: HYPERTENSION

Gāo Xuè Yā

1. Vacuity of Yin and Exuberance of Yang - 2. Exuberant Liver Fire - 3. Obstruction by Phlegm-Dampness - 4. Yin and Yang Vacuity

In Chinese, dizziness and vertigo is known as *xuàn yūn*. *Xuàn* means blurred vision or blackouts and *yūn* means dizziness or vertigo, the subjective sensation that the body or the environment is spinning. Since these two phenomena are often seen together, *xuàn* and *yūn* have been compounded as *xuàn yūn*.

Mild cases of dizziness and vertigo may be relieved simply by closing the eyes. More severe cases are characterized by sensations of rocking and spinning without relief to the point that standing upright is difficult. Symptoms of nausea, vomiting, perspiration and even fainting often accompany dizziness and vertigo in these severe cases.

Dizziness and vertigo may be present in a variety of biomedical conditions such as hypertension, arteriosclerosis, anemia, labyrinthitis and Menière's disease.

ETIOLOGY AND PATHOGENESIS

Dizziness and vertigo are usually due either to vacuity topatterns, or to patterns of root vacuity and branch repletion. There are a variety of etiological factors leading to dizziness and vertigo. Emotional depression or anger can damage liver yin and result in the ascendancy of liver yang. Extended illness, stress, anxiety, pensiveness or a weak heart and spleen can cause vacuity of qi and blood. Overindulgent sexual activity, extended illness or advancing years can lead to vacuity of kidney essence. Improper diet and eating habits, stress and taxation can damage the spleen and stomach, allowing obstruction of the middle burner by phlegm-dampness or phlegm-fire.

Although the pathogenesis of dizziness and vertigo is complex, all cases may be categorized either as wind, fire, phlegm or as vacuity. Each type of dizziness and vertigo may occur alone, or or may be combined with the other types.

1. ASCENDANT HYPERACTIVITY OF LIVER YANG

Clinical Manifestations: Dizziness and vertigo, tinnitus, distending headache, sore weak lower back and knees, aggravation of symptoms with anger, irritability, bitter taste in the mouth, insomnia, dream-troubled sleep.

Tongue: Red.

Pulse: Wiry.

Treatment Method: Settle the liver, subdue yang, nourish and supplement the liver and kidney.

PRESCRIPTION

Gastrodia and Uncaria Beverage *tiān-má gōu-téng yǐn*

tiān má	gastrodia [root]	Gastrodiae Rhizoma	9 g.
gōu téng	uncaria [stem and thorn] (abbreviated decoction)	Uncariae Ramulus cum Unco	12 g.
shí jué míng	abalone [shell] (extended decoction)	Haliotidis Concha	12 g.
shān zhī zǐ	gardenia [fruit]	Gardeniae Fructus	9 g.
huáng qín	scutellaria [root]	Scutellariae Radix	9 g.
chuān niú xī	cyathula [root]	Cyathulae Radix	12 g.
dù zhòng	eucommia [bark]	Eucommiae Cortex	9 g.
yì mǔ cǎo	leonurus	Leonuri Herba	9 g.
sāng jì shēng	mistletoe	Loranthi seu Visci Ramus	9 g.
yè jiāo téng	flowery knotweed [stem]	Polygoni Multiflori Caulis	9 g.
fú shén	root poria	Poria cum Pini Radice	9 g.

MODIFICATIONS

To enhance subduing the liver, add:

jú huā	chrysanthemum [flower]	Chrysanthemi Flos	9 g.
bái jí	tribulus [fruit]	Tribuli Fructus	9 g.
xià kū cǎo	prunella [spike]	Prunellae Spica	9 g.

In cases tending toward exuberance of liver fire, with symptoms including flushed complexion, bloodshot eyes, red tongue with dry yellow coating and wiry rapid pulse, the prescription is modified to clear the liver and drain heat. Add:

lóng dǎn cǎo	gentian [root]	Gentianae Radix	6 g.
mǔ dān pí	moutan [root bark]	Moutan Radicis Cortex	9 g.

In cases accompanied by constipation, the given prescription is reinforced to drain the liver and free the stool. Use in conjunction with the prepared medicine TANGKUEI, GENTIAN AND ALOE PILL *(dāng-guī lóng huì wán)*.

In cases of liver yang transforming into internal wind, with symptoms of severe dizziness and vertigo accompanied by nausea, vomiting, numbness, trembling of the hands and feet or muscle twitching, the prescription is modified to suppress the liver and extinguish wind.

Add:

lóng gǔ	dragon bone (extended decoction)	Mastodi Ossis Fossilia	30 g.
mǔ lì	oyster shell (extended decoction)	Ostreae Concha	30 g.
líng yáng jiǎo	antelope horn (filed to a powder and stirred in)	Antelopis Cornu	0.5 g.

In cases of vacuity of liver and kidney yin with ascendancy of liver yang, with symptoms of weak aching lower back and legs, seminal emission, tiredness, red tongue with little coating and thready rapid wiry pulse, the prescription is changed to foster yin and subdue yang.

Use:

Major Wind-Stabilizing Pill *dà dìng fēng zhū*

bái sháo yào	white peony [root]	Paeoniae Radix Alba	18 g.
ē jiāo	ass hide glue (dissolved and stirred in)	Asini Corii Gelatinum	9 g.
guī bǎn	tortoise plastron (extended decoction)	Testudinis Plastrum	12 g.
shēng dì huáng	rehmannia [root] dried/fresh	Rehmanniae Radix Exsiccata seu Recens	18 g.
huǒ má rén	hemp seed	Cannabis Semen	6 g.
wǔ wèi zǐ	schisandra [berry]	Schisandrae Fructus	6 g.
mǔ lì	oyster shell (extended decoction)	Ostreae Concha	12 g.
mài mén dōng	ophiopogon [tuber]	Ophiopogonis Tuber	18 g.
biē jiǎ	turtle shell (extended decoction)	Amydae Carapax	12 g.
zhì gān cǎo	licorice [root] (honey-fried)	Glycyrrhizae Radix	12 g.
jī zǐ huáng	egg yolk	Galli Vitelus	2 pc.

If symptoms are alleviated after administration of this medication, the prescription is changed to consolidate the therapeutic results.

Use:

Lycium Berry, Chrysanthemum and Rehmannia Decoction *qǐ jú dì huáng tāng*

shú dì huáng	cooked rehmannia [root]	Rehmanniae Radix Conquita	24 g.
shān zhū yú	cornus [fruit]	Corni Fructus	12 g.
shān yào	dioscorea [root]	Dioscoreae Rhizoma	12 g.
zé xiè	alisma [tuber]	Alismatis Rhizoma	9 g.
mǔ dān pí	moutan [root bark]	Moutan Radicis Cortex	9 g.
fú líng	poria	Poria	9 g.
gǒu qǐ zǐ	lycium [berry]	Lycii Fructus	9 g.
jú huā	chrysanthemum [flower]	Chrysanthemi Flos	9 g.

ACUPUNCTURE AND MOXIBUSTION

Main Points:

BL-23	*shèn shū*
KI-03	*tài xī*
BL-18	*gān shū*
GB-20	*fēng chí*
LR-02	*xíng jiān*

Auxiliary points:

For distention of the costal regions, add:

GB-34	*yáng líng quán*

For tinnitus, add:

SI-19	*tīng gōng*

2. VACUITY OF QI AND BLOOD

Clinical Manifestations: Dizziness and vertigo, pale complexion, lusterless nails and lips, tiredness, disinclination to speak, palpitations, insomnia, loss of appetite. These symptoms are often manifest during recovery from severe illness or after a large loss of blood. In severe cases, there is a possibility of fainting.

Tongue: Pale.

Pulse: Weak, thready.

Treatment Method: Fortify the spleen and stomach, supplement qi and blood.

PRESCRIPTION

Spleen-Returning Decoction *guī pí tāng*

huáng qí	astragalus [root]	Astragali (seu Hedysari) Radix	9 g.
rén shēn	ginseng	Ginseng Radix	9 g.
bái zhú	ovate atractylodes [root]	Atractylodis Ovatae Rhizoma	9 g.
fú shén	root poria	Poria cum Pini Radice	9 g.
lóng yǎn ròu	longan [flesh]	Longanae Arillus	9 g.
suān zǎo rén	spiny jujube [kernel]	Ziziphi Spinosi Semen	9 g.
mù xiāng	saussurea [root]	Saussureae Radix (seu Vladimiriae)	6 g.
dāng guī	tangkuei	Angelicae Sinensis Radix	6 g.
yuǎn zhì	polygala [root]	Polygalae Radix	3 g.
zhì gān cǎo	licorice [root] (honey-fried)	Glycyrrhizae Radix	6 g.
shēng jiāng	fresh ginger	Zingiberis Rhizoma Recens	3 g.
dà zǎo	jujube	Ziziphi Fructus	5 pc.

MODIFICATIONS

In cases of vacuity of the spleen and stomach with loss of appetite and loose stools, the prescription is modified to reinforce strengthening of the spleen and stomach.

Adjust ingredients as follows:

dāng guī	tangkuei (stir-baked)	Angelicae Sinensis Radix
mù xiāng	saussurea [root] (roasted in hot ashes)	Saussureae (seu Vladimiriae) Radix

Add:

yì yǐ rén	coix [seed] (stir-baked)	Coicis Semen	30 g.
zé xiè	alisma [tuber]	Alismatis Rhizoma	9 g.
shā rén	amomum [fruit] (abbreviated decoction)	Amomi Semen seu Fructus	6 g.
shén qū	medicated leaven	Massa Medicata Fermentata	12 g.

In cases with chills, cold extremities and dull abdominal pain, the prescription is modified to warm the middle burner and assist yang.

Add:

guì zhī	cinnamon [twig]	Cinnamomi Ramulus	9 g.
gān jiāng	dried ginger [root]	Zingiberis Rhizoma Exsiccatum	6 g.

In cases of severe vacuity of blood, the prescription is modified to reinforce qi and promote blood production.

Add:

shú dì huáng	cooked rehmannia [root]	Rehmanniae Radix Conquita	15 g.
ē jiāo	ass hide glue (dissolved and stirred in)	Asini Corii Gelatinum	9 g.
zǐ hé chē	placenta (powdered and capsulized)	Hominis Placenta	3 g.

Increase the dosage of:

rén shen	ginseng	Ginseng Radix	to 15 g.
huáng qí	astragalus [root]	Astragali (seu Hedysari) Radix	to 15 g.

ACUPUNCTURE AND MOXIBUSTION

Main Points: Needle with supplementation; add moxibustion.

BL-18	*gān shū*
ST-36	*zú sān lǐ*
CV-06	*qì hǎi*
GV-20	*bǎi huì*
BL-17	*gé shū*
SP-06	*sān yīn jiāo*

Auxiliary Points:

For palpitations, add:

PC-06	*nèi guān*

For insomnia, add:

HT-07	*shén mén*

3. VACUITY OF KIDNEY ESSENCE AND YIN

Clinical Manifestations: Dizziness and vertigo, listlessness, insomnia, dream-troubled sleep, forgetfulness, weak aching lower back and knees, seminal emissions and tinnitus, vexing heat in the five hearts.

Tongue: Red with little coating.

Pulse: Thready, rapid, wiry.

Treatment Method: Supplement the kidney and nourish yin.

PRESCRIPTION

Left-Restoring [Kidney Yin] Pill *zuǒ guī wán*

shú dì huáng	cooked rehmannia [root]	Rehmanniae Radix Conquita	24 g.
shān yào	dioscorea [root]	Dioscoreae Rhizoma	12 g.
shān zhū yú	cornus [fruit]	Corni Fructus	12 g.
gǒu qǐ zǐ	lycium [berry]	Lycii Fructus	12 g.
chuān niú xī	cyathula [root]	Cyathulae Radix	9 g.
tù sī zǐ	cuscuta [seed]	Cuscutae Semen	12 g.
lù jiǎo jiāo	deerhorn glue (dissolved and stirred in)	Cervi Gelatinum Cornu	12 g.
guī ban jiǎo	tortoise plastron (dissolved and stirred in)	Testudinis Plastrum	12 g.

MODIFICATIONS

In cases of marked yin vacuity with internal heat, the prescription is modified to nourish kidney yin and clear internal heat. Add:

biē jiǎ	turtle shell (extended decoction)	Amydae Carapax	30 g.
zhī mǔ	anemarrhena [root]	Anemarrhenae Rhizoma	9 g.
huáng bǎi	phellodendron [bark]	Phellodendri Cortex	9 g.
dì gǔ pí	lycium [root bark]	Lycii Radicis Cortex	12 g.

In cases of severe dizziness and vertigo, the prescription is modified to suppress the liver and subdue yang.

Add:

lóng gǔ	dragon bone (extended decoction)	Mastodi Ossis Fossilia	15 g.
mǔ lì	oyster shell (extended decoction)	Ostreae Concha	15 g.
zhēn zhū mǔ	mother-of-pearl (extended decoction)	Concha Margaritifera	15 g.

ACUPUNCTURE AND MOXIBUSTION

Main Points: Needle with supplementation.

GV-20	*bǎi huì*
KI-03	*tài xī*
ST-36	*zú sān lǐ*
BL-18	*gān shū*
BL-23	*shèn shū*
SP-06	*sān yīn jiāo*

4. VACUITY OF KIDNEY ESSENCE AND YANG

Clinical Manifestations: Dizziness and vertigo, listlessness, insomnia, dream-troubled sleep, forgetfulness, weak aching lower back and knees, seminal emissions and tinnitus, physical cold and cold extremities.

Tongue: Pale with white coating.

Pulse: Deep, thready, forceless.

Treatment Method: Supplement the kidney and assist yang.

PRESCRIPTION

Right-Restoring [Kidney Yang] Pill *yòu guī wán*

shú dì huáng	cooked rehmannia [root]	Rehmanniae Radix Conquita	24 g.
shān yào	dioscorea [root]	Dioscoreae Rhizoma	12 g.
shān zhū yú	cornus [fruit]	Corni Fructus	9 g.
gǒu qǐ zǐ2	lycium [berry]	Lycii Fructus	12 g.
lù jiǎo jiāo	deerhorn glue (dissolved and stirred in)	Cervi Gelatinum Cornu	12 g.
tù sī zǐ	cuscuta [seed]	Cuscutae Semen	12 g.
dù zhòng	eucommia [bark]	Eucommiae Cortex	12 g.
dāng guī	tangkuei	Angelicae Sinensis Radix	9 g.
ròu guì	cinnamon [bark] (abbreviated decoction)	Cinnamomi Cortex	6 g.
zhì fù zǐ	aconite [accessory tuber] (processed) (extended decoction)	Aconiti Tuber Laterale Praeparatum	6 g.

MODIFICATIONS

The prescription of Right-Restoring [Kidney Yang] Pill *(yòu guī wán)* includes processed aconite accessory tuber *(zhì fù zǐ)* and cinnamon bark *(ròu guì),* which are warm, pungent, harsh and drying and thus unsuitable for prolonged administration. Warming and moistening medicines, which assist yang without harming yin, should be used.

Delete:

zhì fù zǐ	aconite [accessory tuber] (processed)	Aconiti Tuber Laterale Praeparatum
ròu guì	cinnamon [bark]	Cinnamomi Cortex

Add:

bā jǐ tiān	morinda [root]	Morindae Radix	12 g.
yín yáng huò	epimedium	Epimedii Herba	12 g.

ACUPUNCTURE AND MOXIBUSTION

Main Points: Needle with supplementation; add moxibustion.

GV-20	*bǎi huì*
BL-20	*pí shū*
ST-36	*zú sān lǐ*
BL-18	*gān shū*
BL-23	*shèn shū*
CV-04	*guān yuán*

5. OBSTRUCTION OF THE MIDDLE BURNER BY PHLEGM-DAMPNESS

Clinical Manifestations: Dizziness and vertigo, head heavy as if tightly bound, oppression in the chest, nausea, loss of appetite, sleepiness.

Tongue: White slimy coating.

Pulse: Soggy or slippery.

Treatment Method: Fortify the spleen, harmonize the stomach, dry dampness and dispel phlegm.

PRESCRIPTION

Pinellia, Ovate Atractylodes and Gastrodia Decoction
bàn xià bái zhú tiān má tāng

fǎ bàn xià	pinellia [tuber] (processed)	Pinelliae Tuber Praeparatum	9 g.
tiān má	gastrodia [root]	Gastrodiae Rhizoma	6 g.
fú líng	poria	Poria	6 g.
jú hóng	red tangerine [peel]	Citri Exocarpium Rubrum	6 g.
bái zhú	ovate atractylodes [root]	Atractylodis Ovatae Rhizoma	15 g.
gān cǎo	licorice [root]	Glycyrrhizae Radix	4 g.
shēng jiāng	fresh ginger	Zingiberis Rhizoma Recens	3 g.
dà zǎo	jujube	Ziziphi Fructus	2 pc.

MODIFICATIONS

In cases of relatively severe dizziness and vertigo with frequent vomiting, the prescription is modified to suppress the counterflow ascent of stomach qi and relieve vomiting. Add:

dài zhě shí	hematite (extended decoction)	Haematitum	30 g.
zhú rú	bamboo shavings	Bambusae Caulis in Taeniam	9 g.

In cases of epigastric fullness and loss of appetite, the prescription is modified to harmonize the stomach and disperse food. Add:

bái dòu kòu	cardamom (abbreviated decoction)	Amomi Cardamomi Fructus	6 g.
shā rén	amomum [fruit] (abbreviated decoction)	Amomi Semen seu Fructus	6 g.

In cases of tinnitus and hardness of hearing, the prescription is modified to free yang and open the orifices. Add:

cōng bái	scallion white	Allii Fistulosi Bulbus Recens	6 g.
yù jīn	curcuma [tuber]	Curcumae Tuber	9 g.
shí chāng pú	acorus [root]	Acori Rhizoma	9 g.

ACUPUNCTURE AND MOXIBUSTION

Main Points: Needle with even supplementation, even drainage.

ST-08	*tóu wéi*
ST-40	*fēng lóng*
CV-12	*zhōng wǎn*
PC-06	*nèi guān*
BL-20	*pí shū*
ST-36	*zú sān lǐ*

Auxiliary points:

For severe dizziness and vertigo, add:

GB-20	*fēng chí*

6. OBSTRUCTION OF THE MIDDLE BURNER BY PHLEGM-FIRE

Clinical Manifestations: Dizziness and vertigo, head heavy as if tightly bound, oppression in the chest, nausea, headache, distending sensation of the eyes, irritability, bitter taste in the mouth, thirst without desire for drink.

Tongue: Yellow slimy coating.

Pulse: Slippery, wiry.

Treatment Method: Transform phlegm, drain heat.

PRESCRIPTION

Gallbladder-Warming Decoction *wēn dǎn tāng*

fǎ bàn xià	pinellia [tuber] (processed)	Pinelliae Tuber Praeparatum	6 g.
zhú rú	bamboo shavings	Bambusae Caulis in Taeniam	6 g.
zhǐ shí	unripe bitter orange	Aurantii Fructus Immaturus	6 g.
chén pí	tangerine [peel]	Citri Exocarpium	6 g.
gān cǎo	licorice [root]	Glycyrrhizae Radix	6 g.
fú líng	poria	Poria	9 g.
shēng jiāng	fresh ginger	Zingiberis Rhizoma Recens	2 pc.
dà zǎo	jujube	Ziziphi Fructus	3 pc.

plus:

huáng lián	coptis [root]	Coptidis Rhizoma	9 g.
huáng qín	scutellaria [root]	Scutellariae Radix	9 g.

ACUPUNCTURE AND MOXIBUSTION

Main Points: Needle with draining.

ST-08	*tóu wéi*
ST-40	*fēng lóng*
CV-12	*zhōng wǎn*
PC-06	*nèi guān*
LR-02	*xíng jiān*
GB-20	*fēng chí*

Auxiliary points:

M-HN-3	*yìn táng*	(Hall of Impression)

ALTERNATE THERAPEUTIC METHODS

1. Ear Acupuncture

Main Point: Kidney, *Shén Mén,* Occipital, Inner Ear, Subcortex.

Method: Choose two to three points per session. Needle to elicit a moderate sensation and retain needles twenty to thirty minutes, manipulating at intervals. Treat once daily, five to seven sessions making one course of treatment.

2. Scalp Acupuncture

Location: Bilateral *Yún Tīng Qū* (Vertigo and Hearing Region)

Method: After routine antisepsis, use filiform needles to puncture the above regions to a depth of 2 mm. During needle retention, periodically apply two or three high-speed twirling manipulations. Treat once daily, ten sessions making one course of treatment. Upon completing one course, allow a three-day interval before beginning the following course.

3. Plum-Blossom Needle Therapy

Main Points:

GV-20	*bǎi huì*	
M-HN-3	*yìn táng*	(Hall of Impression)
M-HN-9	*tài yáng*	(Greater Yang)
M-BW-35	*huá tuó jiā jí*	(Hua Tuo's Paravertebrals)

Method: Tap the above points to elicit a moderate sensation once or twice daily; five to ten sessions constitute one therapeutic course.

REMARKS

In middle-aged and older patients there is a distinct possibility that more severe cases of dizziness and vertigo caused by ascendant hyperactivity of liver yang may result in wind stroke. Hence, prevention and prompt treatment of dizziness and vertigo in older patients is very important. Preventative measures include decreasing consumption of rich foods and alcohol, abstaining from hot spicy foods, controlling the temper, moderating sexual activity, engaging in appropriate physical exercise and taking medicine to aid recuperation after attacks of dizziness and vertigo.

SUPPLEMENT:

HYPERTENSION

Gāo Xuè Yā

1. Vacuity of Yin and Exuberance of Yang - 2. Exuberant Liver Fire - 3. Obstruction by Phlegm-Dampness - 4. Yin and Yang Vacuity

Hypertension is an illness exhibiting a sustained increase in arterial blood pressure, particularly diastolic pressure, as its major clinical manifestation. Resting systolic blood pressure of 140 mm Hg or less and diastolic blood pressure of 90 mm Hg or less are considered normal adult blood pressure. Hypertension is thus defined as resting systolic blood pressure of 160 mm Hg and over and diastolic blood pressure of 95 mm Hg and over. Blood pressures between these two ranges are considered borderline hypertension.

Hypertension is clinically divided into essential or primary hypertension and secondary hypertension. Although the causes and pathogenic mechanism of essential hypertension have not been clearly determined, its development is often related to chronic mental or emotional tension, diets with high fat and/or high salt content, obesity, tobacco smoking and heredity and age factors. Ultimately, the regulatory functions of the central nervous and endocrine systems are thrown into confusion, followed by generalized sustained spasm of arterioles resulting in hypertension. This condition is most often presented during middle age onward and involves important organs such as the heart, kidney and brain in its later stages. Hypertension can also develop secondarily to certain preexisting conditions, including urogenital, intracranial and endocrine system disorders. In these cases, attention should be given to the primary disease.

The present discussion centers on essential hypertension. Traditional Chinese medical literature does not contain a term directly equivalent to hypertension. On the basis of clinical manifestations, however, hypertension can be recognized as a pattern within such illnesses as dizziness and vertigo and headache. Cerebral vascular accident because of hypertension would be categorized as wind stroke. Further discussion is addressed in the relevant chapters.

ETIOLOGY AND PATHOGENESIS

Hypertension originates mainly from excesses of the seven affects and improper diet and eating habits. The result is a state of vacuity below and repletion above, beginning with a vacuity of kidney yin in the lower burner, then a vacuity of both liver and kidney yin and finally profusion of liver yang in the upper burner. Prolonged profusion of liver yang in the upper burner allows transformation of wind and fire. When wind and fire fan each other, fluids will begin to dry and produce phlegm. In addition, prolonged yin vacuity can damage yang qi, ultimately causing pathological changes involving vacuity of both yin and yang.

1. VACUITY OF YIN AND EXUBERANCE OF YANG

Clinical Manifestations: Dizziness and vertigo, headache, aching of the lower back and knees, tinnitus, forgetfulness, vexing heat in the five hearts, palpitations, insomnia.

Tongue: Red with little coating.

Pulse: Thready, wiry.

Treatment Method: Foster liver and kidney yin, subdue liver yang.

PRESCRIPTION

Lycium Berry, Chrysanthemum and Rehmannia Pill *qǐ jú dì huáng wán*

shú dì huáng	cooked rehmannia [root]	Rehmanniae Radix Conquita	24 g.
shān yào	dioscorea [root]	Dioscoreae Rhizoma	12 g.
shān zhū yú	cornus [fruit]	Corni Fructus	12 g.
zé xiè	alisma [tuber]	Alismatis Rhizoma	9 g.
mǔ dān pí	moutan [root bark]	Moutan Radicis Cortex	9 g.
fú líng	poria	Poria	9 g.
gǒu qǐ zǐ	lycium [berry]	Lycii Fructus	9 g.
jú huā	chrysanthemum [flower]	Chrysanthemi Flos	9 g.

MODIFICATIONS

In cases of hypertension the prescription is often modified to reinforce the effects of moistening yin, quelling yang and regulating the blood.

Add:

guī bǎn	tortoise plastron (extended decoction)	Testudinis Plastrum	30 g.
mǔ lì	oyster shell (extended decoction)	Ostreae Concha	30 g.
dān shēn	salvia [root]	Salviae Miltiorrhizae Radix	12 g.

In cases where dizziness is relatively severe, with numbness of the limbs, the prescription is modified to calm the liver and extinguish wind. Add:

tiān má	gastrodia [root]	Gastrodiae Rhizoma	9 g.
gōu téng	uncaria [stem and thorn] (abbreviated decoction).	Uncariae Ramulus cum Unco	12 g
dì lóng	earthworm	Lumbricus	12 g.

In cases of hard dry stools, the prescription is modified to lubricate and free the stool. Add:

hēi zhī má	black sesame [seed]	Sesami Semen Atrum	15 g.
bǎi zǐ rén	biota [seed]	Biotae Semen	15 g.

ACUPUNCTURE AND MOXIBUSTION

Main points: Needle with even supplementation, even draining.

BL-18	*gān shū*
SP-06	*sān yīn jiāo*
BL-23	*shèn shū*
GB-20	*fēng chí*
KI-03	*tài xī*
LR-03	*tài chōng*

Auxiliary Points:

For severe dizziness and headache, add:

GV-20	*bǎi huì*

For palpitations and insomnia, add:

HT-07	*shén mén*
PC-06	*nèi guān*

2. EXUBERANCE OF LIVER FIRE

Clinical Manifestations: Dizziness and vertigo, distending pain of the head and eyes, red complexion, bloodshot eyes, irritability, dry bitter taste in the mouth, dark urine, constipation.

Tongue: Red with yellow coating.

Pulse: Rapid, wiry.

Treatment Method: Calm the liver, drain fire.

PRESCRIPTION

Gentian Liver-Draining Decoction *lóng-dǎn xiè gān tāng*

lóng dǎn cǎo	gentian [root]	Gentianae Radix	6 g.
shān zhī zǐ	gardenia [fruit]	Gardeniae Fructus	9 g.
mù tōng	mutong [stem]	Mutong Caulis	9 g.
chē qián zǐ	plantago [seed] (wrapped)	Plantaginis Semen	9 g.

shēng dì huáng	rehmannia [root] (dried/fresh)	Rehmanniae Radix Exsiccata seu Recens	9 g.
gān cǎo	licorice [root]	Glycyrrhizae Radix	6 g.
huáng qín	scutellaria [root]	Scutellariae Radix	9 g.
zé xiè	alisma [tuber]	Alismatis Rhizoma	12 g.
dāng guī	tangkuei	Angelicae Sinensis Radix	3 g.
chái hú	bupleurum [root]	Bupleuri Radixi	6 g.

MODIFICATIONS

In clinical use the prescription is often modified to reinforce its liver-clearing and fire-purging actions.

Delete:

chái hú	bupleurum [root]	Bupleuri Radix	
dāng guī	tangkuei	Angelicae Sinensis Radix	
zé xiè	alisma [tuber]	Alismatis Rhizoma	
chē qián zǐ	plantago [seed]	Plantaginis Semen	

Add:

jú huā	chrysanthemum [flower]	Chrysanthemi Flos	9 g.
xià kū cǎo	prunella [spike]	Prunellae Spica	12 g.
gōu téng	uncaria [stem and thorn] (abbreviated decoction)	Uncariae Ramulus cum Unco	12 g.
mǔ dān pí	moutan [root bark]	Moutan Radicis Cortex	9 g.

In cases where headache and dizziness and vertigo are severe, the prescription is modified to suppress the liver and subdue yang.

Add:

| *zhēn zhū mǔ* | mother-of-pearl (extended decoction) | Concha Margaritifera | 30 g. |
| *shí jué míng* | abalone shell (extended decoction) | Haliotidis Concha | 30 g |

In cases of constipation, the prescription is modified to drain heat and free the stool.

Add:

| *dà huáng* | rhubarb (abbreviated decoction) | Rhei Rhizoma | 9 g. |

In cases of dry mouth and throat, the prescription is modified to nourish yin and drain fire. Add:

| *shí gāo* | gypsum (extended decoction) | Gypsum | 12 g. |
| *xuán shēn* | scrophularia [root] | Scrophulariae Radix | 9 g. |

ACUPUNCTURE AND MOXIBUSTION

Main points: Needle with draining.

LR-02	*xíng jiān*
GB-20	*fēng chí*
M-HN-9	*tài yáng* (Greater Yang)
GB-43	*xiá xī*
LI-11	*qū chí*
SP-06	*sān yīn jiāo*

Auxiliary points:

For constipation, add:

| TB-6 | *zhī gōu* |

3. OBSTRUCTION BY PHLEGM-DAMPNESS

Clinical Manifestations: Dizziness and vertigo, heaviness and pain of the head, irritability, nausea, oppression in the chest, low food intake, numbness and heaviness of the limbs, obesity.

Tongue: Enlarged with white slimy coating.

Pulse: Slippery, wiry.

Treatment Method: Dispel phlegm, transform dampness.

PRESCRIPTION

Pinellia, Ovate Atractylodes and Gastrodia Decoction
bàn-xià bái-zhú tiān má tāng

fǎ bàn xià	pinellia [tuber] (processed)	Pinelliae Tuber Praeparatum	9 g.
jú hóng	red tangerine peel	Citri Exocarpium Rubrum	6 g.
gān cǎo	licorice [root]	Glycyrrhizae Radix	3 g.
dà zǎo	jujube	Ziziphi Fructus	2 pc.
tiān má	gastrodia [root]	Gastrodiae Rhizoma	6 g.
bái zhú	ovate atractylodes [root]	Atractylodis Ovatae Rhizoma	15 g.
shēng jiāng	fresh ginger	Zingiberis Rhizoma Recens	3 g.
fú líng	poria	Poria	6 g.

MODIFICATIONS

In clinical use, the prescription is modified to reinforce the phlegm-dissolving and wind-eradicating effects.

Delete:

| shēng jiāng | fresh ginger | Zingiberis Rhizoma Recens |
| dà zǎo | jujube | Ziziphi Fructus |

Add:

gōu téng	uncaria [stem and thorn] (abbreviated decoction)	Uncariae Ramulus cum Unco	12 g.
shí chāng pú	acorus [root]	Acori Rhizoma	6 g.
bái jiāng cán	silkworm	Bombyx Batryticatus	9 g.

In cases where phlegm is copious, the tongue coating yellow and slimy, and the pulse wiry, slippery and rapid, the prescription is modified to clear heat and transform phlegm.

Add:

dǎn xīng	(bile-processed) arisaema [root]	Arisaematis Rhizoma cum Felle Bovis	6 g.
tiān zhú huáng	bamboo sugar	Bambusae Concretio Silicea	6 g.
xià kū cǎo	prunella [spike]	Prunellae Spica	12 g.

ACUPUNCTURE AND MOXIBUSTION

Main points: Needle with draining; moxibustion may be added.

CV-12	*zhōng wǎn*
SP-09	*yīn líng quán*
ST-40	*fēng lóng*
PC-06	*nèi guān*
ST-36	*zú sān lǐ*
GB-20	*fēng chí*

Auxiliary points:
For slimy yellow tongue coating and rapid pulse, add:
LI-11   *qū chí*

4. YIN AND YANG VACUITY

Clinical Manifestations: Dizziness and vertigo aggravated by movement, blurred vision, headache, tinnitus, palpitations, shortness of breath, weakness and aching of the lower back and legs, lack of strength, numbness of the hands.

Tongue: Light red.

Pulse: Thready, wiry.

Treatment Method: Supplement kidney yin and yang.

PRESCRIPTION
Two Immortals Powder *èr xiān tāng*

xiān máo	curculigo [root]	Curculiginis Rhizoma	12 g.
dāng guī	tangkuei	Angelicae Sinensis Radix	9 g.
huáng bǎi	phellodendron [bark]	Phellodendri Cortex	6 g.
yín yáng huò	epimedium	Epimedii Herba	12 g.
bā jǐ tiān	morinda [root]	Morindae Radix	9 g.
zhī mǔ	anemarrhena [root]	Anemarrhenae Rhizoma	6 g.

MODIFICATIONS

In cases presenting feverish palms and soles, dryness of the mouth and throat, red tongue with little coating and rapid thready pulse, the prescription is modified to foster yin and supplement essence.

Add:

shú dì huáng	cooked rehmannia [root]	Rehmanniae Radix Conquita	12 g.
shí hú	dendrobium [stem] (extended decoction).	Dendrobii Caulis	12 g
guī bǎn	tortoise plastron (extended decoction)	Testudinis Plastrum	30 g.

In cases presenting physical cold and coldness of the limbs, loose stools, frequent nocturnal urination, pale tongue and deep thready pulse, the prescription is modified to warm the kidney and supplement yang.

Delete:

huáng bǎi	phellodendron [bark]	Phellodendri Cortex
zhī mǔ	anemarrhena [root]	Anemarrhenae Rhizoma

Add:

shú dì huáng	cooked rehmannia [root]	Rehmanniae Radix Conquita	12 g.
dù zhòng	eucommia [bark]	Eucommiae Cortex	12 g.
lù jiǎo jiāo	deerhorn glue (dissolve and administer separately)	Cervi Gelatinum Cornu	9 g.

In cases of shortness of breath, add:

huáng qí	astragalus [root]	Astragali (seu Hedysari) Radix	12 g.

ACUPUNCTURE AND MOXIBUSTION

Main points: Needle with supplementation; may accompany with moxibustion.

BL-23	*shèn shū*
ST-36	*zú sān lǐ*
CV-04	*guān yuán*
GV-20	*bǎi huì*
CV-06	*qì hǎi*
BL-20	*pí shū*

Auxiliary points:

For predominance of kidney yin vacuity, add:

KI-03	*tài xī*
SP-06	*sān yīn jiāo*

For predominance of kidney yang vacuity, add

GV-04	*mìng mén*

ALTERNATE THERAPEUTIC METHODS

1. Ear Acupuncture

Main points: Subcortex, *Shén Mén,* Liver, Sympathetic, Heart, Antihypertension Groove, Endocrine, Kidney.

Method: Select three to four points for each session, every one or two days, seven sessions per therapeutic course. Needle to elicit a moderate sensation and retain needles for twenty to thirty minutes. Auricular needle embedding or auricular acupressure plasters may also be used.

2. Plum Blossom Therapy

Treatment sites: Along both sides of the spine, the lumbar and sacral spine in particular, as well as the cervical spine, the forehead, occipital eye region, palms and soles.

Method: Tap to elicit a mild sensation. Tapping generally begins with the spinal areas, moving from higher to lower, from the center to the outside. The same procedure applies to the other treatment sites.

REMARKS

Because hypertension is often accompanied by arteriosclerosis and microcirculation pathologies, the addition of herbs that invigorate the blood and dissolve stasis will increase the therapeutic effectiveness of herbal prescriptions.

Use:

dān shēn	salvia [root]	Salviae Miltiorrhizae Radix	9-15 g.
chì sháo yào	red peony [root]	Paoniae Radix Rubra	9-15 g.
niú xī	achyranthes [root]	Achyranthis Bidentatae Radix	9-15 g.

Patients suffering from hypertension should avoid mental and emotional stress, follow a low-salt, low-fat diet and abstain from alcohol and tobacco. In the event of any of the danger signs of hypertension, immediate and comprehensive medical attention should be used to prevent the occurrence of cerebral vascular accident. These include sudden severe headache, dizziness and vertigo, restlessness, nausea and vomiting, blurred vision or sudden increase in blood pressure. In cases of secondary hypertension, treatment should focus on the primary illness.

LOW BACK PAIN

Yāo Tòng

1. Cold-Dampness - 2. Damp-Heat - 3. Blood Stasis - 4. Kidney Yang Vacuity - 5. Kidney Yin Vacuity

Low back pain, with pain to one or both sides or directly on the lumbar vertebrae, is a frequently encountered clinical presentation. Low back pain may result from numerous disorders named by Western medicine, including renal diseases, rheumatism, rheumatoid conditions, injury to the lower back muscles and vertebral or spinal cord disorders. Reference may be made to this chapter for all cases manifesting marked low back pain.

ETIOLOGY AND PATHOGENESIS

Low back pain can be divided into three etiological categories: invasion of external evils, internal disruption and traumatic injury.

Low back pain from external evils often involves dampness that is characterized by heaviness and turbidity, and that collects in the lower back. This type may be further subdivided as due to cold-dampness or damp-heat. Low back pain from internal disruption usually involves kidney vacuity, as the lower back is the home of the kidney. Traumatic falls, contusions and sprains injuring the channels and connections of the lumbar region will result in stagnation of qi and stasis of blood, causing pain. All three categories of low back pain can mutually affect one another.

1. COLD-DAMPNESS

Clinical Manifestations: Cold pain and heaviness of the lower back, difficulty turning the waist, pain alleviated by applications of heat but not diminished by lying quietly and an increase in pain during cold or rainy weather.

Tongue: White slimy coating.

Pulse: Slow, deep.

Treatment Method: Dispel cold, disinhibit dampness, warm the channels and free the connections.

PRESCRIPTION

Licorice, Dried Ginger, Poria (Hoelen) and Ovate Atractylodes Decoction
gān cǎo gān jiāng líng zhú tāng

fú líng	poria	Poria	12 g.
gān jiāng	dried ginger [root]	Zingiberis Rhizoma Exsiccatum	12 g.
bái zhú	ovate atractylodes [root]	Atractylodis Ovatae Rhizoma	6 g.
gān cǎo	licorice [root]	Glycyrrhizae Radix	6 g.

MODIFICATIONS

This prescription is usually enhanced to warm the channels and free the connections, to supplement the kidney and strengthen the lower back.
Add:

guì zhī	cinnamon [twig]	Cinnamomi Ramulus	9 g.
niú xī	achyranthes [root]	Achyranthis Bidentatae Radix	9 g.
dù zhòng	eucommia [bark]	Eucommiae Cortex	12 g.
sāng jì shēng	mistletoe	Loranthi seu Visci Ramus	12 g.
xù duàn	dipsacus [root]	Dipsaci Radix	9 g.

In cases of severe cold evil with sensations of cold pain, stiffness and tension of the lumbar region, the prescription is modified to warm the kidney and dispel cold.
Add:

zhì fù zǐ	aconite [accessory tuber] (processed) (extended decoction)	Aconiti Tuber Laterale Praeparatum	9 g.

In cases of severe dampness with heaviness and pain of the lower back, accompanied by a thick slimy tongue coating, the prescription is modified to dry damp.
Add:

cāng zhú	atractylodes [root]	Atractylodis Rhizoma	9 g.

In cases accompanied by wind evil with symptoms of low back pain, alternating from side to side, extending to the feet or up the back and shoulders, or accompanied by roving aching joints, the preceding prescription is modified to dispel wind, quicken the connections and supplement the liver and kidney.
Use in conjunction with:

Tuhuo and Mistletoe Decoction *dú-huó jì shēng tāng*

dú huó	tuhuo [angelica root]	Angelicae Duhuo Radix	9 g.
sāng jì shēng	mistletoe	Loranthi seu Visci Ramus	6 g.
dù zhòng	eucommia [bark]	Eucommiae Cortex	6 g.
niú xī	achyranthes [root]	Achyranthis Bidentatae Radix	6 g.
xì xīn	asarum	Asiasari Herba cum Radice	3 g.
qín jiāo	large gentian [root]	Gentianae Macrophyllae Radix	6 g.
fú líng	poria	Poria	6 g.
fáng fēng	ledebouriella [root]	Ledebouriellae Radix	6 g.
chuān xiōng	ligusticum [root]	Ligustici Rhizoma	6 g.
rén shēn	ginseng	Ginseng Radix	6 g.
dāng guī	tangkuei	Angelicae Sinensis Radix	6 g.
bái sháo yào	white peony [root]	Paeoniae Radix Alba	6 g.
shú dì huáng	cooked rehmannia [root]	Rehmanniae Radix Conquita	6 g.
ròu guì	cinnamon [bark] (abbreviated decoction)	Cinnamomi Cortex	6 g.
gān cǎo	licorice [root]	Glycyrrhizae Radix	6 g.

Since yang qi is easily injured by cold and dampness, cases of frail constitution because of old age or extended illness often involve injury to kidney yang. Symptoms include weak aching lower back and knees and deep forceless pulse. Treatment should be directed toward dispersing cold and disinhibiting dampness, accompanied by supplementation of kidney yang.
Add:

tù sī zǐ	cuscuta [seed]	Cuscutae Semen	12 g.
bǔ gǔ zhī	psoralea [seed]	Psoraleae Semen	9 g.

ACUPUNCTURE AND MOXIBUSTION

Main Points: Needle with draining; accompany with moxibustion or cupping therapy.

BL-23	*shèn shū*
BL-40 (54)	*wěi zhōng*
GV-03	*yāo yáng guān*
BL-32	*cì liáo*
GB-34	*yáng líng quán*
BL-25	*dà cháng shū*
CV-04	*guān yuán*

2. DAMP-HEAT

Clinical Manifestations: Low back pain accompanied by a sensation of heat at the location of the pain, increase in pain during hot or rainy weather, in some cases a decrease in pain after exercise and dark scanty urine.

Tongue: Yellow slimy coating.

Pulse: Soft, rapid.

Treatment Method: Clear heat, disinhibit dampness, ease the lower back and relieve pain.

PRESCRIPTION

Mysterious Four Pill *sì miào wán*

cāng zhú	atractylodes [root]	Atractylodis Rhizoma	9 g.
huáng bǎi	phellodendron [bark]	Phellodendri Cortex	9 g.
yì yǐ rén	coix [seed]	Coicis Semen	15 g.
huái niú xī	achyranthes [root]	Achyranthis Bidentatae Radix	9 g.

MODIFICATIONS

To increase the prescription's clearing connections and relieving pain, add:

mù guā	chaenomeles [fruit]	Chaenomelis Fructus	9 g.
luò shí téng	star jasmine [stem]	Trachelospermi Caulis	12 g.

In cases of profuse heat with symptoms of thirst, red tongue and rapid wiry pulse, the prescription is modified to help clear heat and disinhibit dampness.

Add:

shān zhī zǐ	gardenia [fruit]	Gardeniae Fructus	9 g.
zé xiè	alisma [tuber]	Alismatis Rhizoma	9 g.
mù tōng	mutong [stem]	Mutong Caulis	6 g.

Over a period of time, damp-heat may injure the yin fluids, resulting in aching lower back, dry throat and vexing heat in the five hearts. Treatment should be directed toward clearing damp-heat while nourishing kidney yin. Care must be taken, however, to select herbs that nourish yin without promoting an accumulation of dampness.

Use:

nǔ zhēn zǐ	ligustrum [fruit]	Ligustri Fructus	12 g.
hàn lián cǎo	eclipta	Ecliptae Herba	12 g.

ACUPUNCTURE AND MOXIBUSTION

Main Points: Needle with draining.

BL-23	*shèn shū*
GV-03	*yāo yáng guān*
BL-40 (54)	*wěi zhōng*
GB-34	*yáng líng quán*
BL-32	*cì liáo*
SP-06	*sān yīn jiāo*

3. BLOOD STASIS

Clinical Manifestations: Stabbing low back pain of fixed location, aggravation of pain with external pressure, increase in the severity of pain at night, discomfort bending forward and straightening in mild cases and, in severe cases, an inability to twist sideways. Some cases may have histories of traumatic injury to the lumbar region.

Tongue: Dark, purplish, sometimes with stasis macules on the tongue.

Pulse: Rough.

Treatment Method: Quicken the blood, dissolve stasis, rectify qi and relieve pain.

PRESCRIPTION

Generalized Pain Stasis-Expelling Decoction *shēn tòng zhú yū tāng*

dāng guī	tangkuei	Angelicae Sinensis Radix	9 g.
táo rén	peach [kernel]	Persicae Semen	9 g.
hóng huā	carthamus [flower]	Carthami Flosa	9 g.
mò yào	myrrh	Myrrha	6 g.
wǔ líng zhī	flying squirrel droppings (wrapped)	Trogopteri seu Pteromydis Excrementum	6 g.
chuān xiōng	ligusticum [root]	Ligustici Rhizoma	6 g.
niú xī	achyranthes [root]	Achyranthis Bidentatae Radix	9 g.
dì lóng	earthworm	Lumbricus	6 g.
qiāng huó	notopterygium [root]	Notopterygii Rhizoma	3 g.
qín jiāo	large gentian [root]	Gentianae Macrophyllae Radix	3 g.
xiāng fù zǐ	cyperus [root]	Cyperi Rhizoma	3 g.
gān cǎo	licorice [root]	Glycyrrhizae Radix	6 g.

MODIFICATIONS

The prescription is usually modified to reinforce its collateral clearing and stasis dissolving effects.

Add:

zhè chóng	wingless cockroach	Eupolyphaga seu Opisthoplatia	9 g.
wū shāo shé ròu	black-striped snake flesh	Zaocydis Caro	9 g.
chuān shān jiǎ	pangolin scales	Manitis Squama	9 g.

(or, powdered and administered separately, 1.5 g, each time)

In cases accompanied by kidney vacuity, the prescription is modified to supplement the kidney and strengthen the lower back.

Add:

xù duàn	dipsacus [root]	Dipsaci Radix	12 g.
dù zhòng	eucommia [bark]	Eucommiae Cortex	12 g.
sāng jì shēng	mistletoe	Loranthi seu Visci Ramus	12 g.

ACUPUNCTURE AND MOXIBUSTION

Main Points: Needle with draining.

BL-23	*shèn shū*
GV-03	*yāo yáng guān*
BL-40 (54)	*wěi zhōng* (bleed with a three-edged needle)
GV-26	*shuǐ gōu*
N-UE-19a,b,c	*yāo tòng* (Lumbar Pain a,b,c)
A-Shi Points	*ā shì xué* (Ouch Points)

Auxiliary points:

For low back pain extending down the legs, add to the affected side:

GB-30	*huán tiào*
GB-34	*yáng líng quán*
BL-60	*kūn lún*

4. KIDNEY YANG VACUITY

Clinical Manifestations: Slow onset with extended duration, aching of lower back diminished by pressing and rubbing, fatigue, weakness of knees, increase in pain after exertion, decrease in pain while lying quietly, frequent recurrence of symptoms. Kidney yang vacuity also shows physical cold, pale complexion and cold extremities.

Tongue: Pale.

Pulse: Deep, thready.

Treatment Method: Supplement kidney yang, relieve pain.

PRESCRIPTION

Right-Restoring [Kidney Yang] Pill *yòu guī wán*

shú dì huáng	cooked rehmannia [root]	Rehmanniae Radix Conquita	24 g.
shān yào	dioscorea [root]	Dioscoreae Rhizoma	12 g.
shān zhū yú	cornus [fruit]	Corni Fructus	9 g.
gǒu qǐ zǐ	lycium [berry]	Lycii Fructus	12 g.
lù jiǎo jiāo	deerhorn glue (dissolved and stirred in)	Cervi Gelatinum Cornu	12 g.
tù sī zǐ	cuscuta [seed]	Cuscutae Semen	12 g.
dù zhòng	eucommia [bark]	Eucommiae Cortex	12 g.
dāng guī	tangkuei	Angelicae Sinensis Radix	9 g.
ròu guì	cinnamon [bark] (abbreviated decoction)	Cinnamomi Cortex	6 g.
zhì fù zǐ	aconite [accessory tuber] (processed) (extended decoction)	Aconiti Tuber Laterale Praeparatum	6 g.

MODIFICATIONS

In chronic cases of low back pain without obvious predominance of either kidney yin or kidney yang vacuity, the following is used to supplement the kidney and relieve low back pain. Grind the ingredients into a powder and make into pills; take a 9 gram dose twice daily.

PRESCRIPTION
Young Maid Pill *qīng é wán*

bǔ gǔ zhī	psoralea [seed]	Psoraleae Semen	120 g.
dù zhòng	eucommia [bark]	Eucommiae Cortex	120 g.
hú táo rén	walnut [kernel]	Juglandis Semen	120 g.
dà suàn	garlic [bulb]	Allii Sativi Bulbus	120 g.

In chronic cases caused by kidney vacuity accompanied by spleen qi vacuity, symptoms will include short and weak respiration, low weak voice, loss of appetite, loose stools and, in some cases, renal prolapse. Treatment is directed toward supplementation of the kidney accompanied by strengthening spleen qi. The appropriate kidney-oriented prescription may be used in conjunction with:

Center-Supplementing Qi-Boosting Decoction *bǔ zhōng yì qì tāng*

huáng qí	astragalus [root]	Astragali (seu Hedysari) Radix	15 g.
rén shēn	ginseng	Ginseng Radix	9 g.
bái zhú	ovate atractylodes [root]	Atractylodis Ovatae Rhizoma	9 g.
dāng guī	tangkuei	Angelicae Sinensis Radix	9 g.
chén pí	tangerine [peel]	Citri Exocarpium	6 g.
shēng má	cimicifuga [root]	Cimicifugae Rhizoma	3 g.
chái hú	bupleurum [root]	Bupleuri Radix	3 g.
zhì gān cǎo	licorice [root] (honey-fried)	Glycyrrhizae Radix	6 g.

ACUPUNCTURE AND MOXIBUSTION
Main Points: Needle with supplementation; add moxibustion.

BL-23	*shèn shū*
GV-03	*yāo yáng guān*
BL-40 (54)	*wěi zhōng*
BL-32	*cì liáo*
GV-04	*mìng mén*
M-BW-24	*yāo yǎn* (Lumbar Eye)

5. KIDNEY YIN VACUITY

Clinical Manifestations: Slow onset with extended illness duration, aching of lower back diminished by pressing and rubbing, fatigue, weakness of knees, increase in pain after exertion, decrease in pain while lying quietly, frequent recurrence of symptoms. Kidney yin vacuity also shows irritability, insomnia, dry mouth and throat, red cheeks, vexing heat in the five hearts.

Tongue: Red with little coating.

Pulse: Rapid, thready.

Treatment Method: Nourish kidney yin, relieve pain.

PRESCRIPTION
Left-Restoring [Kidney Yin] Pill *zuǒ guī wán*

shú dì huáng	cooked rehmannia [root]	Rehmanniae Radix Conquita	24 g.
shān yào	dioscorea [root]	Dioscoreae Rhizoma	12 g.
shān zhū yú	cornus [fruit]	Corni Fructus	12 g.
gǒu qǐ zǐ	lycium [berry]	Lycii Fructus	12 g.
chuān niú xī	cyathula [root]	Cyathulae Radix	9 g.
tù sī zǐ	cuscuta [seed]	Cuscutae Semen	12 g.
lù jiǎo jiāo	deerhorn glue (dissolved and stirred in)	Cervi Gelatinum Cornu	12 g.
guī bǎn jiāo	tortoise plastron glue (dissolved and stirred in)	Testudinis Plastrum Gelatinum	12 g.

<u>MODIFICATIONS</u>

In cases of marked vacuity fire, the above prescription is used to nourish yin and reduce vacuity fire with:

Major Yin Supplementation Pill *dà bǔ yīn wán*

zhī mǔ	anemarrhena [root]	Anemarrhenae Rhizoma	9 g.
huáng bǎi	phellodendron [bark]	Phellodendri Cortex	9 g.
shú dì huáng	cooked rehmannia [root]	Rehmanniae Radix Conquita	30 g.
guī bǎn	tortoise plastron (extended decoction)	Testudinis Plastrum	30 g.
zhū jǐ suǐ	pig's spine marrow (spinal cord of pig)	Suis Spinae Medulla	30 g.

ACUPUNCTURE AND MOXIBUSTION

Main Points: Needle with supplementation.

BL-23	*shèn shū*
GV-03	*yāo yáng guān*
BL-40 (54)	*wěi zhōng*
BL-32	*cì liáo*
BL-52 (47)	*zhì shì*
KI-03	*tài xī*

ALTERNATE THERAPEUTIC METHODS

1. Ear Acupuncture

Main Points: Lumbar Vertebrae, Sacral Vertebrae, Kidney, *Shén Mén*.

Method: Needle to elicit a strong sensation. Select points on the affected side. After insertion of needles, they should be rapidly twisted, and the patient should be directed to move his or her limbs, bend the back and twist at the waist.

2. Plum-Blossom Needle Therapy and Cupping Therapy

Using a plum-blossom needle, tap the skin over M-BW-35 (Hua Tuo's Paravertebral Points, *huá tuó jiā jí*), emphasizing the area near BL-23 *(shèn shū)*. For patients with a history of twists or sprains, tapping may be harder to dispel stasis and free the connections. Plum-blossom needle therapy may be used in conjunction with cupping therapy.

REMARKS

Pattern recognition in low back pain involves differentiating external and internal, hot and cold and repletion and vacuity. In general, patterns of external evil are external repletion patterns and the onset of the symptoms is rapid. Treatment usually involves dispelling evils and clearing the connections, as well as other measures based on the differentiation of cold-dampness and damp-heat.

Patterns of kidney vacuity are internal and vacuous, generally of slow onset and frequently recurring. Treatment should include supplementation of either kidney yang or kidney yin based on differential diagnosis.

Low back pain as a result of traumatic injury is differentiated on the basis of history. Patterns are usually repletion complicated by vacuity, and treatment involves quickening the blood, dispelling stasis, rectifying qi and clearing the connections. After alleviation of symptoms, measures are taken to conserve kidney qi to consolidate therapeutic effectiveness. Massage, physical therapy, cupping therapy, medicinal fuming therapy and medicinal plasters can be used to increase results.

SEMINAL EMISSION

Yí Jīng

1. Kidney Yin Vacuity with Exuberant Heart Fire - 2. Kidney Yang Vacuity with Failure to Secure the Essence - 3. Qi Vacuity with Failure to Astringe the Essence - 4. Descent of Damp-Heat into the Lower Burner

Seminal emission *(yí jīng)* refers to patterns characterized by the spontaneous ejaculation of semen when unrelated to sexual activity. Seminal emission is divided into two categories: nocturnal emission and spontaneous seminal discharge. In nocturnal emission the patient's condition is relatively mild and the emission generally occurs while dreaming – hence the Chinese name, "dream emission" *(mèng yí)*. Spontaneous seminal discharge, or "seminal efflux" *(huá jīng),* on the other hand, does not coincide with dreaming, and in its more severe form, it occurs while patients are fully conscious. Spontaneous seminal discharge may well be a pathologic development of nocturnal emission, indicating progressive severity.

One or two instances of seminal emission per month is considered physiologically normal in unmarried adult males or in married men who are living apart from their spouses. Seminal emission is considered pathological when it occurs more than twice per week or when spontaneous seminal discharge is accompanied by dizzy spells, listlessness, weak aching lower back and legs, palpitations, insomnia or forgetfulness.

Seminal emission is often observed in biomedical disorders such as neurosis, prostatitis, spermatocystitis and orchitis.

ETIOLOGY AND PATHOGENESIS

Failure of kidney qi to secure the essence is the constant factor in pathogenesis of seminal emission. Etiologically, failure of kidney qi can be caused by a variety of factors that include emotional stress or disturbance, improper diet and eating habits and overindulgent sexual activity. The pathological mechanism of seminal emission can be divided into four categories: kidney yin vacuity leading to exuberant fire; kidney yang vacuity resulting in failure to secure the essence; failure of qi to astringe the essence; and descent of damp-heat into the lower burner.

Patterns may be purely repletion or vacuity, or complicated by both repletion and vacuity. While heart, liver, spleen or kidney might be involved in the development of seminal emission, the pathogenesis is most intimately related to a disharmony between the heart and kidney.

1. KIDNEY YIN VACUITY WITH EXUBERANT HEART FIRE

Clinical Manifestations: Insomnia or frequent dreaming, palpitations, nocturnal emission, dry throat, dizziness and vertigo, vexation in the heart, weak aching lower back and legs, night sweating, tinnitus, forgetfulness, dark scanty urine.

Tongue: Red with little coating.

Pulse: Rapid, thready.

Treatment Method: Nourish kidney yin, clear heart fire, quiet the spirit, secure essence.

PRESCRIPTION

Anemarrhena, Phellodendron and Rehmannia Decoction
zhī bǎi dì huáng tāng

shú dì huáng	cooked rehmannia [root]	Rehmanniae Radix Conquita	24 g.
shān zhū yú	cornus [fruit]	Corni Fructus	12 g.
shān yào	dioscorea [root]	Dioscoreae Rhizoma	12 g.
zé xiè	alisma [tuber]	Alismatis Rhizoma	9 g.
fú líng	poria	Poria	9 g.
mǔ dān pí	moutan [root bark]	Moutan Radicis Cortex	9 g.
zhī mǔ	anemarrhena [root]	Anemarrhenae Rhizoma	9 g.
huáng bǎi	phellodendron [bark]	Phellodendri Cortex	9 g.

MODIFICATIONS

To reinforce clearing heat, calming the spirit and securing essence, add:

huáng lián	coptis [root]	Coptidis Rhizoma	6 g.
suān zǎo rén	spiny jujube [kernel]	Ziziphi Spinosi Semen	12 g.
wǔ wèi zǐ	schisandra [berry]	Schisandrae Fructus	6 g.
duàn lóng gǔ	calcined dragon bone (extended decoction)	Mastodi Ossis Fossilia Calcinatum	15 g.
duàn mǔ lì	calcined oyster shell (extended decoction)	Ostrea Concha Calcinatum	15 g.

In cases also evidencing qi vacuity, the prescription is changed to supplement qi and astringe the essence.

Use:

Heaven, Human and Earth Marrow-Retaining Elixir
*sān cái fēng suí dān**

shú dì huáng	cooked rehmannia [root]	Rehmanniae Radix Conquita	24 g.
tiān mén dōng	asparagus [tuber]	Asparagi Tuber	9 g.
rén shēn	ginseng	Ginseng Radix	9 g.
huáng bǎi	phellodendron [bark]	Phellodendri Cortex	9 g.
shā rén	amomum [fruit] (abbreviated decoction)	Amomi Semen seu Fructus	3 g.
gān cǎo	licorice [root]	Glycyrrhizae Radix	6 g.

plus:

huáng qí	astragalus [root]	Astragali (seu Hedysari) Radix	12 g.
shān yào	dioscorea [root]	Dioscoreae Rhizoma	12 g.
shān zhū yú	cornus [fruit]	Corni Fructus	12 g.

* Author's note: *sān cái*, "three herbs," refers to Heaven (*tiān*), human (*rén*) and earth (*dì*) through an image derived from three herbs in this formula: *tiān mén dōng*, *rén shēn* and *dì huáng*.

ACUPUNCTURE AND MOXIBUSTION

Main Points: Needle with even supplementation, even draining.

BL-15	*xīn shū*
BL-23	*shèn shū*
HT-07	*shén mén*
KI-03	*tài xī*
BL-52 (47)	*zhì shì*
PC-06	*nèi guān*

2. KIDNEY YANG VACUITY WITH FAILURE TO SECURE THE ESSENCE

Clinical Manifestations: Persistent seminal emission and spontaneous seminal discharge accompanied by cold extremities, physical cold, impotence, premature ejaculation, pale complexion.

Tongue: Delicate, pale, with tooth marks; white glossy coating.

Pulse: Deep, thready.

Treatment Method: Supplement kidney yang, secure essence.

PRESCRIPTION
Right-Restoring [Kidney Yang] Pill *yòu guī wán*

shú dì huáng	cooked rehmannia [root]	Rehmanniae Radix Conquita	24 g.
shān yào	dioscorea [root]	Dioscoreae Rhizoma	12 g.
shān zhū yú	cornus [fruit]	Corni Fructus	9 g.
gǒu qǐ zǐ	lycium [berry]	Lycii Fructus	12 g.
lù jiǎo jiāo	deerhorn glue (dissolved and stirred in)	Cervi Gelatinum Cornu	12 g.
tù sī zǐ	cuscuta [seed]	Cuscutae Semen	12 g.
dù zhòng	eucommia [bark]	Eucommiae Cortex	12 g.
dāng guī	tangkuei	Angelicae Sinensis Radix	9 g.
ròu guì	cinnamon [bark] (abbreviated decoction)	Cinnamomi Cortex	6 g.
zhì fù zǐ	aconite [accessory tuber] (processed) (extended decoction)	Aconiti Tuber Laterale Praeparatum	6 g.

MODIFICATIONS

In the treatment of seminal emission, supplementation of the kidney can be accompanied by the astringent medicines. Combine the given prescription with:

Golden Lock Essence-Securing Pill *jīn suǒ gù jīng wán*

shā yuàn zǐ	complanate astragalus [seed]	Astragali Complanati Semen	12 g.
qiàn shí	euryale [seed]	Euryales Semen	12 g.
lián xū	lotus[stamen]	Nelumbinis Stamen	3 g.
lián zǐ	lotus [fruit-seed]	Nelumbinis Fructus seu Semen	9 g.
duàn lóng gǔ	dragon bone (calcined) (extended decoction)	Mastodi Ossis Fossilia Calcinatum	15 g.
duàn mǔ lì	oyster shell (calcined) (extended decoction)	Ostreae Concha Calcinatum	15 g.

or:

Land and Water Two Immortals Elixir *shuǐ lù èr xiān dān*

jīn yīng zǐ	Cherokee rose [fruit]	Rosae Laevigatae Fructus	15 g.
qiàn shí	euryale [seed]	Euryales Semen	15 g.

ACUPUNCTURE AND MOXIBUSTION

Main Points: Needle with supplementation; add moxibustion.

BL-23	*shèn shū*
CV-04	*guān yuán*
SP-06	*sān yīn jiāo*
BL-52 (47)	*zhì shì*
KI-12	*dà hè*
CV-06	*qì hǎi*
GV-04	*mìng mén*

3. Qi Vacuity with Failure to Astringe the Essence

Clinical Manifestations: Palpitations, insomnia, forgetfulness, sallow complexion, fatigue, loss of appetite, loose stools, seminal emission following overwork.

Tongue: Pale with white coating.

Pulse: Weak.

Treatment Method: Rectify and supplement the heart and spleen, boost qi, secure essence.

PRESCRIPTION

Center-Supplementing Qi-Boosting Decoction *bǔ zhōng yì qì tāng*

huáng qí	astragalus [root]	Astragali (seu Hedysari) Radix	15 g.
rén shēn	ginseng	Ginseng Radix	9 g.
bái zhú	ovate atractylodes [root]	Atractylodis Ovatae Rhizoma	9 g.
dāng guī	tangkuei	Angelicae Sinensis Radix	9 g.
chén pí	tangerine [peel]	Citri Exocarpium	6 g.
shēng mā	cimicifuga [root]	Cimicifugae Rhizoma	3 g.
chái hú	bupleurum [root]	Bupleuri Radix	3 g.
zhì gān cǎo	licorice [root] (honey-fried)	Glycyrrhizae Radix	6 g.

MODIFICATIONS

To support the spleen and quiet the spirit, add:

shān yào	dioscorea [root]	Dioscoreae Rhizoma	12 g.
fú líng	poria	Poria	9 g.
yuǎn zhì	polygala [root]	Polygalae Radix	6 g.

ACUPUNCTURE AND MOXIBUSTION

Main Points: Needle with supplementation; add moxibustion.

BL-20	*pí shū*
BL-23	*shèn shū*
CV-06	*qì hǎi*
ST-36	*zú sān lǐ*
BL-52 (47)	*zhì shì*
SP-06	*sān yīn jiāo*

4. Descent of Damp-Heat into Lower Burner

Clinical Manifestations: Frequent seminal emission, escape of a small amount of semen during urination in some cases; dark burning cloudy urine, or difficult urination in some cases; thirst, bitter taste in the mouth, irritability, insomnia, loose foul-smelling stools, tenesmus, fullness and discomfort of the epigastrium and abdomen, nausea.

Tongue: Yellow slimy coating.

Pulse: Soft, rapid.

Treatment Method: Clear heat, disinhibit dampness, secure essence.

PRESCRIPTION

Cheng's Fish Poison Yam Clear-Turbid Separation Beverage
*chéng shì bì xiè fēn qīng yǐn**

bì xiè	fish poison yam	Dioscoreae Hypoglaucae Rhizoma	12 g.
huáng bǎi	phellodendron [bark]	Phellodendri Cortex	9 g.
shí chāng pú	acorus [root]	Acori Rhizoma	6 g.
fú líng	poria	Poria	9 g.
bái zhú	ovate atractylodes [root]	Atractylodis Ovatae Rhizoma	6 g.
dān shēn	salvia [root]	Salviae Miltiorrhizae Radix	9 g.
lián zǐ xīn	lotus [embryo]	Nelumbinis Embryo	3 g.
chē qián zǐ	plantago [seed] (wrapped)	Plantaginis Semen	12 g.

* Author's Note: There are two different prescriptions sharing the name of *Bì Xiè Fēn Qīng Yǐn*. This one is from Chéng Sōnglíng's medical book of the Qing dynasty, *Yī Xué Xīn Wù (Medicine Comprehended)*.

MODIFICATIONS

In cases of prolonged illness with static heat, manifesting as difficult urination with severe lateral lower abdominal distention, the prescription is modified to abduct stagnation and clear heat.

Add:

bài jiàng cǎo	baijiang	Baijiang Herba cum Radice	12 g.
chì sháo yào	red peony [root]	Paeoniae Radix Rubra	9 g.
hóng téng	sargentodoxa [stem]	Sargentodoxae Caulis	15 g.

ACUPUNCTURE AND MOXIBUSTION

Main Points: Needle with draining.

CV-03	*zhōng jí*
BL-34	*xià liáo*
SP-09	*yīn líng quán*
SP-06	*sān yīn jiāo*
LR-03	*tài chōng*
PC-06	*nèi guān*

ALTERNATE THERAPEUTIC METHODS

1. Ear Acupuncture

Main Points: *Jīng Gōng**, Endocrine, *Shén Mén*, Heart, Kidney.

Method: Select two or three points each session, needle to elicit a mild sensation. Manipulate once every ten to fifteen minutes and retain needles for thirty to fifty minutes.

Jīng Gōng – One of the auricular points in the triangular fossa, located in the depression close to the middle point of helix, also known as *zǐ gōng* (Infant's Palace, M-CA-18).

2. Plum-Blossom Needle Therapy

Method: Use a plum-blossom needle to tap lightly over the lower back and sacral regions as well as along the inner legs in a band through SP-06 *(sān yīn jiāo)*. Tap for twenty to thirty minutes until the skin turns slightly red. Treat once daily or once every two days.

REMARKS

To achieve maximum therapeutic results treating seminal emission, patients should foster a healthy mental attitude towards sex by engaging moderately in sexual activity, refraining from masturbation and abstaining from alcohol and rich foods. It is also advisable to engage in suitable physical exercise, such as qigong.

IMPOTENCE
Yáng Wěi
1. Debilitation of Life-Gate Fire - 2. Downpour of Damp-Heat into the Lower Burner

In *yáng wěi*, the Chinese expression for impotence, *yáng* refers to the penis and *wěi* means flaccidity. *Yáng wěi* refers either to the inability of the penis to attain erection or the ability to attain only partial erection; both of these prohibit normal sexual activity. Clinically, impotence is often seen with seminal emission or premature ejaculation and, in most cases, is a functional disorder. In Western medicine, it is often diagnosed as a sexual neurosis.

ETIOLOGY AND PATHOGENESIS

Impotence is generally the result of overindulgent sexual activity, habitual masturbation or emotional disturbances such as anxiety, worry, fear or fright. These can cause weakening of the life-gate fire and loss of sexual capacity. The downpour of damp-heat into the lower burner can also result in impotence, although such cases are relatively rare.

1. DEBILITATION OF LIFE-GATE FIRE

Clinical Manifestations: Complete or partial impotence, frequent spontaneous seminal discharge, dizziness and vertigo, tinnitus, pale complexion, cold extremities, listlessness, weak aching lower back and legs, frequent urination.

Tongue: Pale with white coating.

Pulse: Deep, thready.

Treatment Method: Supplement the kidney, invigorate yang.

PRESCRIPTION

Use Five-Seed Progeny Pill *(wǔ zǐ yǎn zōng wán)* or Procreation Elixir *(zàn yù dān)*.

Five-Seed Progeny Pill *wǔ zǐ yǎn zōng wán*

gǒu qǐ zǐ	lycium [berry]	Lycii fructus	12 g
fù pén zǐ	rubus [berry]	Rubi Fructus	12 g.
tù sī zǐ	cuscuta [seed]	Cuscutae Semen	12 g.
wǔ wèi zǐ	schisandra [berry]	Schisandrae Fructus	6 g.
chē qián zǐ	plantago [seed] (wrapped)	Plantaginis Semen	6 g.

or:

Procreation Elixir *zàn yù dān*

shú dì huáng	cooked rehmannia [root]	Rehmanniae Radix Conquita	24 g
shān zhū yú	cornus [fruit]	Corni Fructus	12 g
gǒu qǐ zǐ	lycium [berry]	Lycii fructus	12 g.
bā jǐ tiān	morinda [root]	Morindae Radix	12 g.
ròu cōng róng	cistanche [stem]	Cistanches Caulis	12 g.
dù zhòng	eucommia [bark]	Eucommiae Cortex	12 g.
shé chuáng zǐ	cnidium [seed]	Cnidii Monnieri Fructus	9 g.
xiān máo	curculigo [root]	Curculiginis Rhizoma	9 g.
yín yáng huò	epimedium	Epimedii Herba	9 g.
dāng guī	tangkuei	Angelicae Sinensis Radix	9 g.
bái zhú	ovate atractylodes [root]	Atractylodis Ovatae Rhizoma	9 g.
zhì fù zǐ	aconite [accessory tuber] (processed and extended)	Aconiti Tuber Laterale Praeparatum	6 g.
ròu guì	cinnamon bark (abbreviated decoction)	Cinnamomi Cortex	6 g.
jiǔ zǐ	Chinese leek [seed]	Allii Tuberosi Semen	9 g.

MODIFICATIONS

To increase the supplementing and invigorating effects of either of the preceding prescriptions, add:

rén shēn	ginseng	Ginseng Radix	9 g.
lù róng	velvet deerhorn	Cervi Cornu Parvum	1-3 g.
	(powdered; administered separately, beginning in small amounts)		

In cases accompanied by injury to the heart and spleen with symptoms of palpitations, anxiety and insomnia, combine the given prescription with:

Spleen-Returning Decoction *guī pí tāng*

huáng qí	astragalus [root]	Astragali (seu Hedysari) Radix	9 g.
rén shēn	ginseng	Ginseng Radix	9 g.
bái zhú	ovate atractylodes [root]	Atractylodis Ovatae Rhizoma	9 g.
fú shén	root poria	Poria cum Pini Radice	9 g.
lóng yǎn ròu	longan [flesh]	Longanae Arillus	9 g.
suān zǎo rén	spiny jujube [kernel]	Ziziphi Spinosi Semen	9 g.
mù xiāng	saussurea [root]	Saussureae Radix (seu Vladimiriae)	6 g.
dāng guī	tangkuei	Angelicae Sinensis Radix	6 g.
yuǎn zhì	polygala [root]	Polygalae Radix	3 g.
zhì gān cǎo	licorice [root] (honey-fried)	Glycyrrhizae Radix	6 g.
shēng jiāng	fresh ginger	Zingiberis Rhizoma Recens	3 g.
dà zǎo	jujube	Ziziphi Fructus	5 pc.

ACUPUNCTURE AND MOXIBUSTION

Main Points: Needle with supplementation; add moxibustion.

CV-04	*guān yuán*
GV-04	*mìng mén*
BL-23	*shèn shū*
KI-03	*tài xī*
GV-20	*bǎi huì*
BL-31/32/33/34	*bā liáo*

Auxiliary points:

For vacuity of the heart and spleen, add:

BL-15	*xīn shū*
HT-07	*shén mén*
SP-06	*sān yīn jiāo*

2. Downpour of Damp-Heat into the Lower Burner

Clinical Manifestations: Flaccidity of the penis with inability to achieve or sustain erection, accompanied by premature ejaculation in the majority of cases. Symptoms also include sweatiness of the scrotum, heavy aching lower limbs, thirst or bitter taste in the mouth, dark burning urine.

Tongue: Yellow slimy coating.

Pulse: Slippery, rapid.

Treatment Method: Clear heat, disinhibit dampness.

PRESCRIPTION

Gentian Liver-Draining Decoction *lóng dǎn xiè gān tāng*

lóng dǎn	gentian [root]	Gentianae Radix	6 g.
huáng qín	scutellaria [root]	Scutellariae Radix	9 g.
shān zhī zǐ	gardenia [fruit]	Gardeniae Fructus	9 g.
zé xiè	alisma [tuber]	Alismatis Rhizoma	12 g.
mù tōng	mutong [stem]	Mutong Caulis	9 g.
dāng guī	tangkuei	Angelicae Sinensis Radix	3 g.
chē qián zǐ	plantago [seed]	Plantaginis Semen	9 g.
shēng dì huáng	rehmannia [root] dried/fresh	Rehmanniae Radix Exsiccata seu recens	9 g.
chái hú	bupleurum [root]	Bupleuri Radix	6 g.
gān cǎo	licorice [root]	Glycyrrhizae Radix	6 g.

MODIFICATIONS

In cases of accompanying vacuity of kidney yin, manifesting weak aching lower back and legs, red tongue with little coating and thready rapid pulse, the strategy is to nourish yin, clear heat and eliminate dampness. Use:

Anemarrhena, Phellodendron and Rehmannia Pill *zhī bǎi dì huáng wán*

shú dì huáng	cooked rehmannia [root]	Rehmanniae Radix Conquita	24 g.
shān zhū yú	cornus [fruit]	Corni Fructus	12 g.
shān yào	dioscorea [root]	Dioscoreae Rhizoma	12 g.
zé xiè	alisma [tuber]	Alismatis Rhizoma	9 g.
fú líng	poria	Poria	9 g.
mǔ dān pí	moutan [root bark]	Moutan Radicis Cortex	9 g.
zhī mǔ	anemarrhena [root]	Anemarrhenae Rhizoma	9 g.
huáng bǎi	phellodendron [bark]	Phellodendri Cortex	9 g.

ACUPUNCTURE AND MOXIBUSTION

Main Points: Needle with supplementation.

CV-03	*zhōng jí*
GV-04	*mìng mén*
SP-06	*sān yīn jiāo*
SP-09	*yīn líng quán*
ST-36	*zú sān lǐ*
LR-05	*lǐ gōu*

Auxiliary points:
For vacuity of kidney yin, add:
     KI-03   *tài xī*

ALTERNATE THERAPEUTIC METHODS

1. Folk Remedy

In cases of impotence from debilitation of life-gate fire, the following prescription can be used. Take two sheep's testicles and add a small amount of old wine. Steam and consume each morning for one month, continuing for a second month if necessary. During treatment patients should abstain from sexual activity.

REMARKS

Apart from herbal and acumoxa therapy, psychotherapy may reinforce therapeutic effectiveness.

WASTING-THIRST

Xiāo Kě

1. Lung Heat with Injury to Fluids · 2. Profusion of Stomach Fire · 3. Depletion of Kidney Yin

Wasting-thirst patterns have excessive thirst, hunger and urination as their characteristic features. They are often accompanied by emaciation and sweet or turbid urine. They may be divided into upper burner, middle burner and lower burner patterns based on the relative severity of the three excessive symptoms. Upper burner wasting-thirst is characterized by the prominence of excessive thirst; middle burner wasting-thirst by excessive hunger; and lower burner wasting-thirst by excessive urination.

In Western medicine, the clinical manifestations of diabetes mellitus and diabetes insipidus are in many ways similar to those of wasting-thirst patterns. Differential diagnosis and treatment of diabetes can be made according to this chapter.

ETIOLOGY AND PATHOGENESIS

Wasting-thirst patterns are related to a constitutional vacuity of yin, improper diet and eating habits, emotional disturbance and overindulgent sexual activity. The pathogenesis of wasting-thirst is attributed to yin vacuity and dryness heat, with yin insufficiency as the root and heat-dryness as the branch. Very often, these two give rise to one another, with severe heat-dryness depleting yin and the depletion of yin allowing exuberant heat-dryness.

Pathological changes occur mainly in the lung, stomach and particularly the kidney. During the initial stages of the disease, dryness heat is generally prominent. Heat-dryness existing with yin vacuity results in a more prolonged illness, with the yin vacuity becoming more prominent as the illness proceeds. Injury to both qi and yin or insufficiency of both yin and yang are possible developments. Yin deficiency coupled with heat-dryness can lead to blood stasis, producing secondary conditions such as pulmonary tuberculosis, cataracts, night blindness, ulcers, stroke and edema. If the yin-fluids are severely depleted, insufficient yang may rise to the surface and escape, producing symptoms of headache, agitation, nausea, vomiting, dry red tongue and lips and deep rapid breathing. In severe cases cold limbs, faint pulse, coma and prostration can occur.

1. Lung Heat with Injury to Fluids

Clinical Manifestations: Excessive thirst, high fluid intake and dry mouth, accompanied by frequent urination and excessive hunger.

Tongue: Dry red tip; thin yellow coating.

Pulse: Rapid.

Treatment Method: Clear heat, moisten the lung, generate liquid, relieve thirst.

PRESCRIPTION

Wasting Thirst Formula *Xiǎo Kě Fāng*

tiān huā fěn	trichosanthes [root]	Trichosanthis Radix	15 g.
huáng lián	coptis [root]	Coptidis Rhizoma	6 g.
shēng dì huáng	rehmannia [root] fresh/dried	Rehmanniae Radix Exsiccata seu Recens	15 g.
shēng jiāng	fresh ginger	Zingiberis Rhizoma Recens	3 g.
xiān ǒu zhī	lotus [root juice] (stirred in)	Nelumbinis Rhizomatis Recentis Succus	50 cc.
fēng mì	honey	Mel	20 g.
rén rǔ zhī	human milk (breast milk or cow's milk, stirred in)	Hominis Lac	50 cc.

MODIFICATIONS

The prescription is often reinforced to generate liquid and relieve thirst.
Add:

gé gēn	pueraria [root]	Puerariae Radix	15 g.
mài mén dōng	ophiopogon [tuber]	Ophiopogonis Tuber	12 g.

In diagnosis of vacuity of lung and kidney qi and yin, there will be symptoms of rapid forceless pulse, unquenchable thirst, frequent urination and lassitude. The prescription is changed to supplement qi and yin.
Use:

Ophiopogon and Asparagus Decoction *èr dōng tāng*

tiān mén dōng	asparagus [tuber]	Asparagi Tuber	12 g.
mài mén dōng	ophiopogon [tuber]	Ophiopogonis Tuber	12 g.
tiān huā fěn	trichosanthes [root]	Trichosanthis Radix	12 g.
huáng qín	scutellaria [root]	Scutellariae Radix	9 g.
zhī mǔ	anemarrhena [root]	Anemarrhenae Rhizoma	9 g.
hé yè	lotus [leaf]	Nelumbinis Folium	3 g.
gān cǎo	licorice [root]	Glycyrrhizae Radix	6 g.
rén shēn	ginseng	Ginseng Radix	12 g.

This prescription is often modified to support qi and yin.
Delete:

rén shēn	ginseng	Ginseng Radix	

Add:

běi shā shēn	glehnia [root]	Glehniae Radix	12 g.

In cases where the lung and stomach have flared up harming qi and yin, there will be symptoms of dry yellow tongue coating, excessive thirst and a surging pulse. The prescription is changed to clear and drain the stomach and lung, to generate liquid and to relieve thirst.

Use:

White Tiger Decoction Plus Ginseng *bái hǔ jiā rén shēn tāng*

shí gāo	gypsum (extended decoction)	Gypsum	30 g.
zhī mǔ	anemarrhena [root]	Anemarrhenae Rhizoma	12 g.
rén shēn	ginseng	Ginseng Radix	9 g.
jīng mǐ	rice	Oryzae Semen	15 g.
zhì gān cǎo	licorice [root] (honey-fried)	Glycyrrhizae Radix	6 g.

ACUPUNCTURE AND MOXIBUSTION

Main Points: Needle with even supplementation, even draining.

HT-08	*shào fǔ*
BL-15	*xīn shū*
LU-09	*tài yuān*
BL-13	*fèi shū*
M-BW-12	*yí shū* (Pancreas Transport)

Auxiliary points:

For dry mouth and tongue, add:

| CV-23 | *lián quán* |
| CV-24 | *chéng jiāng* |

For clamoring stomach and repletion hunger, add:

| CV-12 | *zhōng wǎn* |
| PC-06 | *nèi guān* |

2. PROFUSION OF STOMACH FIRE

Clinical Manifestations: Excessive hunger, high food intake, emaciation, dry stools or constipation, thirst.

Tongue: Yellow coating.

Pulse: Forceful, slippery.

Treatment Method: Clear stomach, drain fire, nourish yin, generate liquid.

PRESCRIPTION

Jade Lady Brew *yù nǚ jiān*

shí gāo	gypsum (extended decoction)	Gypsum	30 g.
shú dì huáng	cooked rehmannia [root]	Rehmanniae Radix Conquita	15 g.
mài mén dōng	ophiopogon [tuber]	Ophiopogonis Tuber	12 g.
zhī mǔ	anemarrhena [root]	Anemarrhenae Rhizoma	9 g.
niú xī	achyranthes [root]	Achyranthis Bidentatae Radix	9 g.

MODIFICATIONS

The prescription is reinforced to increase its heat-clearing and fire-draining effects. Add:

| *huáng lián* | coptis [root] | Coptidis Rhizoma | 6 g. |
| *shān zhī zǐ* | gardenia [fruit] | Gardeniae Fructus | 9 g. |

In cases of constipation, the prescription is changed to moisten dryness and free the stool. Once constipation has been relieved, follow with Jade Lady Brew (*yù nǚ jiān*) as noted above.

Humor-Increasing Qi-Infusing Decoction *zēng yè chéng qì tāng*

xuán shēn	scrophularia [root]	Scrophulariae Radix	30 g.
mài mén dōng	ophiopogon [tuber]	Ophiopogonis Tuber	24 g.
shēng dì huáng	rehmannia [root] fresh/dried	Rehmanniae Radix Exsiccata seu Recens	24 g.
dà huáng	rhubarb (abbreviated decoction)	Rhei Rhizoma	9 g.
máng xiāo	mirabilite (dissolved)	Mirabilitum	6 g.

ACUPUNCTURE AND MOXIBUSTION

Main Points: Needle with even supplementation, even draining.

ST-44	*nèi tíng*
SP-06	*sān yīn jiāo*
BL-20	*pí shū*
BL-21	*wèi shū*
M-BW-12	*yí shū* (Pancreas Transport)

Auxiliary points:

For constipation, add:

BL-25	*dà cháng shū*
ST-37	*shàng jù xū*

3. DEPLETION OF KIDNEY YIN

Clinical Manifestations: Frequent urination, copious turbid milky urine, dry mouth and lips, thirst, high fluid intake, weak aching lower back and knees, dizziness and vertigo, blurred vision, red cheeks.

Tongue: Red with little coating.

Pulse: Deep, rapid, thready.

Treatment Method: Nourish kidney yin, secure the kidney.

PRESCRIPTION

Six-Ingredient Rehmannia Pill *liù wèi dì-huáng wán*

shú dì huáng	cooked rehmannia [root]	Rehmanniae Radix Conquita	24 g.
shān zhū yú	cornus [fruit]	Corni Fructus	12 g.
shān yào	dioscorea [root]	Dioscoreae Rhizoma	12 g.
zé xiè	alisma [tuber]	Alismatis Rhizoma	9 g.
fú líng	poria	Poria	9 g.
mǔ dān pí	moutan [root bark]	Moutan Radicis Cortex	9 g.

MODIFICATIONS

In cases where vacuity of kidney yin leads to vacuity heat with symptoms of agitation, insomnia and seminal emission, the prescription is modified to nourish yin and clear heat. Add:

zhī mǔ	anemarrhena [root]	Anemarrhenae Rhizoma	9 g.
huáng bǎi	phellodendron [bark]	Phellodendri Cortex	6 g.
guī bǎn	tortoise plastron (extended decoction)	Testudinis Plastrum	30 g.
mǔ lì	oyster shell (extended decoction)	Ostreae Concha	30 g.

In cases of secretion of a high volume of turbid urine, the prescription is modified to supplement the kidney and reduce urine. Add:

yì zhì rén	alpinia [fruit]	Alpiniae Oxyphyllae Fructus	6 g.
sāng xiāo	mantis [egg-case]	Mantidis Oötheca	6 g.
wǔ wèi zǐ	schisandra [berry]	Schisandrae Fructus	6 g.

In cases of vacuity of both qi and yin with symptoms of fatigue and shortness of breath, the prescription is modified to benefit qi. Add:

huáng qí	astragalus [root]	Astragali (seu Hedysari) Radix	12 g.
dǎng shēn	codonopsis [root]	Codonopsitis Radix	9 g.

In cases of prolonged illness where vacuity of kidney yin has led to the injury of kidney yang, symptoms may include dull dark complexion, chills, cold limbs, a very high volume of urine, impotence or amenorrhea, pale tongue with white coating and deep thready forceless pulse. The prescription is modified to warm yang and secure kidney function. Add:

zhì fù zǐ	aconite [accessory tuber] (processed) (extended decoction)	Aconiti Tuber Laterale Praeparatum	6 g.
ròu guì	cinnamon [bark] (abbreviated decoction)	Cinnamomi Cortex	6 g.
sāng piāo xiāo	mantis [egg-case]	Mantidis Oötheca	6 g.
jīn yīng zǐ	Cherokee [rose fruit]	Rosae Laevigatae Fructus	9 g.
fù pén zǐ	rubus [berry]	Rubi Fructus	9 g.

If symptoms of blood stasis present in any of the above mentioned wasting-thirst patterns, the prescription is modified to invigorate the blood and dispel stasis. Add:

dān shēn	salvia [root]	Salviae Miltiorrhizae Radix	9 g.
táo rén	peach [kernel]	Persicae Semen	6 g.
hóng huā	carthamus [flower]	Carthami Flos	6 g.
shān zhā	crataegus [fruit]	Crataegi Fructus	12 g.

ACUPUNCTURE AND MOXIBUSTION

Main Points: Needle with even supplementation, even draining.

KI-03	*tài xī*
LR-03	*tài chōng*
BL-18	*gān shū*
BL-23	*hèn shū*
M-BW-12	*yí shū* (Pancreas Transport)

Auxiliary points:

For dizziness and vertigo, add:

GV-23   *shàng xīng*

For blurred vision, add:

GB-37   *guāng míng*

For vacuity of kidney yang, add moxibustion to:

CV-04   *guān yuán*
GV-04   *mìng mén*

For blood stasis, add:

BL-17   *gé shū*

ALTERNATE THERAPEUTIC METHODS

1. Ear Acupuncture:

Main Points: Pancreas, Endocrine, Kidney, *Sān Jiāo*, *Shén Mén*, Heart, Liver.

Method: Select three to five points per session, needle to elicit a mild sensation and retain needles for twenty minutes. Treat once every two days, ten treatments per therapeutic course.

2. Plum Blossom Needle Therapy

Method: Use a plum-blossom needle to tap along both sides of the spine from the level of the seventh to the tenth thoracic vertebrae. Treat once daily or once every two days, five to ten sessions per therapeutic course.

REMARKS

In addition to herbal medicine and acumoxa therapy, treatment of wasting-thirst patterns should include the alleviation of psychological stress and abstinence from sexual activity. Particular attention should be paid to keeping the diet light and bland, and patients should avoid overeating. Diets should include grains and cereals with vegetables, legumes, lean meat and eggs. Hot, spicy and stimulating foods should be prohibited.

The differential diagnosis and treatment of accompanying symptoms or secondary conditions of wasting-thirst patterns may be undertaken with reference to the appropriate chapters.

URINARY STRANGURY

Lín Zhèng

1. Heat Strangury - 2. Stone Strangury - 3A. Qi Strangury – Repletion Patterns - 3B Qi Strangury – Vacuity Patterns - 4A. Blood Strangury – Repletion Patterns - 4B. Blood Strangury – Vacuity Patterns - 5A. Unctuous Strangury – Repletion Patterns - 5B. Unctuous Strangury – Vacuity Patterns - 6. Taxation Strangury

Patterns of urinary strangury are characterized by frequent scanty or difficult urination, dribbling urination, sharp pain in the urethra and lower abdominal spasms or pain radiating to the lower back during urination. On the basis of pathogenesis and clinical manifestations, urinary strangury may be grouped into six categories: damp-heat (*rè lín,* heat strangury); strangury from calculi (*shí lín,* stone strangury); strangury due to stagnation or vacuity of qi (*qì lín,* qi strangury); urinary disruption with hematuria (*xuè lín,* blood strangury); strangury with milky urine (*gāo lín,* unctuous strangury); and urinary disruption due to taxation (*láo lín,* taxation strangury).

In traditional Chinese medicine, the term urinary strangury includes the Western medical conditions of acute and chronic urinary infection, bladder or kidney stones, acute and chronic prostatitis and chyluria (the presence of chyle or lymph in the urine).

ETIOLOGY AND PATHOGENESIS

Strangury can be divided into repletion and vacuity patterns. The pathogenesis of repletion patterns includes excessive consumption of hot spicy or rich sweet foods, excessive indulgence in alcohol or poor genital hygiene. These factors allow invasion of the urinary bladder by foul turbid evils, which give rise to damp-heat manifesting as sharp pain and to burning of the urethra during urination. Over time, damp-heat can form calculi. If damp-heat injures the blood vessels, hematuria will result with an increase in the pain and difficulty of urination. Downpour of damp-heat into the lower burner can interfere with the transformation of qi, allowing lipid fluids to escape and the urine to appear milky.

Urinary disturbance from repletion patterns can also be caused by emotional disturbance, resulting in the stagnation of liver qi. This will affect the normal function of the urinary bladder, giving rise to symptoms of lower abdominal distention and painful difficult urination.

Strangury related to vacuity is also caused by a number of factors. Prolonged urinary disorders can injure correct qi by accumulating damp-heat. Stress, strain or overindulgence in sexual activity, as well a frail constitution in the elderly, can all lead to spleen and kidney qi vacuity or depletion of kidney yin.

Spleen qi vacuity can cause sinking of center qi, with consequent urinary disruption. Kidney qi vacuity can result in an inability to reabsorb essence, causing milky urine. Urinary disturbance following taxation is generally the result of spleen and kidney vacuity. Finally, depletion of kidney yin with frenetic vacuity fire can give rise to strangury with hematuria.

In sum, the pathological changes occur mainly in the bladder and kidney, although the liver and spleen may also be involved. During the initial stages, patterns are usually of repletion, and transform to vacuity patterns in prolonged cases, or to patterns complicated by both repletion and vacuity. Because of the numerous factors influencing urinary disorders, some of the six groupings listed above are discussed as repletion and vacuity types.

1. HEAT STRANGURY

Clinical Manifestations: Frequent urgent difficult urination, dark scanty urine, burning sensation and sharp pain of the urethra, lower abdominal distention and pain; occasional symptoms of aversion to cold, fever, lower back pain, constipation and bitter taste in the mouth.

Tongue: Yellow slimy coating.

Pulse: Soft, rapid.

Treatment Method: Clear heat, disinhibit dampness, free and disinhibit the urine.

PRESCRIPTION

Eight Corrections Powder *bā zhèng sǎn*

chē qián zǐ	plantago [seed] (wrapped)	Plantaginis Semen	12 g.
qū mài	dianthus	Dianthi Herba	9 g.
biǎn xù	knotgrass	Polygoni Avicularis Herba	9 g.
huá shí	talcum (wrapped)	Talcum	15 g.
shān zhī zǐ	gardenia [fruit]	Gardeniae Fructus	9 g.
mù tōng	mutong [stem]	Mutong Caulis	9 g.
shú dà huáng	cooked rhubarb	Rhei Rhizoma Conquitum	9 g.
zhì gān cǎo	licorice [root] (honey-fried)	Glycyrrhizae Radix	6 g.
dēng xīn cǎo	juncus [pith]	Junci Medulla	3 g.

MODIFICATIONS

In cases of constipation and abdominal distention, the prescription is modified to free the stool and drain heat.

Delete:

shú dà huáng	rhubarb (cooked)	Rhei Rhizoma Conquitum

Add:

shēng dà huáng	rhubarb (raw)	Rhei Rhizoma Crudum	9 g.
zhǐ shí	unripe bitter orange	Aurantii Fructus Immaturus	9 g.

In cases accompanied by aversion to cold, fever, bitter taste in the mouth, nausea and vomiting, the prescription is changed to dispel evil and relieve vomiting.

Combine the preceding prescription with:

Minor Bupleurum Decoction *xiǎo chái hú tāng*

chái hú	bupleurum [root]	Bupleuri Radix	12 g.
huáng qín	scutellaria [root]	Scutellariae Radix	9 g.
jiāng bàn xià	(ginger-processed) pinellia [tuber]	Pinelliae Tuber Praeparatum	9 g.
shēng jiāng	fresh ginger	Zingiberis Rhizoma Recens	9 g.
rén shēn	ginseng	Ginseng Radix	6 g.
zhì gān cǎo	licorice [root] (honey-fried)	Glycyrrhizae Radix	6 g.
dà zǎo	jujube	Ziziphi Fructus	4 pc.

In cases of injury to yin humor by damp-heat, the prescription is modified to nourish yin and clear heat.

Delete:

shú dà huáng	rhubarb (cooked)	Rhei Rhizoma Conquitum

Add:

shēng dì huáng	rehmannia [root] fresh/dried	Rehmanniae Radix Exsiccata seu Recens	9 g.
zhī mǔ	anemarrhena [root]	Anemarrhenae Rhizoma	9 g.
bái máo gēn	imperata [root]	Imperatae Rhizoma	15 g.

ACUPUNCTURE AND MOXIBUSTION

Main Points: Needle with draining.

BL-28	*páng guāng shū*
CV-03	*zhōng jí*
SP-09	*yīn líng quán*
SP-06	*sān yīn jiāo*
TB-05	*wài guān*

Auxiliary points:

For aversion to cold and fever, add:

LI-04	*hé gǔ*

2. STONE STRANGURY

Clinical Manifestations: Unilateral lower backache or periodic cramping pains that extend into the lower abdomen and pubic regions, difficult urination, hematuria in severe cases, passage of urinary gravel in some cases.

Tongue: Red with yellow slimy coating.

Pulse: Wiry or slightly rapid.

Treatment Method: Clear heat, disinhibit dampness, free and disinhibit the urine, expel stones.

PRESCRIPTION

Pyrrosia Powder *shí wéi sǎn*

shí wéi	pyrrosia [leaf]	Pyrrosiae Folium	9 g.
qū mài	dianthus	Dianthi Herba	9 g.
chē qián zǐ	plantago [seed] (wrapped)	Plantaginis Semen	12 g.
dōng kuí zǐ	mallow [seed]	Malvae Verticillatae Semen	9 g.
huá shí	talcum (wrapped)	Talcum	15 g.

MODIFICATIONS

To strengthen the prescription's stone-expelling effects, add:

jīn qián cǎo	moneywort	Jinqiancao Herba	30 g.
hǎi jīn shā	lygodium spore (wrapped)	Lygodii Spora	9 g.
jī nèi jīn	gizzard lining	Galli Gigerii Endothelium	9 g.
	(or, powdered and stirred in, 3 g. each time)		

In cases of cramping pain in the lower back and lower abdomen, the prescription is modified to relax tension and relieve pain. Add:

bái sháo yào	white peony [root]	Paeoniae Radix Alba	12 g.
gān cǎo	licorice [root]	Glycyrrhizae Radix	6 g.

In cases of hematuria, the prescription is modified to cool the blood and relieve bleeding. Add:

shēng dì huáng	rehmannia [root] fresh/dried	Rehmanniae Radix Exsiccata seu Recens	12 g.
xiǎo jì	cephalanoplos	Cephalanoploris Herba seu Radix	12 g.
bái máo gēn	imperata [root]	Imperatae Rhizoma	30 g.

In cases accompanied by fever, the prescription is modified to clear heat and drain fire. Add:

pú gōng yīng	dandelion	Taraxaci Herba cum Radice	12 g.
huáng bǎi	phellodendron [bark]	Phellodendri Cortex	9 g.
shú dà huáng	rhubarb (cooked)	Rhei Rhizoma Conquitum	9 g.

In prolonged cases of urinary stones where both qi and blood have been depleted with symptoms of lusterless complexion, tiredness, fatigue, pale tongue with tooth marks and weak thready pulse, the prescription is changed to supplement qi and blood, free and disinhibit the urine and expel stones. Combine Two Spirits Decoction *(èr shén tāng)* with Eight-Gem Decoction *(bā zhēn tāng)*.

Two Spirits Decoction *èr shén tāng*

hǎi jīn shā	lygodium spore (wrapped)	Lygodii Spora	12 g.
huá shí	talcum (wrapped)	Talcum	12 g.

with:

Eight-Gem Decoction *bā zhēn tāng*

shú dì huáng	cooked rehmannia [root]	Rehmanniae Radix Conquita	12 g.
dāng guī	tangkuei	Angelicae Sinensis Radix	9 g.
bái sháo yào	white peony [root]	Paeoniae Radix Alba	9 g.
chuān xiōng	ligusticum [root]	Ligustici Rhizoma	6 g.
rén shēn	ginseng	Ginseng Radix	9 g.
bái zhú	ovate atractylodes [root]	Atractylodis Ovatae Rhizoma	9 g.
fú líng	poria	Poria	12 g.
zhì gān cǎo	licorice [root] (honey-fried)	Glycyrrhizae Radix	6 g.
shēng jiāng	fresh ginger	Zingiberis Rhizoma Recens	3 g.
dà zǎo	jujube	Ziziphi Fructus	3 pc.

In prolonged cases of urinary stones where yin humor has been injured, with symptoms of dull pain in the lower back and lower abdomen, vexing heat in the five hearts, red tongue with little coating and rapid thready pulse, the prescription is changed to nourish kidney yin, free and disinhibit the urine and expel stones.

Combine the preceding prescription with Six-Ingredient Rehmannia Pill *(liù wèi dì huáng wán)*.

Six-Ingredient Rehmannia Pill *liù wèi dì huáng wán*

shú dì huáng	cooked rehmannia [root]	Rehmanniae Radix Conquita	24 g.
shān zhū yú	cornus [fruit]	Corni Fructus	12 g.
shān yào	dioscorea [root]	Dioscoreae Rhizoma	12 g.
zé xiè	alisma [tuber]	Alismatis Rhizoma	9 g.
fú líng	poria	Poria	9 g.
mǔ dān pí	moutan [root bark]	Moutan Radicis Cortex	9 g.

ACUPUNCTURE AND MOXIBUSTION

Main Points: Needle with draining.

BL-28	*páng guāng shū*
CV-03	*zhōng jí*
SP-09	*yīn líng quán*
BL-39 (53)	*wěi yáng*
KI-02	*rán gǔ*

Auxiliary points:

For hematuria, add:

SP-06	*sān yīn jiāo*
SP-10	*xuè hǎi*

In prolonged cases of urinary stones with depletion of both qi and blood, add:

ST-36	*zú sān lǐ*
CV-06	*qì hǎi*
SP-06	*sān yīn jiāo*

Where injury has been done to kidney yin, add:

BL-23	*shèn shū*
KI-03	*tài xī*

3A. QI STRANGURY – REPLETION PATTERNS

Clinical Manifestations: Difficult urination, dripping urine, fullness and pain in the lateral lower abdomen accompanied by oppression in the chest and distention of the hypochondrium.

Tongue: Thin white coating.

Pulse: Wiry.

Treatment Method: Rectify qi, free and disinhibit the urine.

PRESCRIPTION

Aquilaria Powder *chén xiāng sǎn*

chén xiāng	aquilaria [wood] (powdered and stirred in)	Aquilariae Lignum	1.5 g.
shí wéi	pyrrosia [leaf]	Pyrrosiae Folium	9 g.
huá shí	talcum (wrapped)	Talcum	12 g.
dāng guī	tangkuei	Angelicae Sinensis Radix	6 g.
bái sháo yào	white peony [root]	Paeoniae Radix Alba	9 g.
chén pí	tangerine [peel]	Citri Exocarpium	9 g.
dōng kuí zǐ	mallow [seed]	Malvae Verticillatae Semen	9 g.
wáng bù liú xíng	vaccaria [seed]	Vaccariae Semen	9 g.
gān cǎo	licorice [root]	Glycyrrhizae Radix	6 g.

MODIFICATIONS

In cases of distention of the chest and hypochondrium, the prescription is modified to soothe the liver and rectify qi. Add:

qín pí	ash [bark]	Fraxini Cortex	9 g.
wū yào	lindera [root]	Linderae Radix	9 g.

In prolonged cases with stagnation of qi and stasis of blood, the prescription is modified to quicken the blood and remove stasis. Add:

chì sháo yào	red peony [root]	Paeoniae Radix Rubra	9 g.
hóng huā	carthamus [flower]	Carthami Flos	6 g.
chuān niú xī	cyathula [root]	Cyathulae Radix	9 g.

ACUPUNCTURE AND MOXIBUSTION

Main Points: Needle with draining.

BL-28	páng guāng shū
CV-03	zhōng jí
SP-09	yīn líng quán
LR-03	tài chōng
SP-06	sān yīn jiāo

3B. QI STRANGURY – VACUITY PATTERNS

Clinical Manifestations: Lower abdominal heaviness and distention, weak urination, interrupted flow of urination, dribbling urination in severe cases, dripping of urine following urination, pale complexion, aching lower back, tiredness, shortness of breath.

Tongue: Pale with light coating.

Pulse: Weak.

Treatment Method: Supplement the spleen, boost qi.

PRESCRIPTION

Center-Supplementing Qi-Boosting Decoction *bǔ zhōng yì qì tāng*

huáng qí	astragalus [root]	Astragali (seu Hedysari) Radix	15 g.
rén shēn	ginseng	Ginseng Radix	9 g.
bái zhú	ovate atractylodes [root]	Atractylodis Ovatae Rhizoma	9 g.
dāng guī	tangkuei	Angelicae Sinensis Radix	9 g.
chén pí	tangerine [peel]	Citri Exocarpium	6 g.
shēng má	cimicifuga [root]	Cimicifugae Rhizoma	3 g.
chái hú	bupleurum [root]	Bupleuri Radix	3 g.
zhì gān cǎo	licorice [root] (honey-fried)	Glycyrrhizae Radix	6 g.

MODIFICATIONS

In cases accompanied by depletion of blood and kidney vacuity, the prescription is changed to boost qi, nourish the blood and supplement both the spleen and kidney.

Use:

Eight-Gem Decoction *bā zhēn tāng*

shú dì huáng	cooked rehmannia [root]	Rehmanniae Radix Conquita	12 g.
dāng guī	tangkuei	Angelicae Sinensis Radix	9 g.
bái sháo yào	white peony [root]	Paeoniae Radix Alba	9 g.
chuān xiōng	ligusticum [root]	Ligustici Rhizoma	6 g.
rén shēn	ginseng	Ginseng Radix	9 g.
bái zhú	ovate atractylodes [root]	Atractylodis Ovatae Rhizoma	9 g.
fú líng	poria	Poria	9 g.
zhì gān cǎo	licorice [root] (honey-fried)	Glycyrrhizae Radix	6 g.
shēng jiāng	fresh ginger	Zingiberis Rhizoma Recens	3 g.
dà zǎo	jujube	Ziziphi Fructus	3 pc.

To reinforce strengthening the kidney, add:

dù zhòng	eucommia [bark]	Eucommiae Cortex	12 g.
gǒu qǐ zǐ	lycium [berry]	Lycii Fructus	9 g.
tǔ niú xī	native achyranthes [root]	Achyranthis Radix	9 g.

ACUPUNCTURE AND MOXIBUSTION

Main Points: Needle with even supplementation, even draining; add moxibustion.

BL-28	*páng guāng shū*
CV-03	*zhōng jí*
SP-09	*yīn líng quán*
CV-06	*qì hǎi*
ST-36	*zú sān lǐ*

4A. BLOOD STRANGURY – REPLETION PATTERNS

Clinical Manifestations: Frequent urgent urination, sharp burning pain of the urethra, hematuria, dark red urine, blood-streaked urine or passage of blood clots with the urine.

Tongue: Red with yellow coating.

Pulse: Rapid, slippery, forceful.

Treatment Method: Clear heat, free and disinhibit the urine, cool the blood, relieve bleeding.

PRESCRIPTION

Cephalanoplos Drink *xiǎo jì yǐn zǐ*

shēng dì huáng	rehmannia [root] fresh/dried	Rehmanniae Radix Exsiccata seu Recens	30 g.
xiǎo jì	cephalanoplos	Cephalanoploris Herba seu Radix	15 g.
mù tōng	mutong [stem]	Mutong Caulis	6 g.
huá shí	talcum (wrapped)	Talcum	15 g.
chǎo pú huáng	typha pollen (charred)	Typhae Pollen Carbonisatum	9 g.
dàn zhú yè	bamboo [leaf]	Lophatheri Folium	9 g.
ǒu jié	lotus [root node]	Nelumbinis Rhizomatis Nodus	9 g.
dāng guī	tangkuei	Angelicae Sinensis Radix	9 g.
shān zhī zǐ	gardenia [fruit]	Gardeniae Fructus	9 g.
zhì gān cǎo	licorice [root] (honey-fried)	Glycyrrhizae Radix	6 g.

MODIFICATIONS

In cases of profuse hematuria and severe pain, the prescription is modified to dispel stasis, free and disinhibit the urine, relieve bleeding and relieve pain.
Add:

sān qī	notoginseng [root]	Notoginseng Radix	9 g.
	(powdered and administered separately, 15 g. each time)		
hǔ pò	amber	Succinum	3 g.
	(powdered and stirred in)		

ACUPUNCTURE AND MOXIBUSTION

Main Points: Needle with draining.

BL-28	*páng guāng shū*
CV-03	*zhōng jí*
SP-09	*yīn líng quán*
SP-10	*xuè hǎi*
SP-06	*sān yīn jiāo*

4B. BLOOD STRANGURY – VACUITY PATTERNS

Clinical Manifestations: Bloody urine over an extended period, light red urine without pain or difficult urination, accompanied by tiredness, weak aching lower back and knees, vexing heat in the five hearts.

Tongue: Red with little coating.

Pulse: Rapid, thready.

Treatment Method: Nourish yin, clear heat, relieve bleeding.

PRESCRIPTION

Anemarrhena, Phellodendron and Rehmannia Pill *zhī bǎi dì huáng wán*

shú dì huáng	cooked rehmannia [root]	Rehmanniae Radix Conquita	24 g.
shān zhū yú	cornus [fruit]	Corni Fructus	12 g.
shān yào	dioscorea [root]	Dioscoreae Rhizoma	12 g.
zé xiè	alisma [tuber]	Alismatis Rhizoma	9 g.
fú líng	poria	Poria	9 g.
mǔ dān pí	moutan [root bark]	Moutan Radicis Cortex	9 g.
zhī mǔ	anemarrhena [root]	Anemarrhenae Rhizoma	9 g.
huáng bǎi	phellodendron [bark]	Phellodendri Cortex	9 g.

MODIFICATIONS

To reinforce the effects of nourishing vacuity and of stopping bleeding, add:

hàn lián cǎo	eclipta	Ecliptae Herba	12 g.
xiān hè cǎo	agrimony	Agrimoniae Herba	12 g.
ē jiāo	ass hide glue	Asini Corii Gelatinum	9 g.
	(dissolved and stirred in)		

In cases of lower back pain, the prescription is modified to supplement the kidney and strengthen the lower back. Add:

xù duàn	dipsacus [root]	Dipsaci Radix	12 g.
sāng jì shēng	mistletoe	Loranthi seu Visci Ramus	12 g.

ACUPUNCTURE AND MOXIBUSTION

Main Points: Needle with even supplementation, even draining.

BL-28	*páng guāng shū*
CV-03	*zhōng jí*
SP-09	*yīn líng quán*
SP-10	*xuè hǎi*
SP-06	*sān yīn jiāo*

5A. UNCTUOUS STRANGURY – REPLETION PATTERNS

Clinical Manifestations: Cloudy, milky or creamy urine that may contain precipitate or blood; urethral pain and burning.

Tongue: Red with yellow slimy coating.

Pulse: Soft, rapid.

Treatment Method: Clear heat, disinhibit dampness.

PRESCRIPTION

Cheng's Fish Poison Yam Clear-Turbid Separation Beverage
*chéng shì bì xiè fēn qīng yǐn**

bì xiè	fish poison yam	Dioscoreae Hypoglaucae Rhizoma	12 g.
huáng bǎi	phellodendron [bark]	Phellodendri Cortex	9 g.
shí chāng pú	acorus [root]	Acori Rhizoma	6 g.
fú líng	poria	Poria	9 g.
bái zhú	ovate atractylodes [root]	Atractylodis Ovatae Rhizoma	6 g.
dān shēn	salvia [root]	Salviae Miltiorrhizae Radix	9 g.
lián zǐ xīn	lotus [embryo]	Nelumbinis Embryo	3 g.
chē qián zǐ	plantago seed (wrapped)	Plantaginis Semen	12 g.

* Author's Note: There are two different prescriptions sharing the name of *Bì Xiè Fēn Qīng Yǐn*. This one is from Chéng Sōnglíng's medical book of the Qing dynasty, *Yī Xué Xīn Wǔ (Medicine Comprehended)*.

<u>MODIFICATIONS</u>

In cases of lower abdominal distention and difficult urination, the prescription is modified to rectify qi. Add:

wū yào	lindera [root]	Linderae Radix	9 g.
qīng pí	unripe tangerine [peel]	Citri Exocarpium Immaturum	9 g.

In cases accompanied by hematuria, the prescription is modified to relieve bleeding. Add:

xiǎo jì	cephalanoplos	Cephalanoploris Herba seu Radix	9 g.
ǒu jié	lotus [root node]	Nelumbinis Rhizomatis Nodus	9 g.
bái máo gēn	imperata [root]	Imperatae Rhizoma	15 g.

ACUPUNCTURE AND MOXIBUSTION

Main Points: Needle with draining.

BL-28	*páng guāng shū*
CV-03	*zhōng jí*
SP-09	*yīn líng quán*
SP-06	*sān yīn jiāo*
ST-28	*shuǐ dào*

5B. UNCTUOUS STRANGURY – VACUITY PATTERNS

Clinical Manifestations: Prolonged repeated dribbling of milky urine, moderate urethral pain accompanied by emaciation, weakness and aching of the lower back and knees, tiredness, dizziness and vertigo, tinnitus.

Tongue: Pale with slimy coating.

Pulse: Weak, thready.

Treatment Method: Supplement the kidney, secure essence.

PRESCRIPTION

Unctuous Strangury Decoction *gāo lín tāng*

shān yào	dioscorea [root]	Dioscoreae Rhizoma	30 g.
qiàn shí	euryale [seed]	Euryales Semen	15 g.
duàn lóng gǔ	calcined dragon bone	Mastodi Ossis Fossilia Calcinatum	30 g.
duàn mǔ lì	calcined oyster shell	Ostreae Concha Calcinatum	30 g.
shēng dì huáng	rehmannia [root] fresh/dried	Rehmanniae Radix Exsiccata seu Recens	12 g.
dǎng shēn	codonopsis [root]	Codonopsitis Radix	12 g.
bái sháo yào	white peony [root]	Paeoniae Radix Alba	9 g.

MODIFICATIONS

To reinforce kidney supplementation and absorb essence, add:

jīn yīng zǐ	Cherokee rose [fruit]	Rosae Laevigatae Fructus	12 g.
tù sī zǐ	cuscuta [seed]	Cuscutae Semen	12 g.

In cases of vacuity of both the spleen and kidney with sinking of center qi and insecurity of kidney qi, the prescription is changed to supplement the spleen, upbear qi, nourish the kidney and retain essence. Combine Center-Supplementing Qi-Boosting Decoction (*bǔ zhōng yì qì tāng*) with Seven-Ingredient Metropolis Qi Pill (*qī wèi dū qì wán*).

Center-Supplementing Qi-Boosting Decoction *bǔ zhōng yì qì tāng*

huáng qí	astragalus [root]	Astragali (seu Hedysari) Radix	15 g.
rén shēn	ginseng	Ginseng Radix	9 g.
bái zhú	ovate atractylodes [root]	Atractylodis Ovatae Rhizoma	9 g.
dāng guī	tangkuei	Angelicae Sinensis Radix	9 g.
chén pí	tangerine [peel]	Citri Exocarpium	6 g.
shēng má	cimicifuga [root]	Cimicifugae Rhizoma	3 g.
chái hú	bupleurum [root]	Bupleuri Radix	3 g.
zhì gān cǎo	licorice [root] (honey-fried)	Glycyrrhizae Radix	6 g.

with:

Seven-Ingredient Metropolis Qi Pill *qī wèi dū qì wán*

shú dì huáng	cooked rehmannia [root]	Rehmanniae Radix Conquita	24 g.
shān zhū yú	cornus [fruit]	Corni Fructus	12 g.
shān yào	dioscorea [root]	Dioscoreae Rhizoma	12 g.
zé xiè	alisma [tuber]	Alismatis Rhizoma	9 g.
fú líng	poria	Poria	9 g.
mǔ dān pí	moutan [root bark]	Moutan Radicis Cortex	9 g.
wǔ wèi zǐ	schisandra [berry]	Schisandrae Fructus	6 g.

ACUPUNCTURE AND MOXIBUSTION

Main Points: Needle with even supplementation, even draining.

SP-09	*yīn líng quán*
CV-03	*zhōng jí*
BL-28	*páng guāng shū*
BL-23	*shèn shū*
KI-06	*zhào hǎi*

6. TAXATION STRANGURY

Clinical Manifestations: Urine not particularly dark or difficult; periodic involuntary dribbling, urination generally occurring after strain, not easily responding to treatment, lassitude, weak and aching lower back and knees.

Tongue: Pale.

Pulse: Weak.

Treatment Method: Strengthen the spleen, supplement the kidney.

PRESCRIPTION

Matchless Dioscorea Pill *wú bǐ shān-yào wán*

shān yào	dioscorea [root]	Dioscoreae Rhizoma	30 g.
ròu cōng róng	cistanche [stem]	Cistanches Caulis	15 g.
shú dì huáng	cooked rehmannia [root]	Rehmanniae Radix Conquita	12 g.
shān zhū yú	cornus [fruit]	Corni Fructus	12 g.
fú shén	root poria	Poria cum Pini Radice	9 g.
tù sī zǐ	cuscuta [seed]	Cuscutae Semen	9 g.
wǔ wèi zǐ	schisandra [berry]	Schisandrae Fructus	6 g.
chì shí zhī	halloysite (wrapped)	Halloysitum Rubrum	12 g.
bā jǐ tiān	morinda [root]	Morindae Radix	12 g.
zé xiè	alisma [tuber]	Alismatis Rhizoma	9 g.
dù zhòng	eucommia [bark]	Eucommiae Cortex	12 g.
tǔ niú xī	native achyranthes [root]	Achyranthis Radix	9 g.

MODIFICATIONS

In cases of vacuity of the spleen and sinking of qi with lower abdominal heaviness and distention and dribbling following urination, Center-Supplementing Qi-Boosting Decoction *(bǔ zhōng yì qì tāng)* may also be added to boost and upbear qi.

Center-Supplementing Qi-Boosting Decoction *bǔ zhōng yì qì tāng*

huáng qí	astragalus [root]	Astragali (seu Hedysari) Radix	15 g.
rén shēn	ginseng	Ginseng Radix	9 g.
bái zhú	ovate atractylodes [root]	Atractylodis Ovatae Rhizoma	9 g.
dāng guī	tangkuei	Angelicae Sinensis Radix	9 g.
chén pí	tangerine peel	Citri Exocarpium	6 g.
shēng má	cimicifuga [root]	Cimicifugae Rhizoma	3 g.
chái hú	bupleurum [root]	Bupleuri Radix	3 g.
zhì gān cǎo	licorice [root] (honey-fried	Glycyrrhizae Radix	6 g.

In cases of depleted kidney yin with vacuity fire, producing red cheeks, vexing heat in the five hearts, red tongue with little coating and rapid thready pulse, the prescription is modified to nourish yin and downbear fire.

Delete:

bā jǐ tiān	morinda [root]	Morindae Radix
tù sī zǐ	cuscuta [seed]	Cuscutae Semen
ròu cōng róng	cistanche [stem]	Cistanches Caulis

Add:

zhī mǔ	anemarrhena [root]	Anemarrhenae Rhizoma	9 g.
huáng bǎi	phellodendron [bark]	Phellodendri Cortex	9 g.

In cases of depleted kidney yang, the above prescription may be used in conjunction with Right-Restoring [Kidney Yang] Pill *(yòu guī wán)* to warm the kidney and assist yang.

Right-Restoring [Kidney Yang] Pill *yòu guī wán*

shú dì huáng	cooked rehmannia [root]	Rehmanniae Radix Conquita	24 g.
shān yào	dioscorea [root]	Dioscoreae Rhizoma	12 g.
shān zhū yú	cornus [fruit]	Corni Fructus	9 g.
gǒu qǐ zǐ	lycium [berry]	Lycii Fructus	12 g.
lù jiǎo jiāo	deerhorn glue (dissolved and stirred in)	Cervi Gelatinum Cornu	12 g.
tù sī zǐ	cuscuta [seed]	Cuscutae Semen	12 g.
dù zhòng	eucommia [bark]	Eucommiae Cortex	12 g.
dāng guī	tangkuei	Angelicae Sinensis Radix	9 g.
ròu guì	cinnamon [bark] (abbreviated decoction)	Cinnamomi Cortex	6 g.
zhì fù zǐ	aconite [accessory tuber] (processed) (extended decoction)	Aconiti Tuber Laterale Praeparatum	6 g.

ACUPUNCTURE AND MOXIBUSTION

Main Points: Needle with even supplementation, even draining; add moxibustion.

BL-28	*páng guāng shū*
CV-03	*zhōng jí*
SP-09	*yīn líng quán*
CV-06	*qì hǎi*
ST-36	*zú sān lǐ*

ALTERNATE THERAPEUTIC METHODS

1. Ear Acupuncture

Main Points: Urinary Bladder, Kidney, Sympathetic, Adrenal.

Method: Select two to four points each session, needle to elicit a strong sensation and retain needles for twenty to thirty minutes. Treat once daily, ten sessions per therapeutic course.

2. Electro-Acupuncture

Main Points:

BL-23	*shèn shū*
SP-06	*sān yīn jiāo*

Method: Apply high frequency electric pulse for five to ten minutes daily.

REMARKS

The diagnosis and treatment of strangury calls for a clear distinction between the various types of urinary disturbance and the differentiation of repletion and vacuity.

Clinically, repletion patterns are characterized as damp-heat of the lower burner. Treatment emphasizes clearing heat and draining dampness. Vacuity patterns are characterized as vacuity of the spleen and kidney, with treatment emphasizing the strengthening of the spleen and kidney. Presentation of patterns exhibiting both repletion and vacuity requires concurrent draining and supplementation. Cases may be further complicated by presenting two types of strangury simultaneously. Also, mutual transformation between different patterns of urinary disturbance is possible.

In ancient classics, diaphoresis and supplementation are both contraindicated in the treatment of strangury. According to clinical experience, however, this does not always or necessarily apply. In cases of urinary disturbance that present symptoms of external evil, or cases of urinary disturbance that are later exposed to external attack, symptoms can include aversion to cold, fever, stuffy runny nose, cough and sore throat. In these cases, treatment should include cool pungent medicines to relieve the external patterns.

The contraindication of supplementation in treating strangury should only apply to cases exhibiting repletion of damp-heat. Treatment of strangury caused by vacuity of the spleen and kidney requires medicinals to supplement the spleen and kidney and thus the ancient warning does not apply.

DRIBBLING URINARY BLOCK

Lóng Bì

1. Bladder Damp-Heat - 2. Exuberant Lung Heat Congestion - 3. Liver Qi Stagnation - 4. Internal Obstruction by Static Blood - 5. Spleen Qi Vacuity - 6. Exhaustion of Kidney Yang

Dribbling urinary block *(lóng bì)* refers to conditions characterized by diminished volume of urine, dribbling urination and, in its extreme, complete cessation of the passage of urine without accompanying pain. *Lóng* describes milder conditions in which urination is difficult, volume is diminished and the urine dribbles instead of flowing freely. *Bì*, on the other hand, describes more severe cases where there is complete cessation of urination. Although *lóng* and *bì* are distinct from one another, both refer to difficulty in urination, differing as regards severity. Hence the compound *lóng bì*. Clinically, *lóng bì* includes difficulty in urination and retention of urine because of organic and functional pathological changes of the urinary bladder, urethra and prostate gland, as well as weakened kidney function and kidney failure.

ETIOLOGY AND PATHOGENESIS

Dysfunction of the urinary bladder in storing and discharging urine is the principal element in the development of retention of urine, although dysfunction of the lung, spleen, kidney and triple burner can also be involved. Commonly observed patterns include damp-heat of the urinary bladder, exuberant lung heat congestion, spleen qi vacuity and exhaustion of kidney yang. Other causes of urinary retention include liver qi stagnation disrupting the triple burner's function of regulating the waterways, or static blood obstruction blocking the urinary tract.

1. BLADDER DAMP-HEAT

Clinical Manifestations: Dribbling urination or an extremely small volume of dark urine with burning sensation on urination, lower abdominal distention and fullness, sticky bitter taste in the mouth, thirst without desire for drink and, in some cases, difficult bowel movements.

Tongue: Red with yellow slimy coating.

Pulse: Rapid, slippery.

Treatment Method: Clear heat, disinhibit dampness, free and disinhibit the urine.

PRESCRIPTION

Eight Corrections Powder *bā zhèng săn*

chē qián zǐ	plantago [seed] (wrapped)	Plantaginis Semen	12 g.
qū mài	dianthus	Dianthi Herba	9 g.
biăn xù	knotgrass	Polygoni Avicularis Herba	9 g.
huá shí	talcum (wrapped)	Talcum	15 g.
shān zhī zǐ	gardenia [fruit]	Gardeniae Fructus	9 g.
mù tōng	mutong [stem]	Mutong Caulis	9 g.
shú dà huáng	(wine-cooked) rhubarb	Rhei Rhizoma Conquitum	9 g.
zhì gān căo	licorice [root] (honey-fried)	Glycyrrhizae Radix	6 g.
dēng xīn căo	juncus [pith]	Junci Medulla	3 g.

MODIFICATIONS

In cases with yellow thick slimy tongue coating, the prescription is modified to reinforce heat-clearing and dampness-dispelling.
Add:

cāng zhú	atractylodes [root]	Atractylodis Rhizoma	9 g.
huáng băi	phellodendron [bark]	Phellodendri Cortex	9 g.

In cases accompanied by vexation in the heart and sores on the tongue and mouth, the prescription is changed to clear heart fire and drain damp-heat. Combine the preceding prescription with:

Red-Abducting Powder *dăo chì săn*

shēng dì huáng	rehmannia [root] dried/fresh	Rehmanniae Radix Exsiccata seu Recens	15 g.
mù tōng	mutong [stem]	Mutong Caulis	9 g.
zhú yè	black bamboo [leaf]	Bambusae Folium	9 g.
gān căo	licorice [root]	Glycyrrhizae Radix	6 g.

In cases where chronic damp-heat in the lower burner has injured kidney yin, with symptoms of dry mouth and throat, tidal fever, night sweating, vexing heat in the five hearts and shiny red tongue, the prescription is changed to nourish kidney yin, clear heat and disinhibit dampness.
Use:

Kidney Enriching Gate-Opening Pill *zī shèn tōng guān wán*

zhī mŭ	anemarrhena [root]	Anemarrhenae Rhizoma	12 g.
huáng băi	phellodendron [bark]	Phellodendri Cortex	9 g.
ròu guì	cinnamon [bark] (abbreviated decoction)	Cinnamomi Cortex	1.5 g.
Add:			
shēng dì huáng	rehmannia [root] dried/fresh	Rehmanniae Radix Exsiccata seu Recens	12 g.
niú xī	achyranthes [root]	Achyranthis Bidentatae Radix	9 g.
chē qián zǐ	plantago [seed] wrapped)	Plantaginis Semen	12 g.

In cases of congestion of the triple burner with accumulated damp-heat, with symptoms of a very small volume of urine or anuria, dark gloomy complexion, oppression in the chest, agitation, nausea, vomiting, urine-like halitosis and, in severe cases, delirium and mental confusion, the prescription is changed to clear heat, transform dampness, harmonize the stomach and free and disinhibit the urine.

Use:

Coptis Gallbladder-Warming Decoction *huáng lián wēn dǎn tāng*

huáng lián	coptis [root]	Coptidis Rhizoma	6 g.
jiāng bàn xià	(ginger-processed) pinellia [tuber]	Pinelliae Tuber Praeparatum	6 g.
chén pí	tangerine [peel]	Citri Exocarpium	9 g.
fú líng	poria	Poria	9 g.
zhǐ shí	unripe bitter orange	Aurantii Fructus Immaturus	9 g.
zhú rú	bamboo shavings	Bambusae Caulis in Taeniam	6 g.
gān cǎo	licorice [root] (honey-fried)	Glycyrrhizae Radix	6 g.
dà zǎo	jujube	Ziziphi Fructus	2 pc.

Add:

chē qián zǐ	plantago [seed] (wrapped)	Plantaginis Semen	12 g.
bái máo gēn	imperata [root]	Imperatae Rhizoma	30 g.
mù tōng	mutong [stem]	Mutong Caulis	3 g.

ACUPUNCTURE AND MOXIBUSTION

Main points: Needle with draining.

BL-28	*páng guāng shū*
CV-03	*zhōng jí*
SP-06	*sān yīn jiāo*
SP-09	*yīn líng quán*

Auxiliary points:

For mental confusion, add:

GV-26	*shuǐ gōu*
PC-09	*zhōng chōng* (bleed)

2. EXUBERANT LUNG HEAT CONGESTION

Clinical Manifestations: Difficulty in urination or retention of urine, dry throat, excessive thirst, sensation of heat in the chest, short rapid breathing, coughing in some cases.

Tongue: Thin yellow coating.

Pulse: Rapid.

Treatment Method: Clear lung heat, free and disinhibit the urine.

PRESCRIPTION

Lung-Clearing Beverage *qīng fèi yǐn*

fú líng	poria	Poria	12 g.
huáng qín	scutellaria [root]	Scutellariae Radix	9 g.
sāng bái pí	mulberry [root bark]	Mori Radicis Cortex	12 g.
mài mén dōng	ophiopogon [tuber]	Ophiopogonis Tuber	9 g.
chē qián zǐ	plantago [seed] (wrapped)	Plantaginis Semen	12 g.
shān zhī zǐ	gardenia [fruit]	Gardeniae Fructus	9 g.
mù tōng	mutong [stem]	Mutong Caulis	9 g.

MODIFICATIONS

In cases of rising heart fire, with symptoms of vexation in the heart and red tongue tip, the prescription is modified to clear heart fire. Add:

huáng lián	coptis [root]	Coptidis Rhizoma	9 g.
zhú yè	black bamboo [leaf]	Bambusae Folium	12 g.

In cases of lung yin vacuity presenting red tongue with little coating, the prescription is modified to nourish lung yin.

Add:

běi shā shēn	glehnia [root]	Glehniae Radix	12 g.
bǎi hé	lily [bulb]	Lilii Bulbus	12 g.

In cases of constipation, the prescription is modified to diffuse the lung and free the stool.

Add:

dà huáng	rhubarb (abbreviated decoction)	Rhei Rhizoma	9 g.
xìng rén	apricot [kernel] (abbreviated decoction)	Armeniacae Semen	9 g.

In cases manifesting external patterns, with stuffy nose, headache and floating pulse, the prescription is modified to relieve the exterior and diffuse the lung.

Add:

bò hé	mint (abbreviated decoction)	Menthae Herba	6 g.
jié gěng	platycodon [root]	Platycodonis Radix	9 g.

ACUPUNCTURE AND MOXIBUSTION

Main points: Needle with draining.

LU-05	*chǐ zé*
LI-04	*hé gǔ*
CV-03	*zhōng jí*
BL-28	*páng guāng shū*

Auxiliary points:

For irritability, add:

PC-06	*nèi guān*

3. LIVER QI STAGNATION

Clinical Manifestations: Difficulty in urination accompanied by emotional depression or irritability, distention and fullness of the lower abdomen and hypochondrium.

Tongue: Thin white or yellow coating.

Pulse: Wiry.

Treatment Method: Soothe the liver, regulate qi, free and disinhibit the urine.

PRESCRIPTION

Aquilaria Powder *chén xiāng sǎn*

chén xiāng	aquilaria [wood] (powdered and stirred in)	Aquilariae Lignum	1.5 g.
shí wéi	pyrrosia [leaf]	Pyrrosiae Folium	9 g.
huá shí	talcum (wrapped)	Talcum	12 g.
dāng guī	tangkuei	Angelicae Sinensis Radix	6 g.
bái sháo yào	white peony [root]	Paeoniae Radix Alba	9 g.
chén pí	tangerine [peel]	Citri Exocarpium	9 g.
dōng kuí zǐ	mallow [seed]	Malvae Verticillatae Semen	9 g.
wáng bù liú xíng	vaccaria [seed]	Vaccariae Semen	9 g.
gān cǎo	licorice [root]	Glycyrrhizae Radix	6 g.

MODIFICATIONS

To increase the prescription's liver-smoothing and qi regulation, add:

xiāng fù zǐ	cyperus [root]	Cyperi Rhizoma	9 g.
yù jīn	curcuma [tuber]	Curcumae Tuber	9 g.
wū yào	lindera [root]	Linderae Radix	9 g.

In cases of stagnant qi giving rise to fire, the prescription is modified to clear the liver and drain fire. Add:

mǔ dān pí	moutan [root bark]	Moutan Radicis Cortex	9 g.
lóng dǎn cǎo	gentian [root]	Gentianae Radix	6 g.
shān zhī zǐ	gardenia [fruit]	Gardeniae Fructus	9 g.

ACUPUNCTURE AND MOXIBUSTION

Main points: Needle with draining.

LR-03	*tài chōng*
BL-39 (53)	*wěi yáng*
CV-03	*zhōng jí*
BL-28	*páng guāng shū*

Auxiliary points:
For costal pain, add:

GB-34	*yáng líng quán*

4. INTERNAL OBSTRUCTION BY STAGNANT BLOOD

Clinical Manifestations: Retention of urine following traumatic injury or surgery, lower abdominal fullness and distention.

Tongue: Dark, purple; sometimes presenting stasis macules on the tongue.

Pulse: Rough.

Treatment Method: Invigorate the blood, dispel stasis, free and disinhibit the urine.

PRESCRIPTION

Substitute Dead-On Pill *dài dǐ dàng wán*

shú dà huáng	(wine-cooked) rhubarb	Rhei Rhizoma Conquitum	9 g.
dāng guī wěi	tangkuei tail	Angelicae Sinensis Radicis Extremitas	9 g.
shēng dì huáng	rehmannia [root] dried/fresh	Rehmanniae Radix Exsiccata seu Recens	6 g.
chuān shān jiǎ	pangolin [scales]	Manitis Squama	9 g.
táo rén	peach [kernel]	Persicae Semen	9 g.
máng xiāo	mirabilite (stirred in)	Mirabilitum	9 g.
ròu guì	cinnamon [bark] (abbreviated decoction)	Cinnamomi Cortex	3 g.

MODIFICATIONS

To reinforce the ability of the prescription to quicken the blood and dispel stasis, add:

hóng huā	carthamus [flower]	Carthami Flos	6 g.
niú xī	achyranthes [root]	Achyranthis Bidentatae Radix	9 g.

In cases of prolonged illness where both qi and blood have been depleted and the complexion is lusterless, the prescription is modified to supplement qi and nourish the blood.

Add:

| *huáng qí* | astragalus [root] | Astragali (seu Hedysari) Radix | 15 g. |
| *dān shēn* | salvia [root] | Salviae Miltiorrhizae Radix | 12 g. |

In cases of acute and complete cessation of urination, with unbearable distention of the lower abdomen, the prescription is changed to open the orifices and free and disinhibit the urine.

Add:

| *shè xiāng* | musk (stirred in) | Moschus | 0.1 g. |

ACUPUNCTURE AND MOXIBUSTION

Main points: Needle with draining.

CV-03	*zhōng jí*
SP-06	*sān yīn jiāo*
ST-28	*shuǐ dào*
KI-05	*shuǐ quán*

Auxiliary points:

In cases of prolonged illness with vacuity of both qi and blood, add:

| CV-04 | *guān yuán* |
| ST-36 | *zú sān lǐ* |

5. SPLEEN QI VACUITY

Clinical Manifestations: Lower abdominal bearing-down sensation and distention, retention of urine with periodic urge to urinate, passage of small volume of urine and discomfort during urination in some cases, fatigue, tiredness, loss of appetite, shortness of breath, weak voice.

Tongue: Pale with thin coating.

Pulse: Weak, thready.

Treatment Method: Supplement the spleen, boost qi, free and disinhibit the urine.

PRESCRIPTION

Combine Center-Supplementing Qi-Boosting Decoction *(bǔ zhōng yì qì tāng)* with Poria (Hoelen) Five Powder *(wǔ líng sǎn)*.

Center-Supplementing Qi-Boosting Decoction *bǔ zhōng yì qì tāng*

huáng qí	astragalus [root]	Astragali (seu Hedysari) Radix	15 g.
rén shēn	ginseng	Ginseng Radix	9 g.
bái zhú	ovate atractylodes [root]	Atractylodis Ovatae Rhizoma	9 g.
dāng guī	tangkuei	Angelicae Sinensis Radix	9 g.
chén pí	tangerine [peel]	Citri Exocarpium	6 g.
shēng má	cimicifuga [root]	Cimicifugae Rhizoma	3 g.
chái hú	bupleurum [root]	Bupleuri Radix	3 g.
zhì gān cǎo	licorice [root] (honey-fried)	Glycyrrhizae Radix	6 g.

with:

Poria (Hoelen) Five Powder *wǔ líng sǎn*

fú líng	poria	Poria	9 g.
zhū líng	polyporus	Polyporus	9 g.
zé xiè	alisma [tuber]	Alismatis Rhizoma	15 g.
bái zhú	ovate atractylodes [root]	Atractylodis Ovatae Rhizoma	9 g.
guì zhī	cinnamon [twig]	Cinnamomi Ramulus	6 g.

ACUPUNCTURE AND MOXIBUSTION

Main points: Needle with supplementation; add moxibustion.

BL-20	*pí shū*
ST-36	*zú sān lǐ*
SP-09	*yīn líng quán*
CV-03	*zhōng jí*
BL-22	*sān jiāo shū*

Auxiliary points:

For anal prolapse, add:

BL-32	*cì liáo*

6. Exhaustion of Kidney Yang

Clinical Manifestations: Retention of urine or dribbling, uncomfortable urination, weakened force of urinary expulsion, pale complexion, tiredness, physical cold, weakness, aching and cold in the lower back and knees.

Tongue: Pale with white coating.

Pulse: Deep, weak.

Treatment Method: Warm and supplement kidney yang, free and disinhibit the urine.

PRESCRIPTION

Life Saver Kidney Qi Pill *jì shēng shèn qì wán**

shú dì huáng	cooked rehmannia [root]	Rehmanniae Radix Conquita	6 g.
shān yào	dioscorea [root]	Dioscoreae Rhizoma	12 g.
shān zhū yú	cornus [fruit]	Corni Fructus	12 g.
zé xiè	alisma [tuber]	Alismatis Rhizoma	12 g.
fú líng	poria	Poria	12 g.
mǔ dān pí	moutan [root bark]	Moutan Radicis Cortex	12 g.
zhì fù zǐ	aconite [accessory tuber] (processed) (extended decoction)	Processed Aconiti Tuber Laterale	6 g.
ròu guì	cinnamon bark (abbreviated decoction)	Cinnamomi Cortex	6 g.
chuān niú xī	cyathula [root]	Cyathulae Radix	6 g.
chē qián zǐ	plantago [seed] (wrapped)	Plantaginis Semen	12 g.

*Author's note: Life Saver Kidney Qi Pill (*jì shēn shèn qì wán*) is a prescription from *Jì Shēng Fāng* (*Prescriptions for Succoring the Sick*) compiled by Yan Yonghe during the southern Song dynasty.

MODIFICATIONS

In cases of elderly patients with qi vacuity, the prescription is modified to warm yang and boost qi. Add:

rén shēn	ginseng	Ginseng Radix	9 g.
lù jiǎo jiāo	deerhorn glue	Cervi Gelatinum Cornu	9 g.

ACUPUNCTURE AND MOXIBUSTION

Main points: Needle with supplementation; add moxibustion.

BL-23	*shèn shū*
CV-04	*guān yuán*
KI-10	*yīn gǔ*
CV-06	*qì hǎi*
BL-22	*sān jiāo shū*

Auxiliary points:

For elderly patients with weak constitutions where both the spleen and kidney are depleted, add moxibustion to:

GV-20	*bǎi huì*
ST-36	*zú sān lǐ*

ALTERNATE THERAPEUTIC METHODS

1. Ear Acupuncture

Main points: Urinary bladder, Kidney, Urethra, Triple Burner.

Method: Select two or three points per session, needle to elicit a moderate sensation. Retain needle forty to sixty minutes, apply manipulation at ten to fifteen-minute intervals.

2. Electro-Acupuncture

Method: Select bilateral GB-28 *(wéi dào)*. Needle horizontally beneath the skin in the direction of CV-02 *(qū gǔ)*. Apply appropriate electric current for fifteen to thirty minutes.

3. Moxibustion with Acupressure

Method: First, apply moxibustion to CV-04 *(guān yuán)* and CV-06 *(qì hǎi)* for twenty minutes with a moxa roll. Afterward, use the thumb to press and knead lower abdominal acupoints in the region of the urinary bladder. Begin with mild pressure and gradually increase to heavy pressure. The above manipulations will stimulate the circulation of qi and blood, promoting urination.

REMARKS

In the treatment of dribbling urinary block, differentiation should first be made between repletion and vacuity. Repletion patterns call for clearing damp-heat, regulating qi and dispersing blood stasis to open the water passages. Vacuity patterns, on the other hand, require supplementation of the spleen and kidney and restoration of normal water metabolism.

In cases of complete cessation of urination, various physical manipulations are often used, including acumoxa therapy. These techniques are simple and give notable results, making them adaptable to many situations. During acumoxa therapy, however, attention should be paid to the degree of distention of the bladder. Acupoints in the lower abdomen should be needled superficially with an oblique insertion. Deep needling and vertical insertion is contraindicated when distention of the bladder is significant.

DEPRESSION PATTERNS
Yù Zhèng

1. Stagnation of Liver Qi - 2. Transformation of Static Qi into Fire - 3. Obstruction by Static Qi and Phlegm - 4. Vacuity of Yin and Blood

Yù zhèng refers to a class of patterns stemming from emotional disturbance that are characterized by stagnation and obstruction of the flow of qi. Clinical manifestations of depression include despondence, moodiness, a trancelike mental state, melancholy or bouts of crying. There may also be costal pain and distention and an uncomfortable sensation in the throat as if obstructed by some object.

Stagnant qi untreated over a period of time can give rise to stagnation of blood, phlegm, dampness, heat or food matter. Collectively known as *liù yù* (six depressions), all are initiated by stagnation of qi, and correct treatment looks at stagnation of qi as the major pathological change. The scope of such patterns includes the biomedical disorders of neurosis, hysteria, manic-depression (depressive phase) and menopausal pattern.

ETIOLOGY AND PATHOGENESIS

Depression is caused by internal disruption from emotional factors, including internalized anger, anxiety, overthinking or grief. All these can lead to functional disturbance and pathological changes in the viscera and bowels. Dysfunction of the liver in maintaining the free flow of qi, dysfunction of the spleen in transportation and transformation and disturbance of heart spirit constitute the major etiology and pathogenesis of depression.

During the initial stages of illness, patterns are often of repletion and involve accumulation of phlegm-dampness, food matter or heat as a result of the stagnation of qi. Prolonged cases of depression can injure the yin and blood; therefore, depression patterns typically follow a repletion to vacuity development.

1. STAGNATION OF LIVER QI

Clinical Manifestations: Despondence, distention and pain of the chest and hypochondrium, epigastric fullness, belching, frequent sighing, abdominal distention, loss of appetite, vomiting in some cases, abnormal bowel movements or amenorrhea.

Tongue: Thin white coating.

Pulse: Wiry.

Treatment Method: Soothe the liver, regulate qi, relieve depression.

PRESCRIPTION

Bupleurum Liver-Coursing Powder *chái hú shū gān sǎn*

chái hú	bupleurum [root]	Bupleuri Radix	6 g.
bái sháo yào	white peony [root]	Paeoniae Radix Alba	9 g.
xiāng fù zǐ	cyperus [root]	Cyperi Rhizoma	6 g.
chuān xiōng	ligusticum [root]	Ligustici Rhizoma	6 g.
chén pí	tangerine [peel]	Citri Exocarpium	6 g.
zhǐ ké	bitter orange [fruit]	Aurantii Fructus	6 g.
zhì gān cǎo	licorice [root] (honey-fried)	Glycyrrhizae Radix	3 g.

MODIFICATIONS

To assist invigoration of liver qi in relieving depression, add:

yù jīn	curcuma [tuber]	Curcumae Tuber	9 g.
qīng pí	unripe tangerine [peel]	Citri Exocarpium Immaturum	9 g.

In cases of frequent belching accompanied by epigastric and thoracic discomfort, the prescription is modified to soothe the liver and move qi downward. Add:

xuán fù huā	inula [flower] (wrapped)	Inulae Flos	9 g.
dài zhě shí	hematite (extended decoction)	Haematitum	12 g.

In cases accompanied by food stasis and abdominal distention, the prescription is modified to disperse food and remove food stagnation. Add:

shén qū	medicated leaven	Massa Medicata Fermentata	12 g.
shān zhā	crataegus [fruit]	Crataegi Fructus	12 g.
jī nèi jīn	gizzard lining	Galli Gigerii Endothelium	9 g.

In cases of pain of fixed location in the thorax and hypochondrium, sometimes accompanied by amenorrhea in female patients and a rough pulse, the prescription is modified to invigorate the blood and dispel blood stasis. Add:

dāng guī	tangkuei	Angelicae Sinensis Radix	9 g.
dān shēn	salvia [root]	Salviae Miltiorrhizae Radix	12 g.
táo rén	peach [kernel]	Persicae Semen	6 g.
hóng huā	carthamus [flower]	Carthami Flos	6 g.

ACUPUNCTURE AND MOXIBUSTION

Main Points: Needle with even supplementation and draining.

BL-18	*gān shū*
LR-03	*tài chōng*
CV-17	*tǎn zhōng*
CV-12	*zhōng wǎn*
ST-36	*zú sān lǐ*

Auxiliary points:

For oppression in the chest and vomiting, add:

PC-06	*nèi guān*
SP-04	*gōng sūn*

For signs of blood stasis, add:

BL-17	*gé shū*
SP-06	*sān yīn jiāo*

2. Transformation of Static Qi into Fire

Clinical Manifestations: Agitation, irritability, oppression in the chest, distention of the hypochondrium, acid regurgitation, clamoring stomach, dry bitter taste in the mouth, constipation, headache, bloodshot eyes and tinnitus.

Tongue: Red with yellow coating.

Pulse: Rapid, wiry.

Treatment Method: Clear the liver, drain fire, calm the stomach, relieve depression.

PRESCRIPTION

Combine Moutan and Gardenia Free Wanderer Powder *(dān zhī xiāo yáo săn)* with Evodia and Coptis Pill (Left Metal Pill) *(yú lián wán [zuŏ jīn wán])*

Moutan and Gardenia Free Wanderer Powder *dān zhī xiāo yáo săn*

chái hú	bupleurum [root]	Bupleuri Radix	9 g.
bái sháo yào	white peony [root]	Paeoniae Radix Alba	12 g.
dāng guī	tangkuei [root]	Angelicae Sinensis Radix	9 g.
bái zhú	ovate atractylodes [root]	Atractylodis Ovatae Rhizoma	9 g.
fú líng	poria	Poria	9 g.
mŭ dān pí	moutan [root bark]	Moutan Radicis Cortex	9 g.
shān zhī zĭ	gardenia [fruit]	Gardeniae Fructus	9 g.
zhì gān căo	licorice [root] (honey-fried)	Glycyrrhizae Radix	6 g.
shēng jiāng	fresh ginger	Zingiberis Rhizoma Recens	3 g.
bò hé	mint (abbreviated decoction)	Menthae Herba	3 g.

with:

Evodia and Coptis Pill (Left Metal Pill) *yú lián wán (zuŏ jīn wán)*

huáng lián	coptis [root]	Coptidis Rhizoma	180 g.
wú zhū yú	evodia [fruit]	Evodiae Fructus	30 g.

Grind the above herbs into a powder and make into pills. Take a two to three gram dosage twice daily with water. The two herbs may also be decocted in water, the proportion of coptis *(huáng lián)* to evodia *(wú zhū yú)* being six to one.

MODIFICATIONS

In cases of bitter taste in the mouth, yellow tongue coating and constipation, the prescription is modified to drain fire and free the stool. Add:

lóng dăn căo	gentian [root]	Gentianae Radix	6 g.
dà huáng	rhubarb (abbreviated decoction)	Rhei Rhizoma	9 g.

ACUPUNCTURE AND MOXIBUSTION

Main Points: Needle with draining.

LR-02	*xíng jiān*
GB-34	*yáng líng quán*
GB-43	*xiá xī*
CV-13	*shàng wăn*

Auxiliary Points:

For constipation, add:

TB-6	*zhī gōu*

3. Obstruction by Static Qi and Phlegm

Clinical Manifestations: Discomfort in the throat as if obstructed by a plum pit, relief brought neither by coughing nor swallowing, sensation of congestion and blockage in the chest, costal pain.

Tongue: White slimy coating.

Pulse: Wiry, slippery.

Treatment Method: Regulate qi, transform phlegm, dissipate binds, relieve depression.

PRESCRIPTION

Pinellia and Magnolia Bark Decoction *bàn xià hòu pò tāng*

fǎ bàn xià	pinellia [tuber] (processed)	Pinelliae Tuber Praeparatum	12 g.
hòu pò	magnolia [bark]	Magnoliae Cortex	9 g.
fú líng	poria	Poria	12 g.
shēng jiāng	fresh ginger	Zingiberis Rhizoma Recens	9 g.
zǐ sū yè	perilla [leaf] (abbreviated decoction).	Perillae Folium	6 g

MODIFICATIONS

The prescription may be modified to reinforce the effects of regulating qi, dissolving phlegm and relieving depression.

Add:

xiāng fù zǐ	cyperus [root]	Cyperi Rhizoma	9 g.
zhǐ ké	bitter orange	Aurantii Fructus	9 g.
fó shǒu gān	Buddha's hand [fruit]	Citri Sarcodactylidis Fructus	9 g.
xuán fù huā	inula [flower] (wrapped)	Inulae Flos	9 g.
dài zhě shí	hematite (extended decoction)	Haematitum	12 g.

In cases accompanied by vomiting, bitter taste in the mouth and yellow slimy tongue coating, the pattern is one of phlegm-heat and the prescription is changed to transform phlegm and clear heat.

Use:

Gallbladder-Warming Decoction *wēn dǎn tāng*

fǎ bàn xià	pinellia [tuber] (processed)	Pinelliae Tuber Praeparatum	6 g.
zhú rú	bamboo shavings	Bambusae Caulis in Taeniam	6 g.
zhǐ shí	unripe bitter orange	Aurantii Fructus Immaturus	6 g.
chén pí	tangerine [peel]	Citri Exocarpium	6 g.
zhì gān cǎo	licorice [root] (honey-fried)	Glycyrrhizae Radix	6 g.
fú líng	poria	Poria	9 g.
shēng jiāng	fresh ginger	Zingiberis Rhizoma Recens	2 pc.
dà zǎo	jujube	Ziziphi Fructus	3 pc.

Add:

huáng qín	scutellaria [root]	Scutellariae Radix	9 g.
zhè bèi mǔ	Zhejiang fritillaria [bulb]	Fritillariae Verticillatae Bulbus	9 g.
guā lóu pí	trichosanthes [rind]	Trichosanthis Pericarpium	9 g.

ACUPUNCTURE AND MOXIBUSTION

Main Points: Needle with even supplementation, even draining.

CV-17	*tǎn zhōng*
PC-06	*nèi guān*
LR-03	*tài chōng*
ST-40	*fēng lóng*
CV-22	*tiān tú*
CV-12	*zhōng wǎn*

Auxiliary Points:

For costal pain, add:

LR-14	*qī mén*

4. VACUITY OF YIN AND BLOOD

Clinical Manifestations: Hysteria, trance-like mental state, susceptibility to fright, agitation, restlessness, abnormal emotional reactions, suspiciousness, spells of grief and crying without apparent reason, irregular manifestations of happiness and anger, initiation of symptoms by random psychological stimuli (most often observed in female patients), presentation of sudden oppression in the chest, deafness, loss of voice or convulsions and disturbance of consciousness in severe cases.

Tongue: Pale with thin white coating.

Pulse: Thready, wiry.

Treatment Method: Nourish the heart, quiet the spirit.

PRESCRIPTION

Licorice, Wheat and Jujube Decoction *gān mài dà zǎo tāng*

gān cǎo	licorice [root]	Glycyrrhizae Radix	9 g.
xiǎo mài	wheat	Tritici Semen	30 g.
dà zǎo	jujube	Ziziphi Fructus	10 pc.

MODIFICATIONS

The prescription may be modified to increase its effects.

Add:

bǎi zǐ rén	biota [seed]	Biotae Semen	15 g.
suān zǎo rén	spiny jujube [kernel]	Ziziphi Spinosi Semen	15 g.
fú shén	root poria	Poria cum Pini Radice	9 g.
hé huān huā	silk tree [flower]	Albizziae Flos	6 g.

In cases accompanied by epigastric fullness and discomfort, loss of appetite, palpitations, insomnia, tiredness, lusterless complexion, pale tongue and weak thready pulse, the pattern is vacuity of both the heart and spleen. The prescription is changed to fortify the spleen, nourish the heart, quiet the spirit and relieve depression.

Use:

Spleen-Returning Decoction *guī pí tāng*

huáng qí	astragalus [root]	Astragali (seu Hedysari) Radix	9 g.
rén shēn	ginseng	Ginseng Radix	9 g.
bái zhú	ovate atractylodes [root]	Atractylodis Ovatae Rhizoma	9 g.
fú shén	root poria	Poria cum Pini Radice	9 g.
lóng yǎn ròu	longan [flesh]	Longanae Arillus	9 g.
suān zǎo rén	spiny jujube [kernel]	Ziziphi Spinosi Semen	9 g.
mù xiāng	saussurea [root]	Saussureae Radix (seu Vladimiriae)	6 g.
dāng guī	tangkuei [root]	Angelicae Sinensis Radix	6 g.
yuǎn zhì	polygala [root]	Polygalae Radix	3 g.
zhì gān cǎo	licorice [root] (honey-fried)	Glycyrrhizae Radix	6 g.
shēng jiāng	fresh ginger	Zingiberis Rhizoma Recens	3 g.
dà zǎo	jujube	Ziziphi Fructus	5 pc.

plus:

yù jīn	curcuma [tuber]	Curcumae Tuber	9 g.
hé huān huā	silk tree [flower]	Albizziae Flos	6 g.

In cases accompanied by dizziness and vertigo, tinnitus, vexing heat in the five hearts, excessive perspiration, lower backache, forgetfulness, insomnia, red tongue with little coating and rapid thready pulse, the pattern is one of yin vacuity with hyperactive fire. The prescription is changed to nourish yin, clear heat, settle the heart and quiet the spirit. Use:

Water-Enriching Liver-Clearing Beverage *zī shuǐ qīng gān yǐn*

shēng dì huáng	rehmannia [root] dried/fresh	Rehmanniae Radix Exsiccata seu Recens	24 g.
shān zhū yú	cornus [fruit]	Corni Fructus	12 g.
shān yào	dioscorea [root]	Dioscoreae Rhizoma	12 g.
fú líng	poria	Poria	9 g.
mǔ dān pí	moutan [root bark]	Moutan Radicis Cortex	9 g.
zé xiè	alisma [tuber]	Alismatis Rhizoma	9 g.
chái hú	bupleurum [root]	Bupleuri Radix	6 g.
bái sháo yào	white peony [root]	Paeoniae Radix Alba	12 g.
dāng guī	tangkuei	Angelicae Sinensis Radix	9 g.
shān zhī zǐ	gardenia	Gardeniae Fructus	6 g.
suān zǎo rén	spiny jujube [kernel]	Ziziphi Spinosae Semen	15 g.

plus:

zhēn zhū mǔ	mother-of-pearl (extended decoction)	Concha Margaritifera	30 g.
cí shí	loadstone (extended decoction)	Magnetitum	30 g.

ACUPUNCTURE AND MOXIBUSTION

Main Points: Needle with even supplementation, even draining.

CV-14	*jù què*
HT-07	*shén mén*
SP-06	*sān yīn jiāo*
ST-36	*zú sān lǐ*
LI-04	*hé gǔ*

Auxiliary points:

For oppression in the chest, add:

CV-17	*tǎn zhōng*
PC-06	*nèi guān*

For deafness, add:

GB-02   *tīng huì*
TB-03   *zhōng zhǔ*

For sudden loss of voice, add:

HT-05   *tōng lǐ*
CV-23   *lián quán*

For convulsions, add:

LR-03   *tài chōng*
GB-34   *yáng líng quán*

For hiccough, add:

CV-12   *zhōng wǎn*

For lockjaw, add:

ST-06   *jiá chē*

For disturbance or loss of consciousness, add:

GV-26   *shuǐ gōu*
KI-01   *yǒng quán*

For yin vacuity with effulgent fire, add:

BL-23   *shèn shū*
KI-03   *tài xī*

For vacuity of heart and spleen, add:

BL-15   *xīn shū*
BL-20   *pí shū*

ALTERNATE THERAPEUTIC METHODS

1. Ear Acupuncture

Main Points: Heart, Subcortex, Occipital, Brain, Liver, Endocrine, *Shén Mén*, plus points corresponding to site of pathological changes.

Method: When patients are in a state of depression, use filiform needles to puncture selected points of both ears. Needle to elicit a strong sensation and retain needles for twenty minutes. Treat once every two days, five to ten sessions per therapeutic course.

During remission, needle embedding therapy may be used.

REMARKS

Patterns of depression are categorized as repletion or vacuity. Repletion patterns usually present during the initial stages of illness. Treatment is directed at soothing the liver and regulating qi. Depending on the clinical manifestations, this can be accompanied by invigorating blood, dissolving phlegm, transforming dampness, purging heat or removing food stasis.

Prolonged cases are generally vacuous; treatment is to nourish the blood, moisten yin and disinhibit qi. During the later stages of illness, dry fragrant qi-regulating medicines must be used prudently to avoid further injury to yin and blood.

In addition to herbal medicine and acumoxa therapy, psychological therapy is very important in treating depression. The physician should pay attention to the power of suggestion. The language chosen must be such that it helps the patient to relieve apprehension and that establishes an attitude of certain victory over the illness. Such changes in attitude have a definite beneficial effect on therapeutic results.

Mania and Withdrawal

Diān Kuáng

1. Depressive Psychotic Patterns - 1A. Binding Depression of Qi and Phlegm - 1B. Heart and Spleen Vacuity - 2. Manic Psychotic Patterns - 2A. Phlegm-Fire Harassing the Interior - 2B. Exuberant Fire with Injury to Yin

Mania and withdrawal *(diān kuáng)* is characterized by abnormal psychological or emotional behavior. It corresponds to manic-depressive psychosis in Western medicine. The clinical manifestations of *diān* and *kuáng* differ. Depressive psychosis *(diān)* is characterized by introverted behavior, lethargy, muttering to oneself and stupor or giddiness; while manic psychosis *(kuáng)* is characterized by excitability, violent physical behavior, agitation, insomnia and uncontrollable anger. Although *diān* and *kuáng* are distinct, they have a pathological relationship and mutual transformation is possible, hence the compound *diān kuáng.*

This chapter addresses the differential diagnosis and treatment of such conditions as manic-depression, schizophrenia and catatonic psychosis in Western medicine.

Etiology and Pathogenesis

The major etiologic factor in the development of psychotic patterns is internal disruption from disturbance of the seven affects. Emotional disturbance, combined with disharmony of yin and yang, the viscera and bowels, leads to various pathological changes: stagnation of qi and blood, stagnation of phlegm and qi, or internal disturbance by phlegm and fire. These pathological conditions occur mainly in the liver, gallbladder, heart and spleen.

Diān, or depressive psychotic patterns, are generally brought on by stagnation of phlegm and qi leading to vacuity of both heart and spleen and vacuity of qi and blood. *Kuáng,* or manic psychotic patterns, are generally caused by internal disturbance by phlegm and fire, which can lead to depletion of qi and injury to yin in chronic cases. Psychosis typically presents as a repletion pattern during its initial stages and gradually develops into a vacuity pattern or a pattern complicated by both repletion and vacuity.

Heredity can play a strong role in the occurrence of psychosis; many patients show a family history of mental illness.

1A. DEPRESSIVE PSYCHOTIC PATTERNS — BINDING DEPRESSION OF QI AND PHLEGM

Clinical Manifestations: Gradual onset of illness, emotional depression, with increased dullness of the senses during the initial stages, followed by incoherent speech in later stages or muttering to oneself, unprovoked bouts of sadness and crying, loss of ability to differentiate clean from dirty, loss of appetite.

Tongue: White slimy coating.

Pulse: Wiry, slippery.

Treatment Method: Rectify qi, resolve stagnation, transform phlegm, open the orifices.

PRESCRIPTION

Qi-Normalizing Phlegm-Abducting Decoction *shùn qì dǎo tán tāng*

fǎ bàn xià	pinellia [tuber] (processed)	Pinelliae Tuber Praeparatum	9 g.
chén pí	tangerine [peel]	Citri Exocarpium	9 g.
fú líng	poria	Poria	12 g.
dǎn xīng	[bile-processed] arisaema [root]	Arisaematis Rhizoma cum Felle Bovis	6 g.
zhǐ shí	unripe bitter orange	Aurantii Fructus Immaturus	9 g.
mù xiāng	saussurea [root]	Saussureae Radix (seu Vladimiriae)	9 g.
xiāng fù zǐ	cyperus [root]	Cyperi Rhizoma	9 g.
shēng jiāng	fresh ginger	Zingiberis Rhizoma Recens	9 g.
zhì gān cǎo	licorice root (honey-fried)	Glycyrrhizae Radix	6 g.

MODIFICATIONS

To reinforce qi-regulating, phlegm-dissolving and orifice-opening, add:

yuǎn zhì	polygala [root]	Polygalae Radix	9 g.
yù jīn	curcuma [tuber]	Curcumae Tuber	9 g.
shí chāng pú	acorus [root]	Acori Rhizoma	9 g.

Prior to administration of this prescription, the prepared medicine LIQUID STORAX PILL *(sū-hé-xiāng wán)* can first be prescribed to open the orifices.

In cases of phlegm and qi giving rise to heat, there will be symptoms of insomnia, agitation and a tendency toward being easily frightened, accompanied by signs of red tongue with yellow coating and rapid slippery pulse. The prescription is changed to clear heat and transform phlegm. Combine Coptis Gallbladder-Warming Decoction *(huáng-lián wēn dǎn tāng)* with Alum and Curcuma Pill *(bái jīn wán)*.

Coptis Gallbladder-Warming Decoction *huáng lián wēn dǎn tāng*

huáng lián	coptis [root]	Coptidis Rhizoma	6 g.
fǎ bàn xià	pinellia [tuber] (processed)	Pinelliae Tuber Praeparatum	6 g.
chén pí	tangerine [peel]	Citri Exocarpium	9 g.
fú líng	poria	Poria	9 g.
zhǐ shí	unripe bitter orange	Aurantii Fructus Immaturus	9 g.
zhú rú	bamboo shavings	Bambusae Caulis in Taeniam	6 g.
zhì gān cǎo	licorice [root] (honey-fried)	Glycyrrhizae Radix	3 g.
shēng jiāng	ginger [root] (fresh)	Zingiberis Rhizoma Recens	5 pc.
dà zǎo	jujube	Ziziphi Fructus	1 pc.

with:

Alum and Curcuma Pill *bái jīn wán*

| *bái fán* | alum (powdered and stirred in) | Alumen | 3 g. |
| *yù jīn* | curcuma [tuber] | Curcumae Tuber | 9 g. |

ACUPUNCTURE AND MOXIBUSTION

Main points: Needle with even supplementation, even draining; add moxibustion.

HT-07	*shén mén*
LR-03	*tài chōng*
PC-07	*dà líng*
CV-17	*tǎn zhōng*
M-HN-3	*yìn táng* (Hall of Impression)
ST-40	*fēng lóng*
SP-06	*sān yīn jiāo*

Auxiliary points:

For unprovoked bouts of sadness and crying, add:

| LU-09 | *tài yuān* |

1B. DEPRESSIVE PSYCHOTIC PATTERNS — HEART AND SPLEEN VACUITY

Clinical Manifestations: Chronic duration of illness, trance-like mental state, loss of contact with reality, palpitations, tendency to be easily frightened, fatigue, decrease in food intake, lusterless complexion.

Tongue: Pale.

Pulse: Thready, forceless.

Treatment Method: Strengthen spleen qi, nourish heart blood, boost qi, quiet the spirit.

PRESCRIPTION

Combine Heart-Nourishing Decoction *(yǎng xīn tāng)* with Licorice, Wheat and Jujube Decoction *(gān mài dà zǎo tāng)*.

Heart-Nourishing Decoction *yǎng xīn tāng*

huáng qí	astragalus [root]	Astragali (seu Hedysari) Radix	9 g.
rén shēn	ginseng	Ginseng Radix	9 g.
fú líng	poria	Poria	9 g.
fú shén	root poria	Poria cum Pini Radice	9 g.
dāng guī	tangkuei	Angelicae Sinensis Radix	9 g.
chuān xiōng	ligusticum [root]	Ligustici Rhizoma	6 g.
zhì bàn xià	pinellia [tuber] (processed)	Pinelliae Tuber Praeparatum	6 g.
bǎi zǐ rén	biota [seed]	Biotae Semen	9 g.
yuǎn zhì	polygala [root]	Polygalae Radix	6 g.
suān zǎo rén	spiny jujube [kernel]	Ziziphi Spinosi Semen	15 g.
wǔ wèi zǐ	schisandra [berry]	Schisandrae Fructus	6 g.
ròu guì	cinnamon [bark] (abbreviated decoction)	Cinnamomi Cortex	3 g.
zhì gān cǎo	licorice [root] (honey-fried)	Glycyrrhizae Radix	6 g.

with:

Licorice, Wheat and Jujube Decoction *gān mài dà zǎo tāng*

gān cǎo	licorice [root]	Glycyrrhizae Radix	9 g.
xiǎo mài	wheat	Tritici Semen	30 g.
dà zǎo	jujube	Ziziphi Fructus	10 pc.

ACUPUNCTURE AND MOXIBUSTION

Main points: Needle with supplementation; add moxibustion.

BL-15	*xīn shū*
BL-18	*gān shū*
BL-20	*pí shū*
HT-07	*shén mén*
ST-36	*zú sān lǐ*
SP-06	*sān yīn jiāo*

Auxiliary points:

For tendency towards being easily frightened, add:

PC-07	*dà líng*

2A. MANIC PSYCHOTIC PATTERNS — PHLEGM-FIRE HARASSING THE INTERIOR

Clinical Manifestations: Abrupt onset of illness, with initial symptoms of agitation, irritability, headache, insomnia, flushed complexion and bloodshot eyes, followed by sudden manic behavior, lack of judgment, physical aggression, destructive behavior, spells of boisterousness, cessation of food intake and sleep, exhibitionism in severe cases.

Tongue: Yellow slimy coating.

Pulse: Rapid, wiry, slippery.

Treatment Method: Settle the heart, transform phlegm, drain the liver, clear fire.

PRESCRIPTION

Iron Flakes Beverage *shēng tiě luò yǐn*

tiě luò	iron flakes (extended decoction)*	Ferri Frusta	30 g.
tiān mén dōng	asparagus [tuber]	Asparagi Tuber	9 g.
mài mén dōng	ophiopogon [tuber]	Ophiopogonis Tuber	9 g.
zhè bèi mǔ	Zhejiang fritillaria [bulb]	Fritillariae Verticillatae Bulbus	9 g.
dǎn xīng	arisaema [root] [bile-processed]	Arisaematis Rhizoma cum Felle Bovis	3 g.
jú hóng	red tangerine [peel]	Citri Exocarpium Rubrum	3 g.
yuǎn zhì	polygala [root]	Polygalae Radix	3 g.
shí chāng pú	acorus [root]	Acori Rhizoma	3 g.
lián qiào	forsythia [fruit]	Forsythiae Fructus	3 g.
fú líng	poria	Poria	3 g.
fú shén	root poria	Poria cum Pini Radice	3 g.
xuán shēn	scrophularia [root]	Scrophulariae Radix	4.5 g.
dān shēn	salvia [root]	Salviae Miltiorrhizae Radix	4.5 g.
gōu téng	uncaria [stem and thorn] (abbreviated decoction)	Uncariae Ramulus cum Unco	4.5 g.
zhū shā	cinnabar (stirred in)	Cinnabaris	1 g.

* Use 30 grams of iron flakes. Decoct alone in five cups of water, reduce to three cups over 1-1.5 hours, then add the other ingredients.

MODIFICATIONS

In cases of congestion of severe phlegm-fire with extremely slimy yellow tongue coating, the prescription is changed to drain fire and expel phlegm. Use the prepared medicines CHLORITE-MICA PHLEGM-SHIFTING PILL *(méng-shí gǔn tán wán)* followed by PEACEFUL PALACE BOVINE BEZOAR PILL *(ān gōng niú-huáng wán)* to clear the heart and open the orifices.

In cases manifesting profusion of liver and gallbladder fire with a wiry, rapid forceful pulse, use the prepared medicine, TANGKUEI, GENTIAN AND ALOE PILL *(dāng guī lóng huì wán)* to drain the liver and clear fire.

In cases of constipation with rough yellow tongue coating and large forceful pulse, the prescription is changed to clear heat and free the stool. Use:

Qi-Infusing Variant Decoction *jiā jiǎn chéng qì tāng*

dà huáng	rhubarb (abbreviated decoction)	Rhei Rhizoma	12 g.
máng xiāo	mirabilite (stirred in)	Mirabilitum	9 g.
zhǐ shí	unripe bitter orange	Aurantii Fructus Immaturus	9 g.
qīng méng shí	chlorite [schist]	Chloriti Lapis	9 g.
zào jiá	gleditsia [fruit]	Gleditsiae Fructus	3 g.
zhū dǎn zhī	pig's bile	Suis Bilis	9 g.
cù	vinegar (stirred in)	Acetum	20 cc.

When the patient is relatively lucid and phlegm-heat has not been fully expelled, with symptoms of irritability and insomnia, the prescription is changed to transform phlegm and quiet the spirit. Combine Gallbladder-Warming Decoction *(wēn dǎn tāng)* with CINNABAR SPIRIT-QUIETING PILL *(zhū-shā ān shén wán)*.

Gallbladder-Warming Decoction *wēn dǎn tāng*

fǎ bàn xià	pinellia [tuber] (processed)	Pinelliae Tuber Praeparatum	6 g.
zhú rú	bamboo shavings	Bambusae Caulis in Taeniam	6 g.
zhǐ shí	unripe bitter orange	Aurantii Fructus Immaturus	6 g.
chén pí	tangerine [peel]	Citri Exocarpium	6 g.
zhì gān cǎo	licorice [root] (honey-fried)	Glycyrrhizac Radix	6 g.
fú líng	poria	Poria	9 g.
shēng jiāng	fresh ginger	Zingiberis Rhizoma Recens	5 pc.
dà zǎo	jujube	Ziziphi Fructus	1 pc.

ACUPUNCTURE AND MOXIBUSTION

Main points: Needle with draining.

GV-14	*dà zhuī*
GV-26	*shuǐ gōu*
GV-16	*fēng fǔ*
ST-40	*fēng lóng*
PC-06	*nèi guān*

Auxiliary points:

For acute exuberant heat with manic behavior, bleed the twelve essence-well points of the hands:

LU-11	*shào shāng*
PC-09	*zhōng chōng*
HT-09	*shào chōng*
LI-01	*shāng yáng*
TB-01	*guān chōng*
SI-01	*shào zé*

For mania with constipation, add:

| LR-03 | *tài chōng* |
| TB-06 | *zhī gōu* |

2B. MANIC PSYCHOTIC PATTERNS — EXUBERANT FIRE WITH INJURY TO YIN

Clinical Manifestations: Prolonged illness with moderate symptoms such as irritability, tendency to be easily frightened, insomnia, emaciation, tiredness.

Tongue: Red with little coating.

Pulse: Rapid, thready.

Treatment Method: Nourish yin, downbear fire, quiet the spirit, stabilize emotions.

PRESCRIPTION

Two Yin Brew *èr yīn jiān*

shēng dì huáng	rehmannia [root] dried/fresh	Rehmanniae Radix Exsiccata seu Reccns	12 g.
mài mén dōng	ophiopogon [tuber]	Ophiopogonis Tuber	12 g.
xuán shēn	scrophularia [root]	Scrophulariae Radix	9 g.
huáng lián	coptis [root]	Coptidis Rhizoma	6 g.
mù tōng	mutong [stem]	Mutong Caulis	6 g.
zhú yè	black bamboo [leaf]	Bambusae Folium	9 g.
fú shén	root poria	Poria cum Pini Radice	9 g.
dēng xīn cǎo	juncus [pith]	Junci Medulla	3 g.
suān zǎo rén	spiny jujube [kernel]	Ziziphi Spinosi Semen	12 g.
gān cǎo	licorice [root]	Glycyrrhizae Radix	6 g.

ACUPUNCTURE AND MOXIBUSTION

Main points: Needle with even supplementation, even draining.

HT-07	*shén mén*
SP-06	*sān yīn jiāo*
KI-04	*dà zhōng*
PC-07	*dà líng*
BL-15	*xīn shū*
BL-23	*shèn shū*

ALTERNATE THERAPEUTIC METHODS

1. Ear Acupuncture

Main points: Heart, Subcortex, Kidney, Occiput, Forehead, *Shén Mén*.

Method: Select three or four points per session and needle to elicit a mild sensation for depressive patterns and a strong sensation for manic patterns. Retain the needles for thirty minutes.

REMARKS

Mania and withdrawal are often accompanied by internal obstruction of static blood. In addition to the clinical manifestations mentioned above, patients can also present dark dull complexion, dark purple tongue, distention of the sublingual veins and deep rough, pulse. Appropriate treatment should include medicinals to quicken the blood and dissolve stasis. In addition to medicinal treatment, attention should be paid to conserving the patient's health and psychological condition. Install special nursing care to prevent unforeseen accidents.

EPILEPSY PATTERNS

Xián Zhèng

1. Obstruction by Wind-Phlegm - 2. Internal Profusion of Phlegm-Fire - 3. Vacuity of Liver and Kidney Yin - 4. Vacuity of Spleen and Stomach Qi

Epilepsy is a nervous disorder presenting convulsive seizures as its major symptom. In Chinese, epilepsy is popularly known as *yáng xián fēng,* or "bleating epileptic wind," since during seizures victims often produce sounds similar to the bleating of sheep. Characteristics of epilepsy include momentary trance-like states or, in more severe cases, loss of consciousness, foaming at the mouth, bleating sounds, rolling back of the eyes and violent involuntary movements of the limbs. This is followed by regaining consciousness without lingering symptoms.

Although the symptoms of epilepsy are relatively uniform, cases differ in acuteness, severity, length and frequency of seizures. The epilepsy patterns of traditional Chinese medicine correspond to both the idiopathic and symptomatic epilepsies of Western medicine, including the grand mal and petit mal, as well as psychomotor and focal epilepsies.

ETIOLOGY AND PATHOGENESIS

Major etiological factors in the development of epilepsy include constitutional factors, emotional disturbances, improper diet and eating habits, stress, overstrain and traumatic injury. These can cause disharmony of yin and yang of the viscera and bowels and disturb normal qi movement, allowing phlegm-turbidity to obstruct the channels and connections. This can obscure the opening of the orifices and give rise to epileptic seizures.

Injury to the liver, kidney, heart and spleen is common in the pathogenesis of epilepsy. In addition, the development of epilepsy can be caused by stagnation of qi and blood, especially following traumatic injury.

1. OBSTRUCTION BY WIND-PHLEGM

Clinical Manifestations: Symptoms of dizziness and vertigo, oppression in the chest and loss of strength prior to seizures, although seizures can arise without warning. Seizures are characterized by sudden falling to the ground, loss of consciousness, convulsions, foaming at the mouth, screaming and possible incontinence of urine and stool. In other cases, seizures may manifest only as a temporary clouding of consciousness or trance-like mental state without convulsions.

Tongue: White slimy coating.

Pulse: Wiry and slippery.

Treatment Method: Expel phlegm, extinguish wind, open the orifices, stabilize epilepsy.

PRESCRIPTION

Epilepsy-Stabilizing Pill *dìng xián wán*

tiān má	gastrodia [root]	Gastrodiae Rhizoma	30 g.
chuān bèi mǔ	Sichuan fritillaria [bulb]	Fritillariae Cirrhosae Bulbus	30 g.
fǎ bàn xià	pinellia [tuber] (processed)	Pinelliae Tuber Praeparatum	30 g.
fú líng	poria	Poria	30 g.
fú shén	root poria	Poria cum Pini Radice	30 g.
dǎn xīng	arisaema [root] [bile-processed]	Arisaematis Rhizoma cum Felle Bovis	15 g.
shí chāng pú	acorus [root]	Acori Rhizoma	15 g.
quán xiē	scorpion	Buthus	15 g.
bái jiāng cán	silkworm	Bombyx Batryticatus	15 g.
hǔ pò	amber	Succinum	15 g.
dēng xīn cǎo	juncus [pith]	Junci Medulla	15 g.
chén pí	tangerine peel	Citri Exocarpium	20 g.
yuǎn zhì	polygala [root]	Polygalae Radix	20 g.
dān shēn	salvia [root]	Salviae Miltiorrhizae Radix	60 g.
mài mén dōng	ophiopogon [tuber]	Ophiopogonis Tuber	60 g.
zhū shā	cinnabar	Cinnabaris	9 g.
gān cǎo	licorice [root]	Glycyrrhizae Radix	12 g.
zhú lì	dried bamboo sap	Bambusae Succus Exsiccatus	100 ml.
jiāng zhī	ginger juice	Zingiberis Rhizomatis Succus	50 ml.

Grind the ingredients into a powder and make into pills. Take a 6 g. dosage twice daily with water.

MODIFICATIONS

In cases of chronic epilepsy, with frequent seizures and resultant depletion of qi, the prescription is modified to reinforce and assist qi. Add:

rén shēn	ginseng	Ginseng Radix	9 g.

ACUPUNCTURE AND MOXIBUSTION

Main points: Needle with draining.

CV-15	*jiū wěi*
M-BW-29	*yāo qí* (Lumbar Extra)
PC-05	*jiān shǐ*
LR-03	*tài chōng*
ST-40	*fēng lóng*
LR-03	*tài chōng*

Auxiliary points:

During seizures, add:

GV-26	*shuǐ gōu*
ST-06	*jiá chē*
HT-07	*shén mén*

For prolonged epilepsy with vacuity of qi, add acupuncture and moxibustion on:

CV-04	*guān yuán*
ST-36	*zú sān lǐ*

2. INTERNAL PROFUSION OF PHLEGM-FIRE

Clinical Manifestations: Seizures that are characterized by sudden loss of consciousness, falling to the ground, convulsions, foaming at the mouth and sometimes screaming. Between seizures, symptoms may include an agitated emotional state, irritability, insomnia, difficult expectoration of yellow phlegm, dry bitter taste in mouth and, in some cases, constipation.

Tongue: Red with yellow slimy coating.

Pulse: Rapid, wiry, slippery.

Treatment Method: Clear the liver, drain fire, transform phlegm, open the orifices.

PRESCRIPTION

Combine Gentian Liver-Draining Decoction *(lóng-dǎn xiè gān tāng)* with Phlegm-Flushing Decoction *(dí tán tāng)*.

Gentian Liver-Draining Decoction *lóng dǎn xiè gān tāng*

lóng dǎn cǎo	gentian [root]	Gentianae Radix	6 g.
huáng qín	scutellaria [root]	Scutellariae Radix	9 g.
shān zhī zǐ	gardenia [fruit]	Gardeniae Fructus	9 g.
zé xiè	alisma [tuber]	Alismatis Rhizoma	12 g.
mù tōng	mutong [stem]	Mutong Caulis	9 g.
dāng guī	tangkuei	Angelicae Sinensis Radix	3 g.
chē qián zǐ	plantago [seed] (wrapped)	Plantaginis Semen	9 g.
shēng dì huáng	rehmannia [root] dried/fresh	Rehmanniae Radix Exsiccata seu Recens	9 g.
chái hú	bupleurum [root]	Bupleuri Radix	6 g.
gān cǎo	licorice [root]	Glycyrrhizae Radix	6 g.

with:

Phlegm-Flushing Decoction *dí tán tāng*

fǎ bàn xià	pinellia [tuber] (processed)	Pinelliae Tuber Praeparatum	9 g.
zhì tiān nán xīng	arisaema [root] (prepared)	Arisaematis Rhizoma Praeparatum	6 g.
chén pí	tangerine [peel]	Citri Exocarpium	9 g.
zhǐ shí	unripe bitter orange	Aurantii Fructus Immaturus	9 g.
fú líng	poria	Poria	12 g.
rén shēn	ginseng	Ginseng Radix	6 g.
shí chāng pú	acorus [root]	Acori Rhizoma	9 g.
zhú rú	bamboo shavings	Bambusae Caulis in Taeniam	9 g.
shēng jiāng	fresh ginger [root]	Zingiberis Rhizoma Recens	6 g.
gān cǎo	licorice [root]	Glycyrrhizae Radix	3 g.

<u>MODIFICATIONS</u>

To reinforce subduing the liver, eradicating wind, dissolving phlegm and relieving epilepsy, add:

shí jué míng	abalone [shell] (extended decoction)	Haliotidis Concha	15 g.
gōu téng	uncaria [stem and thorn] (abbreviated decoction)	Uncariae Ramulus cum Unco	9 g.
zhú lì	dried bamboo sap	Bambusae Succus Exsiccatus	30 g.
dì lóng	earthworm	Lumbricus	9 g.

In cases accompanied by constipation, the prescription is modified to drain fire and free the stool. Add:

| *dà huáng* | rhubarb (abbreviated decoction) | Rhei Rhizoma | 9 g. |
| *máng xiāo* | mirabilite (stirred in) | Mirabilitum | 9 g. |

ACUPUNCTURE AND MOXIBUSTION

Main points: Needle with draining.

CV-15	*jiū wěi*
M-BW-29	*yāo qí2* (Lumbar Extra)
LR-03	*tài chōng*
GB-13	*běn shén*
ST-40	*fēng lóng*
GV-14	*dà zhuī*

Auxiliary points:

During seizures, add:

GV-26	*shuǐ gōu*
ST-06	*jiá chē*
SI-03	*hòu xī*

For constipation, add:

| TB-06 | *zhī gōu* |

3. VACUITY OF LIVER AND KIDNEY YIN

Clinical Manifestations: Prolonged epilepsy accompanied by dizziness and vertigo, insomnia, forgetfulness, weak aching lower back and knees and, in some cases, dry stools.

Tongue: Red with little coating.

Pulse: Rapid, thready.

Treatment Method: Nourish and supplement liver and kidney yin, subdue yang, quiet the spirit.

PRESCRIPTION

Left-Restoring [Kidney Yin] Pill *zuǒ guī wán*

shú dì huáng	cooked rehmannia [root]	Rehmanniae Radix Conquita	24 g.
shān yào	dioscorea [root]	Dioscoreae Rhizoma	12 g.
shān zhū yú	cornus [fruit]	Corni Fructus	12 g.
gǒu qǐ zǐ	lycium [berry]	Lycii Fructus	12 g.
chuān niú xī	cyathula [root]	Cyathulae Radix	9 g.
tù sī zǐ	cuscuta [seed]	Cuscutae Semen	12 g.
lù jiǎo jiāo	deerhorn glue (dissolved)	Cervi Gelatinum Cornu	12 g.
guī bǎn jiāo	tortoise plastron glue (dissolved)	Testudinis Plastrum Gelatinum	12 g.

MODIFICATIONS

To reinforce the effects of nourishing yin and subduing yang, add:

| *mǔ lì* | oyster shell (extended decoction) | Ostreae Concha | 30 g. |
| *biē jiǎ* | turtle shell (extended decoction) | Amydae Carapax | 30 g. |

To reinforce the effects of settling the heart and calming the spirit, add:

| *bǎi zǐ rén* | biota [seed] | Biotae Semen | 12 g. |
| *cí shí* | loadstone (extended decoction) | Magnetitum | 30 g. |

In cases accompanied by constipation, the prescription is modified to moisten and free the stool. Add:

xuán shēn	scrophularia [root]	Scrophulariae Radix	12 g.
huŏ má rén	hemp [seed]	Cannabis Semen	15 g.

In cases presenting trance, fearfulness, depression and anxiety, the prescription is modified to nourish the heart and moisten dryness. Combine with Licorice, Wheat and Jujube Decoction *(gān mài dà-zăo tāng)*.

Licorice, Wheat and Jujube Decoction *gān mài dà-zăo tāng*

gān căo	licorice [root]	Glycyrrhizae Radix	9 g.
fú xiăo mài	light wheat [grain]	Tritici Semen Leve	30 g.
dà zăo	jujube	Ziziphi Fructus	10 pc.

ACUPUNCTURE AND MOXIBUSTION

Main points: Needle with even supplementation, even draining.

BL-23	*shèn shū*
BL-18	*gān shū*
KI-03	*tài xī*
SP-06	*sān yīn jiāo*
M-BW-29	*yāo qí2* (Lumbar Extra)
CV-15	*jiū wĕi*

Auxiliary points:

During nighttime seizures, add:

KI-01	*yŏng quán*
KI-06	*zhào hăi*

For daytime seizures, add:

BL-62	*shēn mài*

For trance-like state, add:

BL-15	*xīn shū*
HT-07	*shén mén*
M-HN-3	*yìn táng* (Hall of Impression)

4. VACUITY OF SPLEEN AND STOMACH QI

Clinical Manifestations: Prolonged epilepsy accompanied by tiredness, fatigue, dizziness and vertigo, poor appetite, lusterless complexion, loose stools, possibly nausea and vomiting.

Tongue: Pale.

Pulse: Soft, weak.

Treatment Method: Strengthen the spleen, boost qi, calm the stomach, transform turbidity.

PRESCRIPTION

Six Gentlemen Decoction *liù jūn zĭ tāng*

rén shēn	ginseng	Ginseng Radix	9 g.
bái zhú	ovate atractylodes [root]	Atractylodis Ovatae Rhizoma	9 g.
fú líng	poria	Poria	9 g.
jiāng bàn xià	(ginger-processed) pinellia [tuber]	Pinelliae Tuber Praeparatum	6 g.
chén pí	tangerine [peel]	Citri Exocarpium	6 g.
zhì gān căo	licorice [root] (honey-fried)	Glycyrrhizae Radix	6 g.

MODIFICATIONS

To reinforce expelling phlegm and settling spirit, add:

shí chāng pú	acorus [root]	Acori Rhizoma	9 g.
yuǎn zhì	polygala [root]	Polygalae Radix	6 g.
dǎn xīng	arisaema [root] (bile-processed)	Arisaematis Rhizoma cum Felle Bovis	4.5 g.
bái jiāng cán	silkworm	Bombyx Batryticatus	9 g.

ACUPUNCTURE AND MOXIBUSTION

Main points: Needle with supplementation; add moxibustion.

M-BW-29	*yāo qí2* (Lumbar Extra)
CV-15	*jiū wěi*
BL-20	*pí shū*
CV-12	*zhōng wǎn*
SP-06	*sān yīn jiāo*
ST-36	*zú sān lǐ*

Auxiliary points:

In cases where seizures manifest as prolonged periods of unconsciousness, add:

KI-01	*yǒng quán*

plus moxibustion to:

CV-06	*qì hǎi*

For dizziness and vertigo, add:

GV-20	*bǎi huì*

ALTERNATE THERAPEUTIC METHODS

1. Ear Acupuncture

Main points: Stomach, Subcortex, *Shén Mén,* Heart, Occiput, Brain.

Method: Select two to three points each session, needle to elicit a strong sensation and retain needles for thirty minutes, manipulating periodically. Treat once every two days, ten sessions per therapeutic course. Needle implantation therapy can also be used, intradermal needles being implanted for three to five day periods, ten implantations per therapeutic course.

REMARKS

The treatment of epilepsy is based on the differentiation of root from branch and repletion from vacuity. During periods of frequent seizures, treat the branch manifestations, since controlling the seizures is the highest priority. This is generally accomplished by expelling phlegm, regulating the flow of qi, extinguishing wind and opening the orifices. Acupuncture is often used to promote regaining of consciousness, after which internal treatment can be initiated. Between seizures, treatment is aimed at the root of the illness and generally involves fortifying the spleen, transforming phlegm, supplementing the liver and kidney, nourishing the heart and settling the spirit.

Since epilepsy patterns are often related to qi stagnation and blood stasis, treatment often includes methods to rectify qi, quicken the blood and abduct stagnation. Clinical practice has proven that entomological medicines such as scorpion *(quán xiē)* and centipede *(wú gōng)* effectively extinguish wind and release spasms, increasing the therapeutic effect in all epilepsy patterns. These are generally administered in the form of a powder at a dose of 1 g. twice daily. If *quán xiē* and *wú gōng* are used together, the dosage of each is reduced to 0.5 g. twice daily. Doses for children should be reduced appropriately.

Regulating daily habits plays an important role in the treatment of epilepsy. Patients should avoid stress, strain and emotional disturbance. The emotional state should be tranquil and any factors known to induce seizures should be strictly avoided. Foods such as lamb and liquor can induce seizures and should be prohibited. To avoid accidents, epileptics should not drive or ride bicycles, or be employed at jobs on boats or at heights. During seizures, dentures should be removed and measures taken to protect the tongue. In patients whose seizures are relatively long, special attention should be paid to sanitation of the oral cavity and removing obstructions to the expulsion of phlegm from the mouth.

Bi Patterns

Bì Zhèng

1. Wind Dominant Bi – 2. Cold Dominant Bi – 3. Dampness Dominant Bi – 4. Heat Dominant Bi – 5. Bi with Blood Stasis and Phlegm-Turbidity – 6. Bi with Depletion of Qi and Blood, Kidney and Liver Vacuity – 7. Bi with Heart Vacuity

Bì means obstruction or blockage. Bi pattern describes a set of patterns in which the invasion of external evils such as wind, cold, dampness and heat obstruct the flow of qi and blood through the channels and connections. This affects the muscles, bones, tendons and joints, presenting symptoms of aching, pain, heaviness, numbness, difficulty of movement or redness and swelling.

Bì patterns include several disorders known in Western medicine as osteoarthritis, rheumatoid arthritis, rheumatic fever, fibrositis, gout and sciatica.

ETIOLOGY AND PATHOGENESIS

The etiology of bi patterns usually combines an internal or pre-existing vacuity of correct qi with external evils entering the body: wind, cold, dampness or heat. Simultaneous invasion by wind, cold and dampness is the most common. Bi patterns are considered in four classes based on the specific external evil and the differing clinical manifestations.

Wind bi *(fēng bì)*, also known as wandering bi *(xíng bì)*, is characterized by wind evil with pain roving through various locations.

Cold bi *(hán bì)*, also known as painful bi *(tòng bì)*, is characterized by the accumulation of cold with severe pain.

Damp bi *(shī bì)*, also known as fixed bi *(zháo bì)*, is characterized by the accumulation of dampness with muscular and joint numbness, aching, heaviness, swelling and pain of fixed location.

Heat bi *(rè bì)*, is characterized by fever and red swollen painful joints. Its causes include invasion by heat evil; untreated and chronic wind-cold dampness bi that has transformed into heat; or constitutions of either profuse yang or vacuous yin, that have transformed external evils to heat.

All bi patterns involve obstruction of the channels and connections inhibiting the flow of qi and blood. Chronic cases of bi, regardless of a particular evil's dominance, present three major categories of pathological change.

The first includes manifestations of blood stasis and phlegm-turbidity such as stasis macules on the tongue, nodes in the area of affected joints and swelling and difficulty moving the joints.

The second involves symptoms of vacuous qi and blood. The severity will vary according to the injury and depletion of qi and blood during the illness.

The third includes pathological changes from the progress of evils from the channels and connections into the viscera and bowels. Most commonly observed is heart bi with palpitations, cyanosis, asthma and edema.

1. WIND-DOMINANT BI

Clinical Manifestations: Roving pain in the joints and limbs, pain of indeterminate location, difficulty in flexion and extension of joints, aversion to cold and in some cases, fever.

Tongue: Thin white coating.

Pulse: Wiry, floating.

Treatment Method: Dispel wind, clear the connections, dissipate cold, dispel dampness.

PRESCRIPTION

Ledebouriella Decoction *fáng fēng tāng*

fáng fēng	ledebouriella [root]	Ledebouriellae Radix	9 g.
dāng guī	tangkuei	Angelicae Sinensis Radix	9 g.
fú líng	poria	Poria	9 g.
xìng rén	apricot [kernel]	Armeniacae Semen	6 g.
qín jiāo	large gentian [root]	Gentianae Macrophyllae Radix	9 g.
má huáng	ephedra	Ephedrae Herba	9 g.
gé gēn	pueraria [root]	Puerariae Radix	9 g.
huáng qín	scutellaria [root]	Scutellariae Radix	3 g.
ròu guì	cinnamon [bark] (abbreviated decoction)	Cinnamomi Cortex	6 g.
shēng jiāng	fresh ginger [root]	Zingiberis Rhizoma Recens	6 g.
gān cǎo	licorice [root]	Glycyrrhizae Radix	6 g.
dà zǎo	jujube	Ziziphi Fructus	3 pc.

MODIFICATIONS

In cases where pain of the upper limbs is predominant, the prescription is modified to relieve upper limb pain. Add:

qiāng huó	notopterygium [root]	Notopterygii Rhizoma	9 g.
bái zhǐ	angelica [root]	Angelicae Dahuricae Radix	6 g.
wēi líng xiān	clematis [root]	Clematidis Radix	9 g.
jiāng huáng	turmeric	Curcumae Longae Rhizoma	9 g.
chuān xiōng	ligusticum [root]	Ligustici Rhizoma	6 g.

In cases where pain of the lower limbs is predominant, the prescription is modified to relieve lower limb pain. Add:

dú huó	tuhuo angelica [root]	Angelicae Duhuo Radix	9 g.
niú xī	achyranthes [root]	Achyranthis Bidentatae Radix	9 g.
fáng jǐ	fangji [root]	Fangji Radix	6 g.
bì xiè	fish poison yam	Dioscoreae Hypoglaucae Rhizoma	6 g.

In cases where pain of the lower back is predominant, the pattern often involves vacuity of kidney qi. The prescription is modified to warm the kidney and strengthen the lower back.

Add:

dù zhòng	eucommia [bark]	Eucommiae Cortex	12 g.
sāng jì shēng	mistletoe	Loranthi seu Visci Ramus	12 g.
yín yáng huò	epimedium	Epimedii Herba	9 g.
bā jǐ tiān	morinda [root]	Morindae Radix	9 g.
xù duàn	dipsacus [root]	Dipsaci Radix	9 g.

In cases presenting swollen painful joints, dry sore throat, and a thin yellow tongue coating, the evils are undergoing transformation to heat. The prescription is changed to dispel wind-dampness, clear heat and relieve pain.

Use:

Cinnamon Twig, Peony and Anemarrhena Decoction
guì zhī sháo yào zhī mǔ tāng

guì zhī	cinnamon [twig]	Cinnamomi Ramulus	6 g.
bái sháo yào	white peony [root]	Paeoniae Radix Alba	9 g.
má huáng	ephedra	Ephedrae Herba	6 g.
bái zhú	ovate atractylodes [root]	Atractylodis Ovatae Rhizoma	9 g.
zhī mǔ	anemarrhena [root]	Anemarrhenae Rhizoma	9 g.
fáng fēng	ledebouriella [root]	Ledebouriellae Radix	9 g.
zhì fù zǐ	aconite [accessory tuber] (processed) (extended decoction)	Aconiti Tuber Laterale Praeparatum	6 g.
shēng jiāng	fresh ginger	Zingiberis Rhizoma Recens	6 g.
zhì gān cǎo	licorice [root] (honey-fried)	Glycyrrhizae Radix	6 g.

ACUPUNCTURE AND MOXIBUSTION

Main Points: Needle with draining, add moxibustion or cupping therapy.

BL-12	*fēng mén*
BL-17	*gé shū*
SP-10	*xuè hǎi*

Auxiliary Points:

For pain of the shoulder joint, add:

LI-15	*jiān yú*
TB-14	*jiān liáo*
SI-10	*nào shū*

For pain of the scapular region, add:

SI-11	*tiān zōng*
SI-12 -	*bǐng fēng*
SI-14	*jiān wài shū*
BL-43 (38)	*gāo huāng shū*

For pain of the elbow, add:

LI-11	*qū chí*
LU-05	*chǐ zé*
LI-04	*hé gǔ*
TB-10	*tiān jǐng*
TB-05	*wài guān*

For pain of the wrist, add:

TB-04	*yáng chí*
LI-05	*yáng xī*
TB-05	*wài guān*
GB-12	*wán gǔ*

For stiffness of the fingers, add:

SI-05	*yáng gǔ*
LI-04	*hé gǔ*
SI-03	*hòu xī*

For numbness and pain of the fingers, add:

SI-03	*hòu xī*
LI-03	*sān jiān*
M-UE-22	*bā xié* (Eight Evils)

For pain of the lumbar region, add:

GV-26	*shuǐ gōu* or *rén zhōng*
GV-12	*shēn zhù*
GV-03	*yāo yáng guān*

For pain of the hip joint, add:

GB-30	*huán tiào*
GB-29	*jū liáo*
GB-39	*xuán zhōng*

For pain of the thigh, add:

BL-54 (49)	*zhì biān*
BL-36 (50)	*chéng fú*
GB-34	*yáng líng quán*

For pain of the knee joint, add:

ST-35	*dú bí*
GB-34	*yáng líng quán*
ST-34	*liáng qiū*
GB-33	*xī yáng guān*
M-LE-16a	*nèi xī yǎn* (Inner Eye of the Knee)
SP-09	*yīn líng quán*

For pain of the ankle, add:

BL-62	*shēn mài*
KI-06	*zhào hǎi*
ST-41	*jiě xī*
BL-60	*kūn lún*
GB-40	*qiū xū*
SP-05	*shāng qiū*

For numbness and pain of the calf, add:

| BL-57 | *chéng shān* |
| BL-58 | *fēi yáng* |

For numbness and pain of the toes, add:

SP-04	*gōng sūn*
BL-65	*shù gǔ*
M-LE-8	*bā fēng* (Eight Winds)

For general pain over the entire body, add:

SI-03	*hòu xī*
BL-62	*shēn mài*
SP-21	*dà bāo*
LI-15	*jiān yú*
LI-11	*qū chí*
LI-04	*hé gǔ*
TB-04	*yáng chí*
GB-30	*huán tiào*
GB-34	*yáng líng quán*
GB-39	*xuán zhōng*
ST-41	*jiě xī*

2. COLD-DOMINANT BI

Clinical Manifestations: Severe pain of the joints and limbs, pain of fixed location accompanied by sensation of cold, decrease in pain with application of heat, increase in pain upon exposure to cold, without redness or feverishness of joints, with difficulty moving the affected parts.

Tongue: Thin white coating.

Pulse: Tight, wiry.

Treatment Method: Dissipate cold, warm the connections, dispel wind, dispel dampness.

PRESCRIPTION

Aconite Main Tuber Decoction *wū tóu tāng*

zhì chuān wū tóu	aconite [main tuber] (processed) (extended decoction)	Aconiti Tuber Praeparatum	6 g.
má huáng	ephedra	Ephedrae Herba	9 g.
bái sháo yào	white peony [root]	Paeoniae Radix Alba	9 g.
huáng qí	astragalus [root]	Astragali (seu Hedysari) Radix	12 g.
zhì gān cǎo	licorice [root] (honey-fried)	Glycyrrhizae Radix	9 g.

MODIFICATIONS

In cases where pain of the elbow and shoulder joints is predominant, the prescription is modified to relieve this pain. Add:

qiāng huó	notopterygium [root]	Notopterygii Rhizoma	9 g.
wēi líng xiān	clematis [root]	Clematidis Radix	9 g.
jiāng huáng	turmeric	Curcumae Longae Rhizoma	9 g.

In cases where pain of the knee and ankle joints is predominant, the prescription is modified to relieve these pains. Add:

niú xī	achyranthes [root]	Achyranthis Bidentatae Radix	9 g.
dú huó	tuhuo [angelica root]	Angelicae Duhuo Radix	9 g.
mù guā	chaenomeles [fruit]	Chaenomelis Fructus	9 g.

With a predominance of lumbar pain the prescription is modified to warm the kidney, strengthen the lower back, and relieve lumbar pain. Add:

dù zhòng	eucommia [bark]	Eucommiae Cortex	12 g.
sāng jì shēng	mistletoe	Loranthi seu Visci Ramus	12 g.
xù duàn	dipsacus [root]	Dipsaci Radix	9 g.

Herbal medicines to invigorate the blood and free the connections may also be added, these include:

jī xuè téng	millettia [root and stem]	Millettiae Radix et Caulis	12 g.
dāng guī	tangkuei	Angelicae Sinensis Radix	9 g.
luò shí téng	star jasmine [stem]	Trachelospermi Caulis	6 g.

ACUPUNCTURE AND MOXIBUSTION

Main Points: Needle with draining and moxibustion. Warming needle moxibustion and cupping therapy may also be employed.

BL-23	*shèn shū*
CV-04	*guān yuán*

Auxiliary points:
    See "Wind Dominant Bi."

3. DAMPNESS-DOMINANT BI

Clinical Manifestations: Heaviness and aching of the joints and limbs, distention and swelling in some cases, pain of fixed location, local numbness or loss of sensation, with symptoms often increasing during overcast or rainy weather.

Tongue: White slimy coating .

Pulse: Soft, tardy.

Treatment Method: Dispel dampness, clear the connections, dispel wind, dissipate cold.

PRESCRIPTION

Coix Decoction *yì yǐ rén tāng*

yì yǐ rén	coix [seed]	Coicis Semen	30 g.
chuān xiōng	ligusticum [root]	Ligustici Rhizoma	9 g.
dāng guī	tangkuei	Angelicae Sinensis Radix	9 g.
qiāng huó	notopterygium [root]	Notopterygii Rhizoma	9 g.
dú huó	tuhuo angelica [root]	Angelicae Duhuo Radix	9 g.
má huáng	ephedra	Ephedrae Herba	6 g.
guì zhī	cinnamon [twig]	Cinnamomi Ramulus	6 g.
fáng fēng	ledebouriella [root]	Ledebouriellae Radix	6 g.
cāng zhú	atractylodes [root]	Atractylodis Rhizoma	6 g.
shēng jiāng	fresh ginger [root]	Zingiberis Rhizoma Recens	6 g.
zhì chuān wū tóu	aconite [main tuber] (processed) (extended decoction)	Aconiti Tuber Praeparatum	3 g.
gān cǎo	licorice [root]	Glycyrrhizae Radix	6 g.

MODIFICATIONS

In cases of joint distention and swelling the prescription is modified to dispel dampness and disperse swelling. Add:

bì xiè	fish poison yam	Dioscoreae Hypoglaucae Rhizoma	9 g.
mù tōng	mutong [stem]	Mutong Caulis	6 g.
jiāng huáng	turmeric	Curcumae Longae Rhizoma	9 g.

In cases of numbness or loss of sensation in the affected areas the prescription is modified to quicken the blood and free the connections. Add:

hǎi tóng pí	erythrina [bark]	Erythrinae Cortex	9 g.
xī xiān cǎo	siegesbeckia	Siegesbeckiae Herba	9 g.
jī xuè téng	millettia [root and stem]	Millettiae Radix et Caulis	12 g.

In cases where the relative predominance of wind, cold or dampness is not apparent, use the following basic prescription:

Bi-Alleviating Decoction *juān bì tāng*

qiāng huó	notopterygium [root]	Notopterygii Rhizoma	9 g.
dú huó	tuhuo [angelica root]	Angelicae Duhuo Radix	9 g.
guì zhī	cinnamon [twig]	Cinnamomi Ramulus	9 g.
qín jiāo	large gentian [root]	Gentianae Macrophyllae Radix	9 g.
dāng guī	tangkuei	Angelicae Sinensis Radix	9 g.

chuān xiōng	ligusticum [root]	Ligustici Rhizoma	9 g.
hǎi fēng téng	kadsura pepper [stem]	Piperis Kadsurae Caulis	9 g.
sāng zhī	mulberry [twig]	Mori Ramulus	15 g.
rǔ xiāng	frankincense	Olibanum	6 g.
mù xiāng	saussurea [root]	Saussureae (seu Vladimiriae) Radix	6 g.
zhì gān cǎo	licorice [root] (honey-fried)	Glycyrrhizae Radix	6 g.

ACUPUNCTURE AND MOXIBUSTION

Main Points: Needle with draining; add moxibustion or cupping therapy.

BL-20	*pí shū*
ST-36	*zú sān lǐ*
SP-09	*yīn líng quán*

Auxiliary Points:
See: "Wind-Dominant Bi."

4. HEAT-DOMINANT BI

Clinical Manifestations: Severe pain, local heat, redness and swelling; difficulty of movement affecting one or more joints accompanied by fever, sore throat, thirst, irritability and dark scanty urine.

Tongue: Yellow coating

Pulse: Rapid, slippery

Treatment Method: Drain heat, clear the connections, dispel wind, dispel dampness.

PRESCRIPTION

White Tiger Decoction Plus Cinnamon Twig *bái hǔ jiā guì zhī tāng*

guì zhī	cinnamon [twig]	Cinnamomi Ramulus	6 g.
zhī mǔ	anemarrhena [root]	Anemarrhenae Rhizoma	9 g.
shí gāo	gypsum (extended decoction)	Gypsum	30 g.
jīng mǐ	rice [seed]	Oryzae Semen	15 g.
zhì gān cǎo	licorice [root] (honey-fried)	Glycyrrhizae Radix	6 g.

MODIFICATIONS

To clear heat and resolve toxin, add:

jīn yín huā	lonicera [flower]	Lonicerae Flos	15 g.
lián qiào	forsythia [fruit]	Forsythiae Fructus	12 g.
huáng bǎi	phellodendron [bark]	Phellodendri Cortex	9 g.

To quicken the blood, free the connections, dispel wind and dispel dampness, add:

hǎi tóng pí	erythrina [bark]	Erythrinae Cortex	9 g.
jiāng huáng	turmeric	Curcumae Longae Rhizoma	9 g.
wēi líng xiān	clematis [root]	Clematidis Radix	6 g.
fáng jǐ	fangji [root]	Fangji Radix	9 g.
sāng zhī	mulberry [twig]	Mori Ramulus	15 g.

In cases of red macules on the tongue, the prescription is modified to clear heat and cool the blood.

Add:

mǔ dān pí	moutan [root bark]	Moutan Radicis Cortex	9 g.
shēng dì huáng	rehmannia [root] dried/fresh	Rehmanniae Radix Exsiccata seu Recens	12 g.
dì fū zǐ	kochia [fruit]	Kochiae Fructus	9 g.
chì sháo yào	red peony [root]	Paeoniae Radix Rubra	9 g.

In cases where heat bi has given rise to fire with injury to yin, the prescription is altered to clear heat, resolve toxin, cool the blood, nourish yin, and relieve pain. Symptoms include severe pain, redness and swelling of the joints, an increase in pain during the night, high fever, thirst, red tongue with little coating, and a rapid wiry pulse. Use:

Rhinoceros Horn Powder *xī-jiǎo sǎn*

xī jiǎo	rhinoceros horn* (powdered and stirred in)	Rhinocerotis Cornu	6 g.
huáng lián	coptis [root]	Coptidis Rhizoma	9 g.
shēng má	cimicifuga [root]	Cimicifugae Rhizoma	9 g.
shān zhī zǐ	gardenia	Gardeniae Fructus	9 g.

plus:

shēng dì huáng	rehmannia [root] dried/fresh	Rehmanniae Radix Exsiccata seu Recens	12 g.
xuán shēn	scrophularia [root]	Scrophulariae Radix	9 g.
mài mén dōng	ophiopogon [tuber]	Ophiopogonis Tuber	9 g.
fáng jǐ	fangji [root]	Fangji Radix	9 g.
jiāng huáng	turmeric	Curcumae Longae Rhizoma	9 g.
qín jiāo	large gentian [root]	Gentianae Macrophyllae Radix	9 g.
hǎi tóng pí	erythrina [bark]	Erythrinae Cortex	9 g.

*Use of *xī jiǎo* (rhinoceros horn) is prohibited in North America by the endangered species law. Water Buffalo Horn *(shuǐ niú jiǎo)* may be substituted. Increase the dose to 15 g., extended decoction.)

In cases where damp-heat has descended to the lower burner, resulting in swelling and pain in the lower limbs, dark burning urine, yellow slimy tongue coating and a soft rapid pulse, the prescription is changed to clear heat, dispel dampness, disperse swelling and relieve pain. Use:

Mysterious Three Pill *sān miào wán*

cāng zhú	atractylodes [root]	Atractylodis Rhizoma	9 g.
huáng bǎi	phellodendron [bark]	Phellodendri Cortex	9 g.
chuān niú xī	cyathula [root]	Cyathulae Radix	9 g.

plus:

hǎi tóng pí	erythrina [bark]	Erythrinae Cortex	9 g.
fáng jǐ	fangji [root]	Fangji Radix	9 g.
bì xiè	fish poison yam	Dioscoreae Hypoglaucae Rhizoma	9 g.
mù tōng	mutong [stem]	Mutong Caulis	6 g.

ACUPUNCTURE AND MOXIBUSTION

Main Points: Needle with draining.

GV-14	*dà zhuī*
LI-11	*qū chí*

Auxiliary Points:

See: "Wind Dominant Bi."

5. Bi with Blood Stasis and Phlegm-Turbidity

Clinical Manifestations: In each of the above bi patterns, chronic illnesses that have not been properly treated lead to blood stasis and phlegm-turbidity. This blocks the channels, connections and joints. Symptoms include swelling, stiffness and deformity of the joints, incessant pain and complete immobility.

Tongue: Dark or purple, with white slimy coating.

Pulse: Deep, rough or deep, slippery.

Treatment Method: Dispel stasis, transform phlegm, free the connections, relieve pain.

PRESCRIPTION

Peach Kernel and Carthamus Beverage *táo hóng yǐn*

táo rén	peach [kernel]	Persicae Semen	9 g.
hóng huā	carthamus [flower]	Carthami Flosa	9 g.
chuān xiōng	ligusticum [root]	Ligustici Rhizoma	6 g.
dāng guī wěi	tangkuei tail	Angelicae Sinensis Radicis Extremitas	9 g.
wēi líng xiān	clematis [root]	Clematidis Radix	9 g.

MODIFICATIONS

To quicken the blood and dissolve stasis, add:

chuān shān jiǎ	pangolin scales	Manitis Squama	9 g.
	(or, 1.5 g. each time, powdered and administered separately)		
dì lóng	earthworm	Lumbricus	9 g.
zhè chóng	wingless cockroach	Eupolyphaga seu Opisthoplatia	9 g.

To expel phlegm-turbidity, add:

bái jiè zǐ	white mustard [seed]	Brassicae Albae Semen	9 g.
dǎn xīng	arisaema [root] (bile-processed)	Arisaematis Rhizoma cum Felle Bovis	4.5 g.

To free the connections, add:

quán xiē	scorpion	Buthus	4.5 g.
	(or, 1 g. each time, powdered and administered separately)		
wū shāo shé	black-striped snake	Zaocys	9 g.

6. Bi with Depletion of Qi and Blood, Kidney and Liver Vacuity

Clinical Manifestations: Prolonged cases of bi pattern often present symptoms of depletion of qi and blood as well as vacuity of the liver and kidney. These include aching pain in the lower back and knees, difficulty in the flexion and extension of joints, numbness or loss of sensation in affected areas, palpitations and shortness of breath, in some cases aversion to cold and symptoms relieved by warmth.

Tongue: Pale with white coating.

Pulse: Weak, thready.

Treatment Method: Supplement qi and blood, benefit liver and kidney, dispel wind, cold and dampness.

PRESCRIPTION
Tuhuo and Mistletoe Decoction *dú huó jì shēn tāng*

dú huó	tuhuo [angelica root]	Angelicae Duhuo Radix	9 g.
sāng jì shēng	mistletoe	Loranthi seu Visci Ramus	6 g.
dù zhòng	eucommia [bark]	Eucommiae Cortex	6 g.
niú xī	achyranthes [root]	Achyranthis Bidentatae Radix	6 g.
xì xīn	asarum	Asiasari Herba cum Radice	3 g.
qín jiāo	large gentian [root]	Gentianae Macrophyllae Radix	6 g.
fú líng	poria	Poria	6 g.
fáng fēng	ledebouriella [root]	Ledebouriellae Radix	6 g.
chuān xiōng	ligusticum [root]	Ligustici Rhizoma	6 g.
rén shēn	ginseng	Ginseng Radix	6 g.
dāng guī	tangkuei	Angelicae Sinensis Radix	6 g.
bái sháo yào	white peony [root]	Paeoniae Radix Alba	6 g.
shú dì huáng	cooked rehmannia [root]	Rehmanniae Radix Conquita	6 g.
ròu guì	cinnamon bark (abbreviated decoction)	Cinnamomi Cortex	6 g.
gān cǎo	licorice [root]	Glycyrrhizae Radix	6 g.

or:
Three Bi Decoction *sān bì tāng*

dú huó	tuhuo [angelica root]	Angelicae Duhuo Radix	9 g.
huáng qí	astragalus [root]	Astragali (seu Hedysari) Radix	12 g.
qín jiāo	large gentian [root]	Gentianae Macrophyllae Radix	9 g.
xù duàn	dipsacus [root]	Dipsaci Radix	9 g.
dù zhòng	eucommia [bark]	Eucommiae Cortex	9 g.
fáng fēng	ledebouriella [root]	Ledebouriellae Radix	9 g.
xì xīn	asarum	Asiasari Herba cum Radice	3 g.
dāng guī	tangkuei	Angelicae Sinensis Radix	9 g.
chì sháo yào	red peony [root]	Paeoniae Radix Rubra	9 g.
chuān xiōng	ligusticum [root]	Ligustici Rhizoma	6 g.
shú dì huáng	cooked rehmannia [root]	Rehmanniae Radix Conquita	15 g.
niú xī	achyranthes [root]	Achyranthis Bidentatae Radix	9 g.
rén shēn	ginseng	Ginseng Radix	9 g.
fú líng	poria	Poria	9 g.
guì zhī	cinnamon twig	Cinnamomi Ramulus	6 g.
gān cǎo	licorice [root]	Glycyrrhizae Radix	6 g.

7. BI WITH HEART VACUITY

Clinical Manifestations: Palpitations, oppression in the chest, shortness of breath, edema, aggravation of symptoms with physical activity, lusterless complexion and, in some cases, cyanosis.

Tongue: Pale.

Pulse: Rapid, forceless or intermittent.

Treatment Method: Boost qi, nourish the heart, warm yang, restore the pulse.

PRESCRIPTION
Honey-Fried Licorice Decoction *zhì-gān-cǎo tāng*

zhì gān cǎo	licorice [root] (honey-fried)	Glycyrrhizae Radix	12 g.
rén shēn	ginseng	Ginseng Radix	6 g.
shēng dì huáng	rehmannia [root] dried/fresh	Rehmanniae Radix Exsiccata seu Recens	30 g.
guì zhī	cinnamon twig	Cinnamomi Ramulus	9 g.
ē jiāo	ass hide glue (dissolved and stirred in)	Asini Corii Gelatinum	6 g.

mài mén dōng	ophiopogon [tuber]	Ophiopogonis Tuber	9 g.
huǒ má rén	hemp [seed]	Cannabis Semen	9 g.
shēng jiāng	fresh ginger [root]	Zingiberis Rhizoma Recens	9 g.
dà zǎo	jujube	Ziziphi Fructus	10 pc.
bái jiǔ	white wine	Vinum Alba	10 cc.

ALTERNATE THERAPEUTIC METHODS

1. Ear Acupuncture

Main Points: Tender spots in areas corresponding to affected parts, Sympathetic, *Shén Mén*.

Method: Needle to elicit a strong sensation, and retain needles for ten to twenty minutes. Ear acupuncture is generally used in cases where pain is the major complaint. Treat once daily or once every two days according to severity, ten sessions per therapeutic course.

2. Plum-Blossom Needle Therapy

Used in cases where distention and swelling are the chief complaints.

Method: Use a plum-blossom needle to tap the affected area or the region surrounding the affected joints, as well as along both sides of the vertebral column where the nerves associated with the affected areas originate. Treat once every three days, five sessions per therapeutic course.

REMARKS

During the treatment of bi patterns, prescriptions for wind-cold-dampness with severe pain often use aconite main tuber *(chuān wū tóu)*, 3-9 g., or processed aconite accessory tuber *(zhì fù zǐ)*, 3-15 g. When using these medicinals, begin with small dosages and gradually increase to an appropriate amount for each person. These medicinals should be decocted for longer periods (30-60 minutes) and should be combined with 6-9 g. licorice root *(gān cǎo)* to neutralize their poisonous effects. If patients experience numbness of the lips, tongue, fingers or toes, or have nausea, palpitations and an abrupt pulse, appropriate emergency measures may be necessary. These medicinals should then be omitted from the prescriptions.*

In chronic cases of bi patterns that manifest spasmodic pain and spastic contraction of the limbs, entomological medicines such as scorpion *(quán xie)* (2-5 g.) and centipede *(wú gōng)* (1-3 g.) are used to free the connections and relieve pain. These medicines have strong effects and are poisonous to some degree. Doses should be moderate and administration should be discontinued after improvement of the patient's condition.

In addition to treatment with medicinals, acumoxa therapy and tuina therapy have good effects in the treatment of bi patterns. These methods are especially effective during the earlier stages. Prolonged cases with severe symptoms require long-term comprehensive treatment. Important in the prevention and treatment of bi patterns are increased participation in physical exercise, residing in less damp environments and preventing the invasion of external evils.

---

* There are two kinds of aconite tuber *(wū tóu)* available in the market: aconite main tuber (Aconiti Tuber) *(chuān wū tóu)* and wild aconite tuber (Aconiti Tsao-Wu-Tou Tuber) *(cǎo wū tóu)*. Of the two, the former is less poisonous than the latter. However, both should be detoxified prior to administration.) (Editor's note: *fù zǐ* is detoxified prior to exportation to North America.)

ATONY PATTERNS

Wĕi Zhèng

1. Lung Heat with Injury to Body Fluids - 2. Invasion by Damp-Heat Evils - 3. Spleen and Stomach Qi Vacuity - 4. Depletion of Liver and Kidney Yin

Wĕi zhèng refers to a set of patterns in which the four limbs become atonic – weak, flaccid and unresponsive to voluntary motor control. In prolonged cases, muscular atrophy begins and complete paralysis of the affected limbs can develop. Because weakness and flaccidity of the lower limbs are more commonly observed, *wĕi* are also often termed *wĕi bì*, having the meaning of flaccidity and loss of function of the lower limbs, with the result that patients are unable to walk.

Wĕi patterns include the Western medical conditions of polyneuritis or Guillain Barre's disease, acute myelitis (inflammation of the spinal cord), myasthenia gravis, paralysis, muscular dystrophy, hysterical paralysis, multiple sclerosis and sequelae of infectious diseases of the central nervous system, including polio.

ETIOLOGY AND PATHOGENESIS

The primary etiological classifications in *wĕi* patterns are made according to external and internal evils. External factors include invasion of heat evil or damp-heat. Internal factors include depletion of qi, blood, yin and essence; these are caused by emotional stress, overindulgent sexual activity or weak constitution following prolonged illness. The majority of atony patterns present vacuity rather than repletion and heat rather than cold; patterns of repletion in the midst of vacuity are also common.

The major pathological mechanism is lack of nourishment and moistening of the sinews – muscles, tendons and vessels. These are caused by four basic differentiations: lung heat with injury to fluids, invasion by damp-heat, vacuity of spleen and stomach qi or depletion of liver and kidney yin, which may be complicated by phlegm accumulation or blood stasis. Pathological changes, therefore, can involve the lung, stomach, liver and kidney.

Although the pathogenesis of *wĕi* patterns is usually divided according to these four differentiations, mutual transformation is frequently observed. Prolonged cases of lung heat with injury to fluids can cause injury to the liver and kidney. Vacuity of spleen and stomach qi is conducive to the accumulation of damp-heat and damp-heat may descend to the lower burner, injuring kidney yin. Atony patterns, therefore, rarely involve one viscera or bowel; clinically, it is likely to affect several.

1. LUNG HEAT WITH INJURY TO BODY FLUIDS

Clinical Manifestations: Muscular weakness and flaccidity and motor impairment of the limbs, accompanied by fever, irritability, dry cough, dry throat, thirst, dark scanty urine, dry stools.

Tongue: Red with dry yellow coating.

Pulse: Rapid, thready.

Treatment Method: Clear heat, moisten dryness, nourish the lung, generate liquids.

PRESCRIPTION

Dryness-Clearing Lung-Rescuing Decoction *qīng zào jiù fèi tāng*

sāng yè	mulberry [leaf]	Mori Folium	9 g.
mài mén dōng	ophiopogon [tuber]	Ophiopogonis Tuber	9 g.
shí gāo	gypsum (extended decoction)	Gypsum	15 g.
xìng rén	apricot [kernel] (abbreviated decoction)	Armeniacae Semen	9 g.
pí pá yè	loquat [leaf]	Eriobotryae Folium	9 g.
huǒ má rén	hemp [seed]	Cannabis Semen	9 g.
rén shēn	ginseng	Ginseng Radix	3 g.
ē jiāo	ass hide glue (dissolved and stirred in)	Asini Corii Gelatinum	9 g.
gān cǎo	licorice [root]	Glycyrrhizae Radix	3 g.

MODIFICATIONS

In cases of high fever, excessive thirst and heavy perspiration, the prescription is modified to clear heat evil and generate liquids.

Delete:

rén shēn	ginseng	Ginseng Radix
ē jiāo	ass hide glue	Asini Corii Gelatinum

Increase the dosage of:

shí gāo	gypsum (extended decoction)	Gypsum	30 g.

Add:

běi shā shēn	glehnia [root]	Glehniae Radix	12 g.
zhī mǔ	anemarrhena [root]	Anemarrhenae Rhizoma	9 g.
jīn yín huā	lonicera [flower]	Lonicerae Flos	12 g.
lián qiào	forsythia [fruit]	Forsythiae Fructus	12 g.

In cases of copious phlegm, the prescription is modified to clear the lung and transform phlegm. Add:

zhè bèi mǔ	Zhejiang fritillaria [bulb]	Fritillariae Verticillatae Bulbus	9 g.
guā lóu	trichosanthes [fruit]	Trichosanthis Fructus	12 g.

In cases where fever has abated, with loss of appetite and severe dry mouth and throat, indicating injury to the lung as well as stomach yin, the prescription is changed to boost the stomach and generate liquids. Use:

Stomach-Boosting Decoction *yì wèi tāng*

běi shā shēn	glehnia [root]	Glehniae Radix	9 g.
shēng dì huáng	rehmannia [root] dried/fresh	Rehmanniae Radix Exsiccata seu Recens	12 g.
mài mén dōng	ophiopogon [tuber]	Ophiopogonis Tuber	9 g.
yù zhú	Solomon's seal [root]	Polygonati Yuzhu Rhizoma	9 g.
bīng táng	rock candy	Saccharon Crystallinum	3 g.

plus:

shān yào	dioscorea [root]	Dioscoreae Rhizoma	30 g.
gǔ yá	rice [sprout]	Oryzae Fructus Germinatus	12 g.

ACUPUNCTURE AND MOXIBUSTION

Main Points: Needle with draining.

BL-13	*fèi shū*
LU-05	*chǐ zé*

Auxiliary points:

For flaccidity and motor impairment of the upper limbs, add:

LI-15	*jiān yú*
LI-11	*qū chí*
TB-05	*wài guān*
LI-04	*hé gǔ*

For flaccidity and motor impairment of the lower limbs, add:

ST-31	*bì guān*
GB-30	*huán tiào*
ST-34	*liáng qiū*
ST-36	*zú sān lǐ*
ST-41	*jiě xī*
GB-39	*xuán zhōng*

For incontinence of urine, add:

CV-03	*zhōng jí*
SP-06	*sān yīn jiāo*

For incontinence of stools, add:

BL-25	*dà cháng shū*
BL-32	*cì liáo*

For fever, add:

GV-14	*dà zhuī*

2. INVASION BY DAMP-HEAT EVILS

Clinical Manifestations: Heaviness, weakness and flaccidity of the limbs; occasionally a numbness with slight swelling in the lower limbs, accompanied by fever, congestion and fullness of the chest and epigastrium and dark scanty urine.

Tongue: Yellow slimy coating.

Pulse: Soft, rapid.

Treatment Method: Clear heat, disinhibit dampness.

PRESCRIPTION

Supplemented Mysterious Two Powder (Pill) *jiā wèi èr miào sǎn (wán)*

huáng bǎi	phellodendron [bark]	Phellodendri Cortex	9 g.
cāng zhú	atractylodes [root]	Atractylodis Rhizoma	9 g.
niú xī	achyranthes [root]	Achyranthis Bidentatae Radix	9 g.
fáng jǐ	fangji [root]	Fangji Radix	9 g.
bì xiè	fish poison yam	Dioscoreae Hypoglaucae Rhizoma	9 g.
dāng guī	tangkuei	Angelicae Sinensis Radix	6 g.
guī bǎn	tortoise plastron (extended decoction)	Testudinis Plastrum	6 g.

MODIFICATIONS

The formula may be modified to disinhibit dampness and free the connections.

Delete:

dāng guī	tangkuei	Angelicae Sinensis Radix
guī bǎn	tortoise plastron	Testudinis Plastrum

Add:

yì yǐ rén	coix [seed]	Coicis Semen	30 g.
mù tōng	mutong [stem]	Mutong Caulis	9 g.
cán shā	silkworm droppings	Bombycis Excrementum	9 g.
mù guā	chaenomeles [fruit]	Chaenomelis Fructus	9 g.

In cases of predominance of dampness evil presenting white slimy tongue coating, the prescription is modified to rectify qi and dispel dampness.

Add:

hòu pò	magnolia [bark]	Magnoliae Cortex	9 g.
fú líng	poria	Poria	12 g.
huá shí	talcum (wrapped)	Talcum	12 g.

During rainy summer weather, the prescription is modified to transform dampness. Add:

huò xiāng	agastache/patchouli	Agastaches seu Pogostemi Herba	9 g.
pèi lán	eupatorium	Eupatorii Herba	9 g.

In cases where damp-heat has injured yin with symptoms of emaciation, feverish sensation in the lower limbs, irritability, redness of the sides and tip of the tongue, absence of coating in the center of the tongue and rapid thready pulse, the prescription is modified to clear heat and promote body fluid production.

Delete:

cāng zhú	atractylodes [root]	Atractylodis Rhizoma

Add:

shēng dì huáng	rehmannia [root] dried/fresh	Rehmanniae Radix Exsiccata seu Recens	9 g.
mài mén dōng	ophiopogon [tuber]	Ophiopogonis Tuber	9 g.
tiān huā fěn	trichosanthes [root]	Trichosanthis Radix	12 g.

In cases presenting symptoms of blood stasis including numbness and loss of sensation in the limbs, difficulty in flexion and extension of joints, purplish tongue and rough thready pulse, the prescription is modified to invigorate the blood and free the connections. Add:

chì sháo yào	red peony [root]	Paeoniae Radix Rubra	9 g.
dān shēn	salvia [root]	Salviae Miltiorrhizae Radix	9 g.
táo rén	peach [kernel]	Persicae Semen	6 g.
hóng huā	carthamus [flower]	Carthami Flosa	6 g.

ACUPUNCTURE AND MOXIBUSTION

Main Points: Needle with draining.

BL-20	*pí shū*
SP-09	*yīn líng quán*

Auxiliary points:

See "Lung Heat with Injury to Fluids."

3. SPLEEN AND STOMACH QI VACUITY

Clinical Manifestations: Flaccidity and weakness of the limbs progressing to muscular atrophy, loss of appetite, loose stools, tiredness, fatigue, lusterless complexion, shortness of breath, facial puffiness.

Tongue: Pale with thin white coating.

Pulse: Thready, weak.

Treatment Method: Fortify the spleen and stomach, boost qi.

PRESCRIPTION

Ginseng, Poria and Ovate Atractylodes Powder *shēn líng bái zhú sǎn*

rén shēn	ginseng	Ginseng Radix	12 g.
fú líng	poria	Poria	12 g.
bái zhú	ovate atractylodes [root]	Atractylodis Ovatae Rhizoma	12 g.
shān yào	dioscorea [root]	Dioscoreae Rhizoma	12 g.
biǎn dòu	lablab [bean]	Lablab Semen	9 g.
lián zǐ	lotus [fruit-seed]	Nelumbinis Fructus seu Semen	6 g.
yì yǐ rén	coix [seed]	Coicis Semen	6 g.
shā rén	amomum [fruit] (abbreviated decoction)	Amomi Semen seu Fructus	6 g.
jié gěng	platycodon [root]	Platycodonis Radix	6 g.
zhì gān cǎo	licorice [root] (honey-fried)	Glycyrrhizae Radix	12 g.

MODIFICATIONS

In cases accompanied by food stasis, the prescription is modified to disperse food and dissolve obstruction. Add:

gǔ yá	rice [sprout]	Oryzae Fructus Germinatus	12 g.
mài yá	barley sprout	Hordei Fructus Germinatus	12 g.
shān zhā	crataegus [fruit]	Crataegi Fructus	12 g.
shén qū	medicated leaven	Massa Medicata Fermentata	12 g.

In cases of chills and cold extremities, the prescription is modified to warm spleen yang. Add:

zhì fù zǐ	aconite [accessory tuber] (processed) (extended decoction)	Aconiti Tuber Laterale Praeparatum	6 g.
gān jiāng	dried ginger [root]	Zingiberis Rhizoma Exsiccatum	6 g.

In cases of vacuity of qi and blood, the prescription is modified to reinforce qi and nourish the blood. Add:

huáng qí	astragalus [root]	Astragali (seu Hedysari) Radix	12 g.
dāng guī	tangkuei	Angelicae Sinensis Radix	12 g.

ACUPUNCTURE AND MOXIBUSTION

Main Points: Needle with supplementation; add moxibustion.

CV-12	*zhōng wǎn*
SP-06	*sān yīn jiāo*
BL-20	*pí shū*

Auxiliary Points:

See "Lung Heat with Injury to Fluids."

4. Depletion of Liver and Kidney Yin

Clinical Manifestations: Flaccidity and weakness (most commonly observed in the lower limbs), accompanied by weak aching lower back and knees, dizziness and vertigo, tinnitus, dry throat, fatigue, seminal emission, irregular menstruation

Tongue: Red with little coating.

Pulse: Rapid, thready.

Treatment Method: Reinforce the liver and kidney, nourish yin, clear heat.

PRESCRIPTION

Hidden Tiger Pill *hǔ qián wán*

shú dì huáng	cooked rehmannia [root]	Rehmanniae Radix Conquita	24 g.
zhī mǔ	anemarrhena [root]	Anemarrhenae Rhizoma	12 g.
guī bǎn	tortoise plastron (extended decoction)	Testudinis Plastrum	30 g.
huáng bǎi	phellodendron [bark]	Phellodendri Cortex	9 g.
bái sháo yào	white peony [root]	Paeoniae Radix Alba	9 g.
hǔ gǔ	tiger bone*	Tigris Os	6 g.
chén pí	tangerine [peel]	Citri Exocarpium	6 g.
suǒ yáng	cynomorium [stem]	Cynomorii Caulis	6 g.
gān jiāng	dried ginger [root]	Zingiberis Rhizoma Exsiccatum	3 g.

(Editor's note: *hǔ gǔ* (tiger bone) is prohibited in North America by endangered species laws. Leg bone of pig or dog may be substituted.)

MODIFICATIONS

In cases of strong heat, the prescription is modified to nourish yin and clear heat. Delete:

suǒ yáng	cynomorium [stem]	Cynomorii Caulis
gān jiāng	dried ginger [root]	Zingiberis Rhizoma Exsiccatum

or change the prescription, using:

Anemarrhena, Phellodendron and Rehmannia Pill *zhī bǎi dì huáng wán*

shú dì huáng	cooked rehmannia [root]	Rehmanniae Radix Conquita	24 g.
shān zhū yú	cornus [fruit]	Corni Fructus	12 g.
shān yào	dioscorea [root]	Dioscoreae Rhizoma	12 g.
zé xiè	alisma [tuber]	Alismatis Rhizoma	9 g.
fú líng	poria	Poria	9 g.
mǔ dān pí	moutan [root bark]	Moutan Radicis Cortex	9 g.
zhī mǔ	anemarrhena [root]	Anemarrhenae Rhizoma	9 g.
huáng bǎi	phellodendron [bark]	Phellodendri Cortex	9 g.

In cases with sallow complexion, palpitations, pale tongue and weak thready pulse, the prescription is modified to reinforce qi and nourish the blood. Add:

huáng qí	astragalus [root]	Astragali (seu Hedysari) Radix	12 g.
dǎng shēn	codonopsis [root]	Codonopsitis Radix	9 g.
dāng guī	tangkuei	Angelicae Sinensis Radix	9 g.
jī xuè téng	millettia [root and stem]	Millettiae Radix et Caulis	12 g.

In cases of prolonged illness where injury of yin has led to injury of yang with physical cold, cold extremities, copious clear urine, impotence, pale tongue and deep thready forceless pulse, the prescription is modified to supplement the kidney and assist yang.

Delete:

huáng bǎi	phellodendron [bark]	Phellodendri Cortex
zhī mǔ	anemarrhena [root]	Anemarrhenae Rhizoma

Add:

lù jiǎo jiāo	deerhorn glue (dissolved and stirred in)	Cervi Gelatinum Cornu	9 g.
bǔ gǔ zhī	psoralea [seed]	Psoraleae Semen	9 g.
bā jǐ tiān	morinda [root]	Morindae Radix	9 g.
ròu guì	cinnamon [bark] (abbreviated decoction)	Cinnamomi Cortex	6 g.

ACUPUNCTURE AND MOXIBUSTION

Main Points: Needle with supplementation.

BL-18	*gān shū*
BL-23	*shèn shū*
GB-39	*xuán zhōng*
GB-34	*yáng líng quán*

Auxiliary Points:

See "Lung Heat with Injury to Fluids."

ALTERNATE THERAPEUTIC METHODS

1. Ear Acupuncture

Main Points: Lung, Stomach, Large Intestine, Liver, Kidney, Spleen, *Shén Mén* and points corresponding to affected parts.

Method: Select three to five points each session, needle to elicit a strong sensation and retain needles for ten minutes. Treat once every two days, ten sessions per therapeutic course.

2. Plum-Blossom Needle Therapy

Method: Use a plum-blossom needle to tap lightly over the lung, stomach, liver and spleen back-shu points as well as along the courses of the channels of hand and foot yangming. Treat once every two days, ten sessions per therapeutic course.

REMARKS

Since lung fluids, liver blood and kidney essence all depend upon the functions of the spleen and stomach in digestion and transformation, emphasis on regulation of the spleen and stomach is the guiding principle in the treatment of atony patterns. This applies to the use of both herbal prescriptions and acumoxa therapy. Etiological factors in the development of atony patterns are numerous, however, and pathogenesis can become complex, requiring that treatment be based on a comprehensive differential diagnosis.

Acumoxa therapy, tuina massage and qigong therapy are often combined with herbal medicine for a more comprehensive treatment of atony patterns. Since therapeutic courses are relatively long, patients must be encouraged to persevere in undergoing treatment as well as appropriate therapeutic exercises to improve the tone and function of the muscles of the limbs. Such exercises have a marked effect on the efficacy of treatment, accelerating recovery from atony patterns.

INTERNAL DAMAGE FEVER

Nèi Shāng Fā Rè

1. Qi Stagnation Fever - 2. Blood Stasis Fever - 3. Qi Vacuity Fever - 4. Blood Vacuity Fever - 5. Yin Vacuity Fever

Internal damage fevers are those conditions in which the fever results from internal etiological factors and their pathogenic mechanisms. These involve the depletion of qi, blood, yin or essence, or dysfunction of the viscera and bowels. The progression of illness is generally gradual and the condition is prolonged and often recurrent.

Clinically, internal damage fever occurs intermittently and is usually slight. In some cases it manifests only as the subjective sensation of fever or as five-hearts fever, while the actual body temperature doesn't rise above normal. In the majority of patients, fever does not coincide with aversion to cold; if a chill accompanies internal damage fever, it can often be relieved by simply bundling up. The most common accompanying symptoms of internal damage fever include dizzy spells, fatigue, spontaneous perspiration or night sweating and a weak forceless pulse.

Internal damage fever can also manifest as high fever, although it is clearly distinguishable from external contraction fever in terms of pathogenic mechanism and clinical manifestations. External contraction fever is characterized by abrupt onset, short duration of illness, aversion to cold that is not relieved by bundling up, headache, body aches and pains, nasal congestion, runny nose, coughing and floating pulse.

ETIOLOGY AND PATHOGENESIS

The major etiology in internal damage fevers involve factors such as emotional disruption, stress and taxation, improper diet and eating habits. Certain cases may be caused by externally contracted evils that have been left untreated, bringing about internal damage by weakening the viscera and bowels. The common pathogenesis of internal damage fever is dysfunction of the viscera and bowels and the consequent depletion of qi, blood, yin or essence. Each type of internal damage fever naturally involves different organs.

Clinically, internal damage fever is divided into the following types: qi stagnation fever, which is the result of the stagnation of liver qi and its subsequent transformation into fire; blood stasis fever, where the blockage of the channels and connections by static blood leads to poor circulation of qi and blood; qi vacuity fever, brought on by vacuity of spleen and stomach qi, allowing the internal production of yin fire *(yīn huǒ)*; blood vacuity fever, which can be caused either by depletion of heart and liver blood, or by insufficiency of the spleen leading to poor production of blood; and yin vacuity fever, in which vacuity of lung and kidney yin leads to the inability of water to control fire.

Qi stagnation fever and blood stasis fever are classified as repletion patterns whereas qi, blood and yin vacuity fevers are classified as vacuity patterns. In some patients, internal damage fever can involve two of the above mechanisms: stagnation of qi and stasis of blood, vacuity of both qi and blood, or depletion of both qi and yin. Repletion can also be coupled with vacuity, as in vacuity of qi and stasis of blood, blood vacuity and stasis of blood, or stagnation of qi and depletion of yin. Therefore, care should be taken during clinical differentiation.

1. QI STAGNATION FEVER

Clinical Manifestations: Intermittent sensation of feverishness and agitation generally commencing with changes in mood, accompanied by emotional depression or irritability, sensations of oppression and distention of the chest and hypochondria, frequent sighing, dry bitter taste in the mouth. Female patients can manifest symptoms of irregular menstruation, dysmenorrhea or breast distention.

Tongue: Yellow coating.

Pulse: Rapid, wiry.

Treatment Method: Dredge the liver, resolve stagnation, clear heat.

PRESCRIPTION
Moutan and Gardenia Free Wanderer Powder *dān zī xiāo yáo sǎn*

chái hú	bupleurum [root]	Bupleuri Radix	9 g.
bái sháo yào	white peony [root]	Paeoniae Radix Alba	12 g.
dāng guī	tangkuei	Angelicae Sinensis Radix	9 g.
bái zhú	ovate atractylodes [root]	Atractylodis Ovate Rhizoma	9 g.
fú líng	poria	Poria	9 g.
mǔ dān pí	moutan [root bark]	Moutan Radices Cortex	9 g.
shān zhī zǐ	gardenia [fruit]	Gardeniae Fructus	9 g.
zhì gān cǎo	licorice [root] (honey-fried)	Glycyrrhizae Radix	6 g.
shēng jiāng	fresh ginger [root]	Zingiberis Rhizoma Recens	3 g.
bò hé	mint (abbreviated decoction)	Menthae Herba	3 g.

MODIFICATIONS

In cases where heat is prevalent, with symptoms of red tongue, dry mouth and constipation, the prescription is modified to drain liver fire.
Delete:

bái zhú	ovate atractylodes [root]	Atractylodis Ovate Rhizoma	

Add:

huáng qín	scutellaria [root]	Scutellariae Radix	9 g.
lóng dǎn cǎo	gentian [root]	Gentianae Radix	6 g.

In cases of pain and distention of the chest and costal regions, the prescription is modified to regulate qi and relieve pain. Add:

yù jīn	curcuma [tuber]	Curcumae Tuber	9 g.
chuān liàn zǐ	toosendan [fruit]	Toosendan Fructus	9 g.

In cases of constitutionally vacuous yin coupled with fever from stagnation of liver qi, or cases where qi stagnation fever, left untreated, has done injury to yin, the prescription is changed to nourish kidney yin, course the liver and clear heat. Use:

Water-Enriching Liver-Clearing Beverage *zī shuǐ qīng gān yǐn*

shēng dì huáng	rehmannia [root] dried/fresh	Rehmanniae Radix Exsiccata seu Recens	24 g.
shān zhū yú	cornus [fruit]	Corni Fructus	12 g.
shān yao	dioscorea [root]	Dioscoreae Rhizome	12 g.
fú líng	poria	Poria	9 g.
mǔ dān pí	moutan [root bark]	Moutan Radices Cortex	9 g.
zé xiè	alisma [tuber]	Alismatis Rhizoma	9 g.
chái hú	bupleurum [root]	Bupleuri Radix	6 g.
bái sháo yào	white peony [root]	Paeoniae Radix Alba	12 g.
dāng guī	tangkuei	Angelicae Sinensis Radix	9 g.
shān zhī zǐ	gardenia [fruit]	Gardeniae Fructus	6 g.
suān zǎo rén	spiny jujube [kernel]	Ziziphi Spinosi Semen	15 g.

ACUPUNCTURE AND MOXIBUSTION

Main points: Needle with draining.

GV-14	*dà zhuī*
LI-04	*hé gǔ*
LR-03	*tài chōng*
GB-34	*yáng líng quán*
TB-05	*wài guān*

Auxiliary points:

For pain and distention of the chest and costal regions, add:

LR-14	*qī mén*
CV-17	*tǎn zhōng*

2. BLOOD STASIS FEVER

Clinical Manifestations: Tidal fever in the afternoon or at night; dryness of the throat and mouth (yet fluid intake is not high); painful pressure points of fixed location on the limbs, or the presence of palpable lumps in the body; sallow or ashen complexion with scaling of the skin in more severe cases.

Tongue: Dark, purplish, sometimes presenting stasis macules on the tongue.

Pulse: Thready, rough.

Treatment Method: Quicken the blood, dispel stasis, clear heat.

PRESCRIPTION

House of Blood Stasis-Expelling Decoction *xuè fǔ zhú yū tāng*

táo rén	peach [kernel]	Persicae Semen	12 g.
hóng huā	carthamus [flower]	Carthami Flos	9 g.
dāng guī	tangkuei	Angelicae Sinensis Radix	9 g.
shēng dì huáng	rehmannia [root] dried/fresh	Rehmanniae Radix Exsiccata seu Recens	9 g.
chuān xiōng	ligusticum [root]	Ligustici Rhizoma	4.5 g.
chì sháo yào	red peony [root]	Paeoniae Radix Rubra	6 g.
niú xī	achyranthes [root]	Achyranthis Bidentatae Radix	9 g.
jié gěng	platycodon [root]	Platycodonis Radix	4.5 g.
chái hú	bupleurum [root]	Bupleuri Radix	3 g.
zhǐ ké	bitter orange	Aurantii Fructus	6 g.
gān cǎo	licorice [root]	Glycyrrhizae Radix	3 g.

MODIFICATIONS

To reinforce the effects of clearing heat and cooling the blood, add:

| *bái wéi* | baiwei [cynanchum root] | Cynanchi Baiwei Radix | 9 g. |
| *mǔ dān pí* | moutan [root bark] | Moutan Radicis Cortex | 9 g. |

To reinforce the effects of clearing stagnant heat from the blood, add:

| *zhè chóng* | wingless cockroach | Eupolyphaga seu Opisthoplatia | 6 g. |
| *dà huáng* | rhubarb | Rhei Rhizoma | 6 g. |

In cases with accompanying vacuity of qi, the prescription is modified to benefit qi and move the blood. Add:

| *huáng qí* | astragalus [root] | Astragali (seu Hedysari) Radix 12 g. |

ACUPUNCTURE AND MOXIBUSTION

Main points: Needle with draining.

GV-14	*dà zhuī*
LI-11	*qū chí*
BL-17	*gé shū*
SP-10	*xuè hǎi*
SP-06	*sān yīn jiāo*

Auxiliary points:

For accompanying vacuity of qi, add:

| CV-04 | *guān yuán* |
| ST-36 | *zú sān lǐ* |

3. QI VACUITY FEVER

Clinical Manifestations: Fever generally arising or increasing in severity following overwork, accompanied by dizzy spells, general weakness, shortness of breath, disinclination to speak, spontaneous perspiration, frequent contraction of colds, decreased appetite, loose stools.

Tongue: Pale with thin white coating.

Pulse: Thready, weak.

Treatment Method: Benefit qi, strengthen the spleen, eliminate heat with warm sweet medicines.

PRESCRIPTION

Center-Supplementing Qi-Boosting Decoction *bǔ zhōng yì qì tāng*

huáng qí	astragalus [root]	Astragali (seu Hedysari) Radix	15 g.
rén shēn	ginseng	Ginseng Radix	9 g.
bái zhú	ovate atractylodes [root]	Atractylodis Ovate Rhizoma	9 g.
dāng guī	tangkuei	Angelicae Sinensis Radix	9 g.
chén pí	tangerine [peel]	Citri Exocarpium	6 g.
shēng má	cimicifuga [root]	Cimicifugae Rhizoma	3 g.
chái hú	bupleurum [root]	Bupleuri Radix	3 g.
zhì gān cǎo	licorice [root] (honey-fried)	Glycyrrhizae Radix	6 g.

MODIFICATIONS

In cases of frequent spontaneous perspiration, the prescription is modified to consolidate the body surface and relieve sweating.

Add:

duàn mǔ lì	oyster shell (calcined)	Ostreae Concha Calcinatum	15 g.
duàn lóng gǔ	dragon bone (calcined)	Mastodi Ossis Fossilia Calcinatum	15 g.
fú xiǎo mài	light wheat [grain]	Tritici Semen Leve	15 g.

In cases of fever alternating with chills, as well as perspiration and oversensitivity to drafts, the prescription is modified to harmonize ying and wei. Add:

guì zhī	cinnamon [twig]	Cinnamomi Ramulus	9 g.
bái sháo yào	white peony [root]	Paeoniae Radix Alba	9 g.

In cases presenting oppression in the chest, epigastric fullness and slimy tongue coating, the prescription is modified to fortify the spleen and dry dampness. Add:

cāng zhú	atractylodes [root]	Atractylodis Rhizoma	9 g.
huò xiāng	agastache/patchouli	Agastaches seu Pogostemi Herba	9 g.
hòu pò	magnolia [bark]	Magnoliae Cortex	9 g.

In cases of damp-heat, with bitter taste in the mouth and yellow tongue coating, the prescription is changed to benefit qi, fortify the spleen, clear heat and disinhibit dampness. In place of the preceding decoction use:

Yang-Upbearing Stomach-Boosting Decoction *shēng yáng yì wèi tāng*

huáng qí	astragalus [root]	Astragali (seu Hedysari) Radix	15 g.
rén shēn	ginseng	Ginseng Radix	6 g.
zhì bàn xià	pinellia [tuber] (processed)	Pinelliae Tuber Praeparatum	6 g.
fú líng	poria	Poria	9 g.
chén pí	tangerine [peel]	Citri Exocarpium	6 g.
zhì gān cǎo	licorice [root] (honey-fried)	Glycyrrhizae Radix	3 g.
qiāng huó	notopterygium [root]	Notopterygii Rhizoma	6 g.
dú huó	tuhuo [angelica root]	Angelicae Duhuo Radix	6 g.
fáng fēng	ledebouriella [root]	Ledebouriellae Radix	3 g.
bái sháo yào	white peony [root]	Paeoniae Radix Alba	9 g.
bái zhú	ovate atractylodes [root]	Atractylodis Ovate Rhizoma	9 g.
zé xiè	alisma [tuber]	Alismatis Rhizoma	9 g.
chái hú	bupleurum [root]	Bupleuri Radix	3 g.
huáng lián	coptis [root]	Coptidis Rhizoma	3 g.
shēng jiāng	fresh ginger [root]	Zingiberis Rhizoma Recens	3 g.
dà zǎo	jujube	Ziziphi Fructus	2 pc.

ACUPUNCTURE AND MOXIBUSTION

Main points: Needle with even supplementation, even draining.

CV-04	*guān yuán*
BL-20	*pí shū*
ST-36	*zú sān lǐ*
SP-06	*sān yīn jiāo*
CV-06	*qì hǎi*

Auxiliary points:

For decrease in appetite with loose stools, add:

CV-12	*zhōng wǎn*
ST-25	*tiān shū*

4. BLOOD VACUITY FEVER

Clinical Manifestations: Mild fever accompanied by dizziness and vertigo, physical weakness and fatigue, palpitations, lusterless complexion, pale lips and nails.

Tongue: Pale.

Pulse: Weak, thready.

Treatment Method: Benefit qi, nourish the blood, eliminate heat.

PRESCRIPTION
Spleen-Returning Decoction *guī pí tāng*

huáng qí	astragalus [root]	Astragali (seu Hedysari) Radix	9 g.
rén shēn	ginseng	Ginseng Radix	9 g.
bái zhú	ovate atractylodes [root]	Atractylodis Ovate Rhizoma	9 g.
fú shén	root poria	Poria cum Pini Radice	9 g.
lóng yǎn ròu	longan [flesh]	Longanae Arillus	9 g.
suān zǎo rén	spiny jujube [kernel]	Ziziphi Spinosi Semen	9 g.
mù xiāng	saussurea [root]	Saussureae Radix (seu Vladimiriae)	6 g.
dāng guī	tangkuei	Angelicae Sinensis Radix	6 g.
yuǎn zhì	polygala [root]	Polygalae Radix	3 g.
zhì gān cǎo	licorice [root] (honey-fried)	Glycyrrhizae Radix	6 g.
shēng jiāng	fresh ginger [root]	Zingiberis Rhizoma Recens	3 g.
dà zǎo	jujube	Ziziphi Fructus	5 pc.

<u>MODIFICATIONS</u>

To moisten yin, nourish the blood and eliminate heat, add:

shú dì huáng	cooked rehmannia [root]	Rehmanniae Radix Conquita	12 g.
bái sháo yào	white peony [root]	Paeoniae Radix Alba	9 g.
qīng hāo	sweet wormwood (abbreviated decoction)	Artemisiae Apiaceae seu Annuae Herba	6 g.
bái wēi	baiwei [cynanchum root]	Cynanchi Baiwei Radix	9 g.

In cases of severe palpitations and insomnia, the prescription is modified to nourish the heart and quiet the spirit. Add:

yè jiāo téng	flowery knotweed [stem]	Polygoni Multiflori Caulis	15 g.
wǔ wèi zǐ	schisandra [berry]	Schisandrae Fructus	6 g.
lóng gǔ	dragon bone (extended decoction)	Mastodi Ossis Fossilia	15 g.
mǔ lì	oyster shell (extended decoction)	Ostreae Concha	15 g

ACUPUNCTURE AND MOXIBUSTION

Main points: Needle with even supplementation, even draining.

BL-17	*gé shū*
BL-18	*gān shū*
CV-04	*guān yuán*
ST-36	*zú sān lǐ*
SP-06	*sān yīn jiāo*

Auxiliary points:

For palpitations and insomnia, add:

PC-06	*nèi guān*
HT-07	*shén mén*

5. YIN VACUITY FEVER

Clinical Manifestations: Tidal fever in the afternoon or at night, vexing heat in the five hearts or steaming bone fever, irritability, insomnia, frequent dreaming, flushed cheeks, night sweating, dry mouth and throat, hard dry stools, scanty yellow urine.

Tongue: Red, dry, sometimes with a cracked surface; little or no coating.

Pulse: Thready, rapid.

Treatment Method: Nourish yin, eliminate heat.

PRESCRIPTION

Bone-Clearing Powder *qīng gǔ sǎn*

yín chái hú	lanceolate stellaria [root]	Stellariae Lanceolatae Radix	9 g.
hú huáng lián	picrorhiza [root]	Picrorhizae Rhizoma	6 g.
qín jiāo	large gentian [root]	Gentianae Macrophyllae Radix	6 g.
biē jiǎ	turtle shell (extended decoction)	Amydae Carapax	30 g.
dì gǔ pí	lycium [root bark]	Lycii Radices Cortex	6 g.
qīng hāo	sweet wormwood (abbreviated decoction)	Artemisiae Apiaceae seu Annuae Herba	6 g.
zhī mǔ	anemarrhena [root]	Anemarrhenae Rhizoma	6 g.
zhì gān cǎo	licorice [root] (honey-fried)	Glycyrrhizae Radix	3 g.

MODIFICATIONS

In cases of severe depletion of yin, the prescription is modified to reinforce the moistening of yin and clearing of heat. Add:

shēng dì huáng	rehmannia [root] dried/fresh	Rehmanniae Radix Exsiccata seu Recens	12 g.
xuán shēn	scrophularia [root]	Scrophulariae Radix	9 g.
xī yáng shēn	American ginseng	Panacis Quinquefolii Radix	6 g.

Where night sweating is severe, the prescription is modified to consolidate the body surface and to stop sweating.

Delete:

qīng hāo	sweet wormwood	Artemisiae Apiaceae seu Annuae Herba

Add:

duàn mǔ lì	oyster shell (calcined)	Ostreae Concha Calcinatum	15 g.
fú xiǎo mài	light wheat [grain]	Tritici Semen Leve	15 g.

In cases of insomnia, the prescription is modified to nourish the heart and to quiet the spirit. Add:

suān zǎo rén	spiny jujube [kernel]	Ziziphi Spinosi Semen	12 g.
bǎi zǐ rén	biota [seed]	Biotae Semen	12 g.
yè jiāo téng	flowery knotweed [stem]	Polygoni Multiflori Caulis	15 g.

In cases presenting constipation, the prescription is modified to moisten and free the stool. Add:

huǒ má rén	hemp [seed]	Cannabis Semen	15 g.

In cases accompanied by vacuity of qi and symptoms of dizzy spells, shortness of breath and general fatigue, the prescription is modified to benefit qi and nourish yin. Add:

běi shā shēn	glehnia [root]	Glehniae Radix	9 g.
mài mén dōng	ophiopogon [tuber]	Ophiopogonis Tuber	9 g.
wǔ wèi zǐ	schisandra [berry]	Schisandrae Fructus	6 g.

ACUPUNCTURE AND MOXIBUSTION

Main points: Needle with even supplementation, even draining.

BL-23	*shèn shū*
BL-43 (38)	*gāo huāng shū*
KI-03	*tài xī*
SP-06	*sān yīn jiāo*
KI-01	*yǒng quán*

Auxiliary points:

In cases of insomnia and night sweating, add:

HT-07	*shén mén*
HT-06	*yīn xī*

ALTERNATE THERAPEUTIC METHODS

1. Ear Acupuncture

Main points: Subcortex, Sympathetic, *Shén Mén*, Heart, Liver, Spleen, Kidney.

Method: Needle two or three points once daily or once every two days to elicit a moderate sensation, ten sessions per therapeutic course. Auricular needle embedding can also be employed.

REMARKS

One's first concern in differentiation is between internal damage and external contraction fevers. Once the etiology has been confirmed as internal damage, a clear distinction should be made between repletion and vacuity. Basic treatment methods include the release of stagnation, invigoration of blood, benefit to qi, nourishment of blood and moistening yin. In the clinic, caution must be exercised that pungent and dispersing or bitter and cold prescriptions are not prescribed before conscientious differentiation has been made. Improper use of pungent dispersing prescriptions in cases of internal damage fever can result in the consumption of qi and the injury of fluids, while improper use of cold bitter prescriptions can easily harm spleen and stomach qi, or transform into dryness and injure yin, any of which could further complicate the patient's condition.

It is important in the treatment and prevention of internal damage fevers, that the patient be encouraged to eat appropriately, avoid overwork and maintain an optimistic outlook.

PARASITIC WORM PATTERNS

Chóng Zhèng

1. Roundworm Infection - 2. Pinworm Infection - 3. Tapeworm Infection - 4. Biliary Roundworm (Roundworm Inversion)

This chapter addresses patterns resulting from infection by intestinal parasitic worms, specifically roundworms *(Ascaris lumbricoides)*, pinworms *(Enterobius ver-micularis)* and tapeworms *(Cestoidea)*, and patterns related to biliary roundworm.

ETIOLOGY AND PATHOGENESIS

The major cause of infection by parasitic worms is the consumption of infect-ed foods. Roundworm and pinworm infections generally involve the consumption of raw fruits, melons or vegetables, while tapeworm infection is most often linked to the consumption of undercooked meats containing worm cysts.

The presence of parasitic worms in the intestinal tract obstructs spleen and stomach qi. This leads to the formation of damp-heat and food stasis, causing abdominal distention and pain. Parasitic worms also consume some of the nutrients in the intestinal contents, injuring both qi and blood. This weakens the spleen and stomach and starves the viscera and bowels, causing emaciation and lack of strength.

In biliary roundworm, infestation of roundworms in the small intestine can lead to infestation of the liver and gallbladder through the common biliary duct. This is marked by acute pain in the epigastrium and hypochondrium with nausea or vomiting. Congestion and stagnation can also lead to damp-heat in the liver, with symptoms of jaundice.

1. ROUNDWORM INFECTION

Clinical Manifestations: Intermittent pain in the umbilical region, epigastric discomfort, vomiting of worms when severe and in some cases the desire to eat peculiar or non-food substances. Other symptoms include sallow complexion, emaciation, itching of the nostrils, drooling and grinding of the teeth during sleep, small spots on the inside of the lips or white patches on the face and a history of worms passing with the stool.

Treatment Method: Quiet and expel roundworms, strengthen the spleen and stomach.

PRESCRIPTION

In acute cases with severe abdominal pain, nausea and vomiting, use Mume Pill *(wū-méi wán)* to calm roundworms and relieve pain.

Mume Pill *wū méi wán*

wū méi	mume [fruit]	Mume Fructus	12 g.
zhì fù zǐ	aconite [accessory tuber] (processed) (extended decoction)	Aconiti Tuber Laterale Praeparatum	6 g.
gān jiāng	dried ginger [root]	Zingiberis Rhizoma Exsiccatum	6 g.
huā jiāo	zanthoxylum [husk]	Zanthoxyli Pericarpium	1.5 g.
guì zhī	cinnamon [twig]	Cinnamomi Ramulus	6 g.
xì xīn	asarum	Asiasari Herba cum Radice	1.5 g.
rén shēn	ginseng	Ginseng Radix	9 g.
dāng guī	tangkuei	Angelicae Sinensis Radix	6 g.
huáng lián	coptis [root]	Coptidis Rhizoma	6 g.
huáng bǎi	phellodendron [bark]	Phellodendri Cortex	9 g.

In cases where abdominal pain is mild or absent, use Quisqualis Powder *(shǐ jūn zǐ sǎn)* to expel roundworms.

Quisqualis Powder *shǐ jūn zǐ sǎn*

shǐ jūn zǐ	quisqualis [fruit]	Quisqualis Fructus	9 g.
wú yí	elm cake	Ulmi Fructus Praeparatio	9 g.
chuān liàn zǐ	toosendan [fruit]	Toosendan Fructus	9 g.
gān cǎo	licorice [root]	Glycyrrhizae Radix	6 g.

In cases of prolonged roundworm infection where patients are emaciated and weak, or in cases where spleen and stomach function have not fully recovered following the expulsion of roundworms, use Sassurea and Amomum Six Gentlemen Decoction *(xiāng shā liù jūn zǐ tāng)* to fortify the spleen and stomach.

Sassurea and Amomum Six Gentlemen Decoction *xiāng shā liù jūn zǐ tāng*

rén shēn	ginseng	Ginseng Radix	9 g.
bái zhú	ovate atractylodes [root]	Atractylodis Ovatae Rhizoma	9 g.
fú líng	poria	Poria	9 g.
mù xiāng	saussurea [root]	Saussureae Radix (seu Vladimiriae)	6 g.
shā rén	amomum [fruit] (abbreviated decoction)	Amomi Semen seu Fructus	6 g.
zhì gān cǎo	licorice [root]	Glycyrrhizae Radix	6 g.
chén pí	tangerine [peel]	Citri Exocarpium	6 g.
zhì bàn xià	pinellia [tuber] (processed)	Pinelliae Tuber Praeparatum	6 g.

MODIFICATIONS

To reinforce the expulsion of roundworms, add:

hè shī	carpesium [seed]	Carpesii Fructus	6 g.
bīng láng	areca [nut]	Arecae Semen	9 g.
kǔ liàn pí	chinaberry [root bark]	Meliae Cortex (Radicis)	9 g.

ACUPUNCTURE AND MOXIBUSTION

Main points:

M-UE-9	sì fēng (Four Seams)*
SP-15	dà hèng
CV-06	qì hǎi
ST-36	zú sān lǐ
M-LE-34	bǎi chóng wō (Hundred Worm Nest)

*Use a three-edged or a thick filiform needle to pierce the *sì fēng* points to a depth of 0.3 cm. Withdraw the needle immediately and squeeze a drop of yellow-white fluid from the lesion. Needle the remaining points with even supplementation, even draining.

Auxiliary points:
For emaciation, distention and enlargement of abdomen, add:

        BL-18   *gān shū*
        BL-20   *pí shū*
        SP-06   *sān yīn jiāo*

2. PINWORM INFECTION

Clinical Manifestations: Itching of the anus, especially during the night, restless sleep and the presence of small white worms in the vicinity of the anus during the itching. In chronic cases, symptoms of mild abdominal pain, loss of appetite and emaciation often appear. Pinworm infection is most frequently observed in children.

Treatment Method: Expel worms and relieve itching.

PRESCRIPTION

Quisqualis and Rhubarb Powder *shǐ jūn zǐ dà huáng fěn*

shǐ jūn zǐ	quisqualis [fruit] (powdered)	Quisqualis Fructus Pulveratum
dà huáng	rhubarb (powdered)	Rhei Rhizoma Pulveratum

Method: The daily dosage of quisqualis *(shi jūn zǐ)* is the number of grams equal to the age of the child plus one for children ten years or younger: For example, use 2 grams for a one-year old and 3 grams for a two-year old; for children older than ten years and for adults the dose is 12-15 grams.

The daily dose of rhubarb *(dà huáng)* for children up to six years of age is the number of grams equal to one third of the patient's age plus 0.3 grams. For example, use 0.6 grams for a one-year old and 0.9 grams for a two-year old child. For children older than six years and adult cases, the dosage is 3-6 grams.

Administer the quisqualis *(shǐ jūn zǐ)* dissolved in 50-100 ml boiling water. Divide this into two portions, one-half taken at 2:00 p.m. and the other at 8:00 p.m., for three to six days. Administer the rhubarb *(dà huáng)* steeped in 30-40 ml. boiling water once daily before breakfast for three to six days. A course of treatment begins with the afternoon administration of quisqualis *(shǐ jūn zǐ)* with the initial dose of rhubarb *(dà huáng)* administered the following morning.

ACUPUNCTURE AND MOXIBUSTION

See "Roundworm Infection."

3. TAPEWORM INFECTION

Clinical Manifestations: Mild abdominal pain or distention and discomfort, itching of the anus, diarrhea and the presence of tapeworm segments in the stool. When chronic, symptoms include sallow complexion, emaciation, dizzy spells, fatigue, insomnia.

Tongue: Pale.

Pulse: Thready.

Treatment Method: Expel worms, rectify the spleen and stomach.

PRESCRIPTION

Flushing Expulsion Decoction *qū dí tāng*

nán guā zǐ	pumpkin [seed]	Cucurbitae Semen	60-120 g.
bīng láng	areca [nut]	Arecae Semen	30-60 g.

Method: First shell the pumpkin seed *(nán guā zǐ)* and consume the nutmeat, chewing thoroughly. Two hours later, follow with a concentrated decoction of areca nut *(bīng láng)*. If bowel movements do not commence within four hours of ingesting the areca nut *(bīng láng),* give a 10 g. dose of mirabilite *(máng xiāo)* stirred in boiling water.

These doses should be decreased appropriately for pediatric cases. If the head segment of the tapeworm does not pass with the stool, initiate another treatment, after waiting a minimum of two weeks. After expulsion of tapeworms, give Saussurea and Amomum Six Gentlemen Decoction *(xiāng shā liù jūn zǐ tāng)* to rectify the spleen and stomach and encourage quick recovery.

Saussurea and Amomum Six Gentlemen Decoction *xiāng shā liù jūn zǐ tāng*

rén shēn	ginseng	Ginseng Radix	9 g.
bái zhú	ovate atractylodes [root]	Atractylodis Ovatae Rhizoma	9 g.
fú líng	poria	Poria	9 g.
mù xiāng	saussurea [root]	Saussureae Radix (seu Vladimiriae)	6 g.
shā rén	amomum [fruit] (abbreviated decoction)	Amomi Semen seu Fructus	6 g.
zhì gān cǎo	licorice [root] (honey-fried)	Glycyrrhizae Radix	6 g.
chén pí	tangerine [peel]	Citri Exocarpium	6 g.
zhì bàn xià	pinellia [tuber] (processed)	Pinelliae Tuber Praeparatum	6 g.

4. BILIARY ROUNDWORM (ROUNDWORM INVERSION)

Clinical Manifestations: Sudden acute pain of the epigastrium and right hypochondrium with pain extending through the back and right shoulder, nausea and vomiting, vomiting of worms in some cases and cold extremities. All symptoms seem to disappear with a sudden alleviation of pain, although returning later. On palpation, the abdomen feels soft, with the epigastrium and right hypochondrium sensitive to pressure.

Tongue: Thin white coating.

Pulse: Hidden or wiry, tight. During remissions, normal.

Treatment Method: Quiet and expel worms, relieve pain.

PRESCRIPTION

In acute or early stages of roundworm inversion when the pain is extreme, first administer:

Mume Pill *wū méi wán*

wū méi	mume [fruit]	Mume Fructus	12 g.
zhì fù zǐ	aconite [accessory tuber] (processed) extended decoction)	Aconiti Tuber Laterale Praeparatum	6 g.
gān jiāng	dried ginger [root]	Zingiberis Rhizoma Exsiccatum	6 g.
huā jiāo	zanthoxylum	Zanthoxyli Pericarpium	1.5 g.
guì zhī	cinnamon [twig]	Cinnamomi Ramulus	6 g.

xì xīn	asarum	Asiasari Herba cum Radice	1.5 g.
rén shēn	ginseng	Ginseng Radix	9 g.
dāng guī	tangkuei	Angelicae Sinensis Radix	6 g.
huáng lián	coptis [root]	Coptidis Rhizoma	6 g.
huáng bǎi	phellodendron [bark]	Phellodendri Cortex	9 g.

To reinforce pain relief, the prescription is modified to quicken the blood, rectify qi and relieve pain. Add:

yù jīn	curcuma [tuber]	Curcumae Tuber	9 g.
yán hú suǒ	corydalis [tuber]	Corydalis Tuber	9 g.
bái sháo yào	white peony [root]	Paeoniae Radix Alba	12 g.
gān cǎo	licorice [root]	Glycyrrhizae Radix	6 g.

If accompanied by constipation, the prescription is modified to clear heat and free the stool. Add:

dà huáng	rhubarb (abbreviated decoction)	Rhei Rhizoma	9 g.
bīng láng	areca [nut]	Arecae Semen	9 g.

In cases of severe vomiting, the prescription is modified to harmonize the stomach and downbear qi. Add:

jiāng bàn xià	(ginger-processed) pinellia [tuber]	Pinelliae Tuber Praeparatum	9 g.
chén pí	tangerine [peel]	Citri Exocarpium	9 g.

In cases of biliary roundworm complicated by infection, there will be manifestations of damp-heat, including fever, chills, marked pain upon palpation, jaundice in some cases, yellow slimy tongue coating and rapid slippery pulse. The prescription is modified to clear heat, dispel dampness and regulate gallbladder qi.

Delete:

gān jiāng	dried ginger [root]	Zingiberis Rhizoma Exsiccatum	
zhì fù zǐ	aconite [accessory tuber] (processed) (extended decoction)	Aconiti Tuber Laterale Praeparatum	
guì zhī	cinnamon [twig]	Cinnamomi Ramulus	

Increase the dose of:

huáng lián	coptis [root]	Coptidis Rhizoma	9 g.

and add:

jīn yín huā	lonicera [flower]	Lonicerae Flos	12 g.
lián qiào	forsythia [fruit]	Forsythiae Fructus	12 g.
yīn chén hāo	capillaris	Artemisiae Capillaris Herba	12 g.
shān zhī zǐ	gardenia [fruit]	Gardeniae Fructus	9 g.

After alleviation of the abdominal pain, or in cases where abdominal pain is mild, worms should be expelled.

Use:

Biliary Roundworm-Expelling Decoction *dǎn dào qū huí tāng*

bīng láng	areca [nut]	Arecae Semen	30 g.
shǐ jūn zǐ	quisqualis [fruit]	Quisqualis Fructus	15 g.
yán hú suǒ	corydalis [tuber]	Corydalis Tuber	9 g.
kǔ liàn pí	chinaberry [root bark]	Meliae Cortex (Radicis)	15 g.
dà huáng	rhubarb (abbreviated decoction)	Rhei Rhizoma	9 g.
mù xiāng	saussurea [root]	Saussureae Radix (seu Vladimiriae)	9 g.
hòu pò	magnolia [bark]	Magnoliae Cortex	9 g.

ACUPUNCTURE AND MOXIBUSTION

Main points: Needle with draining; apply strong stimulation.

CV-12	*zhōng wǎn*
CV-13	*shàng wǎn*
GB-34	*yáng líng quán*
ST-36	*zú sān lǐ*
GB-24	*rì yuè*
ST-02	*sì bái*
LI-20	*yíng xiāng*

Auxiliary points:

For abdominal pain, add:

    ST-21   *liáng mén*

For extension of pain through the back and shoulder, add:

    A-Shi Points   *ā shì xué* (Ouch Points)

For vomiting , add:

    PC-06   *nèi guān*

For damp-heat patterns, add:

    SP-09   *yīn líng quán*

ALTERNATE THERAPEUTIC METHODS

1. Ear Acupuncture

Auricular points: Stomach, Small Intestine, Root of Auricle, Vagus Nerve, Sympathetic, *Shén Mén,* Liver, Gallbladder, Spleen.

Method: Select three or four points per session and retain needles 20-30 minutes. Needle to elicit a strong sensation during the attacks of biliary roundworm.

REMARKS

In addition to the particular features of infection by the various parasitic worms mentioned herein, laboratory stool examination will provide valuable diagnostic data by differentiating the intestinal worms. Expulsion of worms is the basic principle in treatment and it is herbal medicine that is most often used. After the worms have been expelled, herbs or acumoxa therapy can be used to regulate spleen and stomach function.

Sanitary eating habits and personal hygiene should both be emphasized in the prevention of infection by parasitic worms.

PULMONARY CONSUMPTION

Fèi Láo

1. Lung Yin Vacuity - 2. Yin Vacuity with Effulgent Fire - 3. Qi and Yin Vacuity - 4. Dual Vacuity of Yin and Yang

Pulmonary consumption *(fèi láo)* is a communicable chronic consumptive disease of the lung, with characteristic symptoms of coughing, spitting blood, tidal fever, night sweating and emaciation.

This chapter discusses treatment of all the types of pulmonary tuberculosis described by Western medicine, including infiltrative pulmonary tuberculosis, focal pulmonary tuberculosis, miliary pulmonary tuberculosis and fibrosa (cavernous pulmonary tuberculosis).

ETIOLOGY AND PATHOGENESIS

The etiology of consumption involves external and internal factors that are mutually causal. Internal factors include weakened constitution, vacuity of both qi and blood, and vacuity of yin and essence. The external factor is invasion of the consumption parasite (*Mycobacterium tuberculosis*). The site of illness is mainly the lung although other visceral organs can also be affected.

The basis of the consumption pathogenesis is depletion of yin. During its initial stages, consumption is most often differentiated as lung yin vacuity. With development, this eventually involves the kidney, heart and liver, ultimately leading to a condition of systemic yin vacuity fire. When damage to the lung involves the spleen, injury to both qi and yin can result. In all cases, advanced stages of the disease show injury to the lung, spleen and kidney, with weakening of both yin and yang.

1. LUNG YIN VACUITY

Clinical Manifestations: Dry cough with scanty phlegm or blood-streaked phlegm in some cases, dull chest pains, afternoon tidal fever, flushed cheeks, night sweating, dry throat and mouth.

Tongue: Dry, thin or peeling coating.

Pulse: Rapid, thready.

Treatment Method: Nourish yin, moisten the lung, relieve coughing, kill worms.

PRESCRIPTION

Lily Bulb Metal-Securing Decoction *bǎi hé gù jīn tāng*

shēng dì huáng	rehmannia [root] dried/fresh	Rehmanniae Radix Exsiccata seu Recens	9 g.
shú dì huáng	cooked rehmannia [root]	Rehmanniae Radix Conquita	9 g.
mài mén dōng	ophiopogon [tuber]	Ophiopogonis Tuber	9 g.
bǎi hé	lily [bulb]	Lilii Bulbus	9 g.
bái sháo yào	white peony [root]	Paeoniae Radix Alba	9 g.
dāng guī	tangkuei	Angelicae Sinensis Radix	6 g.
chuān bèi mǔ	Sichuan fritillaria [bulb]	Fritillariae Cirrhosae Bulbus	9 g.
xuán shēn	scrophularia [root]	Scrophulariae Radix	9 g.
jié gěng	platycodon [root]	Platycodonis Radix	6 g.
gān cǎo	licorice [root]	Glycyrrhizae Radix	6 g.

MODIFICATIONS

To relieve vacuity fever and kill worms, add:

bǎi bù	stemona [root]	Stemonae Radix	9 g.
shí dà gōng láo yè	mahonia [leaf]	Mahoniae Folium	9 g.

In cases of severe lung yin vacuity, the prescription is modified to nourish lung yin. Add:

běi shā shēn	glehnia [root]	Glehniae Radix	12 g.
yù zhú	Solomon's seal [root]	Polygonati Yuzhu Rhizoma	12 g.

In cases of frequent blood expectoration, the prescription is modified to relieve bleeding. Add:

bái jí	bletilla [tuber]	Bletillae Tuber	9 g.
ē jiāo	ass hide glue (dissolved)	Asini Corii Gelatinum	9 g.
xiān hè cǎo	agrimony	Agrimoniae Herba	12 g.
bái máo gēn	imperata [root]	Imperatae Rhizoma	15 g.
ǒu jié	lotus [root node]	Nelumbinis Rhizomatis Nodus	9 g.

For chest pains the prescription is modified to quicken the blood and relieve pain. Add:

yù jīn	curcuma [tuber]	Curcumae Tuber	9 g.
yán hú suǒ	corydalis [tuber]	Corydalis Tuber	9 g.

For tidal fever and vexing heat in the five hearts, the prescription is modified to relieve vacuity fever. Add:

qīng hāo	sweet wormwood (abbreviated decoction)	Artemisiae Apiaceae seu Annuae Herba	9 g.
guī bǎn	tortoise plastron (extended decoction)	Testudinis Plastrum	30 g.
dì gǔ pí	lycium [root bark]	Lycii Radicis Cortex	12 g.

ACUPUNCTURE AND MOXIBUSTION

Main points: Needle with supplementation.

BL-13	*fèi shū*
LU-09	*tài yuān*
BL-43 (38)	*gāo huāng shū*
LU-05	*chǐ zé*

Auxiliary points:
For severe coughing, add:
         LU-07   *liè què*
For blood expectoration, add:
         LU-06   *kǒng zuì*
         BL-17   *gé shū*
For night sweating, add:
         HT-06   *yīn xī*
         KI-07   *fù liū*

2. YIN VACUITY WITH EFFULGENT FIRE

Clinical Manifestations: Choking cough, rapid respiration, sticky scanty yellow phlegm, frequent spitting of bright red blood, steaming bone tidal fever, vexing heat in the five hearts, flushed cheeks, heavy night sweating, irritability, insomnia, frequent dreaming, pulling pains in the chest and hypochondrium, nocturnal emissions, irregular menstruation, emaciation.

Tongue: Red with little coating.

Pulse: Rapid, thready.

Treatment Method: Moisten yin, diminish fire, relieve coughing, kill worms.

PRESCRIPTION

Large Gentian and Turtle Shell Powder *qín jiāo biē jiǎ sǎn*

qín jiāo	large gentian [root]	Gentianae Macrophyllae Radix	9 g.
biē jiǎ	turtle shell (extended decoction)	Amydae Carapax	30 g.
zhī mǔ	anemarrhena [root]	Anemarrhenae Rhizoma	9 g.
dì gǔ pí	lycium [root bark]	Lycii Radicis Cortex	12 g.
chái hú	bupleurum [root]	Bupleuri Radix	6 g.
dāng guī	tangkuei	Angelicae Sinensis Radix	6 g.
qīng hāo	sweet wormwood (abbreviated decoction)	Artemisiae Apiaceae seu Annuae Herba	9 g.
wū méi	mume [fruit]	Mume Fructus	6 g.

MODIFICATIONS

To relieve vacuity fever, delete:
chái hú	bupleurum [root]	Bupleuri Radix

Add:
yín chái hú	lanceolate stellaria [root]	Stellariae Lanceolatae Radix	9 g.

To supplement the lung, relieve coughing and kill worms, add:
bǎi hé	lily [bulb]	Lilii Bulbus	12 g.
chuān bèi mǔ	Sichuan fritillaria [bulb]	Fritillariae Cirrhosae Bulbus	9 g.
bǎi bù	stemona [root]	Stemonae Radix	9 g.

In cases where phlegm is sticky, yellow and turbid, the prescription is modified to clear heat and transform phlegm. Add:
sāng bái pí	mulberry [root bark]	Mori Radicis Cortex	12 g.
mǎ dōu líng	aristolochia [fruit]	Aristolochiae Fructus	9 g.
huáng qín	scutellaria [root]	Scutellariae Radix	9 g.
yú xīng cǎo	houttuynia	Houttuyniae Herba cum Radice	12 g.

In cases of uncontrolled blood expectoration, the prescription is modified to cool the blood and relieve bleeding. Add:

mǔ dān pí	moutan [root bark]	Moutan Radicis Cortex	9 g.
shān zhī zǐ	gardenia	Gardeniae Fructus	9 g.
dà huáng tàn	rhubarb (charred)	Rhei Rhizoma Carbonisata	9 g.

In cases of heavy night sweating, the prescription is modified to moisten yin and control perspiration. Add:

fú xiǎo mài	light wheat [grain]	Tritici Semen Leve	30 g.
wǔ wèi zǐ	schisandra [berry]	Schisandrae Fructus	6 g.
duàn lóng gǔ	dragon bone (calcined)	Mastodi Ossis Fossilia Calcinatum	15 g.
duàn mǔ lì	oyster shell (calcined)	Ostreae Concha Calcinatum	15 g.

In cases of nocturnal emissions, the prescription is modified to nourish the kidney and astringe the essence. Add:

guī bǎn	tortoise plastron (extended decoction)	Testudinis Plastrum	30 g.
shān zhū yú	cornus [fruit]	Corni Fructus	12 g.
qiàn shí	euryale [seed]	Euryales Semen	12 g.
jīn yīng zǐ	Cherokee rose [fruit]	Rosae Laevigatae Fructus	12 g.

In cases of irregular menstruation, the prescription is modified to regulate and rectify the *chōng* and *rèn*. Add:

bái sháo yào	white peony [root]	Paeoniae Radix Alba	12 g.
dān shēn	salvia [root]	Salviae Miltiorrhizae Radix	9 g.
mǔ dān pí	moutan [root bark]	Moutan Radicis Cortex	9 g.
yì mǔ cǎo	leonurus	Leonuri Herba	12 g.

In cases presenting vexation in the heart and insomnia, the prescription is modified to clear heat and quiet the spirit. Add:

shān zhī zǐ	gardenia [fruit]	Gardeniae Fructus	9 g.
yè jiāo téng	flowery knotweed [stem]	Polygoni Multiflori Caulis	15 g.
suān zǎo rén	spiny jujube [kernel]	Ziziphi Spinosi Semen	12 g.
zhēn zhū mǔ	mother-of-pearl (extended decoction)	Concha Margaritifera	30 g.

ACUPUNCTURE AND MOXIBUSTION

Main points: Needle with even supplementation, even draining.

BL-13	*fèi shū*
BL-23	*shèn shū*
BL-43 (38)	*gāo huāng shū*
KI-03	*tài xī*
LU-10	*yú jì*
LR-02	*xíng jiān*

Auxiliary points:

For tidal fever, add:

| GV-14 | *dà zhuī* |
| PC-05 | *jiān shǐ* |

For nocturnal emission, add:

| BL-52 (47) | *zhì shì* |
| SP-06 | *sān yīn jiāo* |

3. Qi and Yin Vacuity

Clinical Manifestations: Weak cough, shortness of breath, weak voice, phlegm occasionally containing light red blood, afternoon tidal fever (although mild), flushed cheeks, night sweating, spontaneous perspiration, pale complexion, tiredness, poor appetite.

Tongue: Tender, red with tooth marks, thin or peeling coating.

Pulse: Rapid, thready, forceless.

Treatment Method: Benefit qi, nourish yin, supplement vacuity, kill worms.

PRESCRIPTION

True-Safeguarding Decoction *bǎo zhēn tāng*

dǎng shēn	codonopsis [root]	Codonopsitis Radix	6 g.
huáng qí	astragalus [root]	Astragali (seu Hedysari) Radix	6 g.
bái zhú	ovate atractylodes [root]	Atractylodis Ovatae Rhizoma	6 g.
fú líng	poria	Poria	6 g.
chì fú líng	red poria	Poria Rubra	6 g.
shú dì huáng	cooked rehmannia [root]	Rehmanniae Radix Conquita	6 g.
shēng dì huáng	rehmannia [root] dried/fresh	Rehmanniae Radix Exsiccata seu Recens	6 g.
dāng guī	tangkuei	Angelicae Sinensis Radix	6 g.
bái sháo yào	white peony [root]	Paeoniae Radix Alba	6 g.
chì sháo yào	red peony [root]	Paeoniae Radix Rubra	6 g.
wǔ wèi zǐ	schisandra [berry]	Schisandrae Fructus	6 g.
tiān mén dōng	asparagus [tuber]	Asparagi Tuber	6 g.
mài mén dōng	ophiopogon [tuber]	Ophiopogonis Tuber	6 g.
chái hú	bupleurum [root]	Bupleuri Radix	6 g.
hòu pò	magnolia [bark]	Magnoliae Cortex	6 g.
dì gǔ pí	lycium [root bark]	Lycii Radicis Cortex	6 g.
zhī mǔ	anemarrhena [root]	Anemarrhenae Rhizoma	6 g.
huáng bǎi	phellodendron [bark]	Phellodendri Cortex	6 g.
chén pí	tangerine [peel]	Citri Exocarpium	6 g.
lián zǐ xīn	lotus [embryo]	Nelumbinis Embryo	3 g.
shēng jiāng	fresh ginger [root]	Zingiberis Rhizoma Recens	3 g.
gān cǎo	licorice [root]	Glycyrrhizae Radix	6 g.
dà zǎo	jujube	Ziziphi Fructus	4 pc.

MODIFICATIONS

In consumption, the prescription is often adjusted as follows:

Delete:

chì sháo yào	red peony [root]	Paeoniae Radix Rubra
chì fú líng	red poria	Poria Rubra
hòu pò	magnolia [bark]	Magnoliae Cortex

Add:

bái jí	bletilla [tuber]	Bletillae Tuber	9 g.
chuān bèi mǔ	Sichuan fritillaria [bulb]	Fritillariae Cirrhosae Bulbus	9 g.
bǎi bù	stemona [root]	Stemonae Radix	9 g.

In cases of coughing blood, the prescription is modified to relieve bleeding. Add:

ē jiāo	ass hide glue (dissolved)	Asini Corii Gelatinum	9 g.
xiān hè cǎo	agrimony	Agrimoniae Herba	12 g.
sān qī	notoginseng [root]	Notoginseng Radix	9 g.
	(or, powdered and stirred in, each time 1.5 g.)		

In cases of vacuity of spleen qi, presenting loose stools, abdominal distention and loss of appetite, the prescription is modified to fortify the spleen and boost qi. Delete moist and sticky medicines such as:

shú dì huáng	cooked rehmannia [root]	Rehmanniae Radix Conquita	
tiān mén dōng	asparagus [tuber]	Asparagi Tuber	
mài mén dōng	ophiopogon [tuber]	Ophiopogonis Tuber	

Add:

shān yào	dioscorea [root]	Dioscoreae Rhizoma	12 g.
biǎn dòu	lablab [bean]	Lablab Semen	12 g.
yì yǐ rén	coix [seed]	Coicis Semen	30 g.

ACUPUNCTURE AND MOXIBUSTION

Main points: Needle with supplementation.

BL-13	*fèi shū*
BL-20	*pí shū*
BL-43 (38)	*gāo huāng shū*
ST-36	*zú sān lǐ*
SP-06	*sān yīn jiāo*

Auxiliary points:

For loss of appetite and abdominal distention, add:

BL-21	*wèi shū*
CV-12	*zhōng wǎn*

4. DUAL VACUITY OF YIN AND YANG

Clinical Manifestations: Choking cough, spitting blood, steaming bone tidal fever, night sweating, loss of voice, frail constitution, physical cold, over-sensitivity to drafts, spontaneous perspiration, difficult respiration, shortness of breath, edema of the face and limbs, diminished food intake, loose stools, spontaneous seminal emission and, in some cases, impotence, diminished menstrual flow or amenorrhea.

Tongue: Red, shiny, lacking moisture; or enlarged, pale with tooth marks.

Pulse: Faint, thready.

Treatment Method: Nourish yin, warm yang, supplement vacuity, kill worms.

PRESCRIPTION

Heaven-Supplementing Great Creation Pill *bǔ tiān dà zào wán*

rén shēn	ginseng	Ginseng Radix	9 g.
huáng qí	astragalus [root]	Astragali (seu Hedysari) Radix	9 g.
bái zhú	ovate atractylodes [root]	Atractylodis Ovatae Rhizoma	9 g.
fú líng	poria	Poria	9 g.
shān yào	dioscorea [root]	Dioscoreae Rhizoma	9 g.
dāng guī	tangkuei	Angelicae Sinensis Radix	6 g.
bái sháo yào	white peony [root]	Paeoniae Radix Alba	9 g.
gǒu qǐ zǐ	lycium [berry]	Lycii Fructus	9 g.
shú dì huáng	cooked rehmannia [root]	Rehmanniae Radix Conquita	9 g.
guī bǎn	tortoise plastron (extended decoction)	Testudinis Plastrum	30 g.
lù jiǎo jiāo	deerhorn glue (dissolved and stirred in)	Cervi Gelatinum Cornu	9 g.
zǐ hé chē	placenta (stirred in)	Hominis Placenta	3 g.
suān zǎo rén	spiny jujube [kernel]	Ziziphi Spinosi Semen	12 g.
yuǎn zhì	polygala [root]	Polygalae Radix	6 g.

MODIFICATIONS

To reinforce the supplementation of vacuity and extermination of parasites, add:

mài mén dōng	ophiopogon [tuber]	Ophiopogonis Tuber	9 g.
ē jiāo	ass hide glue (dissolved)	Asini Corii Gelatinum	9 g.
chuān bèi mǔ	Sichuan fritillaria [bulb]	Fritillariae Cirrhosae Bulbus	9 g.
bǎi bù	stemona [root]	Stemonae Radix	9 g.

In cases where kidney qi vacuity and the consequent counterflow of qi cause labored breathing, the prescription is modified to supplement the kidney and absorb qi and calm panting. Add:

dōng chóng xià cǎo	cordyceps	Cordyceps	9 g.
hē zǐ	chebule	Chebulae Fructus	9 g.

In cases of diarrhea before dawn (cock's crow diarrhea), the prescription is modified to warm and supplement the spleen and kidney, secure the intestines and relieve diarrhea. Add:

ròu dòu kòu	nutmeg (roasted)	Myristicae Semen	9 g.
bǔ gǔ zhī	psoralea [seed]	Psoraleae Semen	9 g.
wú zhū yú	evodia [fruit]	Evodiae Fructus	4.5 g.

ACUPUNCTURE AND MOXIBUSTION

Main points: Needle with supplementation; add moxibustion.

BL-13	*fèi shū*
BL-20	*pí shū*
BL-23	*shèn shū*
BL-43 (38)	*gāo huāng shū*
CV-04	*guān yuán*
ST-36	*zú sān lǐ*

ALTERNATE THERAPEUTIC METHODS

1. Ear Acupuncture

Main points: Lung region *Ā Shì* points, Spleen, Kidney, Endocrine, *Shén Mén*.

Method: Needle to elicit a mild sensation. Treat once every two days, ten days per therapeutic course.

REMARKS

The fundamental principles in the treatment of consumption are supplementing vacuity, fostering correct qi and essence and extermination of the consumption parasite, *Mycobacterium tuberculosis*. Supplementation should be directed primarily at the lung and secondarily at the spleen and kidney. The predominant treatment principle is nourishment of yin, complimented by clearing fire where there is fire, supplementing qi where there is qi vacuity and bolstering both yin and yang when both are vacuous.

When using yin supplements, simultaneous use of sweet bland spleen-strengthening medicinals will serve not only to supplement the spleen and aid the lung, but will also prevent the moist and sticky yin supplementing medicinals from burdening the spleen. These include:

bái zhú	ovate atractylodes [root	Atractylodis Ovatae Rhizoma	9 g.
biǎn dòu	lablab [bean]	Lablab Semen	12 g.
shān yào	dioscorea [root]	Dioscoreae Rhizoma	15 g.
chén pí	tangerine [peel]	Citri Exocarpium	9 g.
gǔ yá	rice [sprout]	Oryzae Fructus Germinatus	12 g.

On the other extreme, the use of medicinals that are too drying or pungent should be avoided, since they tend to consume qi, deplete yin and move the blood. As far as extermination of the parasite is concerned, simultaneous use of Western antituberculosis drugs greatly improves the efficacy of treatment.

Consumption is best treated in its early stages. During treatment, patients should abstain from alcohol and sex, regulate their sleeping habits, avoid emotional stress, take precautions against drastic changes in the weather and participate in some suitable form of physical exercise, such as taijiquan or qigong. Their diet should be rich in nutrients and could include soft shelled turtle, chicken, duck, cow and goat milk, honey, tremella *(bái mù ěr)*, pear, lotus root and loquat fruit. Hot spicy irritating foods should be strictly avoided.

FACIAL PAIN

Miàn Tòng

1. External Wind-Cold - 2. Liver and Stomach Fire

Facial pain refers specifically to spasmodic penetrating pain of the cheek and temple. This pain is of sudden onset and is characteristically paroxysmal, radiating and quite severe.

Facial pain is more common during middle age, and more prevalent among women. The pain persists for only several seconds or minutes before spontaneous remission, with no other symptoms between bouts. Usually, only one side of the face is affected, commonly the upper or lower jaw. Facial pain of the temples and forehead is more rarely observed. In many cases, facial pain can be induced by a specific stimulus, for example, as a result of speaking, chewing, gargling or touching certain points on the face. Cases of facial pain are often prolonged, recurrent and unresponsive to treatment.

In Western medicine, facial pain *(miàn tòng)* corresponds to trigeminal neuralgia.

ETIOLOGY AND PATHOGENESIS

Facial pain is most often the result of wind-cold evil entering the facial portion of the yangming channel, hindering the movement of qi and blood and causes obstruction of the channels, leading to pain. The second cause is liver and stomach fire flaring upward, giving rise to facial pain. This usually results from the transformation of stagnant liver qi to fire, coupled with food stagnation as a consequence of overindulgent eating.

1. EXTERNAL WIND-COLD

Clinical Manifestations: Sudden attacks of facial pain, often occurring with local muscular spasms, aggravation of pain by exposure to cold and alleviation by exposure to heat, runny nose with clear thin mucus, excessive salivation.

Tongue: Thin white coating.

Pulse: Floating, tight.

Treatment Method: Dispel wind, dissipate cold, relieve pain.

PRESCRIPTION

Tea-Blended Ligusticum Powder *chuān xiōng chá tiáo sǎn*

chuān xiōng	ligusticum [root]	Ligustici Rhizoma	9 g.
jīng jiè	schizonepeta (abbreviated decoction)	Schizonepetae Herba et Flos	9 g.
bái zhǐ	angelica [root]	Angelicae Dahuricae Radix	6 g.
qiāng huó	notopterygium [root]	Notopterygii Rhizoma	6 g.
xì xīn	asarum	Asiasari Herba cum Radice	3 g.
fáng fēng	ledebouriella [root]	Ledebouriellae Radix	6 g.
gān cǎo	licorice [root]	Glycyrrhizae Radix	6 g.
bò hé	mint (abbreviated decoction)	Menthae Herba	9 g.

MODIFICATIONS

To reinforce warming the channels and dispersing cold, add:

guì zhī	cinnamon [twig]	Cinnamomi Ramulus	9 g.
gǎo běn	Chinese lovage [root]	Ligustici Sinensis Rhizoma et Radix	9 g.

ACUPUNCTURE AND MOXIBUSTION

Main points: Needle with draining; add moxibustion.

LI-04	*hé gǔ*
GB-20	*fēng chí*
ST-07	*xià guān*
TB-05	*wài guān*

Auxiliary points:

For supraorbital pain, add:

M-HN-6	*yú yāo* (Fish's Lumbus)
BL-02	*zǎn zhú*
GB-14	*yáng bái*
M-HN-9	*tài yáng* (Greater Yang)

For supramaxillary pain, add:

ST-02	*sì bái*
SI-18	*quán liáo*
GB-03	*shàng guān*
LI-20	*yíng xiāng*

For mandibular pain, add:

M-HN-18	*jiā chéng jiāng* (Pinching Sauce Receptacle)
ST-06	*jiá chē*
ST-05	*dà yíng*
TB-17	*yì fēng*

Include *ā shì* points.

2. LIVER AND STOMACH FIRE

Clinical Manifestations: Sudden attacks of facial pain, burning sensation at the site of pain, irritability, bloodshot eyes, tearing of the eyes, thirst, constipation in some cases.

Tongue: Red with yellow coating.

Pulse: Rapid, wiry.

Treatment Method: Clear liver and stomach fire, relieve pain.

PRESCRIPTION

Ligusticum, Dahurican Angelica and Gypsum Decoction
xiōng zhǐ shí gāo tāng

chuān xiōng	ligusticum [root]	Ligustici Rhizoma	6 g.
bái zhǐ	angelica [root]	Angelicae Dahuricae Radix	6 g.
shí gāo	gypsum (extended decoction)	Gypsum	30 g.
jú huā	chrysanthemum [flower]	Chrysanthemi Flos	9 g.
gǎo běn	Chinese lovage [root]	Ligustici Sinensis Rhizoma et Radix	6 g.
qiāng huó	notopterygium [root]	Notopterygii Rhizoma	6 g.

MODIFICATIONS

When using this prescription in cases of facial pain caused by liver and stomach fire, the prescription is modified to drain the liver and stomach, clear heat and relieve pain. Add:

tiān má	gastrodia [root]	Gastrodiae Rhizoma	9 g.
gōu téng	uncaria [stem and thorn]	Uncariae Ramulus cum Unco	9 g.
huáng qín	scutellaria [root]	Scutellariae Radix	9 g.
shān zhī zǐ	gardenia [fruit]	Gardeniae Fructus	9 g.
bái jiāng cán	silkworm	Bombyx Batryticatus	9 g.
quán xiē	scorpion	Buthus	4.5 g.

In cases of yin vacuity with effulgent fire, with symptoms of lower backache, tiredness, emaciation, flushed cheeks, vexing heat in the five hearts, red tongue with little coating, thready rapid pulse and induction or aggravation of pain with stress or strain, the prescription is modified to moisten yin and reduce vacuity fire. Add:

shēng dì huáng	rehmannia [root] dried/fresh	Rehmanniae Radix Exsiccata seu Recens	12 g.
zhī mǔ	anemarrhena [root]	Anemarrhenae Rhizoma	9 g.
gǒu qǐ zǐ	lycium [berry]	Lycii Fructus	9 g.
niú xī	achyranthes [root]	Achyranthis Bidentatae Radix	9 g.

In prolonged cases of facial pain, the prescription is modified to dispel stasis, free the connections and relieve pain. Add:

táo rén	peach kernel	Persicae Semen	9 g.
hóng huā	carthamus [flower]	Carthami Flosa	9 g.
chì sháo yào	red peony [root]	Paeoniae Radix Rubra	9 g.

ACUPUNCTURE AND MOXIBUSTION

Main points: Needle with draining.

LI-04	*hé gǔ*
ST-07	*xià guān*
LR-02	*xíng jiān*
ST-44	*nèi tíng*

Auxiliary points:

For yin vacuity with effulgent fire, add:

KI-03	*tài xī*
SP-06	*sān yīn jiāo*

For supraorbital pain, add:

M-HN-6	*yú yāo* (Fish's Lumbus)
BL-02	*zǎn zhú*
GB-14	*yáng bái*
M-HN-9	*tài yáng* (Greater Yang)

For supramaxillary pain, add:

ST-02	*sì bái*
SI-18	*quán liáo*
GB-03	*shàng guān*
LI-20	*yíng xiāng*

For mandibular pain, add:

M-HN-18	*jiā chéng jiāng* (Pinching Sauce Receptacle)
ST-06	*jiá chē*
ST-05	*dà yíng*
TB-17	*yì fēng*

Include *ā shì* points.

ALTERNATE THERAPEUTIC METHODS

1. Ear Acupuncture

Auricular points: Cheek, Maxilla, Mandible, Forehead, *Shén Mén.*

Method: Needle to elicit a strong sensation and retain needles for twenty to thirty minutes, applying manipulations every five minutes. Needle embedding therapy can also be used.

REMARKS

Acupuncture has been proven in clinical practice to be remarkably effective in alleviating facial pain without side effects. Acupuncture can therefore be considered, at present, a relatively ideal form of treatment for facial pain. In prolonged cases where the patient's constitution is weak, manipulation of the needles should be modified to effect even supplementation, even draining, to support correct qi while dispelling evil.

In cases of facial pain resulting from tooth infection or the development of tumors, emphasis should be placed on treatment of the primary disease.

MALARIAL PATTERNS

Nüè Zhèng

1. Typical Malaria - 2. Taxation Malaria

Malaria is an infectious disease characterized by cycles of recurring chills alternating with high fever. Malaria is most prevalent during the summer and autumn months, although it can occur in any season. The main cause of malaria is infection by malarial evils. In Western medicine, malaria is viewed as caused by the protozoan *Plasmodium,* which is spread by mosquitoes from an infected human host.

Malaria can be classified into twenty-four hour malaria (one cycle per twenty-four hours), forty-eight hour malaria, and seventy-two hour malaria according to the length of the cycle of attacks. Forty-eight hour malaria is most commonly observed clinically.

Malaria is clinically divided according to secondary evils and differing physical constitutions. Classification includes typical malaria, warm malaria, cold malaria, taxation malaria, and miasmic malaria. Typical malaria *(zhèng nüè),* with its alternating chills and fever, is most commonly observed. Warm malaria *(wēn nüè)* describes cases where heat and fever are predominant, and cold malaria *(hán nüè)* describes cases where cold and chills are predominant. In taxation malaria *(láo nüè)* the course of illness is prolonged; qi and blood are depleted, and the symptoms are induced by taxation.

Cases where blood stasis and congealed phlegm have created lumps under the lower border of the rib cage are known as "mother of malaria" *(nüè mǔ).* Miasmic malaria *(zhàng nüè)* is found when pestilence and dampness are involved.

The discussion in this chapter focuses on typical malaria and taxation malaria, as these are the main types, with adjustments according to secondary evils.

ETIOLOGY AND PATHOGENESIS

The major factor in the etiology of malaria is the invasion of malarial evils, although simultaneous invasion of other external evils such as wind, cold, summerheat and dampness are not uncommon. In addition, injury to the spleen and stomach through improper diet and eating habits can result in depletion of qi and blood, accumulation of phlegm and dampness, and malaria.

The etiology of malaria can also involve the invasion of evils when the physical condition has been weakened, for instance, where stress, strain or imprudent sleeping habits have led to the depletion of correct qi or an imbalance between construction and defense. The characteristic chills and fever of malaria are evidence of evils at a half-exterior, half-interior location.

1. TYPICAL MALARIA

Clinical Manifestations: Cyclic bouts of chills and fever characterized by initial yawning and fatigue progressing into chills. Chills are replaced by signs of internal and external heat, exhibiting fever, headache, bloodshot eyes, thirst and a large intake of fluids. The appearance of whole-body perspiration marks the remittance of fever.

Tongue: Red with thin white or yellow slimy coating.

Pulse: Wiry.

Treatment Method: Relieve shao yang symptoms (half-exterior half-interior), dispel evils, terminate malaria.

PRESCRIPTION

Minor Bupleurum Decoction *xiǎo chái hú tāng*

chái hú	bupleurum [root]	Bupleuri Radix	12 g.
huáng qín	scutellaria [root]	Scutellariae Radix	9 g.
zhì bàn xià	pinellia [tuber] (processed)	Pinelliae Tuber Praeparatum	9 g.
shēng jiāng	fresh ginger [root]	Zingiberis Rhizoma Recens	9 g.
rén shēn	ginseng	Ginseng Radix	6 g.
zhì gān cǎo	licorice [root] (honey-fried)	Glycyrrhizae Radix	6 g.
dà zǎo	jujube	Ziziphi Fructus	4 pc.

MODIFICATIONS

To reinforce the effects of dispelling evils and terminating malaria, add:

cháng shān	dichroa [root]	Dichroae Radix	9 g.
cǎo guǒ	tsaoko [fruit]	Amomi Tsao-Ko Fructus	6 g.
qīng hāo	sweet wormwood (abbreviated decoction)	Artemisiae Apiaceae seu Annuae Herba	9 g.

In cases where cold is predominant, with symptoms of severe aversion to cold, little perspiration and a white tongue coating, the prescription is modified to relieve external symptoms and promote perspiration. Add:

guì zhī	cinnamon [twig]	Cinnamomi Ramulus	9 g.
fáng fēng	ledebouriella [root]	Ledebouriellae Radix	9 g.
qiāng huó	notopterygium [root]	Notopterygii Rhizoma	9 g.

In cases where dampness is predominant, with symptoms of fullness and discomfort of the chest and epigastrium, nausea, vomiting and a slimy tongue coating, the prescription is modified to rectify qi and dispel dampness.

Delete:

rén shēn	ginseng	Ginseng Radix

Add:

cāng zhú	atractylodes [root]	Atractylodis Rhizoma	9 g.
hòu pò	magnolia [bark]	Magnoliae Cortex	9 g.
qīng pí	unripe tangerine [peel]	Citri Exocarpium Immaturum	9 g.

In cases of excessive thirst, the prescription is modified to generate liquid and relieve thirst. Add:

gé gēn	pueraria [root]	Puerariae Radix	12 g.
shí hú	dendrobium [stem] (extended decoction)	Dendrobii Caulis	12 g.

In cases where yang is predominant, with symptoms of heat including painful joints, thirst, constipation, dark yellow urine, red tongue with yellow coating and rapid wiry pulse, the prescription is changed to clear heat, dispel evils and relieve malaria.

Use:

White Tiger Decoction Plus Cinnamon Twig *bái hǔ jiā guì zhī tāng*

guì zhī	cinnamon [twig]	Cinnamomi Ramulus	6 g.
zhī mǔ	anemarrhena [root]	Anemarrhenae Rhizoma	9 g.
shí gāo	gypsum (extended decoction)	Gypsum	30 g.
jīng mǐ	rice	Oryzae Semen	15 g.
zhì gān cǎo	licorice [root] (honey-fried)	Glycyrrhizae Radix	6 g.

Add:

| *chái hú* | bupleurum [root] | Bupleuri Radix | 9 g. |
| *qīng hāo* | sweet wormwood (abbreviated decoction) | Artemisiae Apiaceae seu Annuae Herba | 9 g. |

Where heat is present without cold, delete:

| *guì zhī* | cinnamon [twig] | Cinnamomi Ramulus | |

Where damp-heat is predominant, with symptoms of chest oppression, nausea, vomiting and yellow slimy tongue coating, the prescription is modified to clear heat and drain dampness. Add:

huáng qín	scutellaria [root]	Scutellariae Radix	9 g.
huáng lián	coptis [root]	Coptidis Rhizoma	9 g.
huá shí	talcum (wrapped)	Talcum	12 g.
fú líng	poria	Poria	12 g.

In cases of internal invasion of malarial evils, with high fever, loss of consciousness, delirium and convulsions, the prescription is changed to clear the heart and open the orifices. Immediately administer PURPLE SNOW ELIXIR (*zǐ xuě dān*) or SUPREME JEWEL ELIXIR (*zhì bǎo dān*).

ACUPUNCTURE AND MOXIBUSTION

Main points: Needle with draining two hours before onset of symptoms. Where cold is predominant, add moxibustion.

BL-11	*dà zhù*
GV-13	*táo dào*
SI-03	*hòu xī*
PC-05	*jiān shǐ*
TB-02	*yè mén*
PC-06	*nèi guān*

Auxiliary points:

For predominance of heat, add:

| LI-11 | *qū chí* |

For predominance of cold, add:

| LI-04 | *hé gǔ* |

For predominance of phlegm-dampness, add:

| SP-09 | *yīn líng quán* |
| ST-40 | *fēng lóng* |

For loss of consciousness, delirium and convulsions, add:

| GV-26 | *shuǐ gōu* |

Bleed the hand jing-well points *(shí èr jĭng xué)*:

LU-11	*shào shāng*
HT-09	*shào chōng*
PC-09	*zhōng chōng*
LI-01	*shāng yáng*
TB-01	*guān chōng*
SI-01	*shào zé*

2. TAXATION MALARIA

Clinical Manifestations: Prolonged malaria, tiredness, fatigue, shortness of breath, disinclination to speak, poor appetite, sallow complexion, emaciation, spontaneous perspiration, recurrence of malaria symptoms with stress or strain, alternation of fever with chills and, in some cases, presentation of lumps and masses below the lower edge of the rib cage.

Tongue: Pale.

Pulse: Thready, forceless.

Treatment Method: Boost qi, nourish the blood, dispel evils.

PRESCRIPTION
Flowery Knotweed and Ginseng Beverage *hé rén yĭn*

rén shēn	ginseng	Ginseng Radix	12 g.
hé shŏu wū	flowery knotweed [root]	Polygoni Multiflori Radix	30 g.
dāng guī	tangkuei	Angelicae Sinensis Radix	12 g.
chén pí	tangerine [peel]	Citri Exocarpium	9 g.
shēng jiāng	fresh ginger [root]	Zingiberis Rhizoma Recens	9 g.

MODIFICATIONS

The prescription is reinforced to dispel evil and terminate malaria. Add:

cháng shān	dichroa [root]	Dichroae Radix	9 g.
qīng hāo	sweet wormwood (abbreviated decoction)	Artemisiae Apiaceae seu Annuae Herba	9 g.

In cases of formation of lumps and masses below the lower border of the rib cage, the prescription is changed to remove stasis, transform phlegm, soften lumps and dissipate binds. Use the prepared medicine, TURTLE SHELL DECOCTED PILL *(biē jiă jiān wán)*.

Where symptoms of qi and blood vacuity are evident, the prescription is changed to simultaneously address vacuity and repletion. Complement TURTLE SHELL DECOCTED PILL *(biē jiă jiān wán)* with Eight-Gem Decoction *(bā zhēn tāng)*:

Eight-Gem Decoction *bā zhēn tāng*

shú dì huáng	cooked rehmannia [root]	Rehmanniae Radix Conquita	12 g.
dāng guī	tangkuei	Angelicae Sinensis Radix	9 g.
bái sháo yào	white peony [root]	Paeoniae Radix Alba	9 g.
chuān xiōng	ligusticum [root]	Ligustici Rhizoma	6 g.
rén shēn	ginseng	Ginseng Radix	9 g.
bái zhú	ovate atractylodes [root]	Atractylodis Ovatae Rhizoma	9 g.
fú líng	poria	Poria	12 g.
zhì gān căo	licorice [root] (honey-fried)	Glycyrrhizae Radix	6 g.
shēng jiāng	fresh ginger [root]	Zingiberis Rhizoma Recens	3 g.
dà zăo	jujube	Ziziphi Fructus	3 pc.

ACUPUNCTURE AND MOXIBUSTION

Main points: Needle with supplementation; add moxibustion. Apply acupuncture two hours prior to onset of symptoms.

BL-11	*dà zhù*
SI-03	*hòu xī*
PC-05	*jiān shǐ*
TB-02	*yè mén*
BL-20	*pí shū*
ST-36	*zú sān lǐ*

Auxiliary points:

For lumps and masses, add:

LR-13	*zhāng mén*
M-BW-16	*pǐ gēn* (Glomus Root)

ALTERNATE THERAPEUTIC METHODS

1. Ear Acupuncture

Auricular points: Adrenal, Subcortex, Endocrine, Spleen, Liver.

Method: Two hours preceding the onset of symptoms, needle bilaterally to elicit a strong sensation. Retain needles one hour. Treat for three consecutive days.

REMARKS

Acupuncture and moxibustion have been shown to be effective in the treatment of malaria, especially the forty-eight hour type. Not only are the symptoms of malaria brought under control, but *Plasmodium* levels in the blood are seen to drop. The time-frame of the cycle is important in the treatment of malaria. The most effective time to administer medicine or apply acupuncture is about two hours prior to the onset of chills and fever.

Western clinical practice has proven the use of sweet wormwood *(qīng hāo)* to be highly effective in all types of malaria, including miasmic malaria. Results are reliable without toxic reactions or side effects. Administration is either in tablet or injection form, one gram daily over two consecutive days.

In cases of miasmic malaria, a comprehensive treatment involving both traditional and Western therapeutics should be promptly initiated.

PART II

SURGERY

SCROFULA

Luǒ Lì

1. Liver Qi Stagnation - 2. Kidney Yin Depletion

Scrofula is a chronic infectious disease appearing mostly on the neck. Its Chinese name, *luǒ lì,* describes the characteristic arrangement of lumps, much like pearls threaded on a string. Scrofula often affects children and teenagers, with the pathological changes occurring on the neck and behind the ears. In Western medicine, scrofula includes tuberculosis of the cervical lymph nodes.

ETIOLOGY AND PATHOGENESIS

The development of scrofula often involves emotional disturbance. In one etiology, stagnation of liver qi injures the transport function of the spleen. Pathological changes allow the production of internal phlegm-heat; this congeals and obstructs the channels and connections, leading to scrofula.

In a second etiology, which is often a development of the first, stagnation of liver qi gives rise to fire, which descends and scorches kidney yin. The resultant exuberant heat decomposes the tissues and produces pus. Depletion of lung and kidney yin is also seen clinically, giving rise to vacuity fire, which combines with phlegm to form the lumps characteristic of scrofula.

1. LIVER QI STAGNATION

Clinical Manifestations: Generally observed during the initial and intermediate stages of scrofula, symptoms include initial swelling of one or several cervical lymph nodes to the size of a bean. These lumps show no change in the color of the skin and are firm, moveable and painless. During the intermediate stages, symptoms include a gradual increase in size of the lymph nodes, adhesion of lymph nodes to the skin, and, in some cases, the appearance of chains of several lumps that are fixed and tender on palpation. Accompanying symptoms may include emotional depression, distention and pain of the chest and hypochondrium, epigastric fullness and discomfort and poor appetite.

Tongue: Thin tongue coating.

Pulse: Wiry.

Treatment Method: Soothe the liver, strengthen the spleen, transform phlegm, disperse lumps.

PRESCRIPTION

Combine Free Wanderer Powder *(xiāo yáo sǎn)* with Two Matured Ingredients Decoction *(èr chén tāng).*

Free Wanderer Powder *xiāo yáo sǎn*

chái hú	bupleurum [root]	Bupleuri Radix	9 g.
bái sháo yào	white peony [root]	Paeoniae Radix Alba	12 g.
dāng guī	tangkuei	Angelicae Sinensis Radix	9 g.
bái zhú	ovate atractylodes [root]	Atractylodis Ovatae Rhizoma	9 g.
fú líng	poria	Poria	9 g.
zhì gān cǎo	licorice [root] (honey-fried)	Glycyrrhizae Radix	6 g.
bò hé	mint (abbreviated decoction)	Menthae Herba	3 g.
shēng jiāng	fresh ginger [root]	Zingiberis Rhizoma Recens	3 g.

with:

Two Matured Ingredients Decoction *èr chén tāng*

fǎ bàn xià	pinellia [tuber] (processed)	Pinelliae Tuber Praeparatum	12 g.
chén pí	tangerine [peel]	Citri Exocarpium	12 g.
fú líng	poria	Poria	9 g.
zhì gān cǎo	licorice [root] (honey-fried)	Glycyrrhizae Radix	6 g.

MODIFICATIONS

To reinforce the liver-soothing, phlegm-dissolving and lump-dispersing of the given prescription, add:

xuán shēn	scrophularia [root]	Scrophulariae Radix	9 g.
mǔ lì	oyster [shell] (extended decoction)	Ostreae Concha	30 g.
zhè bèi mǔ	Zhejiang fritillaria [bulb]	Fritillariae Verticillatae Bulbus	9 g.
xià kū cǎo	prunella [spike]	Prunellae Spica	12 g.
kūn bù	kelp	Algae Thallus	12 g.

In cases of purulent liquefaction that has not yet ulcerated, with symptoms of dark reddish discoloration and slight rise in temperature of the skin over the enlarged lymph nodes, a slight wave-like motion upon palpation and severe pain, accompanied by slight fever and poor appetite, the prescription is modified to disperse toxins and drain pus. Add:

huáng qí	astragalus [root]	Astragali (seu Hedysari) Radix	12 g.
zào jiǎo cì	gleditsia [thorn]	Gleditsiae Spina	9 g.
chuān shān jiǎ	pangolin scales	Manitis Squama	9 g.
	(or, powdered and administered separately, each time 1.5 g.)		

ACUPUNCTURE AND MOXIBUSTION

Main points: Needle with draining.

LR-13	*zhāng mén*
TB-10	*tiān jǐng*
GB-41	*zú lín qì*

Auxiliary points:

For distention and pain of the chest and hypochondrium, add:

GB-34	*yáng líng quán*
PC-06	*nèi guān*

For epigastric fullness and discomfort and poor appetite, add:

CV-12	*zhōng wǎn*
ST-36	*zú sān lǐ*

2. Kidney Yin Depletion

Clinical Manifestations: Generally observed during the later stages of scrofula, after lancing or spontaneous ulceration, liquefacted lymph nodes release thin clear pus and material resembling decomposing cotton (caseous necrosis), and ulcers fail to heal even after a prolonged period. Accompanying symptoms include tidal fever, coughing, night sweating, irritability, insomnia, dizziness, vertigo and tiredness.

Where etiological factors include depletion of lung and kidney yin, the symptoms of vacuity (listed above) are also presented during the initial stages.

Tongue: Red with little coating.

Pulse: Rapid, thready.

Treatment Method: Nourish yin, downbear vacuity fire.

PRESCRIPTION

Anemarrhena, Phellodendron and Rehmannia Pill *zhī bǎi dì huáng wán*

shú dì huáng	cooked rehmannia [root]	Rehmanniae Radix Conquita	24 g.
shān zhū yú	cornus [fruit]	Corni Fructus	12 g.
shān yào	dioscorea [root]	Dioscoreae Rhizoma	12 g.
zé xiè	alisma [tuber]	Alismatis Rhizoma	9 g.
fú líng	poria	Poria	9 g.
mǔ dān pí	moutan [root bark]	Moutan Radicis Cortex	9 g.
zhī mǔ	anemarrhena [root]	Anemarrhenae Rhizoma	9 g.
huáng bǎi	phellodendron [bark]	Phellodendri Cortex	9 g.

MODIFICATIONS

To reinforce the yin-nourishing and fire-downbearing actions of the above prescription, add:

xià kū cǎo	prunella [spike]	Prunellae Spica	9 g.
mǔ lì	oyster shell (extended decoction)	Ostreae Concha	30 g.
xuán shēn	scrophularia [root]	Scrophulariae Radix	12 g.
tiān huā fěn	trichosanthes [root]	Trichosanthis Radix	12 g.

In cases of marked coughing, the prescription is modified to nourish yin, moisten the lung, clear heat, and relieve cough. Add:

chuān bèi mǔ	Sichuan fritillaria [bulb]	Fritillariae Cirrhosae Bulbus	9 g.
mài mén dōng	ophiopogon [tuber]	Ophiopogonis Tuber	12 g.
dì gǔ pí	lycium root bark	Lycii Radicis Cortex	12 g.

In cases of extended illness where qi and blood are both vacuous, the prescription is modified to regulate and supplement qi and blood. Add:

huáng qí	astragalus [root]	Astragali (seu Hedysari) Radix	12 g.
dǎng shēn	codonopsis [root]	Codonopsitis Radix	9 g.
dāng guī	tangkuei	Angelicae Sinensis Radix	9 g.
shēng dì huáng	rehmannia [root] dried/fresh	Rehmanniae Radix Exsiccata seu Recens	12 g.

ACUPUNCTURE AND MOXIBUSTION

Main points: Needle with supplementation.

TB-10	*tiān jǐng*
HT-03	*shào hǎi*
M-HN-30	*bǎi láo* (Hundred Taxations)
BL-23	*shèn shū*
BL-20	*pí shū*

Auxiliary points:

For night sweating, add:

HT-06	*yīn xī*
BL-43 (38)	*gāo huāng shū*

For coughing, add:

LU-07	*liè quē*
BL-13	*fèi shū*

ALTERNATE THERAPEUTIC METHODS

1. Picking Therapy

Method: First locate the tuberculosis points below the shoulder blades and on both sides of the spine. These points are slightly raised above the surface of the skin and will be red; the color will not fade on external pressure. Use a thicker filiform needle to prick open these points; pick up and snap the glistening white fibers from the underlying tissues.

REMARKS

In prolonged cases accompanied by the formation of fistulas, appropriate surgical methods should be undertaken.

GOITER

Yǐng

1. Liver Qi Stagnation, Static Blood, Congealing Phlegm - 2. Yin Vacuity with Effulgent Fire

In traditional Chinese medicine, there is a class of illness designated by the term *yǐng*. These have as a primary symptom swelling or lumps on the front of the neck bilateral to the Adam's apple. Other symptoms include a gradual increase in the size of the swelling or lumps, no change in local skin color and prolonged course of illness. According to ancient writings, goiter may be classified into groups of qi goiter *(qì yǐng)*, fleshy goiter *(ròu yǐng)* and stone goiter *(shí yǐng)*.

Qi goiter refers to extensive swelling and enlargement of the front part of the neck. The swollen tissue is soft to the touch and may increase or decrease in size depending on the emotional status of the patient. Fleshy goiter refers to unilateral or bilateral presentation of one or several soft but tough round lumps. These resemble masses of muscular tissue and move up and down with the movements of the throat. Stone goiter refers to hard lumps resembling stones appearing bilaterally in a random fashion over the front of the neck. Unlike fleshy goiter, these lumps are unaffected by the swallowing movement of the throat.

The patterns of goiter correspond to the thyroid diseases of Western medicine, of which simple goiter, hyperthyroidism and thyroid tumors are commonly observed.

ETIOLOGY AND PATHOGENESIS

Goiter can be the result of emotional depression or lack of dietary iodine, which can bring about stagnation of qi, static blood and congealed phlegm. When the three coagulate, lumps and masses can form. In addition, vacuity of liver and kidney yin and consequent dysfunction of the *chōng* and *rèn* are also frequently involved in the pathogenesis of goiter.

1. LIVER QI STAGNATION, STATIC BLOOD, CONGEALING PHLEGM

Clinical Manifestations: Qi goiter or fleshy goiter, accompanied by mental depression or irritability, oppression in the chest, distention of the hypochondrium and insomnia.

Pulse: Slippery, wiry.

Tongue: Dark with slimy white coating.

Treatment Method: Regulate qi, dispel stasis, transform phlegm, break masses.

PRESCRIPTION

Sargassum Jade Flask Decoction *hǎi zǎo yù hú tāng*

hǎi zǎo	sargassum	Sargassi Herba	9 g.
kūn bù	kelp	Algae Thallus	9 g.
fǎ bàn xià	pinellia [tuber] (processed)	Pinelliae Tuber Praeparatum	9 g.
chén pí	tangerine [peel]	Citri Exocarpium	6 g.
qīng pí	unripe tangerine [peel]	Citri Exocarpium Immaturum	6 g.
lián qiào	forsythia [fruit]	Forsythiae Fructus	6 g.
dāng guī	tangkuei	Angelicae Sinensis Radix	6 g.
chuān xiōng	ligusticum [root]	Ligustici Rhizoma	6 g.
zhè bèi mǔ	Zhejiang fritillaria [bulb]	Fritillariae Verticillatae Bulbus	9 g.
dú huó	tuhuo [angelica root]	Angelicae Duhuo Radix	6 g.
hǎi dài	eelgrass	Zosterae Marinae Herba	9 g.

MODIFICATIONS

In cases of oppression in the chest and discomfort, the prescription is modified to soothe liver qi. Add:

xiāng fù zǐ	cyperus [root]	Cyperi Rhizoma	9 g.
yù jīn	curcuma [tuber]	Curcumae Tuber	9 g.

During pregnancy or breastfeeding, the prescription is modified to supplement the liver and kidney. Add:

tù sī zǐ	cuscuta [seed]	Cuscutae Semen	12 g.
hé shǒu wū	flowery knotweed [root]	Polygoni Multiflori Radix	12 g.
bǔ gǔ zhī	psoralea [seed]	Psoraleae Semen	9 g.

In cases of stone goiter, a selection from herbal medicines may be added to quicken the blood, dispel stasis, disperse swelling and resolve toxins, including:

chì sháo yào	red peony [root]	Paeoniae Radix Rubra	9 g.
sān léng	sparganium [root]	Sparganii Rhizoma	9 g.
é zhú	zedoary	Zedoariae Rhizoma	9 g.
táo rén	peach [kernel]	Persicae Semen	9 g.
hóng huā	carthamus [flower]	Carthami Flos	9 g.
dān shēn	salvia [root]	Salviae Miltiorrhizae Radix	12 g.
bái huā shé shé cǎo	hedyotis	Hedyotis Herba	30 g.

ACUPUNCTURE AND MOXIBUSTION

Main points: Needle with draining; local encircling needling and perpendicular insertion of one needle at the center of the swelling or masses.

TB-13	*nào huì*
LI-17	*tiān dǐng*
SI-17	*tiān róng*
CV-22	*tiān tú*
LR-03	*tài chōng*
LI-04	*hé gǔ*

Auxiliary points:

For oppression in the chest, add:

CV-17	*tán zhōng*

2. Yin Vacuity with Effulgent Fire

Clinical Manifestations: Most frequently seen in fleshy goiter with accompanying symptoms of emaciation, frequent hunger, large appetite, dry mouth, dry throat, palpitations, excessive perspiration, vexing heat in the five hearts, tidal fever, insomnia, irregular menstruation and trembling of the tongue and hands.

Tongue: Red with little coating.

Pulse: Rapid, thready.

Treatment Method: Moisten yin, downbear fire, break masses.

PRESCRIPTION

Anemarrhena, Phellodendron and Rehmannia Decoction
zhī bǎi dì huáng tāng

shú dì huáng	cooked rehmannia [root]	Rehmanniae Radix Conquita	24 g.
shān zhū yú	cornus [fruit]	Corni Fructus	12 g.
shān yào	dioscorea [root]	Dioscoreae Rhizoma	12 g.
zé xiè	alisma [tuber]	Alismatis Rhizoma	9 g.
fú líng	poria	Poria	9 g.
mǔ dān pí	moutan [root bark]	Moutan Radicis Cortex	9 g.
zhī mǔ	anemarrhena [root]	Anemarrhenae Rhizoma	9 g.
huáng bǎi	phellodendron [bark]	Phellodendri Cortex	9 g.

MODIFICATIONS

In cases of palpitations and insomnia, the prescription is modified to sedate and quiet the spirit. Add:

suān zǎo rén	spiny jujube [kernel]	Ziziphi Spinosi Semen	12 g.
yè jiāo téng	flowery knotweed [stem]	Polygoni Multiflori Caulis	12 g.
fú shén	root poria	Poria cum Pini Radice	9 g.

In cases of trembling of the tongue and hands, the prescription is modified to nourish yin, extinguish wind, and relieve tetany. Add:

gōu téng	uncaria [stem and thorn] (abbreviated decoction)	Uncariae Ramulus cum Unco	12 g.
zhēn zhū mǔ	mother-of-pearl (extended decoction)	Concha Margaritifera	30 g.
bái sháo yào	white peony [root]	Paeoniae Radix Alba	12 g.

In cases of large appetite and frequent hunger, the prescription is modified to clear stomach fire. Add:

shí gāo	gypsum (extended decoction)	Gypsum	15 g.

In cases of irregular menstruation, the prescription is modified to regulate and rectify the *chōng* and *rèn*. Add:

ròu cōng róng	cistanche [stem]	Cistanches Caulis	12 g.
yì mǔ cǎo	leonurus	Leonuri Herba	12 g.
tù sī zǐ	cuscuta [seed]	Cuscutae Semen	12 g.

In cases accompanied by tiredness, fatigue and loose stools, both qi and yin are vacuous. The prescription is modified to boost qi and nourish yin. Add:

bái zhú	ovate atractylodes [root]	Atractylodis Ovatae Rhizoma	9 g.
biǎn dòu	lablab [bean]	Lablab Semen	9 g.

ACUPUNCTURE AND MOXIBUSTION

Main points: Needle with even supplementation, even draining; local encircling needling.

TB-13	*nào huì*
ST-11	*qì shè*
PC-05	*jiān shǐ*
LR-03	*tài chōng*
KI-03	*tài xī*
SP-06	*sān yīn jiāo*

Auxiliary points:

For palpitations, add:

PC-06	*nèi guān*
HT-07	*shén mén*

For protrusion of the eyes, add:

BL-10	*tiān zhù*
GB-20	*fēng chí*
BL-01	*jīng míng*
BL-02	*zǎn zhú*
TB-23	*sī zhú kōng*

For night sweating, add:

HT-06	*yīn xī*
SI-03	*hòu xī*

For loose stools and fatigue, add:

CV-04	*guān yuán*
ST-36	*zú sān lǐ*
BL-20	*pí shū*

Needle with supplementation.

ALTERNATE THERAPEUTIC METHODS

1. Ear Acupuncture

Main points: *Shén Mén*, Subcortex, Endocrine.

In cases of hyperthyroidism, add: Heart, Spleen, Brain point.

Method: Select two to three points each session. Treat once daily.

REMARKS

Surgery should be considered in cases that show little decrease in the size of masses after three months of treatment with Chinese medicines or acupuncture. It should also be considered in cases of hyperthyroidism, or lumps that have become hard and may be malignant. In cases of hyperthyroidism presenting symptoms of a toxic crisis, with high fever, vomiting, delirium and rapid thready pulse, emergency measures should be undertaken immediately.

Intestinal Abscess

Cháng Yōng

**1A. Initial Stage: Qi Stagnation and Blood Stasis with Damp-Heat -
1B. Initial Stage: Blood Stasis with Cold-Dampness - 2. Pyogenic Stage -
3A. Rupture Stage: Heat-Toxin - 3B. Rupture Stage: Cold-Dampness**

Intestinal abscess *(cháng yōng)* refers to swelling and suppuration in the intestinal tract. It is equivalent to appendicitis in Western medicine and is one of the more common acute abdominal conditions treated with surgery. Intestinal abscess may occur at any age, although it is more often seen from teenage to middle-age, with infants and the elderly more rarely presenting the condition.

ETIOLOGY AND PATHOGENESIS

The etiology of intestinal abscess may involve stasis of food matter from improper diet and eating habits, exposure to extremes of temperature, emotional stress or physical exercise directly after eating. These will result in intestinal dysfunction, stagnation of qi and blood stasis, and accumulation of heat and dampness. Blood is destroyed and flesh decomposes to form the abscess.

During the acute stages, intestinal abscesses are repletion heat patterns. Recurring chronic intestinal abscesses are usually the result of coagulation of cold dampness and blood stasis.

1A. Initial Stage : Qi Stagnation and Blood Stasis with Damp-Heat

Clinical Manifestations: Abdominal pain usually beginning in the upper abdomen or umbilical region, then localizing in the right lower abdomen. This pain is dull and constant, periodically becoming severe and sometimes becoming a wrenching pain. Extension of the right leg can aggravate the abdominal pain. Tenderness may be detected in the area of ST-25 *(tiān shū)* on the right side, as well as bilaterally at M-LE-13 (Appendix Point, *lán wěi xué)*. Accompanying symptoms include fever, nausea, poor appetite, dry stools or constipation and dark urine.

Tongue: Yellow slimy coating.

Pulse: Wiry, slippery, or rapid, wiry, slippery.

Treatment Method: Move qi, quicken the blood, free the stool, clear heat, disinhibit dampness.

PRESCRIPTION

Rhubarb and Moutan Decoction *dà huáng mǔ dān pí tāng*

dà huáng	rhubarb (abbreviated decoction)	Rhei Rhizoma	12 g.
mǔ dān pí	moutan [root bark]	Moutan Radicis Cortex	9 g.
táo rén	peach [kernel]	Persicae Semen	12 g.
dōng guā zǐ	wax gourd [seed]	Benincasae Semen	30 g.
máng xiāo	mirabilite (stirred in)	Mirabilitum	9 g.

or:

Sargentodoxa Brewed Formula *hóng-téng jiān jì*

hóng téng	sargentodoxa	Sargentodoxae Caulis	30 g.
zǐ huā dì dīng	Yedo violet	Violae Yedoensis Herba cum Radice	15 g.
rǔ xiāng	frankincense	Olibanum	9 g.
mò yào	myrrh	Myrrha	9 g.
jīn yín huā	lonicera [flower]	Lonicerae Flos	15 g.
lián qiáo	forsythia [fruit]	Forsythiae Fructus	15 g.
dà huáng	rhubarb (abbreviated decoction)	Rhei Rhizoma	12 g.
mǔ dān pí	moutan [root bark]	Moutan Radicis Cortex	9 g.
yán hú suǒ	corydalis [tuber]	Corydalis Tuber	9 g.
gān cǎo	licorice [root]	Glycyrrhizae Radix	6 g.

ACUPUNCTURE AND MOXIBUSTION

Main Points: Needle with draining; retain needles thirty to sixty minutes and manipulate every ten minutes. In severe cases, needle every four to six hours.

ST-37	*hàng jù xū*
ST-25	*tiān shū*
LI-11	*qū chí*
M-LE-13	*lán wěi xué* (Appendix Point)

Auxiliary points:

For fever, add:

GV-14	*dà zhuī*
ST-44	*nèi tíng*

For vomiting, add:

PC-06	*nèi guān*
CV-12	*zhōng wǎn*

For constipation, add:

SP-14	*fù jié*
GB-34	*yáng líng quán*

For abdominal distention, add:

CV-06	*qì hǎi*

1B. INITIAL STAGE: BLOOD STASIS WITH COLD-DAMPNESS

Clinical Manifestations: Mild abdominal pain, absence of fever, loose stools, copious clear urine.

Tongue: White, slimy and sometimes slightly gray tongue coating.

Pulse: Slow, tight.

Treatment Method: Dissipate cold, disinhibit dampness, quicken the blood, free the stool.

PRESCRIPTION

Combine Agastache/Patchouli Qi-Righting Powder *(huò xiāng zhèng qì sǎn)* with Sargentodoxa Brewed Formula *(hóng-téng jiān jì)*.

Agastache/Patchouli Qi-Righting Powder *huò xiāng zhèng qì sǎn*

huò xiāng	agastache/patchouli	Agastaches seu Pogostemi Herba	6 g.
zǐ sū yè	perilla [leaf] (abbreviated decoction)	Perillae Folium	4.5 g.
bái zhǐ	angelica [root]	Angelicae Dahuricae Radix	3 g.
dà fù pí	areca [husk]	Arecae Pericarpium	3 g.
fú líng	poria	Poria	9 g.
bái zhú	ovate atractylodes [root]	Atractylodis Ovatae Rhizoma	6 g.
chén pí	tangerine [peel]	Citri Exocarpium	6 g.
zhì bàn xià	pinellia [tuber] (processed)	Pinelliae Tuber Praeparatum	6 g.
hòu pò	magnolia [bark]	Magnoliae Cortex	3 g.
jié gěng	platycodon [root]	Platycodonis Radix	4.5 g.
zhì gān cǎo	licorice [root] (honey-fried)	Glycyrrhizae Radix	3 g.
shēng jiāng	fresh ginger [root]	Zingiberis Rhizoma Recens	3 g.
dà zǎo	jujube	Ziziphi Fructus	2 pc.

with:

Sargentodoxa Brewed Formula *hóng téng jiān jì*

hóng téng	sargentodoxa	Sargentodoxae Caulis	30 g.
zǐ huā dì dīng	Yedo violet	Violae Yedoensis Herba cum Radice	15 g.
rǔ xiāng	frankincense	Olibanum	9 g.
mò yào	myrrh	Myrrha	9 g.
jīn yín huā	lonicera [flower]	Lonicerae Flos	15 g.
lián qiáo	forsythia [fruit]	Forsythiae Fructus	15 g.
dà huáng	rhubarb (abbreviated decoction)	Rhei Rhizoma	12 g.
mǔ dān pí	moutan [root bark]	Moutan Radicis Cortex	9 g.
yán hú suǒ	corydalis [tuber]	Corydalis Tuber	9 g.
gān cǎo	licorice [root]	Glycyrrhizae Radix	6 g.

ACUPUNCTURE AND MOXIBUSTION

See 1A above, "Initial Stage: Qi Stagnation and Blood Stasis with Damp-Heat."

2. PYOGENIC STAGE

Clinical Manifestations: More severe abdominal pain with marked tenderness and rebound pain, local tightening of the abdominal muscles, presence of a palpable mass in the right lower abdomen, high fever, nausea, vomiting, constipation or diarrhea and dark scanty urine.

Tongue: Thick slimy yellow coating.

Pulse: Surging, rapid.

Treatment Method: Clear heat, resolve toxin, free the stool, discharge pus.

PRESCRIPTION

Sargentodoxa Brewed Formula *hóng téng jiān jì*

hóng téng	sargentodoxa	Sargentodoxae Caulis	30 g.
zǐ huā dì dīng	Yedo violet	Violae Yedoensis Herba cum Radice	15 g.
rǔ xiāng	frankincense	Olibanum	9 g.
mò yào	myrrh	Myrrha	9 g.
jīn yín huā	lonicera [flower]	Lonicerae Flos	15 g.
lián qiáo	forsythia [fruit]	Forsythiae Fructus	15 g.
dà huáng	rhubarb (abbreviated decoction)	Rhei Rhizoma	12 g.
mǔ dān pí	moutan [root bark]	Moutan Radicis Cortex	9 g.
yán hú suǒ	corydalis [tuber]	Corydalis Tuber	9 g.
gān cǎo	licorice [root]	Glycyrrhizae Radix	6 g.

MODIFICATIONS

The prescription is modified to reinforce the clearing of heat and resolving of toxin, discharge of pus, and drain of swelling. Add:

bài jiàng cǎo	baijiang	Baijiang Herba cum Radice	15 g.
tiān huā fěn	trichosanthes [root]	Trichosanthis Radix	15 g.

ACUPUNCTURE AND MOXIBUSTION

See 1A above, "Initial Stage: Qi Stagnation and Blood Stasis with Damp-Heat."

3A. RUPTURE STAGE: HEAT-TOXIN

Clinical Manifestations: Severe abdominal pain spreading from the right lower abdomen to include the entire abdomen, diffuse tenderness, rebounding pain and tightening of the abdominal muscles, abdominal distention, persistent high fever, perspiration, excessive thirst, flushed complexion, bloodshot eyes, dry lips, halitosis, vomiting, loss of appetite, sunken eyes, constipation or mucus-like stools, dark scanty urine or frequent urination.

Tongue: Deep red, with dry thick yellow slimy coating.

Pulse: Rapid, wiry, slippery, or rapid, thready.

Treatment Method: Clear heat, nourish yin, free the stool, discharge pus.

PRESCRIPTION

Combine Rhubarb and Moutan Decoction *(dà huáng mǔ dān pí tāng)* with Humor-Increasing Decoction *(zēng yè tāng)*.

Rhubarb and Moutan Decoction *dà huáng mǔ dān pí tāng*

dà huáng	rhubarb (abbreviated decoction)	Rhei Rhizoma	12 g.
mǔ dān pí	moutan [root bark]	Moutan Radicis Cortex	9 g.
táo rén	peach [kernel]	Persicae Semen	12 g.
dōng guā zǐ	wax gourd [seed]	Benincasae Semen	30 g.
máng xiāo	mirabilite (stirred in)	Mirabilitum	9 g.

with:

Humor-Increasing Decoction *zēng yè tāng*

xuán shēn	scrophularia [root]	Scrophulariae Radix	30 g.
mài mén dōng	ophiopogon [tuber]	Ophiopogonis Tuber	24 g.
shēng dì huáng	rehmannia [root] dried/fresh	Rehmanniae Radix Exsiccata seu Recens	24 g.

MODIFICATIONS

In cases of abdominal distention, the prescription is modified to rectify qi and disperse distention.
Add:

hòu pò	magnolia [bark]	Magnoliae Cortex	9 g.
qín pí	ash [bark]	Fraxini Cortex	6 g.
dà fù pí	areca [husk]	Arecae Pericarpium	6 g.

In cases of severe abdominal pain, the prescription is modified to quicken the blood, move qi, discharge pus and relieve pain.
Add:

yán hú suǒ	corydalis [tuber]	Corydalis Tuber	9 g.
mù xiāng	saussurea [root]	Saussureae seu Vladimiriae Radix	6 g.
jié gěng	platycodon [root]	Platycodonis Radix	9 g.

In cases of dark scanty urine the prescription is modified to free and disinhibit the urine. Add:

fú líng	poria	Poria	9 g.

In cases where stools are mucus-like, the prescription is modified to clear heat, dry dampness and diffuse stagnation.

huáng lián	coptis [root]	Coptidis Rhizoma	6 g.
mù xiāng	saussurea [root]	Saussureae seu Vladimiriae Radix (seu Vladimiriae)	6 g.

In cases of vomiting and loss of appetite, the prescription is modified to nourish the stomach and generate liquid.

xī yáng shēn	American ginseng	Panacis Quinquefolii Radix	6 g.
shí hú	dendrobium [stem] (extended decoction)	Dendrobii Caulis	12 g.
gǔ yá	rice sprout	Oryzae Fructus Germinatus	12 g.

ACUPUNCTURE AND MOXIBUSTION

See 1A above, "Initial Stage: Qi Stagnation and Blood Stasis with Damp-Heat."

3B: RUPTURE STAGE: BLOOD STASIS WITH COLD DAMPNESS

Clinical Manifestations: Abdominal pain, listlessness, cold extremities, spontaneous perspiration, slight fever or absence of fever.

Tongue: Pale with white coating.

Pulse: Deep, rapid, thready.

Treatment Method: Warm yang, disinhibit dampness, invigorate blood, discharge pus.

PRESCRIPTION
Coix, Aconite and Baijiang Powder *yì yǐ fù zǐ bài jiàng sǎn*

yì yǐ rén	coix [seed]	Coicis Semen	30 g.
zhì fù zǐ	aconite [accessory tuber] (processed) (extended decoction)	Aconiti Tuber Laterale Praeparatum	6 g.
bài jiàng cǎo	baijiang	Baijiang Herba cum Radice	15 g.

ACUPUNCTURE AND MOXIBUSTION

See 1A above, "Initial Stage: Qi Stagnation and Blood Stasis with Damp-Heat."

ALTERNATE THERAPEUTIC METHODS

1. Ear Acupuncture
Main Points: Appendix, Sympathetic, *Shén Mén*.

Method: After applying manipulation, retain needles for twenty to thirty minutes. Treat once or twice daily.

2. Enema Treatment
Method: Prepare 200 ml of Rhubarb and Moutan Decoction (*dà huáng mǔ dān pí tāng*) as a retention enema. This enema functions to promote peristalsis, clear heat and resolve toxin.

Rhubarb and Moutan Decoction *dà huáng mǔ dān pí tāng*

dà huáng	rhubarb (abbreviated decoction)	Rhei Rhizoma	12 g.
mǔ dān pí	moutan [root bark]	Moutan Radicis Cortex	9 g.
táo rén	peach [kernel]	Persicae Semen	12 g.
dōng guā zǐ	wax gourd [seed]	Benincasae Semen	30 g.
máng xiāo	mirabilite (stirred in)	Mirabilitum	9 g.

REMARKS

The use of acupuncture in the treatment of early stage intestinal yong, before the formation of pus, has shown highly therapeutic results. After the formation of pus, when symptoms are more severe and there is the possibility of rupture of the appendix, surgery and a more comprehensive treatment with Western medicine may be necessary.

In cases of chronic appendicitis, the acupoints listed may be needled once daily or once every two days, and moxibustion with a moxa stick or indirect ginger moxibustion may be applied at the pain location.

Observation of changes of the tongue coating and pulse are very important in the diagnosis of the severity of intestinal abscesses. Where the tongue coating changes from thin and slimy to thick and greasy, and the pulse changes from slightly rapid to surging rapid, the patient's condition is progressing toward the pyogenic stage. When the opposite changes are observed, the condition has been brought under control and recovery is under way.

During the initial and pyogenic stages (known in Western medicine as acute simple appendicitis, mild suppurative appendicitis, and periappendicular abscess), a liquids or a semi-liquid diet may be administered in accord with the patient's appetite. During the rupture stage, accompanied by peritonitis, foods should be withheld, or the patient restricted to a liquid diet.

HEMORRHOIDS

Zhì Chuāng

1. Stagnation of Blood with Damp-Heat – 2. Qi Vacuity with Prolapse

Small, fleshy protrusions from the anus are known as *zhì*, or hemorrhoids. Hemorrhoids generally occur in adults and present with pain, itching and bleeding of the anus, hence the term *zhì chuāng*, or hemorrhoid lesions. Technically, those appearing within the anus are known as *nèi zhì*, internal hemorrhoids, while those appearing outside the anus are *wài zhì*, external hemorrhoids. Those appearing both within and without are called *hǔn hé zhì*, combined hemorrhoids. Clinically, internal hemorrhoids are most frequently encountered.

ETIOLOGY AND PATHOGENESIS

Hemorrhoids can develop from prolonged sitting, prolonged standing or walking long distances while carrying heavy loads. They can also develop from overindulgence in spicy or rich sweet foods, from chronic dysentery or constipation, from overexertion or following pregnancy and childbirth. All these factors bring about disharmony between the qi and blood of the intestines and anus, causing stagnation of the connections and production of damp-heat promoting the formation of hemorrhoids. If there has been excessive bleeding from hemorrhoids, vacuity of qi and blood can result.

1. STAGNATION OF BLOOD WITH DAMP-HEAT

Clinical Manifestations: Hemorrhoids, anal bleeding, blood dark red in color, swelling, distention, pain and itching of the anus, dry mouth, thirst, dark scanty urine and constipation in some cases.

Tongue: Red with yellow sometimes slimy coating.

Pulse: Rapid, slippery.

Treatment Method: Clear heat, disinhibit dampness, quicken the blood, dispel stasis.

PRESCRIPTION

Divine Pain-Relief Decoction *zhǐ tòng rú shén tāng*

cāng zhú	atractylodes [root]	Atractylodis Rhizoma	9 g.
huáng bǎi	phellodendron [bark]	Phellodendri Cortex	9 g.
zé xiè	alisma [tuber]	Alismatis Rhizoma	9 g.
bīng láng	areca [nut]	Arecae Semen	9 g.
qín jiāo	large gentian [root]	Gentianae Macrophyllae Radix	9 g.
fáng fēng	ledebouriella [root]	Ledebouriellae Radix	6 g.

táo rén	peach [kernel]	Persicae Semen	6 g.
zào jiǎo cì	gleditsia [thorn]	Gleditsiae Spina	6 g.
dāng guī wěi	tangkuei tail	Angelicae Sinensis Radicis Extremitas	6 g.
shú dà huáng	cooked rhubarb	Rhei Rhizoma Conquitum	9 g.

MODIFICATIONS

In cases of constipation, the prescription is modified to free the stool and drain heat.

Delete:

| shú dà huáng | cooked rhubarb | Rhei Rhizoma Conquitum | |

Add:

| dà huáng | rhubarb (abbreviated decoction) | Rhei Rhizoma | 9 g. |
| máng xiāo | mirabilite (stirred in) | Mirabilitum | 9 g. |

In cases where heat is predominant with heavy bleeding of bright red blood, the prescription is changed to clear heat and cool the blood.

Use:

Blood-Cooling Rehmannia Decoction *liáng xuè dì huáng tāng*

shēng dì huáng	rehmannia [root] charred dried	Rehmanniae Radix Carbonisata	15 g.
dì yú	sanguisorba [root]	Sanguisorbae Radix	12 g.
huái jiǎo	sophora [fruit]	Sophorae Fructus	12 g.
tiān huā fěn	trichosanthes [root]	Trichosanthis Radix	12 g.
huáng lián	coptis [root]	Coptidis Rhizoma	9 g.
shēng mā	cimicifuga [root]	Cimicifugae Rhizoma	9 g.
huáng qín	scutellaria [root]	Scutellariae Radix	9 g.
chì sháo yào	red peony [root]	Paeoniae Radix Rubra	6 g.
dāng guī wěi	tangkuei tail	Angelicae Sinensis Radicis Extremitas	3 g.
zhǐ ké	bitter orange	Aurantii Fructus	6 g.
jīng jiè tàn	charred schizonepeta	Schizonepetae Herba et Flos Carbonisatae	6 g.
gān cǎo	licorice [root]	Glycyrrhizae Radix	6 g.

ACUPUNCTURE AND MOXIBUSTION

Main points: Needle with draining.

BL-32	cì liáo
SP-06	sān yīn jiāo
GV-01	cháng qiáng
BL-35	huì yáng
BL-57	chéng shān
M-UE-29	èr bái (Two Whites)

Auxiliary points:

For pain and swelling of the anus, add:

| BL-54 (49) | zhì biān |
| BL-02 | zǎn zhú |

For anal bleeding, add:

| SP-10 | xuè hǎi |
| BL-24 | qì hǎi shū |

For constipation, add:

| BL-25 | dà cháng shū |
| ST-37 | shàng jù xū |

2. Qi Vacuity with Prolapse

Clinical Manifestations: Hemorrhoids, anal bleeding, blood that is abundant and pale in color, protrusion of hemorrhoids from the anus, heavy sensation of the anus, tiredness, fatigue, shortness of breath, disinclination to speak, poor appetite, lusterless complexion.

Tongue: Pale.

Pulse: Weak.

Treatment Method: Boost spleen qi, raise the fallen.

PRESCRIPTION

Center-Supplementing Qi-Boosting Decoction *bǔ zhōng yì qì tāng*

huáng qí	astragalus [root]	Astragali (seu Hedysari) Radix	15 g.
rén shēn	ginseng	Ginseng Radix	9 g.
bái zhú	ovate atractylodes [root]	Atractylodis Ovatae Rhizoma	9 g.
dāng guī	tangkuei	Angelicae Sinensis Radix	9 g.
chén pí	tangerine [peel]	Citri Exocarpium	6 g.
shēng mā	cimicifuga [root]	Cimicifugae Rhizoma	3 g.
chái hú	bupleurum [root]	Bupleuri Radix	3 g.
zhì gān cǎo	licorice [root] (honey-fried)	Glycyrrhizae Radix	6 g.

MODIFICATIONS

In cases of excessive bleeding accompanied by blood vacuity, the prescription is changed to boost qi, supplement the blood and relieve bleeding. Use:

Spleen-Returning Decoction *guī pí tāng*

huáng qí	astragalus [root]	Astragali (seu Hedysari) Radix	9 g.
rén shēn	ginseng	Ginseng Radix	9 g.
bái zhú	ovate atractylodes [root]	Atractylodis Ovatae Rhizoma	9 g.
fú shén	root poria	Poria cum Pini Radice	9 g.
lóng yǎn ròu	longan [flesh]	Longanae Arillus	9 g.
suān zǎo rén	spiny jujube [kernel]	Ziziphi Spinosi Semen	9 g.
mù xiāng	saussurea [root]	Saussureae (seu Vladimiriae) Radix	6 g.
dāng guī	tangkuei	Angelicae Sinensis Radix	6 g.
yuǎn zhì	polygala [root]	Polygalae Radix	3 g.
zhì gān cǎo	licorice [root] (honey-fried)	Glycyrrhizae Radix	6 g.
shēng jiāng	fresh ginger [root]	Zingiberis Rhizoma Recens	3 g.
dà zǎo	jujube	Ziziphi Fructus	5 pc.
Add:			
dì yú tàn	sanguisorba [root] (charred)	Sanguisorbae Radix Carbonisata	12 g
huái huā	sophora flower (charred)	Sophorae Flos	12 g
sān qī	notoginseng [root]	Notoginseng Radix	9 g.

ACUPUNCTURE AND MOXIBUSTION

Main points: Needle with supplementation; add moxibustion.

GV-20	*bǎi huì*
CV-08	*shén què* (indirect ginger or salt moxa - acupuncture prohibited)
BL-20	*pí shū*
ST-36	*zhú sān lǐ*
BL-26	*guān yuán shū*
BL-46 (41)	*gé guān*

Auxiliary points:

For pain and swelling of the anus, add:

BL-58   *fēi yáng*

For anal prolapse, add:

CV-06   *qì hǎi*

BL-32   *cì liáo*

ALTERNATE THERAPEUTIC METHODS

1. Ear Acupuncture

Main points: Lower portion of Rectum, Large Intestine, *Shén Mén*, Brain, Spleen.

Method: Select two to three points each session. Retain needles twenty to thirty minutes. Treat once daily.

2. Pricking Therapy

Method: Locate and prick one hemorrhoid point each session, one session every seven days. Hemorrhoid points are one or several small red papules that appear along the sides of the spine from the level of the seventh thoracic vertebra to the region of the sacrum. Treatment consists of using a thick filiform needle to prick open the papule, then pick up and snap glistening white fibers from within the underlying tissue.

3. Steam Bath

Method: Expose hemorrhoids to the steam of:

Flavescent Sophora Decoction *kǔ shēn tāng*

kǔ shēn	flavescent sophora [root]	Sophorae Flavescentis Radix	60 g.
shé chuáng zǐ	cnidium [seed]	Cnidii Monnieri Fructus	30 g.
bái zhǐ	angelica [root]	Angelicae Dahuricae Radix	15 g.
jīn yín huā	lonicera [flower]	Lonicerae Flos	30 g.
jú huā	chrysanthemum [flower]	Chrysanthemi Flos	60 g.
huáng bǎi	phellodendron [bark]	Phellodendri Cortex	15 g.
dì fū zǐ	kochia [fruit]	Kochiae Fructus	15 g.
shí chāng pú	acorus [root]	Acori Rhizoma	9 g.

After steaming, rinse the hemorrhoids with the decoction.

REMARKS

Patients with hemorrhoids should avoid spicy foods and keep their bowel movements regular. In severe cases, patients may require surgery.

GANGRENE

Tuō Gǔ Jū

1. Qi Stagnation and Blood Stasis - 2. Qi and Blood Vacuity

Necrosis of the fingers and toes, and separation of the digits at the knuckles when severe, is known as gangrene in Western medicine. In traditional Chinese medicine it is called *tuō gǔ jū* (sloughing ju) or bone shedding ulceration. Gangrene is most often observed in young males, more frequently in the lower limbs than in the upper. Also refer to this chapter for cases diagnosed as thromboangitis by Western physicians.

ETIOLOGY AND PATHOGENESIS

The gangrene develops from depletion of spleen and kidney yang, which fails to warm and nourish the extremities. This allows the invasion of cold-damp evils that stagnate qi and blood, obstructing the channels and connections. This stagnation gives rise to heat, leading to the breakdown of tissues and depletion of qi and blood, which furthers the development of gangrene.

1. QI STAGNATION AND BLOOD STASIS

Clinical Manifestations: During the initial and intermediate stages of gangrene, a patient presents with dull lusterless complexion, chills and preference for warmth, accompanied by heaviness, aching and numbness of the affected limb. When a lower limb is affected, many patients present periodic limping, with sudden pain and cramps in the calf when walking. The pulse behind the medial malleolus weakens and the skin over the affected area becomes pale, dry and cool to the touch. With further development, symptoms include purplish discoloration of the skin over the back of the foot, local loss of hair, disappearance of the pulse behind the medial malleolus, thickening of the nails, constant pain of the affected limb increasing in severity at night, muscular atrophy and difficulty in walking.

Tongue: Dark, purplish with white coating.

Pulse: Deep, rough, thready.

Treatment Method: Warm yang, dissipate cold, transform dampness, quicken the blood, clear the connections, relieve pain.

PRESCRIPTION

Combine Harmonious Yang Decoction (*yáng hé tāng*) with Peach Kernel and Carthamus Four Agents Decoction (*táo hóng sì wù tāng*).

Harmonious Yang Decoction *yáng hé tāng*

shú dì huáng	cooked rehmannia [root]	Rehmanniae Radix Conquita	30 g.
ròu guì	cinnamon bark (abbreviated decoction)	Cinnamomi Cortex	3 g.
má huáng	ephedra	Ephedrae Herba	1.5 g.
lù jiǎo jiāo	deerhorn glue (dissolved and stirred in)	Cervi Gelatinum Cornu	9 g.
bái jiè zǐ	white mustard [seed]	Brassicae Albae Semen	6 g.
gān jiāng	dried ginger [root]	Zingiberis Rhizoma Exsiccatum	1.5 g.
gān cǎo	licorice [root]	Glycyrrhizae Radix	3 g.

with:

Peach Kernel and Carthamus Four Agents Decoction *táo hóng sì wù tāng*

shēng dì huáng	rehmannia [root] dried/fresh	Rehmanniae Radix Exsiccata seu Recens	15 g.
chuān xiōng	ligusticum [root]	Ligustici Rhizoma	6 g.
bái sháo yào	white peony [root]	Paeoniae Radix Alba	9 g.
dāng guī	tangkuei	Angelicae Sinensis Radix	12 g.
táo rén	peach [kernel]	Persicae Semen	6 g.
hóng huā	carthamus [flower]	Carthami Flos	6 g.

MODIFICATIONS

In cases coupled with qi vacuity, the prescription is modified to supplement qi and move blood.

Add:

huáng qí	astragalus [root]	Astragali (seu Hedysari) Radix	12 g.
dǎng shēn	codonopsis [root]	Codonopsitis Radix	12 g.

In cases of severe pain, the prescription is modified to quicken the blood, free the connections and relieve pain.

Add:

chuān shān jiǎ	pangolin scales (or, powdered and administered separately, each time 1.5 g.)	Manitis Squama	9 g.
jī xuè téng	millettia [root and stem]	Millettiae Radix et Caulis	15 g.
dì lóng	earthworm	Lumbricus	9 g.
rǔ xiāng	frankincense	Olibanum	6 g.
mò yào	myrrh	Myrrha	6 g.

In cases accompanied by dampness, the prescription is modified to transform dampness. Combine the given prescription with:

Mysterious Two Powder (Pill) *èr miào sǎn (wán)*

huáng bǎi	phellodendron [bark]	Phellodendri Cortex	9 g.
cāng zhú	atractylodes [root]	Atractylodis Rhizoma	9 g.

In cases where prolonged qi stagnation and blood stasis has given rise to heat, with symptoms including dark red discoloration and swelling of the local area, or purplish-black local discoloration, atrophy, ulceration and severe pain preventing sleep, accompanied by fever, dry mouth, loss of appetite, constipation, dark scanty urine, red tongue with yellow slimy coating and surging rapid or rapid thready pulse, the prescription is changed to clear heat, resolve toxin, quicken the blood, dissolve stasis and relieve pain.

Use:

Mysterious Four Resting Hero Decoction *sì miào yǒng ān tāng*

jīn yín huā	lonicera [flower]	Lonicerae Flos	90 g.
xuán shēn	scrophularia [root]	Scrophulariae Radix	90 g.
dāng guī	tangkuei	Angelicae Sinensis Radix	30 g.
gān cǎo	licorice [root]	Glycyrrhizae Radix	15 g.

In severe cases, add:

dān shēn	salvia [root]	Salviae Miltiorrhizae Radix	12 g.
yán hú suǒ	corydalis [tuber]	Corydalis Tuber	9 g.
rǔ xiāng	frankincense	Olibanum	6 g.
mò yào	myrrh	Myrrha	6 g.
zǐ huā dì dīng	Yedo violet	Violae Yedoensis Herba cum Radice	12 g.

ACUPUNCTURE AND MOXIBUSTION

Main points: Needle with draining; may add moxibustion.

BL-17	*gé shū*
BL-26	*guān yuánshu*
CV-06	*qì hǎi*
ST-36	*zú sān lǐ*
SP-06	*sān yīn jiāo*

Auxiliary points:

For gangrene of the fingers, add:

LI-04	*hé gǔ*
PC-06	*nèi guān*
LI-11	*qū chí*
M-UE-22	*bā xié* (Eight Evils)

For gangrene of the toes, add:

SP-05	*shāng qiū*
GB-40	*qiū xū*
KI-06	*zhào hǎi*
M-LE-8	*bā fēng* (Eight Winds)

2. QI AND BLOOD VACUITY

Clinical Manifestations: In the later stages of gangrene, the affected digits may be lost, leaving lesions that fail to heal for an extended time, accompanied by sallow withered complexion, tiredness, fatigue, palpitations, shortness of breath, physical cold, spontaneous perspiration, muscular atrophy, dryness and shedding of the skin of the affected limb.

Tongue: Pale.

Pulse: Deep, thready, forceless.

Treatment Method: Boost qi, supplement the blood.

PRESCRIPTION

Use Perfect Major Supplementation Decoction *(shí quán dà bǔ tāng)* or Ginseng Construction-Nourishing Decoction (Pill) *(rén-shēn yǎng róng tāng [wán])*.

Perfect Major Supplementation Decoction *shí quán dà bǔ tāng*

huáng qí	astragalus [root]	Astragali (seu Hedysari) Radix	9 g.
ròu guì	cinnamon bark (abbreviated decoction)	Cinnamomi Cortex	3 g.
rén shēn	ginseng	Ginseng Radix	9 g.
bái zhú	ovate atractylodes [root]	Atractylodis Ovatae Rhizoma	9 g.
fú líng	poria	Poria	9 g.
zhì gān cǎo	licorice [root] (honey-fried)	Glycyrrhizae Radix	6 g.
shú dì huáng	cooked rehmannia [root]	Rehmanniae Radix Conquita	9 g.
dāng guī	tangkuei	Angelicae Sinensis Radix	9 g.
bái sháo yào	white peony [root]	Paeoniae Radix Alba	6 g.
chuān xiōng	ligusticum [root]	Ligustici Rhizoma	6 g.

or:

Ginseng Construction-Nourishing Decoction *rén shēn yǎng róng tāng*

rén shēn	ginseng	Ginseng Radix	9 g.
bái zhú	ovate atractylodes [root]	Atractylodis Ovatae Rhizoma	9 g.
fú líng	poria	Poria	9 g.
huáng qí	astragalus [root]	Astragali (seu Hedysari) Radix	12 g.
shú dì huáng	cooked rehmannia [root]	Rehmanniae Radix Conquita	9 g.
dāng guī	tangkuei	Angelicae Sinensis Radix	9 g.
bái sháo yào	white peony [root]	Paeoniae Radix Alba	12 g.
chén pí	tangerine [peel]	Citri Exocarpium	9 g.
ròu guì	cinnamon [bark] (abbreviated decoction)	Cinnamomi Cortex	3 g.
wǔ wèi zǐ	schisandra [berry]	Schisandrae Fructus	6 g.
yuǎn zhì	polygala [root]	Polygalae Radix	6 g.
zhì gān cǎo	licorice [root] (honey-fried)	Glycyrrhizae Radix	6 g.
shēng jiāng	fresh ginger [root]	Zingiberis Rhizoma Recens	3 g.
dà zǎo	jujube	Ziziphi Fructus	3 pc.

MODIFICATIONS

In cases accompanied by kidney yang vacuity, the prescription is modified to warm and supplement kidney yang.

Add:

Kidney Qi Pill *shèn qì wán*

shú dì huáng	cooked rehmannia [root]	Rehmanniae Radix Conquita	24 g.
shān yào	dioscorea [root]	Dioscoreae Rhizoma	12 g.
shān zhū yú	cornus [fruit]	Corni Fructus	12 g.
zé xiè	alisma [tuber]	Alismatis Rhizoma	9 g.
fú líng	poria	Poria	9 g.
mǔ dān pí	moutan [root bark]	Moutan Radicis Cortex	9 g.
zhì fù zǐ	aconite [accessory tuber] (processed) (extended decoction)	Processed Aconiti Tuber Laterale	3 g.
ròu guì	cinnamon [bark] (abbreviated decoction)	Cinnamomi Cortex	3 g.

When kidney yin is vacuous, the prescription is modified to moisten and supplement kidney yin.

Delete:

zhì fù zǐ	aconite [accessory tuber] (processed)	Aconiti Tuber Laterale Praeparatum
ròu guì	cinnamon [bark]	Cinnamomi Cortex

ACUPUNCTURE AND MOXIBUSTION

Main points: Needle with supplementation; add moxibustion.

CV-04	*guān yuán*
BL-17	*gé shū*
ST-36	*zú sān lǐ*
LU-09	*tài yuān*
SP-10	*xuè hǎi*
BL-20	*pí shū*

Auxiliary points:

For constipation, add:

KI-06	*zhào hǎi*
GB-34	*yáng líng quán*

For dry mouth, add:

CV-23	*lián quán*

For the kidney vacuity, add:

BL-23	*shèn shū*
KI-03	*tài xī*

ALTERNATE THERAPEUTIC METHODS

1. Ear Acupuncture

Main points: Sympathetic, Kidney, Adrenal, Liver, Endocrine, Occiput, Heart, Subcortex and points corresponding to affected parts.

Method: Select two or three points each session; needle to elicit a strong sensation. Retain needles for thirty minutes. Treat once daily.

2. Folk Remedy

Method: Regardless of whether or not ulceration has occurred, decoct:

chì xiǎo dòu	rice bean	Phaseoli Calcarati Semen	60 g.
dà zǎo	jujube	Ziziphi Fructus	5 pc.
hóng táng	brown sugar	Saccharon Granulatum Rubrum	to taste

Drink as tea once daily.

REMARKS

Acumoxa therapy is appropriate in the treatment of gangrene that has not yet ulcerated. Once ulceration has occurred, acupuncture and moxibustion should be used concurrently with appropriate surgical treatment. Patients with patterns of vacuity cold and static blood should take care to keep warm; the affected part should be exercised to increase local blood circulation. In cases of heat-toxin gangrene where ulceration has occurred, physical exercise of the affected part should be prohibited so as not aggravate the condition. In all cases, patients should abstain from smoking and get plenty of rest.

SPRAIN

Niǔ Shāng

1. Static Qi and Blood Obstruction

The term "sprain" describes injury to the soft tissue surrounding the joints of the limbs or trunk. The soft tissues involved include fascia, tendons, ligaments, parts of muscles, subcutaneous tissues, joint capsules and articular cartilage. Major clinical manifestations are local swelling and pain as well as restricted movement of the injured joint. Damage to the skin, dislocation of the joint, or fracture of bones are not involved in *niǔ shāng*. In traditional Chinese medicine, sprains are collectively known as *shāng jīn*, "damage to sinew."

ETIOLOGY AND PATHOGENESIS

The etiology of sprains can involve strenuous exercise, external blows or collisions, falls, forceful stretching, overburdening or twisting of joints. All these factors can lead to the local stagnation of qi and blood and symptoms of sprain. Conditions of local vacuity following sprains often allow the invasion of external wind, cold and dampness. These evils gradually add to the severity of the injury, prolonging the illness. In extended cases, the viscera and bowels can be affected, blocking complete recovery.

1. STATIC QI AND BLOOD OBSTRUCTION

Clinical Manifestations: Local distention, swelling and pain, sometimes with redness or dark purple discoloration, and restriction of movement. Injury often occurs in joints of the neck, shoulder, elbow, wrist, lower back, hip, knee or ankle. In chronic cases, the symptoms are aggravated by overwork or exposure to cold or draughts.

Treatment Method: Rectify qi, quicken the blood, soothe soft tissues, clear the connections.

PRESCRIPTION

Combine Sinew-Soothing Blood-Quickening Decoction (*shū jīn huó xuè tāng*) with the prepared medicines YUNNAN WHITE (*yún nán bái yào*) or SEVEN PINCHES POWDER (*qī lí sǎn*).

Sinew-Soothing Blood-Quickening Decoction *shū jīn huó xuè tāng*

dú huó	tuhuo [angelica root]	Angelicae Duhuo Radix	9 g.
qiāng huó	notopterygium [root]	Notopterygii Rhizoma	9 g.
fáng fēng	ledebouriella [root]	Ledebouriellae Radix	9 g.

jīng jiè	schizonepeta (abbreviated decoction)	Schizonepetae Herba et Flos	6 g.
dāng guī	tangkuei	Angelicae Sinensis Radix	12 g.
xù duàn	dipsacus [root]	Dipsaci Radix	12 g.
qīng pí	unripe tangerine [peel]	Citri Exocarpium Immaturum	6 g.
niú xī	achyranthes [root]	Achyranthis Bidentatae Radix	9 g.
wǔ jiā pí	acanthopanax [root bark]	Acanthopanacis Radicis Cortex	9 g.
dù zhòng	eucommia [bark]	Eucommiae Cortex	9 g.
hóng huā	carthamus [flower]	Carthami Flosa	6 g.
zhǐ ké	bitter orange [fruit]	Aurantii Fructus	6 g.

MODIFICATIONS

In the later stages of sprains or in cases of chronic sprains where the presence of wind, cold and dampness produce symptoms of local pain and lack of strength, restricted movement, aggravation during damp rainy weather and muscular atrophy or edema, the prescription is changed to dispel wind, dissipate cold, dispel dampness, nourish the blood, harmonize the connections and relieve pain.

Use the prepared medicines MAJOR NETWORK-QUICKENING PILL (*dà huó luò dān*) or MINOR NETWORK-QUICKENING ELIXIR (*xiǎo huó luò dān*).

In cases of sprains in aged patients, the prescription is changed to supplement the liver and kidney as well as dispel wind and dampness.

Use:

Kidney-Supplementing Sinew-Strengthening Decoction
bǔ shèn zhuàng jīn tāng

shú dì huáng	cooked rehmannia [root]	Rehmanniae Radix Conquita	12 g.
dāng guī	tangkuei	Angelicae Sinensis Radix	12 g.
niú xī	achyranthes [root]	Achyranthis Bidentatae Radix	9 g.
shān zhū yú	cornus [fruit]	Corni Fructus	12 g.
fú líng	poria	Poria	12 g.
xù duàn	dipsacus [root]	Dipsaci Radix	12 g.
dù zhòng	eucommia [bark]	Eucommiae Cortex	12 g.
sān qī	notoginseng [root]	Notoginseng Radix	9 g.
qīng pí	unripe tangerine [peel]	Citri Exocarpium Immaturum	6 g.
wǔ jiā pí	acanthopanax [root bark]	Acanthopanacis Radicis Cortex	9 g.

ACUPUNCTURE AND MOXIBUSTION

Main points:

In acute cases, needle with draining; in prolonged cases, needle with supplementation, add moxibustion or employ needle-warming moxibustion.

A-Shi Points   *ā shì xué* (Ouch Points)

Auxiliary points:

For injury to the shoulder, add:

LI-15	*jiān yú*
TB-14	*jiān liáo*
SI-09	*jiān zhēn*

For injury to the elbow, add:

LI-11	*qū chí*
SI-08	*xiǎo hǎi*
TB-10	*tiān jǐng*
LI-04	*hé gǔ*

For injury to the wrist, add:

TB-04	*yáng chí*
LI-05	*yáng xī*
SI-05	*yáng gǔ*
TB-05	*wài guān*

For injury to the lower back, add:

BL-25	*dà cháng shū*
GV-03	*yāo yáng guān*
BL-40 (54)	*wěi zhōng*

For injury to the hip, add:

GB-30	*huán tiào*
BL-54 (49)	*zhì biān*
BL-36 (50)	*chéng fú*
GB-34	*yáng líng quán*

For injury to the knee, add:

ST-35	*dú bí*
ST-34	*liáng qiū*
M-LE-16a	*nèi xī yǎn* (Inner Eye of the Knee)

For injury to the ankle, add:

ST-41	*jiě xī*
BL-60	*kūn lún*
GB-40	*qiū xū*

For injury to the neck, add:

GB-20	*fēng chí*
BL-10	*tiān zhù*
SI-03	*hòu xī*
BL-11	*dà zhù*

ALTERNATE THERAPEUTIC METHODS

1. Ear Acupuncture

Main points: Sensitive points corresponding to the site of injury, Subcortex, *Shén Mén*, Adrenal.

Method: Needle to elicit a moderate sensation and retain needles for ten to thirty minutes once daily or once every second day. This is appropriate in all cases of acute sprains.

2. Bloodletting Cupping Therapy

Method: Use a plum-blossom needle and tap heavily over painful areas until droplets of blood appear on the surface of the skin. Follow with local fire-cupping *(bá huǒ guàn)*.

This treatment is appropriate in cases of recent injury where hematoma is marked as well as in prolonged cases where static blood is evident and cold has invaded the connections.

REMARKS

When using acupuncture in the treatment of sprains, needles should be repeatedly manipulated while having the patient move the injured part. Such a process produces significant results in alleviating pain as well as in the recovery of functional mobility. Corresponding acupoints on the uninjured side can also be selected during treatment. Tuina massage also has high therapeutic value in the treatment of sprains and is often used as an auxiliary treatment. In cases of severe sprains where there is evidence of complete tearing of ligaments or tendons, surgical treatment should be considered. In cases of chronic sprains, refer to the chapter on bi patterns.

CRICK IN THE NECK

Lào Zhĕn

1. Qi Stagnation and Blood Stasis - 2. Invasion by Wind-Cold Evils

Crick in the neck is called *lào zhĕn* in Chinese. This literally means "fallen from the pillow." It describes patterns of acute uncomplicated stiffness and pain of the neck where normal movement is restricted. The majority of cases affect adults, cases in children being rare. Stiff neck is most common during spring and winter, and includes what Western medicine labels torticollis, cervical rheumatism, cervical muscle strain, and cervical fibrositis.

ETIOLOGY AND PATHOGENESIS

The development of crick in the neck often involves improper sleeping posture with either the pillow being too high or too low or excessive rotation or crooking of the neck. This results in excessive stretching and tightening of the cervical muscles. Invasion of the back of the neck by wind-cold evil is also a common etiological factor. These evils obstruct the local flow of qi and blood, causing pain and restriction of movement.

1. QI STAGNATION AND BLOOD STASIS

Clinical Manifestations: Stiffness and pain of the neck, inclination of the head toward the affected side, limited movement of the head in any direction, tightening of the muscles on the back of the neck, local palpable masses sometimes cord-like in shape and local painful pressure points that are relieved by the application of heat. Where wind-cold evil is present, in addition to stiffness and pain of the neck, symptoms can also include aversion to cold and draft, slight fever and headache.

Tongue: Thin coating

Pulse: Wiry.

Treatment Method: Move qi, quicken the blood, soothe soft tissues, harmonize the connections.

PRESCRIPTION

Combine Sinew-Soothing Blood-Quickening Decoction (*shū jīn huó xuè tāng*) with the prepared medicines YUNNAN WHITE (*yún nán bái yào*) or SEVEN PINCHES POWDER (*qī lí săn*).

Sinew-Soothing Blood-Quickening Decoction *shū jīn huó xuè tāng*

dú huó	tuhuo [angelica root]	Angelicae Duhuo Radix	9 g.
qiāng huó	notopterygium [root]	Notopterygii Rhizoma	9 g.
fáng fēng	ledebouriella [root]	Ledebouriellae Radix	9 g.
jīng jiè	schizonepeta	Schizonepetae Herba et Flos	6 g.
	(abbreviated decoction)		
dāng guī	tangkuei	Angelicae Sinensis Radix	12 g.
xù duàn	dipsacus [root]	Dipsaci Radix	12 g.
qīng pí	unripe tangerine [peel]	Citri Exocarpium Immaturum	6 g.
niú xī	achyranthes [root]	Achyranthis Bidentatae Radix	9 g.
wǔ jiā pí	acanthopanax [root bark]	Acanthopanacis Radicis Cortex	9 g.
dù zhòng	eucommia [bark]	Eucommiae Cortex	9 g.
hóng huā	carthamus [flower]	Carthami Flosa	6 g.
zhǐ ké	bitter orange [fruit]	Aurantii Fructus	6 g.

ACUPUNCTURE AND MOXIBUSTION

Main points: Needle affected side with draining; add moxibustion or fire-cupping.

A-Shi Points	*ā shì xué* (Ouch Points)
M-UE-24	*luò zhěn* (Crick in the Neck)
BL-10	*tiān zhù*
SI-03	*hòu xī*
GB-39	*xuán zhōng*

Auxiliary points:

For shoulder pain, add:

SI-13	*qū yuán*
LI-15	*jiān yú*

For back pain, add:

BL-11	*dà zhù*
SI-14	*jiān wài shū*

For restriction in forward-backward movement of the head, add:

BL-60	*kūn lún*
LU-07	*liè quē*

For restriction in left-right movement of the head, add:

SI-07	*zhī zhèng*

2. INVASION BY WIND-COLD EVILS

Clinical Manifestations: Stiffness and pain of the neck, accompanied by external patterns including aversion to cold and draught, slight fever and headache.

Tongue: Thin white coating.

Pulse: Floating, tight.

Treatment Method: Dispel wind, dissipate cold, soothe soft tissues and harmonize the connections.

PRESCRIPTION:

Pueraria Decoction *gé gēn tāng*

gé gēn	pueraria [root]	Puerariae Radix	15 g.
má huáng	ephedra	Ephedrae Herba	6 g.
guì zhī	cinnamon [twig]	Cinnamomi Ramulus	9 g.
bái sháo yào	white peony [root]	Paeoniae Radix Alba	9 g.
zhì gān cǎo	licorice [root] (honey-fried)	Glycyrrhizae Radix	6 g.
shēng jiāng	fresh ginger [root]	Zingiberis Rhizoma Recens	6 g.
dà zǎo	jujube	Ziziphi Fructus	3 pc.

MODIFICATIONS

In cases of severe headache with aversion to cold, the prescription is modified to dissipate cold, dispel wind and relieve pain. Add:

qiāng huó	notopterygium [root]	Notopterygii Rhizoma	9 g.
bái zhǐ	angelica [root]	Angelicae Dahuricae Radix	9 g.
chuān xiōng	ligusticum [root]	Ligustici Rhizoma	9 g.

ACUPUNCTURE AND MOXIBUSTION

Main points: Needle affected side with draining; add moxibustion or fire-cupping.

M-UE-24	*luò zhěn* (Crick in the Neck)
LI-04	*hé gǔ*
A-Shi Points	*ā shì xué* (Ouch Points)
TB-05	*wài guān*
BL-10	*tiān zhù*
SI-03	*hòu xī*
GB-39	*xuán zhōng*

Auxiliary points:
See: 1. "Stagnation of Qi and Blood."

ALTERNATE THERAPEUTIC METHODS

1. Plum Blossom Needle Therapy

Method: Tap over painful and stiff areas of the neck with a plum-blossom needle until the skin is slightly red. Follow with tapping over painful pressure points on the back and shoulders.

2. Ear Acupuncture

Main points: Neck, Cervical Vertebrae, A-Shi points.

Method: Needle to elicit a strong sensation. During two to three minutes of manipulation, have the patient slowly move the neck in all directions. Retain needles for thirty minutes. Treat once daily, performing one or two additional treatments after the pain has been alleviated.

REMARKS

When using acupuncture in the treatment of stiff neck, first needle M-UE-24 (Crick in the Neck, *luò zhěn*), GB-39 *(xuán zhōng)* or SI-03 *(hòu xī)* and have the patient move their neck in a circular fashion. This method has a marked effect in relieving stiffness and pain. Afterward, needle local acupoints and apply needle-warming moxibustion or fire-cupping to acupoints on the shoulders and back to rectify qi, quicken the blood, soothe sinew and dissipate cold. Tuina massage can also expedite recovery.

PART III

DERMATOLOGY

PATCH BALDING

Bān Tū

1. Prevalence of Wind and Dryness in Blood - 2. Qi Stagnation and Blood Stasis

Patch balding, known as *yóu fēng* or "wind gloss scalp" in traditional Chinese medicine, refers to the loss of hair characterized by smooth and shiny (glossy) scalp patches. When severe, patch balding may involve the entire scalp and even the eyebrows, beard and hair of the armpits and pubic region. The presentation of patch balding is unrelated to age and is often observed in cases of stress and strain, insomnia or violent psychological outbursts. In Western medicine this condition is called alopecia areata.

ETIOLOGY AND PATHOGENESIS

Patch balding may develop as a result of liver depression that hinders the harmonious flow of qi. Qi stagnation and stasis of blood then inhibit distribution of nutrients to the hair. In cases of liver and kidney vacuity, blood does not nourish the skin, leading to flaccidity of the pores, wind evil entering the body and loss of hair caused by the prevalence of wind and dryness in the blood.

1. PREVALENCE OF WIND AND DRYNESS IN THE BLOOD

Clinical Manifestations: Sudden loss of hair in patches of round or irregular shape, accompanied by dizziness, insomnia and occasionally mild itching of the scalp.

Tongue: Pale with thin coating.

Pulse: Weak, thready.

Treatment Method: Nourish the blood, dispel wind.

PRESCRIPTION

Wondrous Response True-Nourishing Elixir *shén yìng yǎng zhēn dān*

dāng guī	tangkuei	Angelicae Sinensis Radix	12 g.
shú dì huáng	cooked rehmannia [root]	Rehmanniae Radix Conquita	12 g.
bái sháo yào	white peony [root]	Paeoniae Radix Alba	12 g.
chuān xiōng	ligusticum [root]	Ligustici Rhizoma	9 g.
tiān má	gastrodia [root]	Gastrodiae Rhizoma	9 g.
qiāng huó	notopterygium [root]	Notopterygii Rhizoma	9 g.
mù guā	chaenomeles [fruit]	Chaenomelis Fructus	9 g.
tù sī zǐ	cuscuta [seed]	Cuscutae Semen	12 g.

MODIFICATIONS

In cases of prolonged illness with symptoms of liver and kidney vacuity, the prescription is modified to supplement the liver and kidney, nourish the blood and dispel wind. Combine the prescription given above with the prepared medicine SEVEN JEWEL BEARD-BLACKENING ELIXIR (*qī bǎo měi rán dān*).

ACUPUNCTURE AND MOXIBUSTION

Main points: Needle with even supplementation, even draining.

A-Shi Points	*ā shì xué (Ouch Points)* (along scalp)
GV-20	*bǎi huì*
GB-20	*fēng chí*
BL-17	*gé shū*
SP-06	*sān yīn jiāo*
ST-36	*zú sān lǐ*

Auxiliary points:
For chronic cases with liver and kidney vacuity, add:

BL-18	*gān shū*
BL-23	*shèn shū*

2. QI STAGNATION AND BLOOD STASIS

Clinical Manifestations: Loss of hair occurring over an extended period, dull complexion, headache (in some cases), distention and pain of the chest and costal region.

Tongue: Dark with stasis macules on the tongue.

Pulse: Rough or deep, thready.

Treatment Method: Regulate qi, quicken the blood.

PRESCRIPTION

Combine Free Wanderer Powder (*xiāo yáo sǎn*) with Orifice-Freeing Blood-Quickening Decoction (*tōng qiào huó xuè tāng*).

Free Wanderer Powder *xiāo yáo sǎn*

chái hú	bupleurum [root]	Bupleuri Radix	9 g.
bái sháo yào	white peony [root]	Paeoniae Radix Alba	12 g.
dāng guī	tangkuei	Angelicae Sinensis Radix	9 g.
bái zhú	ovate atractylodes [root]	Atractylodis Ovatae Rhizoma	9 g.
fú líng	poria	Poria	9 g.
zhì gān cǎo	licorice [root] (honey-fried)	Glycyrrhizae Radix	6 g.
bò hé	mint (abbreviated decoction)	Menthae Herba	3 g.
shēng jiāng	fresh ginger [root]	Zingiberis Rhizoma Recens	3 g.

with:

Orifice-Freeing Blood-Quickening Decoction *tōng qiào huó xuè tāng*

chì sháo yào	red peony [root]	Paeoniae Radix Rubra	3 g.
chuān xiōng	ligusticum [root]	Ligustici Rhizoma	3 g.
táo rén	peach [kernel]	Persicae Semen	9 g.
hóng huā	carthamus [flower]	Carthami Flos	9 g.
cōng bái	scallion white	Allii Fistulosi Bulbus Recens	3 g.
dà zǎo	jujube	Ziziphi Fructus	5 pc.
shè xiāng	musk (stirred in)	Moschus	0.1 g.
huáng jiǔ	yellow wine	Vinum Aureum	50 cc.

ACUPUNCTURE AND MOXIBUSTION

Main points: Needle with even supplementation, even draining.

A-Shi Points	*ā shì xué* (Ouch Points)
LI-04	*hé gǔ*
LR-03	*tài chōng*
GV-20	*bǎi huì*
BL-17	*gé shū*
SP-06	*sān yīn jiāo*
ST-36	*zú sān lǐ*

Auxiliary points:

For dizziness and vertigo, add:

GV-23	*shàng xīng*

For insomnia, add:

PC-06	*nèi guān*
HT-07	*shén mén*

ALTERNATE THERAPEUTIC METHODS

1. Plum-Blossom Needle Therapy

Method: Use a plum-blossom needle to tap over the affected patches once daily. When the skin of the bald patches is smooth and shiny, tapping should continue until small droplets of blood appear on the scalp. When sparse growth of new hair is observed in the bald patches, tapping should be light.

2. Moxibustion

Method: Apply moxibustion with a moxa stick to the affected areas until the scalp becomes slightly reddened.

3. External Treatment

Method: Rub the bald patches with fresh ginger or apply aconite main tuber *(chuān wū tóu)*. Powder and mix with dark vinegar; apply to the affected areas twice daily.

CINNABAR TOXIN

Dān Dú

1. Wind-Heat - 2. Damp-Heat - 3. Liver Fire

Dān dú derives its name from the abrupt reddening of the skin, as if smeared with cinnabar, that is characteristic of the disease. Cinnabar toxin is an acute infectious disease spread through direct contact. It is most prevalent during the spring and autumn, commonly infecting the young and the elderly.

Cinnabar toxin is known by different names in traditional Chinese medicine according to the part of the body affected. That occurring on the head and face is known as *bào tóu huǒ dān* (head fire cinnabar), that on the lower legs as *liú huǒ* (fire flow) and that over the entire body as *chì yóu dān* (wandering cinnabar). Cinnabar toxin on the face and lower legs is most commonly seen.

Cinnabar toxin corresponds to erysipelas in Western medicine, and refers to an acute streptococcal cellulitis with a well-demarcated, slightly raised red area with advancing borders. Erysipelas can develop into septicemia.

ETIOLOGY AND PATHOGENESIS

The etiology of cinnabar toxin sore generally involves an external injury where the skin has been broken, allowing the invasion of toxins via the wound. Toxins cause blood heat that stagnates in the superficial tissues resulting in the characteristic redness of the skin. Cinnabar toxin sore occurring on the head and face tends toward wind-heat, that on the lower limbs toward damp-heat and that on the chest and hypochondrium toward liver fire.

1. WIND-HEAT

Clinical Manifestations: Rash mainly on the head and face, appearing as cloud-shaped patches that are bright red in color, slightly raised above the skin surface and clearly defined from the unaffected areas. Affected areas are hot to the touch, painful and drained of color when pressed, quickly resuming a bright red when released. The rash spreads quickly and eventually fades to a dull red with flaky skin. Accompanying symptoms include aversion to wind, fever, painful joints, excessive thirst, constipation and dark concentrated urine.

Tongue: Red with thin yellow coating.

Pulse: Floating, rapid.

Treatment Method: Dispel wind, clear heat, cool the blood, resolve toxins.

PRESCRIPTION

Universal Salvation Toxin-Dispersing Beverage *pǔ jì xiāo dú yǐn*

bǎn lán gēn	isatis [root]	Isatidis Radix	9 g.
huáng qín	scutellaria [root]	Scutellariae Radix	6 g.
huáng lián	coptis [root]	Coptidis Rhizoma	6 g.
xuán shēn	scrophularia [root]	Scrophulariae Radix	6 g.
lián qiáo	forsythia [fruit]	Forsythiae Fructus	6 g.
chái hú	bupleurum [root]	Bupleuri Radix	6 g.
niú bàng zǐ	arctium [seed]	Arctii Fructus	6 g.
bái jiāng cán	silkworm	Bombyx Batryticatus	3 g.
jié gěng	platycodon [root]	Platycodonis Radix	3 g.
shēng má	cimicifuga [root]	Cimicifugae Rhizoma	3 g.
bò hé	mint (abbreviated decoction)	Menthae Herba	3 g.
mǎ bó	puffball	Lasiosphaera seu Calvatia	3 g.
chén pí	tangerine [peel]	Citri Exocarpium	3 g.
gān cǎo	licorice [root]	Glycyrrhizae Radix	3 g.

MODIFICATIONS

In treating cinnabar toxin of the head and face, the prescription is modified to reinforce its wind-dispelling and heat-clearing effects.

Increase:

bái jiāng cán	silkworm	Bombyx Batryticatus	9 g.

Add:

chán tuì	cicada molting	Cicadae Periostracum	6 g.

In cases accompanied by high fever, delirium, oppression in the chest, vomiting, loss of consciousness and convulsions, toxins are attacking internally.

Combine Rhinoceros Horn and Rehmannia Decoction *(xī jiǎo dì huáng tāng)* with Coptis Toxin-Resolving Decoction *(huáng lián jiě dú tāng)*.

Rhinoceros Horn and Rehmannia Decoction *xī jiǎo dì huáng tāng*

xī jiǎo	rhinoceros horn* (powdered and stirred in)	Rhinocerotis Cornu	3 g.
shēng dì huáng	rehmannia [root] dried/fresh	Rehmanniae Radix Exsiccata seu Recens	30 g.
bái sháo yào	white peony [root]	Paeoniae Radix Alba	12 g.
mǔ dān pí	moutan [root bark]	Moutan Radicis Cortex	9 g.

*Use of *xī jiǎo* (rhinoceros horn) is prohibited in North America by the endangered species law. Water Buffalo Horn *(shuǐ niú jiǎo)* may be substituted. Increase the dose to 15 g., extended decoction.)

with:

Coptis Toxin-Resolving Decoction *huáng lián jiě dú tāng*

huáng lián	coptis [root]	Coptidis Rhizoma	9 g.
huáng qín	scutellaria [root]	Scutellariae Radix	6 g.
huáng bǎi	phellodendron [bark]	Phellodendri Cortex	6 g.
shān zhī zǐ	gardenia [fruit]	Gardeniae Fructus	9 g.

Or, the prepared formulas PURPLE SNOW ELIXIR *(zǐ xuě dān)* or PEACEFUL PALACE BOVINE BEZOAR PILL *(ān gōng niú huáng wán)* can be given to clear heat, open the orifices, cool the blood and resolve toxins.

ACUPUNCTURE AND MOXIBUSTION

Main points: Needle with draining.

LI-11	*qū chí*
SP-10	*xuè hǎi*
ST-41	*jiě xī*
BL-40 (54)	*wěi zhōng* (Bleed)
BL-12	*fēng mén*
A-Shi Points	*ā shì xué* (Ouch Points) (Bleed)

Auxiliary points:

For high fever, add:

GV-14	*dà zhuī*
LI-04	*hé gǔ*

For headache, add:

GB-20	*fēng chí*

For constipation, add:

TB-06	*zhī gōu*

For internal attack by evil toxins, bleed the hand jing-well points *(shí èr jǐng xué)*:

LU-11	*shào shāng*
HT-09	*shào chōng*
PC-09	*zhōng chōng*
LI-01	*shāng yáng*
TB-01	*guān chōng*
SI-01	*shào zé*

2. Damp-Heat

Clinical Manifestations: Rash mainly on the lower limbs, sometimes with blistering, accompanied by fever, irritability, thirst, oppression in the chest, vomiting, swollen painful joints, loss of appetite and dark concentrated urine.

Tongue: Yellow slimy coating.

Pulse: Soft, rapid.

Treatment Method: Clear heat, disinhibit dampness, cool the blood, resolve toxins.

PRESCRIPTION

Combine Fish Poison Yam Dampness-Percolating Decoction *(bì xiè shèn shī tāng)* with Five Spirits Decoction *(wǔ shén tāng)*.

Fish Poison Yam Dampness-Percolating Decoction *bì xiè shèn shī tāng*

bì xiè	fish poison yam	Dioscoreae Hypoglaucae Rhizoma	9 g.
yì yǐ rén	coix [seed]	Coicis Semen	30 g.
huáng bǎi	phellodendron [bark]	Phellodendri Cortex	9 g.
fú líng	poria	Poria	12 g.
mǔ dān pí	moutan [root bark]	Moutan Radicis Cortex	9 g.
zé xiè	alisma [tuber]	Alismatis Rhizoma	9 g.
tōng cǎo	rice-paper plant pith	Tetrapanacis Medulla	6 g.
huá shí	talcum (wrapped)	Talcum	15 g.

with:

Five Spirits Decoction *wǔ shén tāng*

fú líng	poria	Poria	12 g.
chē qián zǐ	plantago [seed] (wrapped)	Plantaginis Semen	12 g.
jīn yín huā	lonicera [flower]	Lonicerae Flos	15 g.
niú xī	achyranthes [root]	Achyranthis Bidentatae Radix	12 g.
zǐ huā dì dīng	Yedo violet	Violae Yedoensis Herba cum Radice	15 g.

ACUPUNCTURE AND MOXIBUSTION

Main points: Needle with draining.

LI-04	*hé gǔ*
ST-36	*zú sān lǐ*
SP-10	*xuè hǎi*
LI-11	*qū chí*
SP-09	*yīn líng quán*
A-Shi Points	*ā shì xué* (Ouch Points) (Bleed)

Auxiliary points:

For vomiting, add:

CV-12	*zhōng wǎn*
PC-06	*nèi guān*

3. LIVER FIRE

Clinical Manifestations: Rash mainly over the chest and hypochondria, accompanied by headache, bloodshot eyes, bitter taste in the mouth, distention and pain of the chest and hypochondria, restlessness, irritability and dark concentrated urine.

Tongue: Red with yellow coating.

Pulse: Rapid, wiry.

Treatment Method: Drain liver fire, cool the blood, resolve toxins.

PRESCRIPTION

Gentian Liver-Draining Decoction *lóng dǎn xiè gān tāng*

lóng dǎn cǎo	gentian [root]	Gentianae Radix	6 g.
huáng qín	scutellaria [root]	Scutellariae Radix	9 g.
shān zhī zǐ	gardenia	Gardeniae Fructus	9 g.
zé xiè	alisma [tuber]	Alismatis Rhizoma	12 g.
mù tōng	mutong [stem]	Mutong Caulis	9 g.
dāng guī	tangkuei	Angelicae Sinensis Radix	3 g.
chē qián zǐ	plantago [seed] (wrapped)	Plantaginis Semen	9 g.
shēng dì huáng	rehmannia [root] dried/fresh	Rehmanniae Radix Exsiccata seu Recens	9 g.
chái hú	bupleurum [root]	Bupleuri Radix	6 g.
gān cǎo	licorice [root]	Glycyrrhizae Radix	6 g.

ACUPUNCTURE AND MOXIBUSTION

Main points: Needle with draining.

SP-10	*xuè hǎi*
SP-06	*sān yīn jiāo*
LR-02	*xíng jiān*
BL-40 (54)	*wěi zhōng*
LI-11	*qū chí*
A-Shi Points	*ā shì xué* (Ouch Points) (Bleed)

ALTERNATE THERAPEUTIC METHODS

1. Ear Acupuncture

Main points: *Shén Mén*, Adrenal, Subcortex, Occiput.

Method: Needle to elicit a moderate to strong sensation and retain the needles thirty to sixty minutes.

2. Bloodletting Cupping Therapy

Method: In red swollen areas, let a small amount of blood through multiple needling with a three-edged or a plum-blossom needle, then apply fire-cupping.

3. External Treatment

Method: Mix the prepared medicine GOLDEN YELLOW POWDER *(jīn huáng sǎn)* with cold boiled water and apply to the affected areas.

REMARKS

The spreading of *dān dú* from the limbs or from the face to the chest and abdomen is an unfavorable sign. In newborn infants with wandering cinnabar or elderly patients with head fire cinnabar, because their constitutions are frail or declining, toxins can attack internally; therefore, symptoms are more severe. Additionally, when treating cinnabar toxin with acupuncture, needles should be well sterilized or disposable to prevent cross-infection. In cases of multiple infection leading to ulceration or development of septicemia, comprehensive treatment with Western medicine should be considered.

WIND RASH

Fēng Zhěn

1. Wind-Cold - 2. Wind-Heat - 3. Stomach and Intestine Damp-Heat - 4. Qi and Blood Vacuity - 5. Dysfunction of the *Chōng* and *Rèn*

Wind rash *(fēng zhěn)*, known as urticaria or hives in Western medicine, is a dermatological condition commonly seen in clinical practice. Wind rashes appear in patches, are bright red or pale white in color, and tend to be itchy. They can develop rapidly and likewise disappear rapidly without leaving a scar. Wind rashes can occur at any age, and are generally divided according to acute and chronic, acute cases lasting about one week and chronic cases recurring over several months, or even several years.

ETIOLOGY AND PATHOGENESIS

Wind rash can develop because of a variety of factors. Weakened tone of the pores of the skin can allow invasion of wind-cold evil or wind-heat, leading to disharmony between construction qi *(yíng qì)* and defense qi *(wèi qì)*. Second, the consumption of fish or other seafood such as shrimp or crab, or the presence of intestinal parasites, can give rise to damp-heat in the stomach and intestines; this can stagnate in the superficial tissues, resulting in wind rash. Third, wind rash can develop in cases of vacuity of both qi and blood, either as a consequence of blood depletion giving rise to internal wind, or by invasion of wind evil taking advantage of depleted qi. Finally, vacuity of the liver and kidney and dysfunction of the *chōng* and *rèn* can lead to poor blood nourishment, allowing the development of wind rash.

1. WIND-COLD

Clinical Manifestations: White-colored patchy rash, manifesting or increasing in severity after exposure to cold or wind; some relief with application of heat; most predominant during the winter.

Tongue: Thin white coating.

Pulse: Tardy, floating or tight, floating.

Treatment Method: Course wind and cold, regulate and harmonize construction and defense.

PRESCRIPTION

Use Cinnamon Twig Decoction *(guì zhī tāng)* or Schizonepeta and Ledebouriella Toxin-Vanquishing Powder *(jīng fáng bài dú săn)*.

Cinnamon Twig Decoction *guì zhī tāng*

guì zhī	cinnamon [twig]	Cinnamomi Ramulus	9 g.
bái sháo yào	white peony [root]	Paeoniae Radix Alba	9 g.
zhì gān cǎo	licorice [root] (honey-fried)	Glycyrrhizae Radix	6 g.
shēng jiāng	fresh ginger [root]	Zingiberis Rhizoma Recens	9 g.
dà zǎo	jujube	Ziziphi Fructus	3 pc.

or:

Schizonepeta and Ledebouriella Toxin-Vanquishing Powder *jīng fáng bài dú sǎn*

jīng jiè	schizonepeta (abbreviated decoction)	Schizonepetae Herba et Flos	6 g.
fáng fēng	ledebouriella [root]	Ledebouriellae Radix	6 g.
qiāng huó	notopterygium [root]	Notopterygii Rhizoma	6 g.
dú huó	tuhuo [angelica root]	Angelicae Duhuo Radix	6 g.
chái hú	bupleurum [root]	Bupleuri Radix	6 g.
qián hú	peucedanum [root]	Peucedani Radix	6 g.
chuān xiōng	ligusticum [root]	Ligustici Rhizoma	6 g.
zhǐ ké	bitter orange [fruit]	Aurantii Fructus	6 g.
fú líng	poria	Poria	6 g.
jié gěng	platycodon [root]	Platycodonis Radix	6 g.
gān cǎo	licorice [root]	Glycyrrhizae Radix	3 g.

MODIFICATIONS

To increase dispersion of wind and cold, add to either prescription:

| má huáng | ephedra | Ephedrae Herba | 6 g. |

ACUPUNCTURE AND MOXIBUSTION

Main points: Needle with draining; add moxibustion.

LI-04	hé gǔ
SP-10	xuè hǎi
LU-07	liè quē
LI-11	qū chí
ST-36	zú sān lǐ
GB-20	fēng chí

Auxiliary points:

For asthma, add:

| LU-05 | chǐ zé |
| CV-17 | tǎn zhōng |

2. WIND-HEAT

Clinical Manifestations: Red patchy rash, manifesting or increasing in severity with exposure to heat; some relief of symptoms with application of cold; most predominant during summer; with hot sensation upon palpation of affected area.

Tongue: Thin yellow coating.

Pulse: Rapid, floating.

Treatment Method: Course wind, clear heat.

PRESCRIPTION

Wind Dispersing Powder *xiāo fēng sǎn*

shēng dì huáng	rehmannia [root] dried/fresh	Rehmanniae Radix Exsiccata seu Recens	12 g.
dāng guī	tangkuei	Angelicae Sinensis Radix	9 g.
fáng fēng	ledebouriella [root]	Ledebouriellae Radix	9 g.
chán tuì	cicada molting	Cicadae Periostracum	9 g.
zhī mǔ	anemarrhena [root]	Anemarrhenae Rhizoma	9 g.
kǔ shēn	flavescent sophora [root]	Sophorae Flavescentis Radix	9 g.
huǒ má rén	hemp [seed]	Cannabis Semen	9 g.
jīng jiè	schizonepeta (abbreviated decoction)	Schizonepetae Herba et Flos	9 g.
cāng zhú	atractylodes [root]	Atractylodis Rhizoma	6 g.
niú bàng zǐ	arctium [seed]	Arctii Fructus	9 g.
shí gāo	gypsum (extended decoction)	Gypsum	15 g.
mù tōng	mutong [stem]	Mutong Caulis	6 g.
gān cǎo	licorice [root]	Glycyrrhizae Radix	6 g.

MODIFICATIONS

In cases of blood heat, the prescription is modified to cool the blood and clear heat. Add:

chì sháo yào	red peony [root]	Paeoniae Radix Rubra	9 g.
mǔ dān pí	moutan [root bark]	Moutan Radicis Cortex	9 g.

ACUPUNCTURE AND MOXIBUSTION

Main points: Needle with draining.

LI-11	*qū chí*
LI-04	*hé gǔ*
BL-40 (54)	*wěi zhōng*
SP-10	*xuè hǎi*
SPC-6	*sān yīn jiāo*
GV-14	*dà zhuī*

Auxiliary points:

For sore throat, bleed at:

LU-11	*shào shāng*

3. STOMACH AND INTESTINE DAMP-HEAT

Clinical Manifestations: Red patchy rash accompanied by epigastric and abdominal pain, constipation or diarrhea, poor appetite and, in some cases, nausea and vomiting.

Tongue: Yellow slimy coating.

Pulse: Rapid, slippery.

Treatment Method: Clear heat, disinhibit dampness, free the stool.

PRESCRIPTION

Combine Ledebouriella Sage-Inspired Powder *(fáng fēng tōng shèng sǎn)* with Capillaris Decoction *(yīn-chén-hāo tāng)*.

Ledebouriella Sage-Inspired Powder *fáng fēng tōng shèng sǎn*

fáng fēng	ledebouriella [root]	Ledebouriellae Radix	6 g.
má huáng	ephedra	Ephedrae Herba	3 g.
dà huáng	rhubarb (abbreviated decoction)	Rhei Rhizoma	3 g.
máng xiāo	mirabilite	Mirabilitum	3 g.
jīng jiè	schizonepeta	Schizonepetae Herba et Flos	6 g.
bò hé	mint (abbreviated decoction)	Menthae Herba	6 g.
shān zhī zǐ	gardenia [fruit]	Gardeniae Fructus	6 g.
huá shí	talcum (wrapped)	Talcum	12 g.
shí gāo	gypsum	Gypsum	12 g.
lián qiào	forsythia [fruit]	Forsythiae Fructus	6 g.
huáng qín	scutellaria [root]	Scutellariae Radix	9 g.
jié gěng	platycodon [root]	Platycodonis Radix	9 g.
chuān xiōng	ligusticum [root]	Ligustici Rhizoma	3 g.
dāng guī	tangkuei	Angelicae Sinensis Radix	3 g.
bái sháo yào	white peony [root]	Paeoniae Radix Alba	6 g.
bái zhú	ovate atractylodes [root]	Atractylodis Ovatae Rhizoma	6 g.
gān cǎo	licorice [root]	Glycyrrhizae Radix	9 g.

with:

Capillaris Decoction *yīn chén hāo tāng*

yīn chén hāo	capillaris	Artemisiae Capillaris Herba	18 g.
shān zhī zǐ	gardenia [fruit]	Gardeniae Fructus	12 g.
dà huáng	rhubarb	Rhei Rhizoma	9 g.

MODIFICATIONS

In cases of constipation, the prescription is reinforced to more effectively free the stool. Add:

zhǐ shí	unripe bitter orange [fruit]	Aurantii Fructus Immaturus	9 g.

In cases of diarrhea, the prescription is modified to clear heat, disinhibit dampness and relieve diarrhea.

Delete :

dà huáng	rhubarb	Rhei Rhizoma

Add:

jīn yín huā	lonicera [flower] (charred)	Lonicerae Flos	9 g.
cán shā	silkworm droppings	Bombycis Excrementum	6 g.

In cases of intestinal parasites, the prescription is modified to expel worms. Add:

wū méi	mume [fruit]	Mume Fructus	9 g.
shǐ jūn zǐ	quisqualis [fruit]	Quisqualis Fructus	9 g.
bīng láng	areca [nut]	Arecae Semen	9 g.

ACUPUNCTURE AND MOXIBUSTION

Main points: Needle with draining.

LI-11	*qū chí*
ST-36	*zú sān lǐ*
SP-09	*yīn líng quán*
SP-10	*xuè hǎi*
SP-06	*sān yīn jiāo*
ST-25	*tiān shū*

Auxiliary points:

For intestinal parasites, add:

M-LE-34   *bǎi chóng wō* (Hundred Worm Nest)

4. QI AND BLOOD VACUITY

Clinical Manifestations: Recurring wind rash over several months or several years, manifesting or increasing in severity after strain or when fatigued.

Tongue: Pale with thin coating.

Pulse: Deep, thready or soft, thready.

Treatment Method: Rectify and supplement qi and blood.

PRESCRIPTION

Eight-Gem Decoction *bā zhēn tāng*

shú dì huáng	cooked rehmannia [root]	Rehmanniae Radix Conquita	12 g.
dāng guī	tangkuei	Angelicae Sinensis Radix	9 g.
bái sháo yào	white peony [root]	Paeoniae Radix Alba	9 g.
chuān xiōng	ligusticum [root]	Ligustici Rhizoma	6 g.
rén shēn	ginseng	Ginseng Radix	9 g.
bái zhú	ovate atractylodes [root]	Atractylodis Ovatae Rhizoma	9 g.
fú líng	poria	Poria	9 g.
zhì gān cǎo	licorice [root] (honey-fried)	Glycyrrhizae Radix	6 g.
shēng jiāng	fresh ginger [root]	Zingiberis Rhizoma Recens	3 g.
dà zǎo	jujube	Ziziphi Fructus	3 pc.

MODIFICATIONS

In cases where qi vacuity is predominant, the prescription is modified to boost qi and secure the body surface.

Add:

Jade Wind-Barrier Powder *yù píng fēng sǎn*

huáng qí	astragalus [root]	Astragali (seu Hedysari) Radix	18 g.
bái zhú	ovate atractylodes [root]	Atractylodis Ovatae Rhizoma	6 g.
fáng fēng	ledebouriella [root]	Ledebouriellae Radix	6 g.

In cases where blood vacuity is predominant, the prescription is modified to nourish the blood and dispel wind.

Add:

Tangkuei Beverage *dāng guī yǐn zǐ*

dāng guī	tangkuei	Angelicae Sinensis Radix	12 g.
chuān xiōng	ligusticum [root]	Ligustici Rhizoma	9 g.
bái sháo yào	white peony [root]	Paeoniae Radix Alba	9 g.
shēng dì huáng	rehmannia [root] dried/fresh	Rehmanniae Radix Exsiccata seu Recens	9 g.
fáng fēng	ledebouriella [root]	Ledebouriellae Radix	9 g.
cì jí lí	tribulus [fruit]	Tribuli Fructus	9 g.
jīng jiè	schizonepeta (abbreviated decoction)	Schizonepetae Herba et Flos	9 g.
hé shǒu wū	flowery knotweed [root]	Polygoni Multiflori Radix	12 g.
huáng qí	astragalus [root]	Astragali (seu Hedysari) Radix	12 g.
gān cǎo	licorice [root]	Glycyrrhizae Radix	6 g.

ACUPUNCTURE AND MOXIBUSTION

Main points: Needle with supplementation; add moxibustion.

LI-11	*qū chí*
SP-10	*xuè hǎi*
SP-06	*sān yīn jiāo*
ST-36	*zú sān lǐ*
BL-17	*gé shū*
BL-20	*pí shū*

5. DYSFUNCTION OF THE *CHŌNG* AND *RÈN*

Clinical Manifestations: Wind rash generally occurring several days prior to menstruation and disappearing with the termination of menstruation, recurrence of rash at each period and accompanying dysmenorrhea or irregular menstruation.

Tongue: Pale.

Pulse: Weak or wiry and thready.

Treatment Method: Regulate and rectify the *chōng* and *rèn*.

PRESCRIPTION

Combine Four Agents Decoction *(sì wù tāng)* with Two Immortals Decoction *(èr xiān tāng).*

Four Agents Decoction *sì wù tāng*

shú dì huáng	cooked rehmannia [root]	Rehmanniae Radix Conquita	9 g.
dāng guī	tangkuei	Angelicae Sinensis Radix	9 g.
bái sháo yào	white peony [root]	Paeoniae Radix Alba	9 g.
chuān xiōng	ligusticum [root]	Ligustici Rhizoma	9 g.

with:

Two Immortals Decoction *èr xiān tāng*

xiān máo	curculigo [root]	Curculiginis Rhizoma	12 g.
yín yáng huò	epimedium	Epimedii Herba	12 g.
dāng guī	tangkuei	Angelicae Sinensis Radix	9 g.
bā jǐ tiān	morinda [root]	Morindae Radix	9 g.
huáng bǎi	phellodendron [bark]	Phellodendri Cortex	6 g.
zhī mǔ	anemarrhena [root]	Anemarrhenae Rhizoma	6 g.

MODIFICATIONS

In cases accompanied by stagnation of liver qi, the prescription is modified to soothe the liver and regulate qi. Combine the preceding prescription with:

Free Wanderer Powder *xiāo yáo sǎn*

chái hú	bupleurum [root]	Bupleuri Radix	9 g.
bái sháo yào	white peony [root]	Paeoniae Radix Alba	12 g.
dāng guī	tangkuei	Angelicae Sinensis Radix	9 g.
bái zhú	ovate atractylodes [root]	Atractylodis Ovatae Rhizoma	9 g.
fú líng	poria	Poria	9 g.
zhì gān cǎo	licorice [root] (honey-fried)	Glycyrrhizae Radix	6 g.
bò hé	mint (abbreviated decoction)	Menthae Herba	3 g.
shēng jiāng	fresh ginger	Zingiberis Rhizoma Recens	3 g.

ACUPUNCTURE AND MOXIBUSTION

Main points: Needle with even supplementation, even draining; add moxibustion.

LI-11	*qū chí*
SP-06	*sān yīn jiāo*
SP-10	*xuè hǎi*
CV-03	*zhōng jí*
LI-04	*hé gǔ*
SP-08	*dì jī*

Auxiliary points:

For stagnation of the liver qi, add:

CV-06	*qì hǎi*
LR-03	*tài chōng*

ALTERNATE THERAPEUTIC METHODS

1. Ear Acupuncture

Main Points: *Shén Mén*, Lung, Occiput, Endocrine, Adrenal.

Method: Needle to elicit a moderate sensation. Retain needles for twenty minutes. Treat once daily.

REMARKS

Acute cases of wind rash are usually repletion patterns resulting from external evils. Treatment is mainly to dispel wind, dissipate cold, clear heat, cool the blood or disinhibit dampness according to the symptoms. Chronic cases, on the other hand, are most often vacuity patterns, or patterns complicated by both repletion and vacuity. These generally involve the viscera and bowels, in particular the liver, spleen and kidney. When wind rash involves the throat, laryngeal edema and dyspnea can result, requiring immediate treatment by both traditional and Western medicine.

SNAKE CINNABAR

Shé Dān

1. Liver Fire and Damp-Heat

Snake cinnabar is known as herpes zoster or shingles in Western medicine. It is an acute viral inflammatory disease of the skin, named for red blister-like lesions appearing on the skin in bands much resembling the shape and coloration of a snake. In the majority of cases, the rash is present over the lumbar and costal regions, hence the name *chán yāo huǒ dān* (snake girdle cinnabar). Snake cinnabar is most prevalent during spring and autumn, and mainly affects older adults.

ETIOLOGY AND PATHOGENESIS

The development of snake cinnabar is facilitated by the stagnation of fire in the liver channel simultaneous with latent damp-heat in the spleen channel. In such an internal environment the invasion of external fire-toxins causes liver fire to flare and damp-heat to vaporize, moving through the connecting vessels and superficial tissues, giving rise to blister-like skin lesions.

1. LIVER FIRE AND DAMP-HEAT

Clinical Manifestations: During the initial stages the affected area presents bands of piercing scorching pain and skin redness. Accompanying symptoms include slight fever, fatigue, lack of strength and poor appetite. With continued development, small vesicles the size of mung or soybeans develop. These vesicles quickly develop into blisters that appear in small groups arranged in bands. The skin between blisters remains normal. When the condition is severe, stasis macules or blood blisters may be observed.

Initially, the fluid in the blisters is clear, becoming more turbid after five to six days. The blisters dry after about two weeks, leaving no scars once the crusts have fallen away. Blisters most often occur only on one side of the body, rarely crossing the vertical midline. The lumbar and costal regions are the most common sites of infection, although blistering may also occur on the face, chest, abdomen or lower limbs. In cases of blisters on the face, the condition is more severe and pain is much more acute.

Tongue: Red with yellow slimy coating.

Pulse: Rapid, wiry.

Treatment Method: Clear the liver, drain fire, disinhibit dampness, relieve pain.

PRESCRIPTION

Gentian Liver-Draining Decoction *lóng dǎn xiè gān tāng*

lóng dǎn cǎo	gentian [root]	Gentianae Radix	6 g.
huáng qín	scutellaria [root]	Scutellariae Radix	9 g.
shān zhī zǐ	gardenia [fruit]	Gardeniae Fructus	9 g.
zé xiè	alisma [tuber]	Alismatis Rhizoma	12 g.
mù tōng	mutong [stem]	Mutong Caulis	9 g.
dāng guī	tangkuei	Angelicae Sinensis Radix	3 g.
chē qián zǐ	plantago [seed] (wrapped)	Plantaginis Semen	9 g.
shēng dì huáng	rehmannia [root] dried/fresh	Rehmanniae Radix Exsiccata seu Recens	9 g.
chái hú	bupleurum [root]	Bupleuri Radix	6 g.
gān cǎo	licorice [root]	Glycyrrhizae Radix	6 g.

MODIFICATIONS

For localized rashes, the prescription is reinforced to clear heat, disinhibit dampness and resolve toxins.

In cases of rash occurring on the lumbar and costal regions, add:

bǎn lán gēn	isatis root	Isatidis Radix	9 g.
zǎo xiū	paris [root]	Paridis Rhizoma	6 g.
zǐ cǎo	puccoon [root]	Lithospermi, Macrotomiae, seu Onosmatis Radix	6 g.

In cases of rash occurring on the face, add:

niú bàng zǐ	arctium [seed]	Arctii Fructus	9 g.
yě jú huā	wild chrysanthemum [flower]	Chrysanthemi Indicae seu Borealis Flos	9 g.

In cases of rash occurring on the abdomen and lower limbs, add:

cāng zhú	atractylodes [root]	Atractylodis Rhizoma	9 g.
huáng bǎi	phellodendron [bark]	Phellodendri Cortex	9 g.

In cases where the pain is not alleviated with the disappearance of the rash, treatment is directed to soothe the liver, regulate qi, quicken the blood, and relieve pain.

Use:

Free Wanderer Powder *xiāo yáo sǎn*

chái hú	bupleurum [root]	Bupleuri Radix	9 g.
bái sháo yào	white peony [root]	Paeoniae Radix Alba	12 g.
dāng guī	tangkuei	Angelicae Sinensis Radix	9 g.
bái zhú	ovate atractylodes [root]	Atractylodis Ovatae Rhizoma	9 g.
fú líng	poria	Poria	9 g.
zhì gān cǎo	licorice [root] (honey-fried)	Glycyrrhizae Radix	6 g.
bò hé	mint (abbreviated decoction)	Menthae Herba	3 g.
shēng jiāng	fresh ginger [root]	Zingiberis Rhizoma Recens	3 g.

plus:

dān shēn	salvia [root]	Salviae Miltiorrhizae Radix	12 g.
yán hú suǒ	corydalis [tuber]	Corydalis Tuber	9 g.
zhēn zhū mǔ	mother-of-pearl (extended decoction)	Concha Margaritifera	15 g.
cí shí	loadstone (extended decoction)	Magnetitum	15 g.

ACUPUNCTURE AND MOXIBUSTION

Main Points: Needle with draining, bleed in the area surrounding the blisters and follow with moxibustion. Local encirclement needling: Use a 1 cun filiform needle and insert horizontally from the area surrounding the rash toward the center of the rash. The number of needles used is determined by the extent of the rash, needles generally being spaced at 1-2 cun intervals. Retain the needles thirty to sixty minutes, treating once daily in mild cases and twice daily in more severe cases.

LI-11	*qū chí*
LI-04	*hé gǔ*
LR-03	*tài chōng*
SP-10	*xuè hǎi*
SP-06	*sān yīn jiāo*
Local encirclement needling	

Auxiliary points:

For rash over the chest, hypochondrium and abdomen, add:

GB-34	*yáng líng quán*
TB-06	*zhī gōu*

For rash on the lumbar region, add:

BL-40 (54)	*wěi zhōng*

For rash on the face, add:

ST-44	*nèi tíng*

For irritability, add:

PC-04	*xī mén*
HT-07	*shén mén*

For lingering pain, add:

PC-06	*nèi guān*
GB-38	*yáng fǔ*

ALTERNATE THERAPEUTIC METHODS

1. Ear Acupuncture

Main Points: Liver, *Shén Mén*.

Method: Needle to elicit a strong sensation. Retain needles ten to fifteen minutes, applying manipulations every five minutes. Treat once daily.

2. Plaster Treatment

During the initial stages, apply plasters of Jade Dew Paste *(yù lù gāo)*.

After breaking the blisters apply a plaster of Indigo Paste *(qīng dài gāo)*.

REMARKS

Acupuncture has evident pain-relieving effects in the treatment of snake cinnabar. It has been shown to shorten the length of the illness and prevent lingering pain after the lesions heal. In the few cases compounded with purulent infection, surgery may be necessary.

ECZEMA

Shī Zhěn

1a. Heat-Predominant Damp-Heat - 1b. Dampness Predominant Damp-Heat - 2. Blood Vacuity with Wind-Dryness

Eczema is a Western medical term referring to a commonly observed allergic inflammatory skin condition. Eczema is characterized by itchy polymorphic skin lesions of symmetrical distribution, repeated recurrence and the tendency to develop into a chronic condition. Eczema can be localized or can cover the entire body. It occurs regardless of the season of the year or age of the patient; patients congenitally susceptible to allergic reactions are most commonly affected.

In traditional Chinese medicine, eczema is known by different names based on the location and particular characteristics of the rash. Eczema appearing over the entire body and characterized by an excessive amount of exudate is known as wet spreading sores *(jǐn yín chuāng)*, or as millet sores *(sù chuāng)*. Eczema localized to the ears is known as ear-circling sores *(xuán ěr chuāng)*. Localized in the navel it is known as umbilical sores *(qí chuāng)*; localized in the scrotum it is known as scrotal wind *(yīn náng fēng)*; at the backs of the knees and insides of the elbows it is known as four bends wind *(sì wān fēng)*.

ETIOLOGY AND PATHOGENESIS

Eczema is a result of the obstruction of the channels and connections of the skin by wind, heat or dampness evil. Acute eczema is most often caused by damp-heat; chronic eczema is related to prolonged illness with injury to the blood. This results in the production of internal wind and dryness, with consequent depletion of moisture and nourishment to the superficial tissues.

1A: HEAT PREDOMINANT DAMP-HEAT

Clinical Manifestations: Symptoms are often acute and include redness and itching of the skin. There is rapid eruption of growing patches of papules and vesicles that ulcerate, exude fluid and form scars after being scratched open. Accompanying symptoms may include abdominal pain, constipation or diarrhea, dark scanty urine.

Tongue: Yellow slimy coating.

Pulse: Rapid, slippery.

Treatment Method: Clear heat, drain dampness.

PRESCRIPTION

Combine Gentian Liver-Draining Decoction *(lóng dǎn xǐ gān tāng)* with Mysterious Two Powder *(èr maiò sǎn).*

Gentian Liver-Draining Decoction *lóng dǎn xiè gān tāng*

lóng dǎn cǎo	gentian [root]	Genianae Radix	6 g.
huáng qín	scutellaria [root]	Scutellariae Radix	9 g.
shān zhī zǐ	gardenia [fruit]	Gardeniae Fructus	9 g.
zé xiè	alisma [tuber]	Alismatis Rhizoma	12 g.
mù tōng	mutong [stem]	Mutong Caulis	9 g.
dāng guī	tangkuei	Angelicae Sinensis Radix	3 g.
chě qián zǐ	plantago [seed] (wrapped)	Plantaginis Semen	9 g.
shēng dì huáng	rehmannia [root] (dried/fresh)	Rehmanniae Radix Exsiccata seu Recens	9 g.
chái hú	bupleurum [root]	Bupleuri Radix	6 g.
gān cǎo	licorice [root]	Glycyrrhizae Radix	6 g.

with:

Mysterious Two Powder *èr miào sǎn*

huáng bǎi	phellodendron [bark]	Phellodendri Cortex	9 g.
cāng zhú	atractylodes [root]	Atractylodis Rhizoma	9 g.

MODIFICATIONS

In cases where rash is presented on the upper parts of the body, the prescriptions are modified to reinforce the wind-dispersing and heat-clearing effects. Add:

sāng yè	mulberry [leaf]	Mori Folium	9 g.
yě jú huā	wild crysanthemum [flower]	Chrysanthemi Indicae seu Borealis Flos	12 g.
chán tuì	cicada molting	Cicadae Periostracum	9 g.

In cases of severe itching, the prescription is modified to clear heat, drain dampness, dispel wind and relieve itching. Add:

bái xiān pí	dictamnus [root bark[	Dictamni Radicis Cortes	9 g.
dì fū zǐ	kochia [fruit]	Kochiae Fructus	12 g.
xú cháng qīng	paniculate cynanchum [root]	Cynanchum Paniculatum Herba cum Radix	9 g.

In cases where the skin of the affected areas is bright red and feverish, the prescription is modified to clear heat and cool the blood. Increase:

shēng dì huáng	rehmannia [root] (dried/fresh)	Rehmanniae Radix Exsiccata seu Recens	to 30 g.

and add:

chì sháo yào	red peony [root]	Paeoniae Radix Rubra	9 g.
mǔ dān pí	moutan [root bark]	Moutan Radicis Cortex	9 g.

ACUPUNCTURE AND MOXIBUSTION

Main points: needle with draining.

GV-13	*táo dào*
BL-13	*fèi shū*
SP-09	*yīn líng quán*
LI-11	*qū chí*
HT-07	*shén mén*
SP-10	*xuè hǎi*

Auxiliary points:
For fever, add:

GV-14	*dà zhuī*
LI-04	*hé gǔ*

1A. DAMPNESS PREDOMINANT DAMP-HEAT

Clinical Manifestations: Eczema develops gradually with abundant damp exudate, accompanied by tiredness, fatigue, loss of appetite, loose stools and copious clear urine.

Tongue: White slimy coating.

Pulse: Wiry, slippery.

Treatment Method: Fortify the spleen, drain dampness, clear heat.

PRESCRIPTION

Dampness-Eliminating Stomach-Calming Poria [Hoelen] Five Decoction
chú shī wèi líng tāng

cāng zhú	atractylodes [root]	Atractylodis Rhizoma	9 g.
hòu pò	magnolia [bark]	Magnoliae Cortex	9 g.
chén pí	tangerine [peel]	Citri Exocarpium	9 g.
zhū líng	polyporus	Polyporus	9 g.
zé xiè	alisma [tuber]	Alismatis Rhizoma	12 g.
fú líng	poria	Poria	12 g.
bái zhú	ovate atractylodes [root]	Atractylodis Ovatae Rhizoma	9 g.
huá shí	talcum (wrapped)	Talcum	12 g.
fáng fēng	ledebouriella [root]	Ledebourillae Radix	9 g.
shān zhī zǐ	gardenia [fruit[	Gardeniae Fructus	6 g.
mù tōng	mutong [stem]	Mutong Caulis	6 g.
dēng xīn cǎo	juncus [pith]	Junci Medulla	3 g.
ròu guì	cinnamon [bark] (abbreviated decoction)	Cinnamomi Cortex	3 g.
gān cǎo	licorice [root]	Glycyrrhizae Radix	6 g.

MODIFICATIONS

Main points: Needle with draining.

BL-20	*pí shū*
LI-11	*qū chí*
ST-36	*zú sān lǐ*
HT-07	*shén mén*
SP-09	*yīn líng quán*
SP-10	*xuè hǎi*

Auxiliary points
For excessive exudate, add:

CV-09	*shuǐ fēn*

2. BLOOD VACUITY WITH WIND-DRYNESS

Clinical Manifestations: Symptoms are often chronic, recurring over an extended period of time and including itching, desquamation, crusting, lichenoid thickening and pigmentation. Accompanying symptoms may include dizziness and vertigo, fatigue, lower backache and weakness of the limbs.

Tongue: Pale with thin white coating.

Pulse: Wiry, thready, forceless.

Treatment Method: Nourish the blood, moisten dryness, dispel wind.

PRESCRIPTION

Four Agents Wind-Dispersing Beverage *sì wù xiāo fēng yǐn*

shēng dì huáng	rehmannia [root] (dried/fresh)	Rehmanniae Radix Exsiccata seu Recens	9 g.
dāng quī	tangkuei	Angelicae Sinensis Radix	9 g.
chì sháo yào	red peony [root]	Paeoniae Radix Rubra	9 g.
chuān xiōng	ligusticum [root]	Ligustici Rhizoma	9 g.
jīng jiè	schizonepeta (abbreviated decoction)	Schizonepetae Herba et Flos	9 g.
fáng fēng	ledebouriella [root]	Ledebouriellae Radix	9 g.
dú huó	tuhuo [angelica root]	Agnelicae Duhuo Radix	9 g.
chái hú	bupleurum [root]	Bupleuri Radix	6 g.
bái xiān pí	dictamnus [root bark]	Dictamni Radicis Cortex	9 g.
chán tuì	cicada molting	Cicadae Periostracum	9 g.
bò hé	mint (abbreviated decoction)	Menthae Herba	9 g.
dà zǎo	jujube	Ziziphi Fructus	5 pc.

MODIFICATIONS

In cases of extreme itching that prevents patients from sleeping, the prescription is modified to sedate and quiet the spirit. Add:

zhēn zhū mǔ	mother-of-pearl (extended decoction)	Concha Margaritifera Usta	15 g.
mǔ lì	oyster shell (extended decoction)	Ostreae Concha	15 g.
yè jiāo téng	flowery knotweed [stem]	Polygoni Multiflori Caulis	30 g.
suān zǎo rén	spiny jujube [kernel]	Ziziphi Spinosi Semen	15 g.

In cases with lower backache and weak limbs, the prescription is modified to supplement the kidney and strengthen the lower back. Add:

gǒu jǐ	cibotium [root]	Cibotii Rhizoma	9 g.
yín yáng huò	epimedium	Epimedii Herba	12 g.
tù sī zǐ	cuscuta [seed]	Cuscutae Semen	12 g.

In cases where the skin of the affected area is rough and thickening, the prescription is modified to nourish and quicken the blood. Add:

dān shēn	salvia [root]	Salviae Miltiorrhizae Radix	12 g.
yì mǔ cǎo	leonurus	Leoniuri Herba	12 g.
jī xuè téng	millettia [root and stem]	Millettiae Radix et Caulis	12 g.

ACUPUNCTURE AND MOXIBUSTION

Main points: Needle with supplementation.

ST-36	*zú sān lǐ*
SP-06	*sān yīn jiāo*
LI-11	*qú chí*
SP-10	*xuè hǎi*
PC-04	*xī mén*
BL-17	*gé shū*

Auxiliary points:

After local sterilization, employ a three-edged needle to lightly prick the affected areas until the skin is slightly red or droplets of blood appear. This method is contrainidcated in cases of eczema on the scrotum.

A moxa stick can be used to warm the affected areas until the skin appears red.

ALTERNATE THERAPEUTIC METHODS

1. Ear Acupuncture

Main points: Lung, *Shén Mén,* Adrenal Gland.

Method: Needle to elicit a moderate sensation. Retain needles for one to two hours. For prolonged cases manifesting vacuity patterns, auricular points such as liver and subcortex can be selected.

2. External Treatment

In cases of acute eczema where exudate is abundant, a cool compress can be applied to the affected areas. Employ:

huáng bǎi	phellodendron [bark]	Phellodendri Cortex	10% solution

or a decoction of:

pú gōng yīng	dandelion	Taraxaci Herba cum Radice	30 g.
yě jú huā	wild chrysanthemum [flower]	Chrysanthemi Indicae seu Borealis Flos	15 g.

After the amount of exudate has decreased, apply a mixture of sesame oil and Indigo Powder *(qīng dài sǎn).*

In cases of chronic eczema, spread Indigo Powder *(qīng dài sǎn)* over the affected areas.

REMARKS

In cases of acute eczema, the affected areas should not be washed with hot water or irritants such as soap. Whether acute or chronic, the affected areas should not be scratched. Spicy foods should be avoided, as well as fish, crab, beef and mutton.

Ox-Hide Tinea

Niú Pí Xiǎn

1. External Wind, Heat and Dampness - 2. Blood Vacuity with Wind-Dryness

Ox-hide tinea *(niú pí xiǎn)* is named because the thick leathery skin of affected areas resembles the skin of an ox's neck. It frequently manifests over the neck but can also affect the upper eyelids, sacral region, outsides of the arms and legs, perineum or the entire body.

Ox-hide tinea corresponds to neurodermatitis in Western medicine. It generally presents with periodic itching of the affected areas during the early stages, later developing clusters of round or polygonal flattened papules that may take on a light brown color.

With continued development, papules spread to form large patches, the skin thickens, dries out and becomes crisscrossed by wrinkles, a condition known as lichenification. With scratching of the local area, there is some peeling of the dried skin with periodic bouts of extreme itching. The itching generally increases in severity with emotional stress. Ox-hide tinea is a very persistent condition and prone to recurrence.

ETIOLOGY AND PATHOGENESIS

The development of ox-hide tinea is caused by obstruction of the channels and connections of the skin by external wind, heat and dampness. In prolonged cases, damage to blood gives rise to internal wind and dryness. This leads to a resultant lack of moisture and nourishment to the superficial tissues, causing roughness and peeling of the skin.

1. External Wind, Heat and Dampness

Clinical Symptoms: Relatively short duration, affected area presenting papules, redness, ulceration, moistness and scabs.

Tongue: Slightly red with thin yellow or yellow slimy coating.

Pulse: Soft, rapid.

Treatment Method: Course wind, clear heat, disinhibit dampness.

PRESCRIPTION

Wind-Dispersing Powder *xiāo fēng sǎn*

shēng dì huáng	rehmannia [root] dried/fresh	Rehmanniae Radix Exsiccata seu Recens	12 g.
dāng guī	tangkuei	Angelicae Sinensis Radix	9 g.
fáng fēng	ledebouriella [root]	Ledebouriellae Radix	9 g.
chán tuì	cicada molting	Cicadae Periostracum	9 g.
zhī mǔ	anemarrhena [root]	Anemarrhenae Rhizoma	9 g.
kǔ shēn	flavescent sophora [root]	Sophorae Flavescentis Radix	9 g.
huǒ má rén	hemp [seed]	Cannabis Semen	9 g.
jīng jiè	schizonepeta (abbreviated decoction)	Schizonepetae Herba et Flos	9 g.
cāng zhú	atractylodes [root]	Atractylodis Rhizoma	6 g.
niú bàng zǐ	arctium [seed]	Arctii Fructus	9 g.
shí gāo	gypsum (extended decoction)	Gypsum	15 g.
mù tōng	mutong [stem]	Mutong Caulis	6 g.
gān cǎo	licorice [root]	Glycyrrhizae Radix	6 g.

MODIFICATIONS

In cases with increasing severe symptoms with emotional stress, the prescription is modified to sedate and quiet the spirit. Add:

zhēn zhū mǔ	mother-of-pearl (extended decoction)	Concha Margaritifera	30 g.
yè jiāo téng	flowery knotweed [stem]	Polygoni Multiflori Caulis	30 g.
fú shén	root poria	Poria cum Pini Radice	12 g.

ACUPUNCTURE AND MOXIBUSTION

Main points: Needle with draining.

SP-09	*yīn líng quán*
SP-03	*tài bái*
LU-09	*tài yuān*
GB-20	*fēng chí*
LI-04	*hé gǔ*
A-Shi Points	*ā shì xué* (Ouch Points) (Horizontally insert several needles along the borders of the affected areas toward the center of the pathologic lesions).

Auxiliary points: Select acupoints on the basis of channel pathways associated-with the site of pathological change.

For the neck, add:

LU-07	*liè quē*
BL-40 (54)	*wěi zhōng*

For the insides of the elbows, add:

PC-04	*xī mén*
PC-08	*láo gōng*

For the backs of the knees, add:

BL-37 (51)	*yīn mén*
BL-60	*kūn lún*

For the upper eyelids, add:

ST-08	*tóu wéi*
GV-20	*bǎi huì*

2. BLOOD VACUITY WITH WIND-DRYNESS

Clinical Symptoms: Extended duration of illness, with thickening, dryness and peeling of the skin in the affected areas, insomnia, dizziness and vertigo.

Tongue: Pale with thin coating.

Pulse: Weak, thready.

Treatment Method: Nourish the blood, dispel wind, moisten dryness.

PRESCRIPTION

Four Agents Wind-Dispersing Beverage *(sì wù xiāo fēng yǐn)* or Tangkuei Beverage *(dāng guī yǐn zǐ)*.

Four Agents Wind-Dispersing Beverage *sì wù xiāo fēng yǐn*

shēng dì huáng	rehmannia [root] dried/fresh	Rehmanniae Radix Exsiccata seu Recens	12 g.
dāng guī	tangkuei	Angelicae Sinensis Radix	9 g.
chì sháo yào	red peony [root]	Paeoniae Radix Rubra	9 g.
chuān xiōng	ligusticum [root]	Ligustici Rhizoma	9 g.
jīng jiè	schizonepeta (abbreviated decoction)	Schizonepetae Herba et Flos	9 g.
fáng fēng	ledebouriella [root]	Ledebouriellae Radix	9 g.
dú huó	tuhuo [angelica root]	Angelicae Duhuo Radix	9 g.
chái hú	bupleurum [root]	Bupleuri Radix	6 g.
bái xiān pí	dictamnus [root bark]	Dictamni Radicis Cortex	9 g.
chán tuì	cicada molting	Cicadae Periostracum	9 g.
bò hé	mint (abbreviated decoction)	Menthae Herba	9 g.
dà zǎo	jujube	Ziziphi Fructus	5 pc.

or:

Tangkuei Beverage *dāng guī yǐn zǐ*

dāng guī	tangkuei	Angelicae Sinensis Radix	12 g.
chuān xiōng	ligusticum [root]	Ligustici Rhizoma	9 g.
bái sháo yào	white peony [root]	Paeoniae Radix Alba	9 g.
shēng dì huáng	rehmannia [root] dried/fresh	Rehmanniae Radix Exsiccata seu Recens	9 g.
fáng fēng	ledebouriella [root]	Ledebouriellae Radix	9 g.
cì jí lí	tribulus [fruit]	Tribuli Fructus	9 g.
jīng jiè	schizonepeta (abbreviated decoction)	Schizonepetae Herba et Flos	9 g.
hé shǒu wū	flowery knotweed [root]	Polygoni Multiflori Radix	12 g.
huáng qí	astragalus [root]	Astragali (seu Hedysari) Radix	12 g.
gān cǎo	licorice [root]	Glycyrrhizae Radix	6 g.

MODIFICATIONS

In cases of insomnia, the prescription is modified to sedate and quiet the spirit. Add:

zhēn zhū mǔ	mother-of-pearl (extended decoction)	Concha Margaritifera	30 g.
wǔ wèi zǐ	schisandra [berry]	Schisandrae Fructus	6 g.
yè jiāo téng	flowery knotweed [stem]	Polygoni Multiflori Caulis	30 g.

ACUPUNCTURE AND MOXIBUSTION

Main points: Needle with supplementation; add moxibustion.

LI-11	*qū chí*
SP-10	*xuè hǎi*
SP-06	*sān yīn jiāo*
BL-17	*gé shū*
ST-36	*zú sān lǐ*
A-Shi Points	*ā shì xué* (Ouch Points)

Auxiliary points:

For severe itching that disturbs sleep, add:

KI-06	*zhào hǎi*
HT-07	*shén mén*

ALTERNATE THERAPEUTIC METHODS

1. Ear Acupuncture

Main points: Lung, *Shén Mén*, Adrenal, Liver, Subcortex.

Method: Needle once daily and elicit a moderate sensation. Retain the needles for sixty minutes.

2. Bloodletting Cupping Therapy

Method: Use a plum-blossom needle to tap the affected areas, thoroughly covering the entire site of the lesions; follow with fire cupping. Treat once daily. This method is appropriate for patterns of blood vacuity with wind-dryness.

REMARKS

Ox-hide tinea is a persistent condition; courses of illness are often prolonged and frequently recur. Patients should avoid scratching the affected areas or washing the lesions with hot water. Spicy foods, fish, crab, beef and mutton are best avoided, as is the external application of herbal medicines that might irritate the site of the lesions.

Clove Sores

Dīng Chuāng

1. Exuberant Fire-Toxin

A clove sore is an acute local suppurative inflammation appearing mainly on the skin of the face, hands or feet. Known in Chinese as *dīng chuāng,* the term clove sore describes the nail-like qualities of these clove sores, which are initially small on the surface, deep-rooted and hard at the base.

Clove sores are very diverse and are named on the basis of their location and appearance. For example, clove sores appearing on the philtrum are known as philtrum clove sore *(rén zhōng dīng)*, those appearing on the fingertips as snake's head clove sore *(shé tóu dīng)* and those appearing mainly on the limbs, resembling a red thread and rapidly developing in a line toward the torso, as red thread clove sore *(hóng sī dīng)*.

Clove sores left untreated or treated ineffectively can lead to the development of septicemia. In Western medicine, they are known to be caused by staphylococcal bacteria.

ETIOLOGY AND PATHOGENESIS

Fire-toxin is the common factor in all clove sores. Indulgence in spicy or rich foods and excessive consumption of alcohol can lead to the production of heat in the viscera and bowels, and can bring about the production of internal toxins. As a result of poor hygiene, evil toxins can also invade the body from without, lodging in the pores of the skin and obstructing qi and blood. Critical conditions can result when exuberant fire-toxins move internally to attack the viscus and bowels.

1. EXUBERANT FIRE-TOXIN

Clinical Manifestations: During the initial stages, clove sores are small seed-like lesions, yellow or purple in color, hard at the root and sometimes presenting blisters or pustules. Patients may feel local numbness, itching and slight pain. With continued development, clove sores become red, hot and swollen, swelling expands and pain increases. Accompanying symptoms include fever, thirst, dry stools, dark urine.

Tongue: Yellow, or yellow slimy coating.

Pulse: Rapid, wiry, slippery.

Treatment Method: Clear heat, resolve toxin, relieve pain.

PRESCRIPTION

Coptis Toxin-Resolving Decoction *huáng lián jiě dú tāng*

huáng lián	coptis [root]	Coptidis Rhizoma	9 g.
huáng qín	scutellaria [root]	Scutellariae Radix	6 g.
huáng bǎi	phellodendron [bark]	Phellodendri Cortex	6 g.
shān zhī zǐ	gardenia [fruit]	Gardeniae Fructus	9 g.

MODIFICATIONS

To strengthen the heat-clearing and toxin-resolving actions of the prescription, add:

jīn yín huā	lonicera [flower]	Lonicerae Flos	12 g.
yě jú huā	wild chrysanthemum [flower]	Chrysanthemi Indicae seu Borealis Flos	12 g.
pú gōng yīng	dandelion	Taraxaci Herba cum Radice	12 g.
zǐ huā dì dīng	Yedo violet	Violae Yedoensis Herba cum Radice	12 g.

In cases of high fever and excessive thirst, the prescription is modified to clear heat, generate liquid and relieve thirst. Add:

shí gāo	gypsum (extended decoction)	Gypsum	30 g.
zhī mǔ	anemarrhena [root]	Anemarrhenae Rhizoma	9 g.
zhú yè	black bamboo [leaf]	Bambusae Folium	9 g.

In cases of constipation, the prescription is modified to free the stool and drain heat. Add:

dà huáng	rhubarb (abbreviated decoction)	Rhei Rhizoma	9 g.
máng xiāo	mirabilite (stirred in)	Mirabilitum	9 g.

In cases where suppuration is poor, the prescription is modified to expel toxins and discharge pus. Add:

zào jaiǒ cì	gleditsia [thorn]	Gleditsiae Spina	9 g.

ACUPUNCTURE AND MOXIBUSTION

Main points: Needle with draining; or bleed with a three-edged needle.

GV-12	*shēn zhù*
GV-10	*líng tái*
LI-04	*hé gǔ*
BL-40 (54)	*wěi zhōng*

Auxiliary points: Acupoint selection is according to the location of the clove sores.

For clove sores located on the face along the route of the large intestine channel, add:

LI-11	*qū chí*
LI-01	*shāng yáng*

For clove sores located on the face along the route of the gallbladder channel, add:

GB-34	*yáng líng quán*
GB-44	*zú qiào yīn*

For clove sores located on the tip of the index finger, add:

LI-20	*yíng xiāng*
LI-11	*qū chí*

For clove sores located on the fourth toe, add:

GB-02   *tīng huì*
GB-34   *yáng líng quán*

For red thread clove sores, prick with a three-edged needle to bleed beginning at the terminus and moving along the thread to its beginning.

ALTERNATE THERAPEUTIC METHODS

1. Ear Acupuncture

Main points: *Shén Mén*, Adrenal, Subcortex, Occiput, points corresponding to the location of the boil.

Method: Select two to three points each session; needle to elicit a moderate to strong sensation and the retain needles for thirty to sixty minutes. Treat once or twice daily.

2. Picking Therapy

Locate small papules on the back bilateral to the spine. Employ a thicker filiform needle to prick open such papules, then raise and snap the glistening white fibers in the underlying tissue. Treat once daily.

3. External Treatments

To clear heat and resolve toxin during the initial stages, use the prepared formula JADE DEW POWDER (*yù lù sǎn*).

To promote discharge of pus during the intermediate stages, use the prepared formulas NINE-TO-ONE ELIXIR (*jiǔ yī dān*) and EIGHT-TO-TWO POWDER (*bā èr dān*).

To promote healing during the later stages in cases where pus has been completely expelled, use the prepared formula FLESH-ENGENDERING POWDER (*shēng jī sǎn*).

REMARKS

During the initial stages, local squeezing, scratching, acupuncture and cupping should all be avoided in order to prevent spreading. During the treatment of boils, smoking and alcohol should be prohibited, and spicy foods, fish, shrimp and crab should be eliminated from the diet. Patients presenting generalized or systemic symptoms are best confined to bed.

The appearance of symptoms such as shivering, high fever, restlessness, headache, vomiting, delirium and coma is known as travelling clove sore (*dīng chuāng zǒu huáng*), in Western terms a clove sore complicated by septicemia. This signals an internal attack by the toxins, a critical condition that requires immediate emergency measures.

FLAT WARTS
Biǎn Píng Yóu
1. Wind-Heat - 2. Exuberance of Liver and Dryness of Blood

Wart is a general term referring to a small benign growth in the skin. There are several types including flat warts, common warts, genital warts, plantar warts, etc. The discussion here is confined to flat warts *(verruca plana)*.

Flat warts are small flattish neoplasms that develop in the superficial layers of the skin. Their size can vary from that of a grain of rice to that of a soybean; their surface is generally smooth and their color light brown, if at all different from that of the surrounding skin. Flat warts often appear on the face and the backs of the hands, and can be quite numerous, appearing singly or in clusters. Though they are generally painless, itching may occasionally occur. Flat warts are most prevalent during the teenage years, often in pubescent girls.

ETIOLOGY AND PATHOGENESIS

Flat warts are due, in the main, to wind and heat in the skin. The etiology can also involve exuberance of liver fire causing dryness of the blood.

1. WIND-HEAT

Clinical Manifestations: Flat warts of short duration, often accompanied by aversion to wind, fever.
Tongue: Thin yellow coating.
Pulse: Floating, rapid.
Treatment Method: Course wind, clear heat, resolve toxins, disperse warts.

PRESCRIPTION
Wind-Dispersing Powder *xiāo fēng sǎn*

shēng dì huáng	rehmannia [root] dried/fresh	Rehmanniae Radix Exsiccata seu Recens	12 g.
dāng guī	tangkuei	Angelicae Sinensis Radix	9 g.
fáng fēng	ledebouriella [root]	Ledebouriellae Radix	9 g.
chán tuì	cicada molting	Cicadae Periostracum	9 g.
zhī mǔ	anemarrhena [root]	Anemarrhenae Rhizoma	9 g.
kǔ shēn	flavescent sophora [root]	Sophorae Flavescentis Radix	9 g.
huǒ má rén	hemp [seed]	Cannabis Semen	9 g.
jīng jiè	schizonepeta	Schizonepetae Herba et Flos	9 g.
cāng zhú	atractylodes [root]	Atractylodis Rhizoma	6 g.
niú bàng zǐ	arctium [seed]	Arctii Fructus	9 g.
shí gāo	gypsum (extended decoction)	Gypsum	15 g.
mù tōng	mutong [stem]	Mutong Caulis	6 g.
gān cǎo	licorice [root]	Glycyrrhizae Radix	6 g.

MODIFICATIONS

The prescription can be reinforced by adding herbs to clear heat, resolve toxins, quicken the blood and dispel blood stasis. Choose from the following:

dà qīng yè	isatis [leaf]	Isatidis Folium	12 g.
pú gōng yīng	dandelion	Taraxaci Herba cum Radice	12 g.
yě jú huā	wild chrysanthemum [flower]	Chrysanthemi Indicae seu Borealis Flos	9 g.
dān shēn	salvia [root]	Salviae Miltiorrhizae Radix	9 g.
chì sháo yào	red peony [root]	Paeoniae Radix Rubra	9 g.
é zhú	zedoary	Zedoariae Rhizoma	9 g.

ACUPUNCTURE AND MOXIBUSTION

Main points: Needle with draining; apply moxibustion locally to warts.

LI-11	*qū chí*
LU-10	*yú jì*
GB-20	*fēng chí*
LI-01	*shāng yáng*
A-Shi Points	*ā shì xué* (Ouch Points) (in the area of the flat wart)

2. EXUBERANCE OF LIVER AND DRYNESS OF BLOOD

Clinical Manifestations: Warts of long duration, accompanied by distention of the hypochondrium, bitter taste in the mouth and irritability.

Tongue: Red or normal.

Pulse: Wiry.

Treatment Method: Nourish the blood, soothe the liver, moisten dryness, disperse warts.

PRESCRIPTION

Gastrodia and Uncaria Beverage *tiān má gōu téng yǐn*

tiān má	gastrodia [root]	Gastrodiae Rhizoma	9 g.
gōu téng	uncaria [stem and thorn] (abbreviated decoction)	Uncariae Ramulus cum Unco	12 g.
shí jué míng	abalone [shell] (extended decoction)	Haliotidis Concha	12 g.
shān zhī zǐ	gardenia [fruit]	Gardeniae Fructus	9 g.
huáng qín	scutellaria [root]	Scutellariae Radix	9 g.
chuān niú xī	cyathula [root]	Cyathulae Radix	12 g.
dù zhòng	eucommia [bark]	Eucommiae Cortex	9 g.
yì mǔ cǎo	leonurus	Leonuri Herba	9 g.
sāng jì shēng	mistletoe	Loranthi seu Visci Ramus	9 g.
yè jiāo téng	flowery knotweed [stem]	Polygoni Multiflori Caulis	9 g.
fú shén	root poria	Poria cum Pini Radice	9 g.

MODIFICATIONS

The prescription can be reinforced by choosing from a variety of additional herbs to clear heat, resolve toxins, quicken the blood and dispel blood stasis. Choose from the following:

dà qīng yè	isatis [leaf]	Isatidis Folium	12 g.
pú gōng yīng	dandelion	Taraxaci Herba cum Radice	12 g.
yě jú huā	wild chrysanthemum [flower]	Chrysanthemi Indicae seu Borealis Flos	9 g.
dān shēn	salvia [root]	Salviae Miltiorrhizae Radix	9 g.
chì sháo yào	red peony [root]	Paeoniae Radix Rubra	9 g.
é zhú	zedoary	Zedoariae Rhizoma	9 g.

ACUPUNCTURE AND MOXIBUSTION

Main points: Needle with draining; apply moxibustion locally to warts.

TB-03	*zhōng zhǔ*
GB-40	*qiū xū*
LR-02	*xíng jiān*
GB-43	*xiá xī*

ALTERNATE THERAPEUTIC METHODS

1. Folk Remedy

Purslane Decoction *mǎ chǐ xiàn tāng*

mǎ chǐ xiàn	purslane	Portulacae Herba	30 g.
dà qīng yè	isatis [leaf]	Isatidis Folium	30 g.
bài jiàng cǎo	baijiang	Baijiang Herba cum Radice	30 g.
zǐ cǎo	puccoon [root]	Lithospermi, Macrotomiae, seu Onosmatis Radix	9 g.

Decoct all ingredients, and administer one full prescription each day, two weeks per therapeutic course.

REMARKS

Flat warts often disappear spontaneously, and may also recur spontaneously.

PART IV

GYNECOLOGY

MENSTRUAL IRREGULARITY

Yuè Jīng Bù Tiáo

1. Shortened Menstrual Cycle - 1A. Blood Heat from Ascendant Hyperactivity of Liver Yang - 1B. Blood Heat from Stagnation of Liver Qi - 1C. Blood Heat from Yin Vacuity - 1D. Blood Heat from Qi Vacuity - 2. Lengthened Menstrual Cycle - 2A. Blood Vacuity - 2B. Blood Cold - 2C. Vacuity Cold - 2D. Liver Qi Stagnation - 3. Unpredictable Menstrual Cycle - 3A. Liver Qi Stagnation - 3B. Kidney Vacuity

Irregular menstruation includes all persistent abnormalities in the cycle of the menses, including shortened cycles, lengthened cycles and cycles of unpredictable length. These irregularities are most often accompanied by changes in the length of menstrual periods and in the amount, color and texture of the menstrual discharge. Shortened cycles refer to menstrual cycles terminating seven or more days earlier than twenty-eight days, while lengthened cycles refers to menstrual cycles prolonged for seven or more days longer than this normal length. Unpredictable cycles are those that are at times shortened and at other times lengthened by seven or more days from the normal length.

Temporary changes in the menstrual cycle because of changes in climate, changes in living conditions or emotional factors are not generally considered pathological. Also, indeterminate cycles occurring during menopause or early puberty that are not accompanied by other signs or symptoms are not generally considered pathological. Patterns of irregular menstruation also include menstrual irregularities from functional disturbances of the anterior pituitary or ovaries as diagnosed by Western medicine.

ETIOLOGY AND PATHOGENESIS

Irregular menstruation may be the result of a variety of factors. These include invasion of external heat, cold or dampness evil; internal disruption from emotional upset; improper diet and eating habits; overindulgent sexual activity; prolonged illness; and giving birth to a large number of children. All of these can harm qi and blood and injure the *chōng* and *rèn*, resulting in menstrual irregularities.

Shortened menstrual cycles are most often caused by blood heat or qi vacuity. Lengthened cycles are caused by blood vacuity, blood cold, vacuity cold or qi stagnation. Indeterminate cycles are attributed to stagnation of the liver or depletion of the kidney.

1A. SHORTENED MENSTRUAL CYCLE – BLOOD HEAT FROM ASCENDANT HYPERACTIVITY OF LIVER YANG

Clinical Manifestations: Shortened menstrual cycle, large volume of thick sticky deep red or purplish menstrual discharge, accompanied by irritability, headache, flushed complexion, dry mouth, dark scanty urine, dry stools.

Tongue: Red with yellow coating.

Pulse: Wiry, rapid.

Treatment Method: Clear heat, cool the blood, regulate menstruation.

PRESCRIPTION

Channel-Clearing Powder *qīng jīng sǎn*

mǔ dān pí	moutan [root bark]	Moutan Radicis Cortex	12 g.
dì gǔ pí	lycium [root bark]	Lycii Radicis Cortex	12 g.
bái sháo yào	white peony [root]	Paeoniae Radix Alba	12 g.
shēng dì huáng	rehmannia [root] dried/fresh	Rehmanniae Radix Exsiccata seu Recens	12 g.
qīng hāo	sweet wormwood (abbreviated decoction)	Artemisiae Apiaceae seu Annuae Herba	9 g.
huáng bǎi	phellodendron [bark]	Phellodendri Cortex	9 g.
fú líng	poria	Poria	6 g.

MODIFICATIONS

In cases of very heavy menstrual discharge, the prescription is modified to clear heat, cool the blood and relieve bleeding.

Delete:

fú líng	poria	Poria

Add:

dì yú	sanguisorba [root]	Sanguisorbae Radix	12 g.
huái huā	sophora [flower]	Sophorae Flos	12 g.

ACUPUNCTURE AND MOXIBUSTION

Main points: Needle with draining.

CV-03	*zhōng jí*
LI-11	*qū chí*
SP-10	*xuè hǎi*
LR-03	*tài chōng*

Auxiliary points:

For very heavy menstrual discharge, add:

KI-05	*shuǐ quán*
SP-01	*yǐn bái*

For irritability, add:

PC-05	*jiān shǐ*

1B. SHORTENED MENSTRUAL CYCLE – BLOOD HEAT FROM STAGNATION OF LIVER QI

Clinical Manifestations: Shortened menstrual cycle, heavy or light discharge that is purplish-red in color and contains blood clots, accompanied by pain of the inguinal region, thoracic congestion, distention of the costal regions, distention and pain in the breasts, irritability, bitter taste in the mouth, dry throat.

Tongue: Red with thin yellow coating.

Pulse: Wiry, rapid.

Treatment Method: Clear the liver, resolve stagnation, regulate menstruation.

PRESCRIPTION

Moutan and Gardenia Free Wanderer Powder *dān zhī xiāo yáo săn*

chái hú	bupleurum [root]	Bupleuri Radix	9 g.
dāng guī	tangkuei	Angelicae Sinensis Radix	9 g.
fú líng	poria	Poria	9 g.
shān zhī zĭ	gardenia [fruit]	Gardeniae Fructus	9 g.
bái sháo yào	white peony [root]	Paeoniae Radix Alba	12 g.
bái zhú	ovate atractylodes [root]	Atractylodis Ovatae Rhizoma	9 g.
mŭ dān pí	moutan [root bark]	Moutan Radicis Cortex	9 g.
zhì gān căo	licorice [root] (honey-fried)	Glycyrrhizae Radix	6 g.
bò hé	mint (abbreviated decoction)	Menthae Herba	3 g.
shēng jiāng	fresh ginger [root]	Zingiberis Rhizoma Recens	3 g.

MODIFICATIONS

The prescription contains fresh ginger *(shēng jiāng)*, which is often deleted because of its pungent and warming characteristics.

ACUPUNCTURE AND MOXIBUSTION

Main points: Needle with draining.

CV-03	*zhōng jí*
LI-11	*qū chí*
SP-10	*xuè hăi*
LR-02	*xíng jiān*
SP-08	*dì jī*

Auxiliary points:

For distention and pain of the thorax and hypochondrium, add:

PC-06	*nèi guān*
LR-14	*qī mén*

For distention and pain of the lower abdomen, add:

CV-06	*qì hăi*
KI-13	*qì xué*

1C. SHORTENED MENSTRUAL CYCLE – BLOOD HEAT DUE TO YIN VACUITY

Clinical Manifestations: Shortened menstrual cycle, heavy or light discharge that is red in color and thick in texture, accompanied by flushed cheeks, vexing heat in the five hearts.

Tongue: Red with little coating.

Pulse: Rapid, thready.

Treatment Method: Nourish yin, clear heat, regulate menstruation.

PRESCRIPTION

Rehmannia and Lycium Root Bark Decoction *liǎng dì tāng*

shēng dì huáng	rehmannia [root] dried/fresh	Rehmanniae Radix Exsiccata seu Recens	12 g.
dì gǔ pí	lycium [root bark]	Lycii Radicis Cortex	12 g.
xuán shēn	scrophularia [root]	Scrophulariae Radix	9 g.
bái sháo yào	white peony [root]	Paeoniae Radix Alba	9 g.
ē jiāo	ass hide glue (dissolved and stirred in)	Asini Corii Gelatinum	12 g.
mài mén dōng	ophiopogon [tuber]	Ophiopogonis Tuber	9 g.

ACUPUNCTURE AND MOXIBUSTION

Main points: Needle with supplementation.

CV-03	*zhōng jí*
SP-10	*xuè hǎi*
KI-02	*rán gǔ*
SP-06	*sān yīn jiāo*

Auxiliary points:

For night sweating, add:

HT-06	*yīn xī*
SI-03	*hòu xī*

For lower backache, add:

BL-23	*shèn shū*
M-BW-24	*yāo yǎn* (Lumbar Eye)

1D. SHORTENED MENSTRUAL CYCLE – QI VACUITY

Clinical Manifestations: Shortened menstrual cycle, large volume of thin light-colored menstrual discharge that is accompanied by tiredness, fatigue, empty and "bearing down" sensation in the lower abdomen (in some cases), loss of appetite, loose stools.

Tongue: Pale with white coating.

Pulse: Thready, forceless.

Treatment Method: Supplement qi, contain blood, regulate menstruation.

PRESCRIPTION

Center-Supplementing Qi-Boosting Decoction *bǔ zhōng yì qì tāng*

huáng qí	astragalus [root]	Astragali (seu Hedysari) Radix	15 g.
rén shēn	ginseng	Ginseng Radix	9 g.
bái zhú	ovate atractylodes [root]	Atractylodis Ovatae Rhizoma	9 g.
dāng guī	tangkuei	Angelicae Sinensis Radix	9 g.
chén pí	tangerine [peel]	Citri Exocarpium	6 g.
shēng má	cimicifuga [root]	Cimicifugae Rhizoma	3 g.
chái hú	bupleurum [root]	Bupleuri Radix	3 g.
zhì gān cǎo	licorice [root] (honey-fried)	Glycyrrhizae Radix	6 g.

MODIFICATIONS

In cases with vacuity of both the heart and spleen, with symptoms of palpitations, insomnia and frequent dreaming, the prescription is modified to supplement the heart and spleen.

Delete:

shēng mā	cimicifuga [root]	Cimicifugae Rhizoma
chái hú	bupleurum [root]	Bupleuri Radix
chén pí	tangerine [peel]	Citri Exocarpium

Add:

fú shén	root poria	Poria cum Pini Radice	9 g.
suān zǎo rén	spiny jujube [kernel]	Ziziphi Spinosi Semen	15 g.
yuǎn zhì	polygala [root]	Polygalae Radix	6 g.
lóng yǎn ròu	longan flesh	Longanae Arillus	15 g.
mù xiāng	saussurea [root]	Saussureae Radix (seu Vladimiriae)	6 g.
shēng jiāng	fresh ginger	Zingiberis Rhizoma Recens	3 g.
dà zǎo	jujube	Ziziphi Fructus	8 pc.

In cases where both spleen and kidney qi are depleted with symptoms of thin scanty dull-colored menstrual discharge, lumbar and sacral pain and copious urination and (in some cases) loose stools, with pale tender tongue, the prescription is modified by adding medicinals to warm the kidney and supplement the spleen.

Delete:

shēng mā	cimicifuga [root]	Cimicifugae Rhizoma
chái hú	bupleurum [root]	Bupleuri Radix
chén pí	tangerine [peel]	Citri Exocarpium

Add:

lù jiǎo jiāo	deerhorn glue (dissolved and stirred in)	Cervi Gelatinum Cornu	9 g.
tù sī zǐ	cuscuta [seed]	Cuscutae Semen	9 g.
dù zhòng	eucommia [bark]	Eucommiae Cortex	9 g.
zhì fù zǐ	aconite [accessory tuber] (processed) (extended decoction)	Aconiti Tuber Laterale Praeparatum	6 g.
yì zhì rén	alpinia [fruit]	Alpiniae Oxyphyllae Fructus	6 g.
bǔ gǔ zhī	psoralea [seed]	Psoraleae Semen	9 g.

ACUPUNCTURE AND MOXIBUSTION

Main points: Needle with supplementation; add moxibustion.

CV-06	*qì hǎi*
ST-36	*zú sān lǐ*
BL-20	*pí shū*
SP-06	*sān yīn jiāo*
SP-10	*xuè hǎi*

Auxiliary points:

For vacuity of the spleen and kidney, add:

BL-23	*shèn shū*
CV-04	*guān yuán*

2A. LENGTHENED MENSTRUAL CYCLE – BLOOD VACUITY

Clinical Manifestations: Lengthened menstrual cycle, small volume of light-colored discharge without blood clots that is accompanied by empty sensation and pain in the lower abdomen, dizziness and vertigo, blurred vision, palpitations, insomnia, pale or sallow complexion.

Tongue: Pale.

Pulse: Weak, thready.

Treatment Method: Supplement blood, regulate menstruation.

PRESCRIPTION

Major Origin-Supplementing Brew *dà bǔ yuán jiān*

shú dì huáng	cooked rehmannia [root]	Rehmanniae Radix Conquita	24 g.
shān yào	dioscorea [root]	Dioscoreae Rhizoma	12 g.
rén shēn	ginseng	Ginseng Radix	9 g.
zhì gān cǎo	licorice [root] (honey-fried)	Glycyrrhizae Radix	6 g.
shān zhū yú	cornus [fruit]	Corni Fructus	12 g.
gǒu qǐ zǐ	lycium [berry]	Lycii Fructus	12 g.
dāng guī	tangkuei	Angelicae Sinensis Radix	9 g.

MODIFICATIONS

In cases of vacuity of the spleen with dysfunction in its role of transportation, manifesting in loss of appetite and loose stools, the prescription is modified to supplement the spleen and regulate the stomach.

Delete:

dāng guī	tangkuei	Angelicae Sinensis Radix

Add:

bái zhú	ovate atractylodes [root]	Atractylodis Ovatae Rhizoma	9 g.
bái biǎn dòu	lablab seed	Lablab Semen	15 g.
shā rén	amomum [fruit] (abbreviated decoction)	Amomi Semen seu Fructus	6 g.

In cases of palpitations and insomnia, the prescription is modified to settle the heart and quiet the spirit.

Add:

yuǎn zhì	polygala [root]	Polygalae Radix	6 g.
wǔ wèi zǐ	schisandra [berry]	Schisandrae Fructus	6 g.

In cases of vacuity of blood and depletion of yin, presenting symptoms of tidal fever, night sweating and irritability, the prescription is modified to nourish yin and clear vacuity heat.

Add:

nǚ zhēn zǐ	ligustrum [fruit]	Ligustri Fructus	12 g.
hàn lián cǎo	eclipta	Ecliptae Herba	12 g.
hé shǒu wū	flowery knotweed [root]	Polygoni Multiflori Radix	12 g.
dì gǔ pí	lycium root bark	Lycii Radicis Cortex	9 g.

ACUPUNCTURE AND MOXIBUSTION

Main points: Needle with supplementation; add moxibustion.

BL-20	*pí shū*
ST-36	*zú sān lǐ*
BL-17	*gé shū*
SP-06	*sān yīn jiāo*
CV-06	*qì hǎi*

Auxiliary points:

For dizziness, vertigo, and blurred vision, add:

GV-20	*bǎi huì*

For palpitations and insomnia, add:

HT-07	*shén mén*

2B. LENGTHENED MENSTRUAL CYCLE – BLOOD COLD

Clinical Manifestations: Lengthened menstrual cycle, small volume of dark-colored menstrual discharge that contains blood clots and that is accompanied by lower abdominal coldness and pain decreased by the external application of heat; also cold of the extremities and aversion to cold.

Tongue: White coating.

Pulse: Deep, tight, or slow, deep.

Treatment Method: Warm channels, dispel cold, regulate menstruation.

PRESCRIPTION

Channel-Warming (Menses-Warming) Decoction* *wēn jīng tāng*

dāng guī	tangkuei	Angelicae Sinensis Radix	12 g.
bái sháo yào	white peony [root]	Paeoniae Radix Alba	9 g.
chuān xiōng	ligusticum [root]	Ligustici Rhizoma	9 g.
rén shēn	ginseng	Ginseng Radix	9 g.
mǔ dān pí	moutan [root bark]	Moutan Radicis Cortex	6 g.
é zhú	zedoary	Zedoariae Rhizoma	9 g.
ròu guì	cinnamon [bark] (abbreviated decoction)	Cinnamomi Cortex	6 g.
niú xī	achyranthes [root]	Achyranthis Bidentatae Radix	9 g.
gān cǎo	licorice [root]	Glycyrrhizae Radix	6 g.

*There are two formulas sharing the name "Channel-Warming (Menses-Warming) Decoction *(wēn jīng tāng)* (See Dysmenorrhea, p. 389; Amenorrhea, p 398.) This prescription was first recorded in the book entitled *Jiào Zhù Fù Rén Liáng Fāng (Effective Formulas for Women – A Revised and Annotated Edition).*

MODIFICATIONS

In cases of heavy menstrual discharge, the prescription is modified to warm the channels and relieve bleeding.

Delete:

é zhú	zedoary	Zedoariae Rhizoma
niú xī	achyranthes [root]	Achyranthis Bidentatae Radix

Add:

pào jiāng	blast-fried ginger (charred)	Zingiberis Rhizoma Tostum	6 g.
ài yè	mugwort [leaf] (charred)	Artemisiae Argyi Folium	9 g.

In cases presenting abdominal pain aggravated by external pressure and occasional discharge of blood clots, the prescription is modified to resolve stagnation and relieve pain. Add:

pú huáng	typha pollen (wrapped)	Typhae Pollen	9 g.
wǔ líng zhī	flying squirrel droppings (wrapped)	Trogopteri seu Pteromydis Excrementum	9 g.

ACUPUNCTURE AND MOXIBUSTION

Main points: Needle with even supplementation, even draining; add moxibustion.

CV-04	*guān yuán*
CV-06	*qì hǎi*
SP-06	*sān yīn jiāo*
ST-29	*guī lái*

ST-25   *tiān shū*

Auxiliary points:

For a large number of blood clots, add:

CV-03   *zhōng jí*
KI-14   *sì mǎn*

2C. LENGTHENED MENSTRUAL CYCLE – VACUITY COLD

Clinical Manifestations: Lengthened menstrual cycle, small volume of pale red thin menstrual discharge without blood clots that is accompanied by indistinct lower abdominal pain relieved by external warmth or pressure, weak aching lower back, copious clear urine, loose runny stools.

Tongue: Pale with white coating.

Pulse: Slow, deep or weak, thready.

Treatment Method: Reinforce yang, dispel cold, regulate menstruation.

PRESCRIPTION

Mugwort and Cyperus Palace-Warming Pill *ài fù nuǎn gōng wán*

ài yè	mugwort [leaf]	Artemisiae Argyi Folium	9 g.
xiāng fù zǐ	cyperus [root]	Cyperi Rhizoma	9 g.
dāng guī	tangkuei	Angelicae Sinensis Radix	9 g.
xù duàn	dipsacus [root]	Dipsaci Radix	12 g.
wú zhū yú	evodia [fruit]	Evodiae Fructus	6 g.
chuān xiōng	ligusticum [root]	Ligustici Rhizoma	6 g.
bái sháo yào	white peony [root]	Paeoniae Radix Alba	6 g.
huáng qí	astragalus [root]	Astragali (seu Hedysari) Radix	12 g.
shēng dì huáng	rehmannia [root] dried/fresh	Rehmanniae Radix Exsiccata seu Recens	6 g.
ròu guì	cinnamon [bark] (abbreviated decoction)	Cinnamomi Cortex	6 g.

MODIFICATIONS

In cases presenting loose stools the prescription is modified to warm the kidney and supplement the spleen. Add:

bǔ gǔ zhī	psoralea [seed]	Psoraleae Semen	9 g.
bái zhú	ovate atractylodes [root]	Atractylodis Ovatae Rhizoma	9 g.

ACUPUNCTURE AND MOXIBUSTION

Main points: Needle with supplementation; add moxibustion.

CV-04   *guān yuán*
CV-06   *qì hǎi*
SP-06   *sān yīn jiāo*
GV-04   *mìng mén*
KI-03   *tài xī*

Auxiliary points:

For weak aching lower back, add:

BL-23   *shèn shū*

2D. Lengthened Menstrual Cycle – Liver Qi Stagnation

Clinical Manifestations: Lengthened menstrual cycle, small volume of dark menstrual discharge containing blood clots and accompanied by lower abdominal distention and pain, mental depression, distended sensation of the thorax and hypochondria and breasts.

Tongue: Thin white coating.

Pulse: Wiry.

Treatment Method: Soothe the liver, rectify qi, regulate menstruation.

PRESCRIPTION

Lindera Powder *wū yào sǎn*

wū yào	lindera [root]	Linderae Radix	9 g.
xiāng fù zǐ	cyperus [root]	Cyperi Rhizoma	9 g.
mù xiāng	saussurea [root]	Saussureae Radix	9 g.
dāng guī	tangkuei	Angelicae Sinensis Radix (seu Vladimiriae)	12 g.
zhì gān cǎo	licorice [root] (honey-fried)	Glycyrrhizae Radix	6 g.

MODIFICATIONS

In cases with light menstrual discharge containing blood clots, the prescription is modified to invigorate the blood and regulate menstruation. Add:

chuān xiōng	ligusticum [root]	Ligustici Rhizoma	9 g.

In cases of severe costal pain, the prescription is modified to soothe the liver and relieve pain. Add:

chái hú	bupleurum [root]	Bupleuri Radix	9 g.
yù jīn	curcuma [tuber]	Curcumae Tuber	9 g.

In cases of severe abdominal pain, the prescription is modified to move qi, quicken the blood and relieve pain. Add:

yán hú suǒ	corydalis [tuber]	Corydalis Tuber	9 g.
chuān liàn zǐ	toosendan [fruit]	Toosendan Fructus	9 g.

In cases of stagnation of qi giving rise to fire, manifesting as heavy bright-red menstrual discharge, red tongue and rapid wiry pulse, the prescription is modified to cool the blood and clear heat. Add:

mǔ dān pí	moutan [root bark]	Moutan Radicis Cortex	9 g.
shān zhī zǐ	gardenia [fruit]	Gardeniae Fructus	9 g.

ACUPUNCTURE AND MOXIBUSTION

Main points: Needle with draining.

ST-25	*tiān shū*
KI-13	*qì xué*
SP-08	*dì jī*
SP-06	*sān yīn jiāo*
LR-03	*tài chōng*

Auxiliary points:

For distention and pain of hypochondria and breasts, add:

LR-04	*zhōng fēng*

For fullness and discomfort of the chest, add:

PC-06	*nèi guān*

3A. UNPREDICTABLE MENSTRUAL CYCLE – LIVER QI STAGNATION

Clinical Manifestations: Unpredicatable menstrual cycle with heavy or light discharge, thick sticky purplish-red discharge containing blood clots, discomfort during menstruation that is accompanied by distention and pain of the thorax, hypochondria, breasts and lateral lower abdomen, mental depression, frequent sighing, belching and loss of appetite.

Tongue: Thin white or yellow coating.

Pulse: Wiry.

Treatment Method: Soothe the liver, rectify qi, regulate menstruation.

PRESCRIPTION

Free Wanderer Powder *xiāo yáo sǎn*

chái hú	bupleurum [root]	Bupleuri Radix	9 g.
bái sháo yào	white peony [root]	Paeoniae Radix Alba	12 g.
dāng guī	tangkuei	Angelicae Sinensis Radix	9 g.
bái zhú	ovate atractylodes [root]	Atractylodis Ovatae Rhizoma	9 g.
fú líng	poria	Poria	9 g.
zhì gān cǎo	licorice [root] (honey-fried)	Glycyrrhizae Radix	6 g.
bò hé	mint (abbreviated decoction)	Menthae Herba	3 g.
shēng jiāng	fresh ginger [root]	Zingiberis Rhizoma Recens	3 g.

MODIFICATIONS

In cases of depletion of liver blood and comparative repletion of liver yang, manifesting as dizziness and vertigo, red tongue and dry mouth, remove the pungent and dispersing medicinals.

Delete:

shēng jiāng	fresh ginger [root]	Zingiberis Rhizoma Recens
bò hé	mint	Menthae Herba

In cases where stagnation of liver qi has led to blood stasis, causing lower abdominal distention and pain during menstruation with menstrual discharge containing blood clots, the prescription is modified to quicken the blood and resolve stagnation.

Add:

dān shēn	salvia [root]	Salviae Miltiorrhizae Radix	12 g.
yì mǔ cǎo	leonurus	Leonuri Herba	12 g.
yán hú suǒ	corydalis [tuber]	Corydalis Tuber	9 g.
pú huáng	typha pollen (wrapped)	Typhae Pollen	9 g.

In cases where stagnation of liver qi has transformed to fire, causing heavy thick red menstrual discharge, the prescription is modified to clear heat and cool the blood. Add:

mǔ dān pí	moutan [root bark]	Moutan Radicis Cortex	9 g.
shān zhī zǐ	gardenia [fruit]	Gardeniae Fructus	9 g.

In cases where stagnation of liver qi retards the dispersion of wood to earth, with symptoms including loss of appetite and epigastric fullness, the prescription is modified to rectify qi and aid splenic transportation.

Add:

hòu pò	magnolia [bark]	Magnoliae Cortex	9 g.
chén pí	tangerine [peel]	Citri Exocarpium	9 g.

ACUPUNCTURE AND MOXIBUSTION

Main points: Needle with even supplementation, even draining.

LR-03	*tài chōng*
SP-08	*dì jī*
CV-06	*qì hǎi*
SP-06	*sān yīn jiāo*
LR-14	*qī mén*

Auxiliary points:

For hindered menstrual flow, add:

LR-05	*lǐ gōu*
PC-05	*jiān shǐ*

For menstrual discharge containing blood clots, add:

KI-14	*sì mǎn*

3B. UNPREDICTABLE MENSTRUAL CYCLE – KIDNEY VACUITY

Clinical Manifestations: Indeterminate menstrual cycle with small volume of thin pale-colored menstrual discharge that is accompanied by lumbar and sacral pain, dizziness, vertigo and, in some cases, tinnitus, frequent night urination, unformed stools.

Tongue: Pale.

Pulse: Thready, weak in kidney position.

Treatment Method: Supplement the kidney, regulate menstruation.

PRESCRIPTION

Yin-Securing Brew *gù yīn jiān*

shú dì huáng	cooked rehmannia [root]	Rehmanniae Radix Conquita	24 g.
shān zhū yú	cornus [fruit]	Corni Fructus	12 g.
shān yào	dioscorea [root]	Dioscoreae Rhizoma	12 g.
tù sī zǐ	cuscuta [seed]	Cuscutae Semen	12 g.
rén shēn	ginseng	Ginseng Radix	9 g.
yuǎn zhì	polygala [root]	Polygalae Radix	6 g.
wǔ wèi zǐ	schisandra [berry]	Schisandrae Fructus	6 g.
zhì gān cǎo	licorice [root] (honey-fried)	Glycyrrhizae Radix	6 g.

MODIFICATIONS

In cases accompanied by liver qi stagnation, the prescription is modified to soothe the liver and resolve stagnation. Add:

chái hú	bupleurum [root]	Bupleuri Radix	6 g.
bái sháo yào	white peony [root]	Paeoniae Radix Alba	9 g.
dāng guī	tangkuei	Angelicae Sinensis Radix	9 g.

ACUPUNCTURE AND MOXIBUSTION

Main points: Needle with supplementation; add moxibustion.

CV-04	*guān yuán*
SP-06	*sān yīn jiāo*
BL-23	*shèn shū*
KI-03	*tài xī*
KI-05	*shuǐ quán*

Auxiliary points:

For weak aching lower back and knees, add:

KI-10   *yīn gǔ*

M-BW-24   *yāo yǎn* (Lumbar Eye)

For distention and pain of the thorax and hypochondria, add:

TB-06   *zhī gōu*

LR-03   *tài chōng*

ALTERNATE THERAPEUTIC METHODS

1. Ear Acupuncture

Main points: Uterus, Endocrine, Ovary, Liver, Kidney.

Method: Select two to three points each session, needle to elicit a moderate sensation and retain the needles for fifteen to twenty minutes. Treat once every two days. Auricular embedding therapy may also be used.

REMARKS

Patients suffering from irregular menstruation must pay particular attention to personal hygiene during the menstrual period as well as to regulation of their daily habits. Maintenance of a relaxed psychological state, avoidance of negative emotional stimuli during menstruation, abstention from raw, cold and spicy foods, ample rest and avoidance of chills and draughts are all recommended.

DYSMENORRHEA

Tòng Jīng

1. Coagulation of Cold and Dampness - 2. Stagnation of Liver Qi - 3. Descent of Damp-Heat - 4. Vacuity of Yang with Internal Cold - 5. Vacuity of Liver and Kidney - 6. Vacuity of Qi and Blood

Dysmenorrhea is a gynecological disorder characterized by cramping pains in the lower abdomen preceding, during or following menstruation. At times the pain may extend through to the lower back and sacral region, or, in severe cases, it can be so extreme that it causes fainting. Dysmenorrhea is a disorder most frequently observed in young women.

Dysmenorrhea caused by the displacement of the uterus, a narrow cervical canal, endometrial hyperplasia, pelvic inflammation or endometriosis may all be treated according to the instructions found in this chapter.

ETIOLOGY AND PATHOGENESIS

Impediment of the flow of qi and blood is the major pathological mechanism in dysmenorrhea; it has a number of causes. Frequently there is coagulation of blood from cold and dampness in the *chōng* and *rèn* during the menstrual period. Stagnation of liver qi can result in the impairment of blood flow, leading to a stasis of menstrual blood in the uterus. Invasion of external damp-heat and its subsequent entry into the *chōng* and *rèn* during the menstrual period may also lead to the stagnation of qi and blood, resulting in dysmenorrhea.

Cases of dysmenorrhea from vacuity are also observed, all giving rise to pain. These include vacuity of kidney yang giving rise to internal cold; vacuity of the liver and kidney with depletion of essence and blood; and vacuity of qi and blood resulting in a loss of nourishment to the *chōng* and *rèn*.

Cases of severe abdominal pain occurring before and during menstruation and aggravated by external pressure are generally related to repletion, while those of dull abdominal pain occurring after menstruation, and only somewhat relieved by external pressure, are generally related to vacuity. Although cases of dysmenorrhea include both cold and heat, repletion and vacuity, heat patterns seldom give rise to this disorder.

1. COAGULATION OF COLD AND DAMPNESS

Clinical Manifestations: Cold and pain of the lower abdomen either preceding or during menstruation; aggravation of pain upon external pressure and some relief with external application of heat; scanty menstrual discharge that is dark in color and contains blood clots; aversion to cold and, occasionally, body aches and pains.

Tongue: White slimy coating.

Pulse: Deep, tight.

Treatment Method: Warm the vessels, dissipate cold, dispel dampness, dispel blood stasis, relieve pain.

PRESCRIPTION

Lesser Abdomen Stasis-Expelling Decoction *shào fù zhú yū tāng*

dāng guī	tangkuei	Angelicae Sinensis Radix	9 g.
chì sháo yào	red peony [root]	Paeoniae Radix Rubra	6 g.
pú huáng	typha pollen (wrapped)	Typhae Pollen	9 g.
mò yào	myrrh	Myrrha	6 g.
chuān xiōng	ligusticum [root]	Ligustici Rhizoma	3 g.
wǔ líng zhī	flying squirrel droppings (wrapped)	Trogopteri seu Pteromydis Excrementum	6 g.
yán hú suǒ	corydalis [tuber]	Corydalis Tuber	3 g.
gān jiāng	dried ginger [root]	Zingiberis Rhizoma Exsiccatum	3 g.
ròu guì	cinnamon [bark] (abbreviated decoction)	Cinnamomi Cortex	3 g.
xiǎo huí xiāng	fennel [fruit]	Foeniculi Fructus	3 g.

MODIFICATIONS

To fortify the spleen and dispel dampness routinely, add:

cāng zhú	atractylodes [root]	Atractylodis Rhizoma	9 g.
fú líng	poria	Poria	12 g.

In cases of severe pain and fainting where the extremities are cold or the body is covered in cold sweat, the prescription is modified to revitalize yang. Add:

zhì fù zǐ   aconite [accessory tube]r   Aconiti Tuber Laterale Praeparatum   9 g.
           (processed) (extended decoction)

ACUPUNCTURE AND MOXIBUSTION

Main Points: Needle with draining.

     CV-03   *zhōng jí*
     ST-28   *shuǐ dào*
     SP-08   *dì jī*

Auxiliary points:

For severe pain, add:

     BL-32   *cì liáo*
     ST-29   *guī lái*

For abdominal pain extending through the lower back, add:

     GV-04   *mìng mén*
     BL-23   *shèn shū*

2. STAGNATION OF LIVER QI

Clinical Manifestations: Distending pain in the lower abdomen preceding or during menstruation, aggravation of pain on external pressure, difficult menstruation, scanty menstrual discharge that is dark purple in color and contains blood clots, decrease in pain upon expulsion of clots and disappearance of pain with termination of the menstrual period. Some cases may be accompanied by a distended sensation in the chest, hypochondria and breasts.

Tongue: Dark with thin white coating.

Pulse: Deep, wiry, or slippery, wiry.

Treatment Method: Soothe the liver, rectify qi, dispel blood stasis, relieve pain.

PRESCRIPTION

Infradiaphragmatic Stasis-Expelling Decoction *gé xià zhú yū tāng*

wǔ líng zhī	flying squirrel's droppings (wrapped)	Trogopterui seu Pteromydis Excrementum	9 g.
dāng guī	tangkuei	Angelicae Sinensis Radix	9 g.
táo rén	peach [kernel]	Persicae Semen	9 g.
hóng huā	carthamus [flower]	Carthami Flosa	9 g.
chuān xiōng	ligusticum [root]	Ligustici Rhizoma	6 g.
mǔ dān pí	moutan [root bark]	Moutan Radicis Cortex	6 g.
wū yào	lindera [root]	Linderae Radix	6 g.
xiāng fù zǐ	cyperus [root]	Cyperi Rhizoma	4.5 g.
chì sháo yào	red peony [root]	Paeoniae Radix Rubra	6 g.
zhǐ ké	bitter orange [fruit]	Aurantii Fructus	4.5 g.
yán hú suǒ	corydalis [tuber]	Corydalis Tuber	3 g.
gān cǎo	licorice [root]	Glycyrrhizae Radix	9 g.

MODIFICATIONS

In cases of stagnation of liver qi giving rise to heat, the patient reporting a bitter taste in the mouth, tongue with yellow coating and a lengthened menstrual period with blackish-purple thick sticky menstrual discharge, the prescription is modified to clear liver heat and relieve pain. Add:

shān zhī zǐ	gardenia [fruit]	Gardeniae Fructus	9 g.
xià kū cǎo	prunella [spike]	Prunellae Spica	12 g.
yì mǔ cǎo	leonurus	Leonuri Herba	12 g.

In cases of heaviness and distention in the urethral and anal regions, the prescription is modified to increase the strength of liver qi regulation. Add:

chuān liàn zǐ	toosendan [fruit]	Toosendan Fructus	9 g.
chái hú	bupleurum [root]	Bupleuri Radix	9 g.

In cases where liver depression attacks the spleen, with oppression in the chest and loss of appetite, the prescription is modified to supplement spleen qi. Add:

bái zhú	ovate atractylodes [root]	Atractylodis Ovatae Rhizoma	9 g.
fú líng	poria	Poria	12 g.
chén pí	tangerine [peel]	Citri Exocarpium	9 g.

In cases of severe pain accompanied by nausea and vomiting, the prescription is modified to harmonize the stomach and downbear qi. Add:

wú zhū yú	evodia [fruit]	Evodiae Fructus	1.5 g.
huáng lián	coptis [root]	Coptidis Rhizoma	9 g.
shēng jiāng	fresh ginger [root]	Zingiberis Rhizoma Recens	6 g.

ACUPUNCTURE AND MOXIBUSTION

Main Points: Needle with draining.

CV-06	*qì hǎi*
LR-03	*tài chōng*
SP-06	*sān yīn jiāo*

Auxiliary points:

For abdominal distention and fullness, add:

ST-25	*tiān shū*
KI-13	*qì xué*
SP-08	*dì jī*

For pain in the costal regions, add:

GB-34	*yáng líng quán*
GB-37	*guāng míng*

For oppression in the chest, add:

PC-06	*nèi guān*

3. DESCENT OF DAMP-HEAT

Clinical Manifestations: Lower abdominal pain preceding menstruation, aggravation of pain with external pressure accompanied by a burning sensation or distending pain in the lower back and sacrum. In some cases, there is a recurrent pain in the lower abdomen that becomes more severe with the onset of menstruation. Accompanying symptoms include thick blackish-red menstrual discharge containing blood clots, thick yellowish leukorrhea, scanty concentrated urine and, in many cases, a mild fever.

Tongue: Red with yellow slimy coating.

Pulse: Rapid, wiry, or rapid, slippery.

Treatment Method: Clear heat, dispel dampness, dispel blood stasis, relieve pain.

PRESCRIPTION
Heat-Clearing Blood-Regulating Decoction *qīng rè tiáo xuè tāng*

mǔ dān pí	moutan [root bark]	Moutan Radicis Cortex	12 g.
shēng dì huáng	rehmannia [root] dried/fresh	Rehmanniae Radix Exsiccata seu Recens	12 g.
bái sháo yào	white peony [root]	Paeoniae Radix Alba	12 g.
huáng lián	coptis [root]	Coptidis Rhizoma	9 g.
dāng guī	tangkuei	Angelicae Sinensis Radix	9 g.
chuān xiōng	ligusticum [root]	Ligustici Rhizoma	6 g.
hóng huā	carthamus [flower]	Carthami Flosa	6 g.
táo rén	peach [kernel]	Persicae Semen	6 g.
é zhú	zedoary [rhizome]	Zedoariae Rhizoma	6 g.
xiāng fù zǐ	cyperus [root]	Cyperi Rhizoma	6 g.
yán hú suǒ	corydalis [tuber]	Corydalis Tuber	9 g.

MODIFICATIONS

To reinforce the effect of clearing heat and dispelling dampness, add:

hóng téng	sargentodoxa [stem]	Sargentodoxae Caulis	15 g.
bài jiàng cǎo	baijiang	Baijiang Herba cum Radice	15 g.
yì yǐ rén	coix [seed]	Coicis Semen	30 g.

ACUPUNCTURE AND MOXIBUSTION

Main Points: Needle with draining.

CV-03	*zhōng jí*
SP-08	*dì jī*
ST-29	*guī lái*
LR-03	*tài chōng*
BL-32	*cì liáo*
LI-04	*hé gǔ*

4. VACUITY OF YANG WITH INTERNAL COLD

Clinical Manifestations: Cold and pain of the lower abdomen either during or following menstruation, some relief from pain with external pressure or the application of heat, small volume of dark-colored menstrual discharge, weak aching lower back and legs, copious clear urine.

Tongue: White moist coating.

Pulse: Deep.

Treatment Method: Warm the channels, warm the uterus, relieve pain.

PRESCRIPTION
Channel-Warming (Menses-Warming) Decoction* *wēn jīng tāng*

wú zhū yú	evodia [fruit]	Evodiae Fructus	9 g.
dāng guī	tangkuei	Angelicae Sinensis Radix	9 g.
bái sháo yào	white peony [root]	Paeoniae Radix Alba	6 g.
chuān xiōng	ligusticum [root]	Ligustici Rhizoma	6 g.
rén shēn	ginseng	Ginseng Radix	6 g.
shēng jiāng	fresh ginger [root]	Zingiberis Rhizoma Recens	6 g.
mài mén dōng	ophiopogon [tuber]	Ophiopogonis Tuber	9 g.
mǔ dān pí	moutan [root bark]	Moutan Radicis Cortex	6 g.
zhì bàn xià	pinellia [tuber] (processed)	Processed Pinelliae Tuber	6 g.
guì zhī	cinnamon [twig]	Cinnamomi Ramulus	6 g.
ē jiāo	ass hide glue (dissolved and stirred in)	Asini Corii Gelatinum	9 g.
gān cǎo	licorice [root]	Glycyrrhizae Radix	6 g.

Two formulas share the name Channel-Warming (Menses Warming) Decoction *(wēn jīng tāng).* (See Menstrual Irregularity, p. 379, and Amenorrhea, p. 398.) This prescription was first recorded in the book entitled, *Jīn Guì Yaò Luè Fāng Lùn (Synopsis of Prescriptions of the Golden Chamber).*

MODIFICATIONS

To increase the ability of the prescription to warm the kidney and uterus, dissipate cold, and relieve pain, add:

zhì fù zǐ	aconite [accessory tuber] (processed) extended decoction)	Aconiti Tuber Laterale Praeparatum	6 g.
ài yè	mugwort [leaf]	Artemisiae Argyi Folium	9 g.
xiǎo huí xiāng	fennel [fruit]	Foeniculi Fructus	6 g.

In cases where the extremities are cold, the face pale and greenish and the tongue tender and pale, the prescription is modified to avoid obstructing yang and retarding the blood. Delete:

mài mén dōng	ophiopogon [tuber]	Ophiopogonis Tuber
ē jiāo	ass hide glue	Asini Corii Gelatinum

ACUPUNCTURE AND MOXIBUSTION

Main Points: Needle with supplementation; add moxibustion.

BL-23	*shèn shū*
CV-04	*guān yuán*
ST-36	*zú sān lǐ*
SP-06	*sān yīn jiāo*
CV-03	*zhōng jí*
SP-08	*dì jī*

5. VACUITY OF THE LIVER AND KIDNEY

Clinical Manifestations: Indistinct lower abdominal pain either preceding or following menstruation, some relief from pain with external pressure, thin light-colored menstrual discharge, aching of the lower back and spine, general fatigue, dizzy spells and tinnitus and in some cases tidal fever.

Tongue: Pale.

Pulse: Deep, thready, or weak, thready.

Treatment Method: Supplement the liver and kidney, regulate and rectify the *chōng* and *rèn*, relieve pain.

PRESCRIPTION

Liver-Regulating Decoction *tiáo gān tāng*

dāng guī	tangkuei	Angelicae Sinensis Radix	12 g.
bái sháo yào	white peony [root]	Paeoniae Radix Alba	9 g.
shān zhū yú	cornus [fruit]	Corni Fructus	12 g.
bā jǐ tiān	morinda [root]	Morindae Radix	12 g.
shān yào	dioscorea [root]	Dioscoreae Rhizoma	30 g.
zhì gān cǎo	licorice [root] (honey-fried)	Glycyrrhizae Radix	6 g.
ē jiāo	ass hide glue (dissolved and stirred in)	Asini Corii Gelatinum	9 g.

MODIFICATIONS

In cases of pain extending through the lower back and sacrum, the prescription is modified to supplement the kidney. Add:

xù duàn	dipsacus [root]	Dipsaci Radix	12 g.
dù zhòng	eucommia [bark]	Eucommiae Cortex	12 g.

In cases of distending pain in the costal or lateral lower abdomen, the prescription is modified to rectify qi and relieve pain. Add:

chuān liàn zǐ	toosendan [fruit]	Toosendan Fructus	9 g.
yán hú suǒ	corydalis [tuber]	Corydalis Tuber	9 g.
xiǎo huí xiāng	fennel [fruit]	Foeniculi Fructus	6 g.
yù jīn	curcuma [tuber]	Curcumae Tuber	9 g.

ACUPUNCTURE AND MOXIBUSTION

Main Points: Needle with supplementation.

BL-18	*gān shū*
BL-23	*shèn shū*
CV-04	*guān yuán*
ST-36	*zú sān lǐ*
KI-06	*zhào hǎi*

Auxiliary points:

For dizziness and tinnitus, add:

GB-39	*xuán zhōng*
KI-03	*tài xī*

For lower abdominal pain, add:

KI-12	*dà hè*
KI-13	*qì xué*

6. VACUITY OF QI AND BLOOD

Clinical Manifestations: Indistinct lower abdominal pain either during or following menstruation, some relief from pain with external pressure, empty and bearing down sensation in the lower abdominal and pubic regions, scanty menstrual discharge that is light in color and thin in texture, tiredness, fatigue and occasionally dull complexion, loss of appetite or diarrhea.

Tongue: Pale.

Pulse: Weak, thready.

Treatment Method: Supplement qi and blood, relieve pain.

PRESCRIPTION

Sagely Cure Decoction *shèng yù tāng*

huáng qí	astragalus [root]	Astragali (seu Hedysari) Radix	12 g.
rén shēn	ginseng	Ginseng Radix	9 g.
dāng guī	tangkuei	Angelicae Sinensis Radix	12 g.
chuān xiōng	ligusticum [root]	Ligustici Rhizoma	9 g.
shú dì huáng	cooked rehmannia [root]	Rehmanniae Radix Conquita	12 g.
shēng dì huáng	rehmannia [root] dried/fresh	Rehmanniae Radix Exsiccata seu Recens	12 g.

MODIFICATIONS

The prescription is often modified to increase its pain relieving effects.

Delete:

shēng dì huáng	rehmannia [root] dried/fresh	Rehmanniae Radix Exsiccata seu Recens

Add:

bái sháo yào	white peony [root]	Paeoniae Radix Alba	12 g.
xiāng fù zǐ	cyperus [root]	Cyperi Rhizoma	9 g.
yán hú suǒ	corydalis [tuber]	Corydalis Tuber	9 g.

In cases of vacuity of blood and stagnation of the liver, characterized by pain in the costal regions, distending sensation in the breasts and distending pain in the lower abdomen, the prescription is modified to rectify qi and relieve pain. Add:

chái hú	bupleurum [root]	Bupleuri Radix	6 g.
chuān liàn zǐ	toosendan [fruit]	Toosendan Fructus	9 g.
xiǎo huí xiāng	fennel [fruit]	Foeniculi Fructus	6 g.
wū yào	lindera [root]	Linderae Radix	9 g.

In cases of severe vacuity of blood, characterized by dizziness and vertigo, palpitations, and insomnia, the prescription is modified to settle the heart and quiet the spirit. Add:

jī xuè téng	millettia [root and stem]	Millettiae Radix et Caulis	15 g.
suān zǎo rén	spiny jujube [kernel]	Ziziphi Spinosi Semen	15 g.
dà zǎo	jujube	Ziziphi Fructus	10 pc.

In cases accompanied by kidney vacuity, characterized by weak aching lower back and legs, the prescription is modified to supplement the kidney. Add:

tù sī zǐ	cuscuta [seed]	Cuscutae Semen	12 g.
xù duàn	dipsacus [root]	Dipsaci Radix	12 g.
sāng jì shēng	mistletoe	Loranthi seu Visci Ramus	12 g.

ACUPUNCTURE AND MOXIBUSTION

Main Points: Needle with supplementation; add moxibustion.

BL-23	*shèn shū*
CV-04	*guān yuán*
ST-36	*zú sān lǐ*
SP-06	*sān yīn jiāo*

ALTERNATE THERAPEUTIC METHODS

1. Ear Acupuncture

Main points: Uterus, Endocrine, Sympathetic, Kidney.

Method: Needle to elicit a moderate sensation and retain the needles for fifteen to twenty minutes. Auricular needle embedding therapy may also be used.

REMARKS

In the treatment of dysmenorrhea, common pain-relieving medicines may be chosen on the basis of differential diagnosis and added to the basic prescriptions to enhance the pain-dispelling effects.

In cases of cold, add herbs that warm the channels and relieve pain, including:

ài yè	mugwort [leaf]	Artemisiae Argyi Folium	9 g.
ziǎo huí xiāng	fennel [fruit]	Foeniculi Fructus	6 g.
gān jiāng	dried ginger [root]	Zingiberis Rhizoma Exsiccatum	6 g.
ròu guì	cinnamon [bark] (abbreviated decoction)	Cinnamomi Cortex	6 g.
wū yào	lindera [root]	Linderae Radix	9 g.
wú zhū yú	evodia [fruit]	Evodiae Fructus	6 g.

In cases of stagnation of qi, add herbs to activate qi and relieve pain, including:

xiāng fù zǐ	cyperus [root]	Cyperi Rhizoma	9 g.
chuān liàn zǐ	toosendan [fruit]	Toosendan Fructus	9 g.
yán hú suǒ	corydalis [tuber]	Corydalis Tuber	9 g.
jiāng huáng	turmeric [rhizome]	Curcumae Longae Rhizoma	9 g.
mù xiāng	saussurea [root]	Saussureae (seu Vladimiriae) Radix	9 g.
zhǐ ké	bitter orange [fruit]	Aurantii Fructus	9 g.

In cases of stagnation of blood, add herbs to quicken the blood and relieve pain, including:

chuān xiōng	ligusticum [root]	Ligustici Rhizoma	9 g.
rǔ xiāng	frankincense	Olibanum	9 g.
sān qī	notoginseng [root]	Notoginseng Radix	9 g.
mò yào	myrrh	Myrrha	9 g.
pú huáng	typha pollen	Typhae Pollen	9 g.
wǔ líng zhī	flying squirrel's droppings (wrapped)	Trogopteri seu Pteromydis Excrementum	9 g.

For symptoms of heat, use heat clearing herbal medicines, including:

chuān liàn zǐ	toosendan [fruit]	Toosendan Fructus	9 g.
mǔ dān pí	moutan [root bark]	Moutan Radicis Cortex	9 g.
chì sháo yào	red peony [root]	Paeoniae Radix Rubra	9 g.

Patients should be advised to avoid strong emotional upsets, stress and overwork. Effort should be made to avoid catching cold and to limit consumption of raw and cold foods during menstruation.

AMENORRHEA

Jìng Bì

1. Vacuity of Liver and Kidney - 2. Depletion of Yin and Dryness of Blood - 3. Vacuity of Qi and Blood - 4. Stagnation of Qi and Stasis of Blood - 5. Obstruction by Phlegm-Dampness

In traditional Chinese medicine, menstrual block *(jìng bì)* indicates blockage of the normal bodily discharge, termed amenorrhea in Western medicine. In practice, amenorrhea constitutes gynecological disorders where menstruation has not begun by eighteen years of age, or where the menstrual cycle has been interrupted for three months or longer.

Certain normal physiological phenomena are not included in the clinical perception of amenorrhea. These include the cessation of menstruation during pregnancy and while breastfeeding, the termination of menstruation at menopause and, in some young women, the absence of menstruation for a period following their first menses. Also, some women experience an interruption of one or two menstrual periods after a sudden change of environment. When no other pathological manifestations are present, treatment is not given in these cases.

Absence of menstruation because of congenital underdevelopment or malformation of the reproductive organs, or organic injury to the reproductive organs, cannot be affected by herbal medicine or acumoxa therapy, and also are not included in this discussion.

Endocrine, nervous and psychological factors may all play a part in the onset of amenorrhea. Certain biomedical conditions, including anemia, tuberculosis, nephritis and heart disease, can also lead to amenorrhea.

ETIOLOGY AND PATHOGENESIS

Although the etiology and pathogenesis of amenorrhea is complex, patterns may be divided into the categories of vacuity and repletion. In vacuity patterns, essence and blood are insufficient, the sea of blood *(xuè hǎi)* is empty and no blood can be discharged as menses. In repletion patterns, obstruction of the channels by evil prevents the downward passage of blood during menstruation.

Amenorrhea caused by vacuity may involve vacuity of the liver and kidney, qi and blood vacuity or depletion of yin and dryness of the blood. Amenorrhea caused by repletion is brought on by stagnation of qi and blood or obstruction by phlegm and dampness.

1. VACUITY OF LIVER AND KIDNEY

Clinical Manifestations: Absence of initial menstruation by 18 years of age, or late menstruation where the menstrual discharge gradually decreases to the point where menstruation does not occur; accompanying symptoms include weak physical constitution, lower backache, weakness of the legs, dizziness and vertigo, and tinnitus.

Tongue: Pale red with little coating.

Pulse: Deep, weak or rough, thready.

Treatment Method: Supplement the kidney, nourish the liver, regulate menstruation.

PRESCRIPTION

Kidney-Returning Pill *guī shèn wān*

tù sī zǐ	cuscuta [seed]	Cuscutae Semen	12 g.
dù zhòng	eucommia [bark]	Eucommiae Cortex	9 g.
dì gǔ pí	lycium [root bark]	Lycii Radicis Cortex	12 g.
shān zhū yú	cornus [fruit]	Corni Fructus	12 g.
dāng guī	tangkuei	Angelicae Sinensis Radix	12 g.
shú dì huáng	cooked rehmannia [root]	Rehmanniae Radix Conquita	15 g.
shān yào	dioscorea [root]	Dioscoreae Rhizoma	12 g.
fú líng	poria	Poria	9 g.

MODIFICATIONS

To enhance liver blood supplementation, add:

jī xuè téng	millettia [root and stem]	Millettiae Radix et Caulis	15 g.
hé shǒu wū	flowery knotweed [root]	Polygoni Multiflori Radix	15 g.

In cases presenting with tidal fever, vexing heat in the five hearts and night sweating, vacuity of liver and kidney yin has given rise to vacuity heat. Treatment should be given according to "Depletion of Yin and Dryness of Blood," which follows.

ACUPUNCTURE AND MOXIBUSTION

Main points: Needle with supplementation; add moxibustion.

BL-18	*gān shū*
BL-23	*shèn shū*
BL-17	*gé shū*
CV-04	*guān yuán*
SP-06	*sān yīn jiāo*

Auxiliary points:

For aching of the lower back and knees, add:

GV-04	*mìng mén*
KI-10	*yīn gǔ*
M-BW-24	*yāo yǎn* (Lumbar Eye)

2. DEPLETION OF YIN AND DRYNESS OF BLOOD

Clinical Manifestations: Gradual decrease in menstrual discharge until menstruation no longer occurs, vexing heat in the five hearts, flushed cheeks, dry mouth and throat, night sweating, bone steaming fever, or, in some cases, coughing with blood-streaked phlegm.

Tongue: Red with little coating.

Pulse: Rapid, thready.

Treatment Method: Nourish yin, clear heat, regulate menstruation.

PRESCRIPTION

Yin-Boosting Variant Brew *jiā jiǎn yī yīn jiān*

shēng dì huáng	rehmannia, [root] dried/fresh	Rehmanniae Radix Exsiccata seu Recens	12 g.
shú dì huáng	cooked rehmannia [root]	Rehmanniae Radix Conquita	12 g.
bái sháo yào	white peony [root]	Paeoniae Radix Alba	12 g.
mài mén dōng	ophiopogon [tuber]	Ophiopogonis Tuber	9 g.
zhī mǔ	anemarrhena [root]	Anemarrhenae Rhizoma	9 g.
dì gǔ pí	lycium [root bark]	Lycii Radicis Cortex	12 g.
zhì gān cǎo	licorice [root] (honey-fried)	Glycyrrhizae Radix	6 g.

MODIFICATIONS

The prescription is often modified to nourish yin and rectify qi and blood.
Add:

huáng jīng	polygonatum [root]	Polygonati Huangjing Rhizoma	12 g.
dān shēn	salvia [root]	Salviae Miltiorrhizae Radix	12 g.
zhǐ ké	bitter [orange]	Aurantii Fructus	9 g.

In cases of pronounced restlessness and tidal fever, the prescription is modified to nourish yin and clear vacuity heat.
Add:

biē jiǎ	turtle shell (extended decoction)	Amydae Carapax	30 g.
qīng hāo	sweet wormwood (abbreviated decoction)	Artemisiae Apiaceae seu Annuae Herba	9 g.

In cases where menstrual block is accompanied by coughing with blood-streaked phlegm, the prescription is modified to nourish yin, moisten the lung and relieve coughing.
Add:

chuān bèi mǔ	Sichuan fritillaria [bulb]	Fritillariae Cirrhosae Bulbus	9 g.
wǔ wèi zǐ	schisandra [berry]	Schisandrae Fructus	6 g.
bǎi hé	lily [bulb]	Lilii Bulbus	12 g.
ē jaiō	ass hide glue (dissolved and stirred in)	Asini Corii Gelatinum	9 g.

In cases of menstrual block accompanied by restlessness, insomnia and palpitations, the prescription is modified to nourish the heart and quiet the spirit.
Add:

bǎi zǐ rén	biota [seed]	Biotae Semen	12 g.
yè jaiō téng	flowery knotweed [stem]	Polygoni Multiflori Caulis	15 g.

In cases where repletion heat has scorched yin resulting in dryness of the blood and amenorrhea, the prescription is modified to clear heat and nourish yin.
Add:

xuán shēn	scrophularia [root]	Scrophulariae Radix	9 g.
huáng bǎi	phellodendron [bark]	Phellodendri Cortex	9 g.

ACUPUNCTURE AND MOXIBUSTION

Main points: Needle with supplementation.

BL-18	*gān shū*
BL-23	*shèn shū*
BL-17	*gé shū*
SP-06	*sān yīn jiāo*
KI-06	*zhào hǎi*

Auxiliary Points:

For tidal fever, coughing and night sweating, add:

BL-43 (38)	*gāo huāng shū*
KI-02	*rán gǔ*

3. Vacuity of Qi and Blood

Clinical Manifestations: Gradual lengthening of the menstrual cycle, light menstrual discharge of pale color and thin consistency, with the menses eventually ceasing. Accompanying symptoms include dizziness and vertigo, blurred vision, palpitations, shortness of breath, tiredness, fatigue, loss of appetite, loose stools, loss of luster of the hair (or in some cases, loss of hair), emaciation, sallow complexion.

Tongue: Pale with white coating.

Pulse: Weak, thready.

Treatment Method: Supplement qi, nourish the blood, regulate menstruation.

PRESCRIPTION

Ginseng Construction-Nourishing Decoction (Pill)
rén shēn yǎng róng tāng (wán)

rén shēn	ginseng	Ginseng Radix	9 g.
bái zhú	ovate atractylodes [root]	Atractylodis Ovatae Rhizoma	9 g.
fú líng	poria	Poria	9 g.
huáng qí	astragalus [root]	Astragali (seu Hedysari) Radix	12 g.
shú dì huáng	cooked rehmannia [root]	Rehmanniae Radix Conquita	9 g.
dāng guī	tangkuei	Angelicae Sinensis Radix	9 g.
bái sháo yào	white peony [root]	Paeoniae Radix Alba	12 g.
chén pí	tangerine peel	Citri Exocarpium	9 g.
ròu guì	cinnamon bark (abbreviated decoction)	Cinnamomi Cortex	3 g.
wǔ wèi zǐ	schisandra [berry]	Schisandrae Fructus	6 g.
yuǎn zhì	polygala [root]	Polygalae Radix	6 g.
zhì gān cǎo	licorice [root] (honey-fried)	Glycyrrhizae Radix	6 g.
shēng jiāng	fresh ginger	Zingiberis Rhizoma Recens	3 g.
dà zǎo	jujube	Ziziphi Fructus	3 pc.

MODIFICATIONS

In cases of amenorrhea because of a post-partum loss of blood, symptoms of qi and blood vacuity are accompanied by apathy, lack of vaginal mucus, loss of pubic hair, a decrease in libido and atrophy of the reproductive organs. This indicates exhaustion of essence and blood, insufficiency of kidney qi and degeneration of the *chōng* and *rèn*. The preceding prescription may be administered on a long-term basis in these cases, with the addition of:

lù róng	velvet deerhorn	Cervi Cornu Parvum	1 g.
	(1 g., each time, powdered and stirred in)		
lù jiǎo jiāo	deerhorn glue	Cervi Gelatinum Cornu	12 g.
zǐ hé chē	placenta (powdered and capsulized)	Hominis Placenta	3 g.

ACUPUNCTURE AND MOXIBUSTION

Main points: Needle with supplementation; add moxibustion.

CV-04	*guān yuán*
BL-20	*pí shū*
ST-36	*zú sān lǐ*
SP-06	*sān yīn jiāo*
SP-10	*xuè hǎi*

Auxiliary points:

For loss of appetite and loose stools, add:

| CV-12 | *zhōng wǎn* |
| ST-25 | *tiān shū* |

4. STAGNATION OF QI AND STASIS OF BLOOD

Clinical Manifestations: Cessation of menstruation, psychological depression, irritability, distention and fullness in the chest and costal region, lower abdominal distention with pain that is aggravated by external pressure.

Tongue: Dark, purplish; sometimes with stasis macules on the tongue body.

Pulse: Deep, wiry, or deep, rough.

Treatment Method: Rectify qi, quicken the blood, dispel stasis, free menstruation.

PRESCRIPTION

House of Blood Stasis-Expelling Decoction *xuè fŭ zhú yū tāng*

táo rén	peach [kernel]	Persicae Semen	12 g.
hóng huā	carthamus [flower]	Carthami Flosa	9 g.
dāng guī	tangkuei	Angelicae Sinensis Radix	9 g.
shēng dì huáng	rehmannia [root] dried/fresh	Rehmanniae Radix Exsiccata seu Recens	9 g.
chuān xiōng	ligusticum [root]	Ligustici Rhizoma	4.5 g.
chì sháo yào	red peony [root]	Paeoniae Radix Rubra	6 g.
niú xī	achyranthes [root]	Achyranthis Bidentatae Radix	9 g.
jié gěng	platycodon [root]	Platycodonis Radix	4.5 g.
chái hú	bupleurum [root]	Bupleuri Radix	3 g.
zhǐ ké	bitter orange [fruit]	Aurantii Fructus	6 g.
gān cǎo	licorice [root]	Glycyrrhizae Radix	3 g.

MODIFICATIONS

In cases where stagnation of qi is predominant, manifesting as severe distention of the chest, costal and lower abdominal regions, the prescription is modified to rectify qi and relieve distention. Add:

qīng pí	unripe tangerine [peel]	Citri Exocarpium Immaturum	9 g.
é zhú	zedoary	Zedoariae Rhizoma	9 g.
mù xiāng	saussurea [root]	Saussureae (seu Vladimiriae) Radix	9 g.

In cases where stasis of blood is predominant, manifesting as severe lower abdominal pain aggravated by external pressure, the prescription is modified to quicken the blood and relieve pain.

Add:

jiāng huáng	turmeric	Curcumae Longae Rhizoma	9 g.
sān léng	sparganium [root]	Sparganii Rhizoma	9 g.

In cases of coagulation of cold and stasis of blood, with symptoms including lack of warmth in the limbs, lower abdominal cold and pain, white tongue coating and deep tight pulse, treatment is directed at warming the channels, dissipating cold, invigorating the blood and freeing menstruation.

Use:

Channel-Warming (Menses-Warming) Decoction *wēn jīng tāng*

wú zhū yú	evodia [fruit]	Evodiae Fructus	9 g.
dāng guī	tangkuei	Angelicae Sinensis Radix	9 g.
bái sháo yào	white peony [root]	Paeoniae Radix Alba	6 g.
chuān xiōng	ligusticum [root]	Ligustici Rhizoma	6 g.
rén shēn	ginseng	Ginseng Radix	6 g.
shēng jiāng	fresh ginger [root]	Zingiberis Rhizoma Recens	6 g.
mài mén dōng	ophiopogon [tuber]	Ophiopogonis Tuber	9 g.
mǔ dān pí	moutan [root bark]	Moutan Radicis Cortex	6 g.
zhì bàn xià	pinellia [tuber] (processed)	Pinelliae Tuber Praeparatum	6 g.
guì zhī	cinnamon [twig]	Cinnamomi Ramulus	6 g.
ē jiāo	ass hide glue (dissolved and stirred in)	Asini Corii Gelatinum	9 g.
gān cǎo	licorice [root]	Glycyrrhizae Radix	6 g.

In cases where the accumulation of repletion heat has led to blood stasis, with symptoms of burning sensation and pain in the lower abdomen, yellow vaginal discharge, yellow tongue coating and rapid pulse, the prescription is modified to clear heat and dissolve stasis.

Add:

huáng bǎi	phellodendron [bark]	Phellodendri Cortex	9 g.
bài jiàng cǎo	baijiang	Baijiang Herba cum Radice	12 g.
mǔ dān pí	moutan [root bark]	Moutan Radicis Cortex	9 g.

ACUPUNCTURE AND MOXIBUSTION

Main points: Needle with draining.

CV-03	*zhōng jí*
SP-08	*dì jī*
LI-04	*hé gǔ*
SP-06	*sān yīn jiāo*
LR-03	*tài chōng*
SP-10	*xuè hǎi*

Auxiliary points:

For lower abdominal distention, or pain that is increased on external pressure, accompanied by internal mass, Add:

CV-06	*qì hǎi*
KI-14	*sì mǎn*

For distention and fullness of the chest and costal regions, Add:

LR-14	*qī mén*
TB-06	*zhī gōu*

5. OBSTRUCTION BY PHLEGM-DAMPNESS

Clinical Manifestations: Cessation of menstruation, obesity, fullness and oppression in the chest and costal regions, nausea and vomiting, excessive phlegm, tiredness, fatigue, excessive white vaginal discharge, edema of the face and feet.

Tongue: White greasy coating.

Pulse: Slippery.

Treatment Method: Expel phlegm, dispel dampness, rectify qi, quicken the blood, free menstruation.

PRESCRIPTION

Combine Atractylodes and Cyperus Phlegm-Abducting Decoction *(cāng fù dǎo tán tāng)* with Hand-of-Buddha Powder *(fó shǒu sǎn)*.

Atractylodes and Cyperus Phlegm-Abducting Decoction
cāng fù dǎo tán tāng

cāng zhú	atractylodes [root]	Atractylodis Rhizoma	9 g.
xiāng fù zǐ	cyperus [root]	Cyperi Rhizoma	9 g.
fú líng	poria	Poria	12 g.
fǎ bàn xià	pinellia [tuber] (processed)	Pinelliae Tuber Praeparatum	9 g.
chén pí	tangerine [peel]	Citri Exocarpium	9 g.
dǎn xīng	bile-processed arisaema [root]	Arisaematis Rhizoma cum Felle Bovis	6 g.
zhǐ ké	bitter orange [fruit]	Aurantii Fructus	6 g.
spirit2 qū	medicated leaven	Massa Medicata Fermentata	12 g.
shēng jiāng	fresh ginger [root]	Zingiberis Rhizoma Recens	9 g.
zhì gān cǎo	licorice [root] (honey-fried)	Glycyrrhizae Radix	6 g.

with:

Hand-of-Buddha Powder *fó shǒu sǎn*

fó shǒu gān	Buddha's hand [fruit]	Citri Sarcodactylidis Fructus	9 g.
dāng guī	tangkuei	Angelicae Sinensis Radix	12 g.
chuān xiōng	ligusticum [root]	Ligustici Rhizoma	9 g.

ACUPUNCTURE AND MOXIBUSTION

Main points: Needle with even supplementation, even draining; add moxibustion.

CV-03	*zhōng jí*
SP-08	*dì jī*
ST-40	*fēng lóng*
SP-06	*sān yīn jiāo*
LI-04	*hé gǔ*
ST-36	*zú sān lǐ*

Auxiliary points:

For excessive white vaginal discharge, add:

BL-32	*cì liáo*

ALTERNATE THERAPEUTIC METHODS

1. Ear Acupuncture

Main points: Uterus, Endocrine, Subcortex, Ovary, Liver, Kidney, *Sān Jiāo*, Stomach, Spleen.

Method: Select three to four points per session and needle to elicit a moderate sensation. Treat once every two days, ten treatments per therapeutic course. Auricular needle embedding therapy may also be used.

2. Plum Blossom Needle Therapy

Main points: Governing Vessel, lumbar and sacral portions of the Bladder Channel.

Method: Tap with light or moderate force over these areas once every two days.

REMARKS

During the clinical investigation of amenorrhea, the patient's medical history must be thoroughly investigated, in addition to the completion of other relevant examinations. Diagnosis should first determine that the amenorrhea is not caused by normal physiological phenomena, with special attention to distinguishing amenorrhea from pregnancy.

An understanding of the patient's physical development, nutrition, secondary sexual characteristics and psychological state must be achieved. Inquiry as to whether medication has been taken incorrectly, whether the patient has detrimental eating habits or whether the patient suffers from a contributing illnesses, provide valuable information that aids the elucidation of amenorrhea's cause. Examination of the reproductive organs should also be included in a clinical examination.

After amenorrhea is diagnosed, a clear distinction must be made as to whether the problem is associated with repletion or vacuity. Generally speaking, absence of the onset of menstruation by the age of eighteen years, or gradual lengthening of the menstrual cycle until it ceases altogether, accompanied by symptoms of vacuity, are classified as vacuity patterns. Abrupt termination of menstruation in patients whose menstrual cycle was ordinarily normal, and accompanied by symptoms of repletion, are classified as repletion patterns.

Treatment of vacuity should serve to supplement and free menstruation, while treatment of repletion should dispel evils and promote menstruation. When amenorrhea is the result of other illnesses, first treat the primary illness, or treat the root and branch pattern simultaneously.

UTERINE BLEEDING

Bēng Lòu

1. Spleen Qi Vacuity - 2. Kidney Yang Vacuity - 3. Kidney Yin Vacuity - 4. Blood Heat - 5. Blood Stasis

Uterine bleeding *(bēng lòu)* can refer to either a heavy discharge of blood from the vagina or a constant dribbling of blood from the vagina that occurs during or beyond the regular menstrual period. *Bēng* means an abrupt onset of heavy uterine bleeding, while *lòu* means the gradual onset of uterine bleeding, with a continuous dribbling of a small amount of blood. Although *bēng* and *lòu* describe different degrees of bleeding, during the course of the illness they often undergo mutual transformation or manifest alternately; hence, the compound *bēng lòu*.

Functional uterine bleeding, as well as uterine bleeding from other etiological factors, may be diagnosed and treated according to this chapter.

ETIOLOGY AND PATHOGENESIS

The major pathological mechanism involved in the onset of uterine bleeding is injury to the *chōng* and *rèn*, with weakening of the functions of consolidation and retention. Factors leading to injury of the *chōng* and *rèn* fall into the categories of vacuity and repletion.

Vacuity patterns apply to both the spleen and kidney. Spleen qi vacuity can be caused by poor physical constitution, improper dietary and eating habits or taxation. This results in insufficient spleen qi with an inability to secure the blood, coupled with weakening of the *chōng* and *rèn*. Debilitation of kidney yang, with the consequent failure of the *chōng* and *rèn* to secure and retain, can also cause uterine bleeding. Vacuity of kidney yin with accompanying frenetic vacuity fire and failure to hold the blood also leads to this condition.

Uterine bleeding resulting from repletion can be caused by an excessively yang physical constitution, by invasion of heat evil, by overindulgence in spicy foods or by depression of liver qi transforming into fire. All these cause heat injury to the *chōng* and *rèn*, allowing blood to leave its proper course.

Uterine bleeding may also be a result of internal disruption by the seven affects, or invasion of external heat or cold during menstrual or postpartum bleeding. These can lead to obstruction of the *chōng* and *rèn* by static blood, allowing blood to escape the channels.

In summary, the etiology and pathogenesis of uterine bleeding can be classified according to spleen vacuity, kidney vacuity, blood heat or blood stasis. Prolonged injury to blood and depletion of qi may in turn lead to vacuity of both qi and blood, depletion of both qi and yin or vacuity of both yin and yang. Regardless of where in the viscera and bowels the pathogenesis began, involvement of the kidney is inevitable.

1. SPLEEN QI VACUITY

Clinical Manifestations: Uterine bleeding with thin light-colored discharge, accompanied by pale complexion, fatigue, shortness of breath, disinclination to speak, loss of appetite, loose stools, edema of the face and limbs in some cases and lack of warmth in the extremities.

Tongue: Pale with white coating.

Pulse: Weak, thready.

Treatment Method: Supplement the spleen, boost qi, secure the blood and relieve bleeding.

PRESCRIPTION

Root-Securing Uterine Bleeding Decoction *gù běn zhǐ bēng tāng*

huáng qí	astragalus [root]	Astragali (seu Hedysari) Radix	30 g.
rén shēn	ginseng	Ginseng Radix	9 g.
bái zhú	ovate atractylodes [root]	Atractylodis Ovatae Rhizoma	9 g.
shú dì huáng	cooked rehmannia [root]	Rehmanniae Radix Conquita	9 g.
dāng guī	tangkuei	Angelicae Sinensis Radix	6 g.
pào jiāng	blast-fried ginger [root]	Zingiberis Rhizoma Tostum	6 g.

MODIFICATIONS

In cases of uterine bleeding the prescription is often modified to supplement and upbear spleen qi, secure retention and relieve bleeding.

Delete:

dāng guī	tangkuei	Angelicae Sinensis Radix

Add:

shān yào	dioscorea [root]	Dioscoreae Rhizoma	30 g.
hǎi piāo xiāo	cuttlefish [bone]	Sepiae seu Sepiellae Os	9 g.
shēng mā	cimicifuga [root]	Cimicifugae Rhizoma	3 g.
dà zǎo	jujube	Ziziphi Fructus	8 pc.

With signs of blood vacuity the prescription is modified to supplement the blood.
Add:

hé shǒu wū	flowery knotweed [root]	Polygoni Multiflori Radix	9 g.
bái sháo yào	white peony [root]	Paeoniae Radix Alba	9 g.
sāng jì shēng	mistletoe	Loranthi seu Visci Ramus	12 g.

In cases of prolonged uterine bleeding accompanied by blood stasis, with lower abdominal distention and pain, the prescription is modified to rectify qi, quicken the blood and relieve bleeding.
Add:

jīng jiè tàn	schizonepeta (charred)	Schizonepetae Herba et Flos Carbonisatae	9 g.
yì mǔ cǎo	leonurus	Leonuri Herba	12 g.
mù xiāng	saussurea [root]	Saussureae (seu Vladimirae) Radix	9 g.

ACUPUNCTURE AND MOXIBUSTION

Main points: Needle with supplementation; add moxibustion.

CV-04	*guān yuán*
BL-20	*pí shū*
ST-36	*zú sān lǐ*
SP-06	*sān yīn jiāo*
GV-20	*bǎi huì*

Auxiliary points:

For loose stools, add:

ST-25	*tiān shū*

2. KIDNEY YANG VACUITY

Clinical Manifestations: Uterine bleeding with thin light-colored discharge that is accompanied by physical cold, dull complexion, cold extremities, weak aching lower back and legs, frequent urination, lower abdominal cold and pain.

Tongue: Pale with white coating.

Pulse: Deep, thready.

Treatment Method: Warm and supplement kidney yang, relieve bleeding.

PRESCRIPTION

Right-Restoring [Kidney Yang] Pill *yòu guī wán*

shú dì huáng	cooked rehmannia [root]	Rehmanniae Radix Conquita	24 g.
shān yào	dioscorea [root]	Dioscoreae Rhizoma	12 g.
shān zhū yú	cornus [fruit]	Corni Fructus	9 g.
gǒu qǐ zǐ	lycium [berry]	Lycii Fructus	12 g.
lù jiǎo jiāo	deerhorn glue (dissolved and stirred in)	Cervi Gelatinum Cornu	12 g.
tù sī zǐ	cuscuta [seed]	Cuscutae Semen	12 g.
dù zhòng	eucommia [bark]	Eucommiae Cortex	12 g.
dāng guī	tangkuei	Angelicae Sinensis Radix	9 g.
ròu guì	cinnamon [bark] (abbreviated decoction)	Cinnamomi Cortex	6 g.
zhì fù zǐ	aconite [accessory tuber] (processed) (extended decoction)	Aconiti Tuber Laterale Praeparatum	6 g.

MODIFICATIONS

In cases of uterine bleeding, the prescription is often modified to supplement qi, secure the kidney and secure the blood.

Delete:

ròu guì	cinnamon [bark]	Cinnamomi Cortex
dāng guī	tangkuei	Angelicae Sinensis Radix

Add:

huáng qí	astragalus [root]	Astragali (seu Hedysari) Radix	12 g.
fù pén zǐ	rubus [berry]	Rubi Fructus	9 g.
chì shí zhī	halloysite (wrapped)	Halloysitum Rubrum	12 g.

In cases of young patients with kidney qi vacuity, the prescription is modified to reinforce kidney supplementation and qi boosting. Add:

xiān máo	curculigo [root]	Curculiginis Rhizoma	9 g.
yín yáng huò	epimedium	Epimedii Herba	9 g.
zǐ hé chē	placenta (powdered and capsulized)	Hominis Placenta	3 g.

In cases of vacuity of spleen and kidney yang with symptoms of loss of appetite, loose stools and edema, the prescription is modified to supplement the spleen and warm the middle burner. Add:

fú líng	poria	Poria	12 g.
shā rén	amomum [fruit] (abbreviated decoction)	Amomi Semen seu Fructus	3 g.
gān jiāng	dried ginger [root]	Zingiberis Rhizoma Exsiccatum	6 g.

In cases caused by coagulation of cold with blood stasis, there will be symptoms of vaginal discharge with a large volume of blackish-red blood containing clots and severe lower abdominal pain. The prescription is modified to warm the channels, invigorate the blood and relieve bleeding. Add:

rǔ xiāng	frankincense	Olibanum	6 g.
mò yào	myrrh	Myrrha	6 g.
wǔ líng zhī	flying squirrel droppings (wrapped)	Trogopteri seu Pteromydis Excrementum	6 g.

ACUPUNCTURE AND MOXIBUSTION

Main points: Needle with supplementation; add moxibustion.

CV-04	*guān yuán*
BL-23	*shèn shū*
CV-06	*qì hǎi*
SP-06	*sān yīn jiāo*
GV-04	*mìng mén*

Auxiliary points:

For vacuity of spleen yang, add:

ST-36	*zú sān lǐ*

For weak aching lower back and legs, add:

M-BW-24	*yāo yǎn*	(Lumbar Eye)

3. KIDNEY YIN VACUITY

Clinical Manifestations: Uterine bleeding with a relatively thick bright red discharge, accompanied by dizziness, vertigo, tinnitus, weak aching lower back and knees, tidal fever, night sweating, dry throat, irritability, insomnia and dark scanty urine.

Tongue: Red with little coating.

Pulse: Rapid, thready, forceless.

Treatment Method: Nourish and supplement kidney yin, relieve bleeding.

PRESCRIPTION

Left-Restoring [Kidney Yin] Pill *zuǒ guī wán*

shú dì huáng	cooked rehmannia [root]	Rehmanniae Radix Conquita	24 g.
shān yào	dioscorea [root]	Dioscoreae Rhizoma	12 g.
shān zhū yú	cornus [fruit]	Corni Fructus	12 g.
gǒu qǐ zǐ	lycium [berry]	Lycii Fructus	12 g.
chuān niú xī	cyathula [root]	Cyathulae Radix	9 g.
tù sī zǐ	cuscuta [seed]	Cuscutae Semen	12 g.
lù jiǎo jiāo	deerhorn glue (dissolved and stirred in)	Cervi Gelatinum Cornu	12 g.
guī bǎn jiāo	tortoise plastron glue (dissolved and stirred in)	Testudinis Plastrum Gelatinum	12 g.

MODIFICATIONS

In cases of uterine bleeding, the prescription is modified to nourish the liver and kidney. Delete:

niú xī	achyranthes [root]	Achyranthis Bidentatae Radix

Add:

nǚ zhēn zǐ	ligustrum [fruit]	Ligustri Fructus	12 g.
hàn lián cǎo	eclipta	Ecliptae Herba	12 g.

In cases of vacuity of liver yin and ascendant hyperactivity of liver yang, with symptoms of dizziness and vertigo, the prescription is modified to nourish yin and subdue yang. Add:

xià kū cǎo	prunella [spike]	Prunellae Spica	9 g.
mǔ lì	oyster shell (extended decoction)	Ostreae Concha	30 g.

In cases of vacuity of heart yin with symptoms of insomnia, the prescription is modified to nourish the heart and quiet the spirit. Add:

wǔ wèi zǐ	schisandra [berry]	Schisandrae Fructus	6 g.
yè jiāo téng	flowery knotweed [stem]	Polygoni Multiflori Caulis	30 g.

In cases of yin vacuity with signs of vacuity fire, the prescription is changed to nourish yin, clear heat and relieve bleeding. Use:

Yin-Safeguarding Brew *bǎo yīn jiān*

shēng dì huáng	rehmannia [root] dried/fresh	Rehmanniae Radix Exsiccata seu Recens	12 g.
shú dì huáng	cooked rehmannia [root]	Rehmanniae Radix Conquita	12 g.
huáng qín	scutellaria [root]	Scutellariae Radix	9 g.
huáng bǎi	phellodendron [bark]	Phellodendri Cortex	9 g.
bái sháo yào	white peony [root]	Paeoniae Radix Alba	12 g.
shān yào	dioscorea [root]	Dioscoreae Rhizoma	12 g.
xù duàn	dipsacus [root]	Dipsaci Radix	9 g.
gān cǎo	licorice [root]	Glycyrrhizae Radix	6 g.

plus:

běi shā shēn	glehnia [root]	Glehniae Radix	9 g.
mài mén dōng	ophiopogon [tuber]	Ophiopogonis Tuber	9 g.
wǔ wèi zǐ	schisandra [berry]	Schisandrae Fructus	6 g.
ē jiāo	ass hide glue (dissolved and stirred in)	Asini Corii Gelatinum	9 g.

In cases of vacuity of both kidney yin and kidney yang, prescriptions included in sections on "Kidney Yang Vacuity" and "Kidney Yin Vacuity" may be combined, with appropriate additions and deletions to suit the individual case.

ACUPUNCTURE AND MOXIBUSTION

Main points: Needle with supplementation.

CV-04	*guān yuán*
BL-23	*shèn shū*
SP-06	*sān yīn jiāo*
KI-03	*tài xī*
KI-08	*jiāo xìn*

Auxiliary points:

For night sweating, add:

HT-06	*yīn xī*

For insomnia, add:

HT-07	*shén mén*

4. Blood Heat

Clinical Manifestations: Uterine bleeding with thick concentrated deep-red discharge, accompanied by flushed complexion, irritability, dry mouth, thirst, dark-urine and, in some cases, hard dry stools.

Tongue: Red with yellow coating.

Pulse: Rapid.

Treatment Method: Clear heat, cool the blood, relieve bleeding.

PRESCRIPTION
Heat-Clearing Channel-Securing Decoction *qīng rè gù jīng tāng*

huáng qín	scutellaria [root]	Scutellariae Radix	9 g.
shān zhī tàn	gardenia [fruit] (charred)	Gardeniae Fructus Carbonisata	9 g.
shēng dì huáng	rehmannia [root] dried/fresh	Rehmanniae Radix Exsiccata seu Recens	12 g.
dì gǔ pí	lycium [root bark]	Lycii Radicis Cortex	12 g.
dì yú	sanguisorba [root]	Sanguisorbae Radix	9 g.
ē jiāo	ass hide glue (dissolved and stirred in)	Asini Corii Gelatinum	9 g.
ǒu jié	lotus [root node]	Nelumbinis Rhizomatis Nodus	9 g.
guī bǎn	tortoise plastron (extended decoction)	Testudinis Plastrum	15 g.
gān cǎo	licorice [root]	Glycyrrhizae Radix	6 g.
mǔ lì	oyster [shell] (extended decoction)	Ostreae Concha	15 g.
zōng lǘ tàn	trachycarpus [stipule fiber] (charred)	Trachycarpi Stipulae Fibra Carbonisata	9 g.

MODIFICATIONS

In cases with distention and pain of the chest, costal and internal lower abdominal regions, irritability and rapid wiry pulse, the prescription is modified to clear the liver and drain heat. Add:

chái hú	bupleurum [root]	Bupleuri Radix	6 g.
xià kū cǎo	prunella [spike]	Prunellae Spica	12 g.

In cases where the discharged blood is dark red and accompanied by foul-smelling leukorrhea, slimy yellow tongue coating and soft rapid pulse, the prescription is modified to clear heat and dispel dampness. Add:

huáng bǎi	phellodendron [bark]	Phellodendri Cortex	9 g.
cán shā	silkworm droppings	Bombycis Excrementum	9 g.

In cases accompanied by tiredness and disinclination to speak, the prescription is modified to supplement and boost qi and yin. Add:

běi shā shēn	glehnia [root]	Glehniae Radix	12 g.
dǎng shēn	codonopsis [root]	Codonopsitis Radix	9 g.

ACUPUNCTURE AND MOXIBUSTION

Main points: Needle with draining.

CV-03	*zhōng jí*
SP-06	*sān yīn jiāo*
SP-10	*xuè hǎi*
SP-01	*yǐn bái*
KI-05	*shuǐ quán*

Auxiliary points:

For severe heat, add:

GV-14	*dà zhuī*
LI-11	*qū chí*

For irritability add:

PC-05	*jiān shǐ*

For distention and pain of the chest and costal regions, add:

LR-03	*tài chōng*
GB-34	*yáng líng quán*

For leukorrhea, add:

BL-32	*cì liáo*
SP-09	*yīn líng quán*

5. BLOOD STASIS

Clinical Manifestations: Uterine bleeding with blackish-purple discharge containing blood clots, accompanied by lower abdominal pain that is aggravated by pressure; decrease in pain after expulsion of the clots.

Tongue: Dark purplish, sometimes with stasis macules on the tongue.

Pulse: Deep, rough.

Treatment Method: Quicken the blood, dispel stasis, relieve bleeding.

PRESCRIPTION

Combine Four Agents Decoction *(sì wù tāng)* with Sudden Smile Powder *(shī xiào sǎn)*.

Four Agents Decoction *sì wù tāng*

shú dì huáng	cooked rehmannia [root]	Rehmanniae Radix Conquita	9 g.
dāng guī	tangkuei	Angelicae Sinensis Radix	9 g.
bái sháo yào	white peony [root]	Paeoniae Radix Alba	9 g.
chuān xiōng	ligusticum [root]	Ligustici Rhizoma	9 g.

with:

Sudden Smile Powder *shī xiào sǎn*

wǔ líng zhī	flying squirrel droppings (wrapped)	Trogopteri seu Pteromydis Excrementum	9 g.
pú huáng	typha pollen (wrapped)	Typhae Pollen	9 g.

MODIFICATIONS

In the treatment of uterine bleeding from blood stasis, the prescription is modified to dispel stasis and relieve bleeding. Add:

sān qī	notoginseng [root] (or, powdered and administered separately, 1.5 g. each time)	Notoginseng Radix	9 g.
qiàn cǎo gēn	madder [root] (charred)	Rubiae Radix Carbonisata	9 g.
hǎi piāo xiāo	cuttlefish [bone]	Sepiae seu Sepiellae Os	9 g.

In cases with symptoms of qi stagnation, including severe distention of the hypochondrium and abdomen, the prescription is modified to rectify qi and relieve pain. Add:

chuān liàn zǐ	toosendan [fruit]	Toosendan Fructus	9 g.
xiāng fù zǐ	cyperus [root]	Cyperi Rhizoma	9 g.

In prolonged cases of gradual onset of light uterine bleeding, accompanied by blood stasis, the prescription is modified to quicken the blood and dispel stasis. Add:

táo rén	peach [kernel]	Persicae Semen	6 g.
hóng huā	carthamus [flower]	Carthami Flosa	6 g.
yì mǔ cǎo	leonurus	Leonuri Herba	12 g.

In cases presenting symptoms of transformation of stasis to fire such as dry bitter taste in mouth and heavy discharge of bright red blood, the prescription is modified to clear heat, cool the blood and relieve bleeding. Add:

xiān hè cǎo	agrimony	Agrimoniae Herba	12 g.
dì yú	sanguisorba [root]	Sanguisorbae Radix	9 g.
xià kū cǎo	prunella [spike]	Prunellae Spica	9 g.
qiàn cǎo gēn	madder [root]	Rubiae Radix	9 g.

ACUPUNCTURE AND MOXIBUSTION

Main points: Needle with draining.

CV-03	zhōng jí
SP-06	sān yīn jiāo
SP-10	xuè hǎi
SP-01	yǐn bái
ST-30	qì chōng

Auxiliary points:

For severe lower abdominal pain aggravated by external pressure, add:

| KI-14 | sì mǎn |
| SP-08 | dì jī |

ALTERNATE THERAPEUTIC METHODS

1. Ear Acupuncture

Main points: Uterus, Ovary, Endocrine, Liver, Kidney, *Shén Mén.*

Method: Select three to four points each session, needle to elicit a moderate sensation and retain the needles for thirty to sixty minutes. Treat once daily or once every two days. Auricular needle embedding therapy may also be employed.

2. Plum-Blossom Needle Therapy

Main points:

BL-17	gé shū
BL-18	gān shū
BL-20	pí shū
BL-21	wèi shū
BL-31	shàng liáo
BL-32	cì liáo
BL-33	zhōng liáo
BL-34	xià liáo
BL-43 (38)	gāo huāng shū
GV-20	bǎi huì
ST-36	zú sān lǐ
CV-04	guān yuán
SP-10	xuè hǎi
SP-06	sān yīn jiāo
M-BW-35	huá tuó jiā jí (Hua Tuo's Paravertebrals)

Method: Use a plum-blossom needle to tap over the above acupoints to elicit a moderate sensation. Treat once daily or once every two days.

REMARKS

Among gynecological disorders, patterns of uterine bleeding are considered both serious and difficult to treat. During clinical diagnosis a clear distinction must be made between uterine bleeding and other disorders including threatened miscarriage, ectopic pregnancy, postpartum disorders, pinkish leukorrhea, abdominal masses *(zhēng jiǎ)*, and vaginal bleeding from external injury.

Generally speaking, in the differential diagnosis and treatment of uterine bleeding, patterns are more often a result of vacuity than of repletion, and more often caused by heat than by cold. Cases of prolonged abrupt onset of heavy uterine bleeding *(bēng)* generally manifest as vacuity, while those of prolonged gradual onset of light uterine bleeding *(lòu)* manifest as blood stasis.

The patient's age is an important factor during differential diagnosis as well as during treatment. Uterine bleeding in teenage patients is most often caused by a congenital vacuity of kidney qi. With these cases treatment should emphasize supplementation of kidney qi and strengthening of the *chōng* and *rèn* vessels. During the reproductive years, uterine bleeding is usually from stagnation of liver qi and blood heat, calling for treatment that soothes the liver and clears heat. Uterine bleeding in menopausal patients is most frequently caused by insufficiency of the liver and kidney, or spleen qi vacuity. Here, treatment is directed at nourishing the liver and kidney and supplementing spleen qi.

The severity of bleeding must be considered in every case. Treatment is best undertaken according to the following principle: "In emergency cases, treat acute symptoms; in chronic cases, treat the root of illness."

In cases of abrupt onset of heavy uterine bleeding *(bēng)*, immediate measures should be taken to relieve bleeding and prevent prostration or collapse. The prescription is oriented to secure qi and contain the blood.

Use:

Pulse-Engendering Beverage *shēng mài yǐn*

rén shēn	ginseng	Ginseng Radix	9 g.
mài mén dōng	ophiopogon [tuber]	Ophiopogonis Tuber	15 g.
wǔ wèi zǐ	schisandra [berry]	Schisandrae Fructus	6 g.

MODIFICATIONS

In cases presenting cold extremities and a faint barely perceptible pulse, the prescription is modified to warm yang.

Delete:

| *mài mén dōng* | ophiopogon [tuber] | Ophiopogonis Tuber |

Add:

| *zhì fù zǐ* | aconite [accessory tuber] (processed) (extended decoction) | Aconiti Tuber Laterale Praeparatum | 9 g. |

In more severe cases, use:

Ginseng and Aconite Decoction *shēn fù tāng*

rén shēn	ginseng	Ginseng Radix	30 g.
zhì fù zǐ	aconite [accessory tuber] (processed)	Aconiti Tuber Laterale Praeparatum	15 g.

Plus:

pào jiāng	blast-fried ginger [root]	Zingiberis Rhizoma Tostum	9 g.

ACUPUNCTURE AND MOXIBUSTION

Main points: Needle with supplementation.

GV-26	*shuǐ gōu*
LI-04	*hé gǔ*
GV-20	*bǎi huì* (apply moxibustion)

In cases where no decrease in bleeding is observed after the above treatments, blood transfusion should be initiated.

Once the severity of the bleeding has lessened and the uterine bleeding has been brought under control, treatment should be undertaken according to a differential diagnosis of the root cause. The overall therapeutic effect can be reinforced through supplementation of the kidney, regulation of the liver, strengthening the spleen and securing the *chōng* and *rèn* vessels. In addition, patients should pay attention to diet, abstaining from cold or raw food, and avoid stress and strain.

For post-menopausal patients with repeated uterine bleeding, gynecological examinations should be performed to eliminate the possibility of a malignant uterine tumor.

Further discussion and special considerations can be found in opening and closing remarks for the chapter on Menstrual Irregularity.

Morbid Vaginal Discharge

Dài Xià

1. Spleen Qi Vacuity - 2. Kidney Yang Vacuity - 3. Kidney Yin Vacuity - 4. Downpour of Damp-Heat

Vaginal discharge, in Chinese *dài xià,* refers to gynecological disorders involving increased volume of vaginal discharge, with changes in color, texture and odor. These symptoms may be accompanied by other local or general symptoms. A slight increase in vaginal discharge prior to and during menstruation or during pregnancy is considered normal and requires no treatment.

The vaginitis, cervicitis and pelvic inflammation conditions described by Western medicine each give rise to vaginal discharge. Differential diagnosis and treatment of these conditions is covered in this chapter.

ETIOLOGY AND PATHOGENESIS

The development of vaginal discharge is often because of spleen qi vacuity with liver depression, descent of damp-heat to the lower burner or kidney vacuity. All these conditions can lead to dysfunction of the *rèn* and *dài,* allowing the development of vaginal discharge. Common etiological factors include internal disruption by the seven affects, improper diet and eating habits, stress and invasion by external dampness.

1. SPLEEN QI VACUITY

Clinical Manifestations: Heavy vaginal discharge that is white in color, thin in texture, with no foul odor; sallow complexion, loss of appetite, loose stools, tiredness, fatigue, edema of the upper surfaces of the feet.

Tongue: Pale with white sometimes slimy coating.

Pulse: Weak, tardy.

Treatment Method: Strengthen the spleen, boost qi, disinhibit dampness, relieve vaginal discharge.

PRESCRIPTION

Discharge-Ceasing Decoction *wán dài tāng*

bái zhú	ovate atractylodes [root]	Atractylodis Ovatae Rhizoma	30 g.
shān yào	dioscorea [root]	Dioscoreae Rhizoma	30 g.
rén shēn	ginseng	Ginseng Radix	9 g.
bái sháo yào	white peony [root]	Paeoniae Radix Alba	12 g.

cāng zhú	atractylodes [root]	Atractylodis Rhizoma	9 g.
chén pí	tangerine [peel]	Citri Exocarpium	6 g.
chē qián zǐ	plantago [seed] (wrapped)	Plantaginis Semen	12 g.
chái hú	bupleurum [root]	Bupleuri Radix	3 g.
jīng jiè suì tàn	schizonepeta [spike] (charred)	Schizonepetae Herba et Flos Carbonisata	3 g.
gān cǎo	licorice [root]	Glycyrrhizae Radix	3 g.

MODIFICATIONS

In cases accompanied by kidney vacuity with lower back pain, the prescription is modified to supplement the kidney and strengthen the lower back. Add:

| dù zhòng | eucommia [bark] | Eucommiae Cortex | 12 g. |
| tù sī zǐ | cuscuta [seed] | Cuscutae Semen | 12 g. |

In cases of congealed cold marked by abdominal pain, the prescription is modified to warm the channels, rectify qi and relieve pain. Add:

| xiāng fù zǐ | cyperus [root] | Cyperi Rhizoma | 9 g. |
| ài yè | mugwort [leaf] | Artemisiae Argyi Folium | 9 g. |

In cases of prolonged incontinent vaginal discharge, the prescription is modified to strengthen retention and relieve vaginal discharge. Add:

jīn yīng zǐ	Cherokee rose [fruit]	Rosae Laevigatae Fructus	12 g.
duàn lóng gǔ	dragon bone (calcined)	Mastodi Ossis Fossilia Calcinatum	15 g.
qiàn shí	euryale [seed]	Euryales Semen	12 g.
hǎi piāo xiāo	cuttlefish [bone]	Sepiae seu Sepiellae Os	9 g.

In cases where dampness has given rise to heat with symptoms of thick sticky yellow vaginal discharge, the prescription is changed to clear heat, disinhibit dampness and relieve vaginal discharge. Use:

Transforming Yellow Decoction *yì huáng tāng*

bái sháo yào	white peony [root]	Paeoniae Radix Alba	30 g.
qiàn shí	euryale [seed]	Euryales Semen	12 g.
chē qián zǐ	plantago [seed] (wrapped)	Plantaginis Semen	12 g.
huáng bǎi	phellodendron [bark]	Phellodendri Cortex	9 g.
bái guǒ	ginkgo [nut]	Ginkgo Semen	9 g.

ACUPUNCTURE AND MOXIBUSTION

Main points: Needle with supplementation; add moxibustion.

CV-06	*qì hǎi*
GB-26	*dài mài*
BL-30	*bái huán shū*
SP-06	*sān yīn jiāo*
ST-36	*zú sān lǐ*

Auxiliary points:

For continuous vaginal discharge, add:

SP-12	*chōng mén*
ST-30	*qì chōng*
CV-03	*zhōng jí*

For loss of appetite and loose stools, add:

| CV-12 | *zhōng wǎn* |
| ST-25 | *tiān shū* |

2. KIDNEY YANG VACUITY

Clinical Manifestations: Continuous dribbling of a large volume of thin white vaginal mucus, severe lower back pain, cold sensation in the lower abdomen, frequent urination especially during the night, copious clear urine, and, in some cases, loose stools.

Tongue: Pale with thin white coating.

Pulse: Slow, deep.

Treatment Method: Warm and supplement kidney yang, strengthen functions of retention, relieve vaginal discharge.

PRESCRIPTION

Internal Supplementation Pill *nèi bŭ wán*

lù róng	velvet deerhorn (powdered and stirred in)	Cervi Cornu Parvum	1.5 g.
huáng qí	astragalus [root]	Astragali (seu Hedysari) Radix	12 g.
tù sī zĭ	cuscuta [seed]	Cuscutae Semen	12 g.
shā yuàn zĭ	complanate astragalus [seed]	Astragali Complanati Semen	12 g.
zĭ wăn	aster [root]	Asteris Radix et Rhizoma	9 g.
ròu guì	cinnamon [bark] (abbreviated decoction)	Cinnamomi Cortex	6 g.
sāng piāo xiāo	mantis [egg-case]	Mantidis Oötheca	9 g.
cì jí lí	tribulus [fruit]	Tribuli Fructus	9 g.
ròu cōng róng	cistanche [stem]	Cistanches Caulis	12 g.
zhì fù zĭ	aconite [accessory tuber] (processed) (extended decoction)	Processed Aconiti Tuber Laterale	6 g.

MODIFICATIONS

In cases of loose stools, the prescription is adjusted to warm the spleen and normalize stools.

Delete:

ròu cōng róng	cistanche [stem]	Cistanches Caulis

Add:

bŭ gŭ zhī	psoralea [seed]	Psoraleae Semen	9 g.
ròu dòu kòu	nutmeg (roasted)	Myristicae Semen	9 g.

ACUPUNCTURE AND MOXIBUSTION

Main points: Needle with supplementation; add moxibustion.

CV-04	*guān yuán*
GB-26	*dài mài*
BL-23	*shèn shū*
BL-32	*cì liáo*
KI-06	*zhào hăi*

Auxiliary points:

For heavy vaginal discharge, add:

KI-12	*dà hè*
KI-13	*qì xué*

For loose stools, add:

ST-36	*zú sān lĭ*

3. KIDNEY YIN VACUITY

Clinical Manifestations: Reddish white vaginal discharge that is slightly sticky and without odor; burning sensation in the vagina, dizzy spells, malar flush, vexing heat in the five hearts, insomnia, frequent dreaming, difficult bowel movements, yellow or dark urine.

Tongue: Red with little coating.

Pulse: Thready, rapid.

Treatment Method: Supplement and boost kidney yin, clear vacuity heat, relieve vaginal discharge.

PRESCRIPTION

Anemarrhena, Phellodendron and Rehmannia Pill *zhī bǎi dì huáng wán*

shú dì huáng	cooked rehmannia [root]	Rehmanniae Radix Conquita	24 g.
shān zhū yú	cornus [fruit]	Corni Fructus	12 g.
shān yào	dioscorea [root]	Dioscoreae Rhizoma	12 g.
zé xiè	alisma [tuber]	Alismatis Rhizoma	9 g.
fú líng	poria	Poria	9 g.
mǔ dān pí	moutan [root bark]	Moutan Radicis Cortex	9 g.
zhī mǔ	anemarrhena [root]	Anemarrhenae Rhizoma	9 g.
huáng bǎi	phellodendron [bark]	Phellodendri Cortex	9 g.

MODIFICATIONS

To enhance kidney supplementation, strengthen retention and relieve vaginal discharge, add:

qiàn shí	euryale [seed]	Euryales Semen	12 g.
jīn yīng zǐ	Cherokee rose [fruit]	Rosae Laevigatae Fructus	12 g.

ACUPUNCTURE AND MOXIBUSTION

Main points: Needle with even supplementation, even draining.

GB-26	*dài mài*
BL-23	*shèn shū*
SP-06	*sān yīn jiāo*
KI-06	*zhào hǎi*
BL-32	*cì liáo*

Auxiliary points:

For irritability, add:

PC-05	*jiān shǐ*

For insomnia, add:

HT-07	*shén mén*

4. DOWNPOUR OF DAMP-HEAT

Clinical Manifestations: Heavy vaginal discharge that is yellow, yellowish-white or yellow tinged with red in color, thick and sticky in texture and foul smelling; vaginal itching, dark scanty urine, oppression in the chest, slimy sensation in the mouth and loss of appetite.

Tongue: Slimy yellow coating.

Pulse: Soft, rapid.

Treatment Method: Clear heat, disinhibit dampness, relieve vaginal discharge.

PRESCRIPTION

Discharge-Checking Formula *zhǐ dài fāng*

zhū líng	polyporus	Polyporus	9 g.
fú líng	poria	Poria	9 g.
zé xiè	alisma [tuber]	Alismatis Rhizoma	9 g.
chē qián zǐ	plantago [seed] (wrapped)	Plantaginis Semen	12 g.
yīn chén hāo	capillaris	Artemisiae Capillaris Herba	15 g.
chì sháo yào	red peony [root]	Paeoniae Radix Rubra	9 g.
mǔ dān pí	moutan [root bark]	Moutan Radicis Cortex	9 g.
huáng bǎi	phellodendron [bark]	Phellodendri Cortex	9 g.
shān zhī zǐ	gardenia [fruit]	Gardeniae Fructus	9 g.
niú xī	achyranthes [root]	Achyranthis Bidentatae Radix	6 g.

MODIFICATIONS

In cases of damp-heat of the liver channel descending to the lower burner, there will be symptoms of vaginal discharge that is heavy, yellow or yellowish-green, sticky, sometimes foamy and foul-smelling; pain and itching of the vagina, irritability, yellow coating on the tongue and a wiry pulse. The prescription is changed to clear the liver, disinhibit dampness and relieve vaginal discharge. Use:

Gentian Liver-Draining Decoction *lóng dǎn xiè gān tāng*

lóng dǎn cǎo	gentian [root]	Gentianae Radix	6 g.
huáng qín	scutellaria [root]	Scutellariae Radix	9 g.
shān zhī zǐ	gardenia [fruit]	Gardeniae Fructus	9 g.
zé xiè	alisma [tuber]	Alismatis Rhizoma	12 g.
mù tōng	mutong [stem]	Mutong Caulis	9 g.
dāng guī	tangkuei [root]	Angelicae Sinensis Radix	3 g.
chē qián zǐ	plantago [seed] (wrapped)	Plantaginis Semen	9 g.
shēng dì huáng	rehmannia [root] dried/fresh	Rehmanniae Radix Exsiccata seu Recens	9 g.
chái hú	bupleurum [root]	Bupleuri Radix	6 g.
gān cǎo	licorice [root]	Glycyrrhizae Radix	6 g.

ACUPUNCTURE AND MOXIBUSTION

Main points: Needle with draining.

GB-26	*dài mài*
CV-03	*zhōng jí*
BL-32	*cì liáo*
SP-09	*yīn líng quán*
SP-06	*sān yīn jiāo*

Auxiliary points:

For severe heat, add:

LI-11	*qū chí*

For vaginal itching, add:

LR-05	*lǐ gōu*
LR-02	*xíng jiān*

For reddish vaginal discharge, add:

SP-10	*xuè hǎi*

ALTERNATE THERAPEUTIC METHODS

1. Ear Acupuncture

Main points: Uterus, Urinary Bladder, Liver, Spleen, Kidney, Endocrine, *Shén Mén, Sān Jiāo*.

Method: Select three to five points each session, needle to elicit a moderate sensation and retain needles for fifteen to twenty minutes. Treat once daily, or once every two days.

REMARKS

Patients suffering from vaginal discharge should be advised to limit sexual intercourse and to pay close attention to the cleanliness of the vaginal area, especially during menstruation. In women over forty years of age presenting with a heavy vaginal discharge that is pinkish-yellow in color with a foul smell, the possibility of uterine or ovarian cancer should be evaluated.

GENITAL PROLAPSE

Yīn Tǐng

1. Spleen Qi Vacuity - 2. Kidney Vacuity

Genital prolapse is characterized by protrusion of a light red mass from or into the vagina. The mass resembles a goose egg in size and shape. If left untreated, friction, injury or infection may lead to ulceration. Patterns of uterine prolapse include prolapse of the uterus and coleoptosis (prolapse of the vaginal wall) as diagnosed by Western medicine.

ETIOLOGY AND PATHOGENESIS

The major etiological factors causing genital prolapse are spleen qi vacuity or kidney vacuity with loss of retention. Possible causes include weak physical constitution with vacuity of spleen qi, bearing down too early during labor, participating in heavy physical work too soon after childbirth, prolonged constipation and prolonged coughing. Any of these can lead to spleen qi vacuity and prolapse by causing the uterine network vessels to slacken and lose their ability to hold the uterus or vagina in place.

In addition, bearing a large number of children or overindulgent sexual activity with injury to the kidney, may result in weakening of the *chōng* and *rěn* and dysfunction of the *dài mài,* which in turn leads to an inability to restrain the uterus and vagina, resulting in prolapse.

1. SPLEEN QI VACUITY

Clinical Manifestations: Protrusion of a fleshy mass into the vagina, or, in severe cases, protrusion of a hanging fleshy mass outside the vagina; increase in severity of symptoms with overwork, bearing down sensation in the lower abdomen, loss of strength in the limbs, shallow respiration, disinclination to speak, lusterless complexion, frequent urination, large volume of thin white vaginal discharge.

Tongue: Pale with thin coating.

Pulse: Weak, thready.

Treatment Method: Supplement spleen qi, raise the fallen.

PRESCRIPTION

Center-Supplementing Qi-Boosting Decoction *bǔ zhōng yì qì tāng*

huáng qí	astragalus [root]	Astragali (seu Hedysari) Radix	15 g.
rén shēn	ginseng	Ginseng Radix	9 g.
bái zhú	ovate atractylodes [root]	Atractylodis Ovatae Rhizoma	9 g.
dāng guī	tangkuei	Angelicae Sinensis Radix	9 g.
chén pí	tangerine [peel]	Citri Exocarpium	6 g.
shēng mā	cimicifuga [root]	Cimicifugae Rhizoma	3 g.
chái hú	bupleurum [root]	Bupleuri Radix	3 g.
zhì gān cǎo	licorice [root] (honey-fried)	Glycyrrhizae Radix	6 g.

MODIFICATIONS

To enhance supplementation of the kidney and strengthen retention, the prescription is modified in all cases. Add:

xù duàn	dipsacus [root]	Dipsaci Radix	12 g.
jīn yīng zǐ	Cherokee rose [fruit]	Rosae Laevigatae Fructus	12 g.

In cases showing infection with a large volume of yellow sticky foul-smelling vaginal discharge, the prescription is modified to clear heat and disinhibit dampness.

Delete:

dǎng shēn	codonopsis [root]	Codonopsitis Radix
jīn yīng zǐ	Cherokee rose [fruit]	Rosae Laevigatae Fructus

Add:

huáng bǎi	phellodendron [bark]	Phellodendri Cortex	9 g.
bài jiàng cǎo	baijiang	Baijiang Herba cum Radice	12 g.
yì yǐ rén	coix [seed]	Coicis Semen	30 g.

ACUPUNCTURE AND MOXIBUSTION

Main points: Needle with supplementation; add moxibustion.

GV-20	*bǎi huì*
CV-06	*qì hǎi*
GB-28	*wéi dào*
ST-36	*zú sān lǐ*
SP-06	*sān yīn jiāo*

Auxiliary points:

For bearing down sensation in the lower abdomen, add:

CV-12	*zhōng wǎn*
BL-20	*pí shū*

2. KIDNEY VACUITY

Clinical Manifestations: Protrusion of a fleshy mass into the vagina or protrusion of a hanging fleshy mass from the vagina, lower backache, weakness of the knees, bearing down sensation in the lower abdomen, lack of vaginal secretion, frequent urination especially during the night, dizziness, vertigo, tinnitus.

Tongue: Pale red.

Pulse: Deep, weak.

Treatment Method: Supplement the kidney, strengthen retention.

PRESCRIPTION

Major Origin-Supplementing Brew *dà bǔ yuán jiān*

shú dì huáng	cooked rehmannia [root]	Rehmanniae Radix Conquita	24 g.
shān zhū yú	cornus [fruit]	Corni Fructus	12 g.
shān yào	dioscorea [root]	Dioscoreae Rhizoma	12 g.
gǒu qǐ zǐ	lycium [berry]	Lycii Fructus	12 g.
rén shēn	ginseng	Ginseng Radix	9 g.
dāng guī	tangkuei	Angelicae Sinensis Radix	9 g.
zhì gān cǎo	licorice [root] (honey-fried)	Glycyrrhizae Radix	6 g.

MODIFICATIONS

To reinforce the supplementing and consolidating effects, add:

jīn yīng zǐ	Cherokee rose [fruit]	Rosae Laevigatae Fructus	12 g.
qiàn shí	euryale [seed]	Euryales Semen	12 g.
lù jiǎo jiāo	deerhorn glue (dissolved and stirred in)	Cervi Gelatinum Cornu	9 g.
zǐ hé chē	placenta (powdered and capsulized)	Hominis Placenta	3 g.

Where infection develops with descent of damp-heat, symptoms include redness, swelling and ulceration of the vaginal protrusion; large volume of yellow pus-like foul-smelling vaginal discharge; anal swelling and pain; fever, thirst, concentrated urine and painful burning urination. The prescription is modified to clear heat and disinhibit dampness, followed by supplementation of the kidney.

In mild cases, add:

huáng bǎi	phellodendron [bark]	Phellodendri Cortex	9 g.
cāng zhú	atractylodes [root]	Atractylodis Rhizoma	9 g.
tǔ fú líng	smooth greenbrier [root]	Smilacis Glabrae Rhizoma	30 g.
chē qián cǎo	plantago	Plantaginis Herba	12 g.

In severe cases, add:

Gentian Liver-Draining Decoction *lóng dǎn xiè gān tāng*

lóng dǎn cǎo	gentian [root]	Gentianae Radix	6 g.
huáng qín	scutellaria [root]	Scutellariae Radix	9 g.
shān zhī zǐ	gardenia [fruit]	Gardeniae Fructus	9 g.
zé xiè	alisma [tuber]	Alismatis Rhizoma	12 g.
mù tōng	mutong [stem]	Mutong Caulis	9 g.
dāng guī	tangkuei	Angelicae Sinensis Radix	3 g.
chē qián zǐ	plantago [seed] (wrapped)	Plantaginis Semen	9 g.
shēng dì huáng	rehmannia [root] dried/fresh	Rehmanniae Radix Exsiccata seu Recens	9 g.
chái hú	bupleurum [root]	Bupleuri Radix	6 g.
gān cǎo	licorice [root]	Glycyrrhizae Radix	6 g.

ACUPUNCTURE AND MOXIBUSTION

Main points: Needle with supplementation; add moxibustion.

CV-04	*guān yuán*
M-CA-18	*zǐ gōng* (Infant's Palace)
KI-12	*dà hè*
KI-06	*zhào hǎi*

Auxiliary points:

For weak aching lower back and knees, add:

BL-23	*shèn shū*
LR-08	*qū quán*

For vertigo and tinnitus, add:

| GV-20 | *bǎi huì* |
| BL-23 | *shèn shū* |

For accompanying infection, add:

SP-09	*yīn líng quán*
CV-03	*zhōng jí*
BL-34	*xià liáo*

ALTERNATE THERAPEUTIC METHODS

1. Electro-Acupuncture

Main points: M-CA-18 (Infant's Palace, *zǐ gōng*), ST-36 (*zú sān lǐ*).

Method: Needle with supplementation at ST-36 *(zú sān lǐ)*. Using a 2 cun needle, puncture Infant's Palace (*zǐ gōng*) obliquely in the direction of the uterus. Insert to the point where patient reports a feeling of the uterus twitching upward as well as a sensation of aching and distention in the lower back and pubic region. Apply appropriate electric current for fifteen to twenty minutes.

2. Scalp Acupuncture

Location: Bilateral *Zū Yùn Gǎn Qū* (Pedal Motor-Sensory Zone), *Shēng Zhí Qū* (Reproduction Zone).

Method: Needle once daily, ten sessions per therapeutic course. Rest three to five days between courses.

3. EXTERNAL TREATMENT

Prepare as a steam bath:

dān shēn	salvia [root]	Salviae Miltiorrhizae Radix	15 g.
wǔ bèi zǐ	sumac gallnut	Rhois Galla	9 g.
kē zǐ	chebule [fruit]	Chebulae Fructus	9 g.

or:

| *shé chuáng zǐ* | cnidium [seed] | Cnidii Monnieri Fructus | 60 g. |
| *wū méi* | mume [fruit] | Mume Fructus | 60 g. |

Treat at frequent intervals.

In cases of uterine prolapse complicated with infection, prepare a steam and immersion bath where the infected area is first steamed over the herbal bath and then immersed in the herbal bath when it is cool enough to do so. Use:

jīn yín huā	lonicera [flower]	Lonicerae Flos	30 g.
zǐ huā dì dīng	Yedo violet	Violae Yedoensis Herba cum Radice	30 g.
pú gōng yīng	dandelion	Taraxaci Herba cum Radice	30 g.
huáng lián	coptis [root]	Coptidis Rhizoma	9 g.
kǔ shēn	flavescent sophora [root]	Sophorae Flavescentis Radix	15 g.
huáng bǎi	phellodendron [bark]	Phellodendri Cortex	9 g.
bái fán	alum	Alumen	9 g.

REMARKS

To consolidate therapeutic effects during treatment, patients must avoid carrying heavy loads, and practice anus-lifting exercises once daily for ten to fifteen minutes (contract, lift, relax, with repetition). In cases unresponsive to the above treatments, surgical treatment may be necessary and should be considered.

GENITAL ITCH

Yīn Yǎng

1. Downpour of Damp-Heat - 2. Liver and Kidney Yin Vacuity

Patterns of genital itching are characterized by intravaginal itching or itching of the vulva that may be painful or even unbearable in severe cases. Vaginal itching is often associated with vaginal discharge, and is frequently observed in cases diagnosed by Western medicine as trichomonas vaginitis, colpitis (vaginal inflammation), senile vaginitis, leukoplakia vulvae (thickening of vulva epithelium) and pruritis vulvae.

ETIOLOGY AND PATHOGENESIS

The development of genital itching is closely related to disturbances of the liver, kidney and spleen. Some vaginal itching is the result of stagnation of liver qi with transformation into heat and concurrent vacuity of the spleen. This condition allows the generation of dampness and the accumulation of damp-heat that flows downward into the lower burner. Another causative factor is poor hygiene of the genitalia, allowing the invasion of parasites, giving rise to vaginal itching. Other factors responsible for the development of vaginal itching include vacuity of liver and kidney yin, resulting in the transformation of wind and dryness.

1. DOWNPOUR OF DAMP-HEAT

Clinical Manifestations: Vaginal itching with constant agitation, accompanied by pain in severe cases; increased vaginal discharge, yellow in color, fishy-smelling and sometimes foamy; irritability, insomnia, slimy bitter taste in the mouth, thoracic congestion and discomfort and loss of appetite.

Tongue: Yellow slimy coating.

Pulse: Soft, rapid.

Treatment Method: Clear heat, disinhibit dampness, kill worms, relieve itching.

PRESCRIPTION

Fish Poison Yam Dampness-Percolating Decoction *bì xiè shèn shī tāng*

bì xiè	fish poison yam	Dioscoreae Hypoglaucae Rhizoma	9 g.
yì yǐ rén	coix [seed]	Coicis Semen	30 g.
huáng bǎi	phellodendron [bark]	Phellodendri Cortex	9 g.
fú líng	poria	Poria	12 g.
mǔ dān pí	moutan [root bark]	Moutan Radicis Cortex	9 g.
zé xiè	alisma [tuber]	Alismatis Rhizoma	9 g.
tōng cǎo	rice-paper plant pith	Tetrapanacis Medulla	6 g.
huá shí	talcum (wrapped)	Talcum	15 g.

MODIFICATIONS

To enhance dampness-draining, exterminate parasites, and relieve itching, add:

cāng zhú	atractylodes [root]	Atractylodis Rhizoma	9 g.
kǔ shēn	flavescent sophora [root]	Sophorae Flavescentis Radix	9 g.
bái xiān pí	dictamnus [root bark]	Dictamni Radicis Cortex	9 g.

In cases of damp-heat of the liver channel, manifesting as heavy vaginal discharge, unbearable vaginal itching, irritability, distention and pain of the thorax and costal region, dry bitter taste in the mouth, constipation, dark scanty urine, red tongue with thin yellow coating and rapid wiry pulse, the prescription is changed to clear heat and disinhibit dampness.

Use:

Gentian Liver-Draining Decoction *lóng dǎn xiè gān tāng*

lóng dǎn cǎo	gentian [root]	Gentianae Radix	6 g.
huáng qín	scutellaria [root]	Scutellariae Radix	9 g.
shān zhī zǐ	gardenia [fruit]	Gardeniae Fructus	9 g.
zé xiè	alisma [tuber]	Alismatis Rhizoma	12 g.
mù tōng	mutong [stem]	Mutong Caulis	9 g.
dāng guī	tangkuei	Angelicae Sinensis Radix	3 g.
chē qián zǐ	plantago [seed] (wrapped)	Plantaginis Semen	9 g.
shēng dì huáng	rehmannia [root] dried/fresh	Rehmanniae Radix Exsiccata seu Recens	9 g.
chái hú	bupleurum [root]	Bupleuri Radix	6 g.
gān cǎo	licorice [root]	Glycyrrhizae Radix	6 g.

ACUPUNCTURE AND MOXIBUSTION

Main points: Needle with draining.

CV-03	*zhōng jí*
BL-34	*xià liáo*
LR-05	*lǐ gōu*
SP-06	*sān yīn jiāo*
SP-10	*xuè hǎi*
SP-09	*yīn líng quán*

Auxiliary points:

For irritability and insomnia, add:

PC-05	*jiān shǐ*

For excruciating itching, add:

CV-12	*zhōng wǎn*
LR-01	*dà dūn*

2. LIVER AND KIDNEY YIN VACUITY

Clinical Manifestations: Dryness, burning sensation and itching of the vulva, decreased vaginal discharge that is yellow in color or resembling blood in severe cases, vexing heat in the five hearts, dizziness, vertigo, occasional hot flashes with perspiration, dryness of the mouth with no desire for drink, lower backache, tinnitus.

Tongue: Red with little coating.

Pulse: Rapid, thready, forceless.

Treatment Method: Supplement liver and kidney yin, relieve itching.

PRESCRIPTION

Anemarrhena, Phellodendron and Rehmannia Pill *zhī bǎi dì huáng wán*

shú dì huáng	cooked rehmannia [root]	Rehmanniae Radix Conquita	24 g.
shān zhū yú	cornus [fruit]	Corni Fructus	12 g.
shān yào	dioscorea [root]	Dioscoreae Rhizoma	12 g.
zé xiè	alisma [tuber]	Alismatis Rhizoma	9 g.
mǔ dān pí	moutan [root bark]	Moutan Radicis Cortex	9 g.
fú líng	poria	Poria	9 g.
zhī mǔ	anemarrhena [root]	Anemarrhenae Rhizoma	9 g.
huáng bǎi	phellodendron [bark]	Phellodendri Cortex	9 g.

MODIFICATIONS

When treating vaginal itching, the following are added for further relief:

dāng guī	tangkuei	Angelicae Sinensis Radix	9 g.
hé shǒu wū	flowery knotweed [root]	Polygoni Multiflori Radix	12 g.
bái xiān pí	dictamnus [root bark]	Dictamni Radicis Cortex	9 g.

ACUPUNCTURE AND MOXIBUSTION

Main points: Needle with supplementation.

CV-03	*zhōng jí*
SP-10	*xuè hǎi*
SP-06	*sān yīn jiāo*
KI-06	*zhào hǎi*
BL-23	*shèn shū*
BL-18	*gān shū*

Auxiliary points:

For irritability and insomnia, add:

LR-03	*tài chōng*

ALTERNATE THERAPEUTIC METHODS

1. Ear Acupuncture

Main Points: *Shén Mén*, Spleen, Liver, Ovary, External Genitalia.

Method: Select two to three points each session; needle to elicit a strong sensation and retain the needles for fifteen to thirty minutes. Treat once daily. Auricular needle embedding therapy may also be used.

2. Sitz Bath

Method: Decoct the following prescription and prepare as an herbal steam bath followed by an immersion bath once daily, ten times per therapeutic course.

Cnidium Seed Powder *shé chuáng zǐ sǎn*

shé chuáng zǐ	cnidium [seed]	Cnidii Monnieri Fructus	9 g.
huā jiāo	zanthoxylum	Zanthoxyli Pericarpium	9 g.
bái fán	alum	Alumen	9 g.
kǔ shēn	flavescent sophora [root[	Sophorae Flavescentis Radix	9 g.
bǎi bù	stemona [root]	Stemonae Radix	9 g.

REMARKS

In cases of excruciating itching or where the condition is prolonged, therapeutic effectiveness may be enhanced through the use of topical Western medications in conjunction with the treatments described in this chapter.

PRE- AND POSTMENOPAUSAL PATTERNS

Jīng Jué Qián Hòu Zhū Zhèng

1. Kidney Yin Vacuity - 2. Kidney Yang Vacuity

Pre- and postmenopausal patterns refer to patterns occurring just prior to or just following the onset of menopause in women. Symptoms are numerous and include periodic hot flashes marked by flushed complexion and perspiration, dizziness and vertigo, blurred vision, tinnitus, palpitations, insomnia, chest oppression, irritability, menstrual disturbances, occasional edema of the face and lower limbs, loss of appetite, loose stools, over-sensitivity, agitation, emotional instability and, when severe, depression, anxiety and suspiciousness.

The climacteric pattern described by Western medicine can be treated according to this chapter.

ETIOLOGY AND PATHOGENESIS

The development of menopausal patterns is mainly a result of kidney vacuity, although the liver, heart and spleen are also often involved. Pathogenesis includes yin vacuity, yang vacuity and vacuity of both yin and yang.

Patients whose constitution tends toward yin vacuity, or who have given birth to many children or who have a history of overindulgence in sexual activity can be prone to menopausal patterns of kidney yin vacuity. As *tiān guǐ* (literally, "celestial water") gradually dissipates during menopause, kidney yin becomes depleted to an even greater extent. If kidney yin is unable to rise and combine with heart fire, disruption of the interchange between the heart and kidney can result.

When kidney yin is vacuous, there is failure to nourish and moisten liver wood. In this case, liver qi can stagnate and transform to fire, further damaging yin and causing ascendant hyperactivity of liver yang. Stagnation of liver qi can also be from a history of emotional stress, resulting in the same consequences.

Kidney yang vacuity can also aggravate the normal menopausal transition. This can be caused by the gradual decline of kidney qi during menopause or constitutional factors, or overuse of herbal medicines that are cool or cold in nature. If the life-gate fire diminishes to the point that it fails to warm spleen yang, or if taxation has injured spleen yang, vacuity of both spleen and kidney yang can develop.

Finally, prolonged cases of yin or yang vacuity can mutually transform, resulting in vacuity of both yin and yang.

1. KIDNEY YIN VACUITY

Clinical Manifestations: Dizziness and vertigo, tinnitus, periodic hot flashes over the head and face, perspiration, vexing heat in the five hearts, aching lower back and knees, shortened or irregular menstrual cycle, menstrual discharge that is sometimes heavy, sometimes light and bright red in color; and (in some cases) dry itchy skin, dry mouth, dry hard stools and scanty yellow urine.

Tongue: Red with little coating.

Pulse: Rapid, thready.

Treatment Method: Nourish and moisten kidney yin, subdue liver yang.

PRESCRIPTION

Left-Restoring [Kidney Yin] Beverage *zuǒ guī yǐn*

shú dì huáng	cooked rehmannia [root]	Rehmanniae Radix Conquita	24 g.
shān yào	dioscorea [root]	Dioscoreae Rhizoma	12 g.
gǒu qǐ zǐ	lycium [berry]	Lycii Fructus	12 g.
shān zhū yú	cornus [fruit]	Corni Fructus	12 g.
fú líng	poria	Poria	9 g.
zhì gān cǎo	licorice [root] (honey-fried)	Glycyrrhizae Radix	6 g.

MODIFICATIONS

To reinforce the effects of nourishing yin and subduing yang, add:

guī bǎn	tortoise plastron (extended decoction)	Testudinis Plastrum	30 g.
hé shǒu wū	flowery knotweed [root]	Polygoni Multiflori Radix	15 g.

In cases of dry itchy skin, the prescription is modified to moisten dryness, course wind and relieve itching. Add:

chán tuì	cicada molting	Cicadae Periostracum	6 g.
fáng fēng	ledebouriella [root]	Ledebouriellae Radix	9 g.
hǎi tóng pí	erythrina [bark]	Erythrinae Cortex	9 g.
yù zhú	Solomon's seal [root]	Polygonati Yuzhu Rhizoma	12 g.

In vacuity of liver and kidney yin with ascendant hyperactivity of liver yang, symptoms include irritability, costal pain, bitter taste in the mouth, insomnia, dream-disturbed sleep, headache, dizziness and vertigo. The prescription is modified to moisten the kidney, soothe the liver, foster yin and subdue yang. Add:

nǚ zhēn zǐ	ligustrum [fruit]	Ligustri Fructus	9 g.
hàn lián cǎo	eclipta	Ecliptae Herba	9 g.
tiān má	gastrodia [root]	Gastrodiae Rhizoma	9 g.
gōu téng	uncaria [stem and thorn] (abbreviated decoction)	Uncariae Ramulus cum Unco	12 g.
shí jué míng	abalone shell (extended decoction)	Haliotidis Concha	30 g.
sāng jì shēng	mistletoe	Loranthi seu Visci Ramus	12 g.

In addition, the prescription is modified to direct the movement of blood downward. Add:

niú xī	achyranthes [root]	Achyranthis Bidentatae Radix	9 g.

In cases of disruption of the interchange between the heart and kidney, there are symptoms of palpitations, insomnia, dream-disturbed sleep, forgetfulness and anxiety. The prescription is adjusted to nourish the kidney, settle the heart and quiet the spirit. Substitute:

Celestial Emperor Heart-Supplementing Elixir *tiān wáng bǔ xīn dān*

shēng dì huáng	rehmannia [root] dried/fresh	Rehmanniae Radix Exsiccata seu Recens	30 g.
tiān mén dōng	asparagus [tuber]	Asparagi Tuber	12 .g
mài mén dōng	ophiopogon [tuber]	Ophiopogonis Tuber	12 g.
suān zǎo rén	spiny jujube [kernel]	Ziziphi Spinosi Semen	12 g.
dāng guī	tangkuei	Angelicae Sinensis Radix	9 g.
dān shēn	salvia [root]	Salviae Miltiorrhizae Radix	9 g.
xuán shēn	scrophularia [root]	Scrophulariae Radix	9 g.
rén shēn	ginseng	Ginseng Radix	6 g.
fú líng	poria	Poria	6 g.
wǔ wèi zǐ	schisandra [berry]	Schisandrae Fructus	6 g.
yuǎn zhì	polygala [root]	Polygalae Radix	6 g.
jié gěng	platycodon [root]	Platycodonis Radix	6 g.
bǎi zǐ rén	biota [seed]	Biotae Semen	12 g.
zhū shā	cinnabar (powdered and stirred in)	Cinnabaris	0.5 g.

ACUPUNCTURE AND MOXIBUSTION

Main Points: Needle with even supplementation, even draining.

BL-23   *shèn shū*
KI-03   *tài xī*
SP-06   *sān yīn jiāo*
LR-03   *tài chōng*

Auxiliary points:

For dizziness and vertigo, add:

GV-20   *bǎi huì*
GB-20   *fēng chí*

For palpitations and insomnia, add:

BL-15   *xīn shū*
HT-07   *shén mén*

2. KIDNEY YANG VACUITY

Clinical Manifestations: Dull complexion, listlessness, physical cold, cold extremities, cold and aching lower back and knees, loss of appetite, abdominal distention, loose stools, occasional heavy menstrual discharge, pale menstrual discharge that is sometimes dark in color and contains blood clots, edema of the face and limbs, increased nighttime urination and, in some cases, urinary incontinence or thin clear vaginal discharge.

Tongue: Pale, sometimes tender, flaccid with tooth impressions along the edges; thin white coating.

Pulse: Deep, thready, forceless.

Treatment Method: Supplement kidney yang, warm the spleen.

PRESCRIPTION

Combine Right-Restoring [Kidney Yang] Pill *(yòu guī wán)* with Center-Rectifying Decoction *(lǐ zhōng tāng)*.

Right-Restoring [Kidney Yang] Pill *yòu guī wán*

shú dì huáng	cooked rehmannia [root]	Rehmanniae Radix Conquita	24 g.
shān yào	dioscorea [root]	Dioscoreae Rhizoma	12 g.
shān zhū yú	cornus [fruit]	Corni Fructus	9 g.
gǒu qǐ zǐ	lycium [berry]	Lycii Fructus	12 g.
lù jiǎo jiāo	deerhorn glue (dissolved and stirred in)	Cervi Gelatinum Cornu	12 g.
tù sī zǐ	cuscuta [seed]	Cuscutae Semen	12 g.
dù zhòng	eucommia [bark]	Eucommiae Cortex	12 g.
dāng guī	tangkuei	Angelicae Sinensis Radix	9 g.
ròu guì	cinnamon [bark] (abbreviated decoction)	Cinnamomi Cortex	6 g.
zhì fù zǐ	aconite [accessory tuber] (processed) (extended decoction)	Aconiti Tuber Laterale Praeparatum	6 g.

with:

Center-Rectifying Decoction *lǐ zhōng tāng*

rén shēn	ginseng	Ginseng Radix	12 g.
bái zhú	ovate atractylodes [root]	Atractylodis Ovatae Rhizoma	9 g.
gān jiāng	dried ginger [root]	Zingiberis Rhizoma Exsiccatum	9 g.
zhì gān cǎo	licorice [root] (honey-fried)	Glycyrrhizae Radix	6 g.

MODIFICATIONS

In cases presenting loose stools, the prescription is modified to relieve diarrhea.
Delete:

dāng guī	tangkuei	Angelicae Sinensis Radix	

Add:

ròu dòu kòu	nutmeg	Myristicae Semen	9 g.

To reinforce warming kidney yang, add:

bǔ gǔ zhī	psoralea [seed]	Psoraleae Semen	9 g.
xiān máo	curculigo [root]	Curculiginis Rhizoma	12 g.
yín yáng huò	epimedium	Epimedii Herba	12 g.
fù pén zǐ	rubus [berry]	Rubi Fructus	9 g.

Delete:

ròu guì	cinnamon [bark]	Cinnamomi Cortex	
zhì fù zǐ	aconite [accessory tuber] (processed)	Aconiti Tuber Laterale Praeparatum	

In cases of dual kidney yin and yang vacuity, there are symptoms of physical cold, alternating hot flashes and perspiration, dizziness, vertigo, tinnitus, weak aching lower back, thin tongue coating and thready pulse. The prescription is changed to supplement kidney yin, warm kidney yang and nourish, regulate and rectify the *chōng* and *rèn*. Use:

Two Immortals Decoction *èr xiān tāng*

xiān máo	curculigo [root]	Curculiginis Rhizoma	12 g.
yín yáng huò	epimedium	Epimedii Herba	12 g.
dāng guī	tangkuei	Angelicae Sinensis Radix	9 g.
bā jǐ tiān	morinda [root]	Morindae Radix	9 g.
huáng bǎi	phellodendron [bark]	Phellodendri Cortex	6 g.
zhī mǔ	anemarrhena [root]	Anemarrhenae Rhizoma	6 g.

plus:

nǚ zhēn zǐ	ligustrum [fruit]	Ligustri Fructus	12 g.
hàn lián cǎo	eclipta	Ecliptae Herba	12 g.
shú dì huáng	cooked rehmannia [root]	Rehmanniae Radix Conquita	24 g.

ACUPUNCTURE AND MOXIBUSTION

Main Points: Needle with supplementation; add moxibustion.

BL-20	*pí shū*
BL-23	*shèn shū*
ST-36	*zú sān lǐ*
CV-04	*guān yuán*
SP-06	*sān yīn jiāo*

Auxiliary points:

For loose stools, add:

ST-25	*tiān shū*
SP-09	*yīn líng quán*

For edema, add:

CV-09	*shuǐ fēn*
CV-06	*qì hǎi*

ALTERNATE THERAPEUTIC METHODS

1. Ear Acupuncture

Main Points: Ovary, Endocrine, *Shén Mén,* Sympathetic, Subcortex, Heart, Liver, Spleen.

Method: Select three to four points each session and needle to elicit a moderate sensation. Treat once every two days. Auricular needle embedding therapy may also be used.

REMARKS

Menopausal patterns show a high degree of variation in the severity of symptoms and persistence of the condition. The majority of cases, however, present disruption of menstruation occurring just prior to or just following the onset of menopause. Conscientious diagnosis must distinguish menopause patterns from patterns of dizziness and vertigo, palpitations or edema.

ABDOMINAL MASSES

Zhēng Jiǎ

1. Stagnation of Qi - 2. Blood Stasis - 3. Phlegm-Dampness

Abdominal masses refer to a gynecological condition characterized by the occurrence of lumps or masses in the lower abdomen, accompanied at times by pain, distention, vaginal bleeding or vaginal discharge. In Chinese, abdominal masses are known as *zhēng jiǎ*.

Specifically, *zhēng* describes masses (concretions) with defined physical form and fixed location, accompanied by pain in a specific location. In these cases, pathological changes have taken place in the visceral organs; thus these patterns usually involve the blood. *Jiǎ*, on the other hand, describes masses without a distinct physical form (conglomerations), manifesting and dispersing without apparent pattern. Accompanying pain is not fixed in location. In these cases, pathological changes have taken place in the bowel organs. Hence these patterns involve qi. Despite the differences between *zhēng* and *jiǎ*, the two are closely related in terms of pathogenesis and are difficult to differentiate, hence the use of the compound *zhēng jiǎ*.

Abdominal masses include the Western medical conditions of uterine fibroid, ovarian cyst and endometriosis.

ETIOLOGY AND PATHOGENESIS

The development of *zhēng jiǎ* is usually from vacuity of qi and disharmony between qi and blood. Emotional depression, internal injury because of improper diet and eating habits and invasion of wind-cold during menstruation or following childbirth may all cause disharmony within the viscera and bowels, as can the internal obstruction and stagnation of phlegm-dampness, qi and blood stasis.

1. STAGNATION OF QI

Clinical Manifestations: Lower abdominal distention and fullness, soft conglomerations that move upon palpation, pain of indeterminate location.

Tongue: Thin white coating.

Pulse: Deep, wiry.

Treatment Method: Move qi, quicken the blood.

PRESCRIPTION

Cyperus and Sparganium Pill *xiāng léng wán*

mù xiāng	saussurea [root]	Saussureae seu Vladimiriae Radix	9 g.
dīng xiāng	clove	Caryophylli Flos	3 g.
zhǐ ké	bitter orange [fruit]	Aurantii Fructus	9 g.
qīng pí	unripe tangerine [peel]	Citri Exocarpium Immaturum	9 g.
xiǎo huí xiāng	fennel [fruit]	Foeniculi Fructus	6 g.
sān léng	sparganium [root]	Sparganii Rhizoma	6 g.
é zhú	zedoary	Zedoariae Rhizoma	6 g.
chuān liàn zǐ	toosendan [fruit]	Toosendan Fructus	9 g.

MODIFICATIONS

In cases of irregular menstruation, the prescription is modified to regulate menstruation. Add:

dān shēn	salvia [root]	Salviae Miltiorrhizae Radix	12 g.
xiāng fù zǐ	cyperus [root]	Cyperi Rhizoma	9 g.

In cases presenting an excessive vaginal discharge, the prescription is modified to relieve vaginal discharge. Add:

fú líng	poria	Poria	12 g.
yì yǐ rén	coix [seed]	Coicis Semen	30 g.
bái zhǐ	angelica [root]	Angelicae Dahuricae Radix	9 g.

In cases of severe abdominal pain, the prescription is modified to relieve pain. Add:

yán hú suǒ	corydalis [tuber]	Corydalis Tuber	9 g.
sān qī	notoginseng [root]	Notoginseng Radix	9 g.
	(or, powdered and administered separately, each time 1.5 g.)		

ACUPUNCTURE AND MOXIBUSTION

Main points: Needle with draining; add moxibustion.

CV-02	*qū gǔ*
CV-06	*qì hǎi*
KI-11	*héng gǔ*
LR-03	*tài chōng*
M-CA-18	*zǐ gōng* (Infant's Palace)
SP-06	*sān yīn jiāo*

Auxiliary points:

For heavy menstrual discharge, add:

SP-10	*xuè hǎi*

2. BLOOD STASIS

Clinical Manifestations: Lower abdominal masses that are hard in texture and immobile with pain aggravated upon palpation; dull complexion, loss of luster of the skin, heavy menstruation, lengthened menstrual cycles in some cases, dryness of the mouth without desire to drink.

Tongue: Dark, purplish, sometimes presenting stasis macules on the tongue.

Pulse: Deep, rough.

Treatment Method: Quicken the blood, move qi, dispel blood stasis.

PRESCRIPTION

Cinnamon Twig and Poria (Hoelen) Pill *guì zhī fú líng wán*

guì zhī	cinnamon [twig]	Cinnamomi Ramulus	9 g.
fú líng	poria	Poria	9 g.
mǔ dān pí	moutan [root bark]	Moutan Radicis Cortex	9 g.
chì sháo yào	red peony [root]	Paeoniae Radix Rubra	9 g.
táo rén	peach [kernel]	Persicae Semen	9 g.

<u>MODIFICATIONS</u>

In cases of heavy menstruation and uterine bleeding, the prescription is modified to relieve bleeding.

Add:

wǔ líng zhī	flying squirrel's droppings (wrapped)	Trogopteri seu Pteromydis Excrementum	9 g.
xuè yú tàn	charred hair	Hominis Crinis Carbonisatus	9 g.
pú huáng	typha pollen (wrapped)	Typhae Pollen	9 g.

In cases of excessive vaginal discharge, the prescription is modified to relieve vaginal discharge. Add:

yì yǐ rén	coix [seed]	Coicis Semen	30 g.
bái zhǐ	angelica [root]	Angelicae Dahuricae Radix	9 g.

In cases of severe abdominal pain, the prescription is modified to relieve pain. Add:

yán hú suǒ	corydalis [tuber]	Corydalis Tuber	9 g.
rǔ xiāng	frankincense	Olibanum	6 g.
mò yào	myrrh	Myrrha	6 g.

In cases of scanty menstrual discharge or amenorrhea, the prescription is modified to free menstruation.

Add:

niú xī	achyranthes [root]	Achyranthis Bidentatae Radix	9 g.
zé lán	lycopus	Lycopi Herba	12 g.

In cases where evils are replete and the patient's constitution is relatively strong, the prescription is changed to quicken the blood and remove stasis. Use the prepared medicine RHUBARB AND WINGLESS COCKROACH PILL (*dà huáng zhè chóng wán*)

ACUPUNCTURE AND MOXIBUSTION

Main points: Needle with draining; add moxibustion.

CV-02	*qū gǔ*
SP-06	*sān yīn jiāo*
KI-11	*héng gǔ*
CV-06	*qì hǎi*
M-CA-18	*zǐ gōng* (Infant's Palace)
SP-10	*xuè hǎi*

Auxiliary points:

For emotional stress, add:

LR-03	*tài chōng*

3. PHLEGM-DAMPNESS

Clinical Manifestations: Lower abdominal masses that are soft in texture and periodically painful; heavy vaginal discharge that is white in color, thick and sticky in texture; congestion and discomfort of the chest and costal regions; scanty urine.

Tongue: Dark purple tongue with white slimy coating.

Pulse: Soft, thready, or deep, slippery.

Treatment Method: Rectify qi, transform phlegm, quicken the blood.

PRESCRIPTION

Depression-Opening Two Matured Ingredients Decoction
kāi yù èr chén tāng

fǎ bàn xià	pinellia [tuber] (processed)	Pinelliae Tuber Praeparatum	12 g.
chén pí	tangerine (peel)	Citri Exocarpium	9 g.
fú líng	poria	Poria	9 g.
qīng pí	unripe tangerine [peel]	Citri Exocarpium Immaturum	9 g.
xiāng fù zǐ	cyperus [root]	Cyperi Rhizoma	9 g.
chuān xiōng	ligusticum [root]	Ligustici Rhizoma	9 g.
é zhú	zedoary	Zedoariae Rhizoma	9 g.
mù xiāng	saussurea [root]	Saussureae seu Vladimiriae Radix	9 g.
bīng láng	areca [nut]	Arecae Semen	9 g
cāng zhú	atractylodes [root]	Atractylodis Rhizoma	9 g.
shēng jiāng	fresh ginger	Zingiberis Rhizoma Recens	6 g.
zhì gān cǎo	licorice [root] (honey-fried)	Glycerrhizae Radix	6.g

MODIFICATIONS

In cases of vacuity of the spleen and stomach, presenting with loss of appetite and tiredness, the prescription is modified to fortify the spleen and boost the stomach.

Delete:

bīng láng	areca [nut]	Arecae Semen

Add:

bái zhú	ovate atractylodes [root]	Atractylodis Ovatae Rhizoma	9 g.
dǎng shēn	codonopsis [root]	Codonopsitis Radix	12 g.

In cases where the vaginal discharge is thick, sticky, yellow and foul-smelling, sometimes resembling pus, accompanied by spasmodic abdominal pain, thoracic congestion, irritability, fever, thirst, scanty yellow urine and red tongue with a yellow slimy coating (especially at the root of the tongue) and a rapid slippery pulse, the prescription is changed to clear heat, disinhibit dampness, dispel blood stasis and disperse lumps. Use:

Rhubarb and Moutan Decoction *dà huáng mǔ dān pí tāng*

dà huáng	rhubarb	Rhei Rhizoma	12 g.
mǔ dān pí	moutan [root bark]	Moutan Radicis Cortex	9 g.
táo rén	peach [kernel]	Persicae Semen	12 g.
dōng guā zǐ	wax gourd [seed]	Benincasae Semen	30 g.
máng xiāo	mirabilite (stirred in)	Mirabilitum	9 g.

Add:

hóng téng	sargentodoxa	Sargentodoxae Caulis	15 g.
bài jiàng cǎo	baijiang	Baijiang Herba cum Radice	15 g.
chuān shān jiǎ	pangolin scales	Manitis Squama	9 g.

ACUPUNCTURE AND MOXIBUSTION

Main points: Needle with even supplementation, even draining; add moxibustion.

CV-02	*qū gǔ*
KI-11	*héng gǔ*
M-CA-18	*zǐ gōng* (Infant's Palace)
SP-06	*sān yīn jiāo*
BL-20	*pí shū*
ST-30	*qì chōng*

Auxiliary points:

For aching lower back and vaginal discharge, add:

CV-04	*guān yuán*
KI-03	*tài xī*

ALTERNATE THERAPEUTIC METHODS

1. Ear Acupuncture

Main points: Endocrine, Subcortex, Uterus, Kidney, Spleen, Abdomen.

Method: Select two or three points each session. Needle to elicit a moderate or strong sensation once every two days, twenty sessions per therapeutic course. Auricular needle embedding therapy may also be used.

REMARKS

In the differential diagnosis of *zhēng jiǎ,* the all-important step is the distinction between patterns involving qi and those involving blood, taking into account recent conditions and prolonged illnesses. For patterns involving qi, treatment is aimed at regulating qi, and is complemented by the invigoration of blood. In those involving the blood, treatment mainly invigorates the blood, complemented by the regulation of qi.

In recently developed conditions, where the patient's constitution is still relatively strong, methods of attacking evils and breaking stasis are employed, while in more prolonged cases where the constitution is weakened, supplementation and attack are used together, or in succession.

Patterns of abdominal masses accompanied by abdominal pain, prolonged vaginal bleeding, dark foul-smelling vaginal discharge, emaciation and dull complexion are often signs of malignant growths; the prognosis is poor. According to the circumstances, surgical treatment may be required.

Mammary Nodules

Rŭ Pì

1. Stagnation of Liver Qi and Accumulation of Phlegm - 2. Liver and Kidney Vacuity with Accumulation of Phlegm

The appearance of solid breast lumps or masses of varying sizes and shapes is known as *rŭ pì* (mammary nodules). The character *pì* refers to lumps or masses in the breasts that are difficult to detect or elusive. *Rŭ pì* includes both breast fibroids and polycystic breast disease in Western medicine. Breast fibroids are most commonly found in the upper outer quadrant of the breast. They are spherical, variable in size, smooth and solid, with well-defined edges. They may be moved by palpation. The color of the skin over the fibroid nodules is normal and there is no evident pain. Breast fibroids generally occur singularly, although several may be found in either one or both breasts. They most commonly occur in women between twenty and twenty-five years of age.

Polycystic breast disease is a non-inflammatory disease of the breast that is characterized by the bilateral development of irregularly-sized masses, sometimes spherical and sometimes flattened in shape, with unclear borders. The masses are not connected to the skin and show movement with palpation. Three to four days prior to menstruation, these masses become painful and increase in size. After menstruation, the pain diminishes or disappears altogether and the masses shrink. Yellowish-green or brownish bloody discharges may escape from the nipples. Polycystic breast disease is most commonly found in women between the ages of thirty and forty, and is one of the most frequently observed diseases of the breast.

ETIOLOGY AND PATHOGENESIS

Mammary nodules are often a result of emotional stress that causes stagnation of liver qi and phlegm, leading to the formation of masses. A second potential cause is liver and kidney vacuity with a subsequent dysfunction of the *chōng* and *rèn*, allowing the accumulation of phlegm under conditions of vacuous yang, giving rise to lumps or masses in the breasts.

1. STAGNATION OF LIVER QI AND ACCUMULATION OF PHLEGM

Clinical Manifestations: Lumps or masses in the breasts accompanied by irritability, impatience, dizziness and vertigo, oppression in the chest, insomnia, dream-troubled sleep, distention and pain of the breasts and inguinal regions and, in some cases, difficult menstruation.

Tongue: Thin sometimes greasy coating.

Pulse: Wiry, slippery.

Treatment Method: Soothe the liver, resolve stagnation, transform phlegm, dissipate binds.

PRESCRIPTION

Free Wanderer Trichosanthes and Fritillaria Powder *xiāo yáo lóu bèi sǎn*

chái hú	bupleurum [root]	Bupleuri Radix	9 g.
dāng guī	tangkuei	Angelicae Sinensis Radix	9 g.
bái sháo yào	white peony [root]	Paeoniae Radix Alba	12 g.
fú líng	poria	Poria	12 g.
bái zhú	ovate atractylodes [root]	Atractylodis Ovatae Rhizoma	9 g.
guā lóu	trichosanthes [fruit]	Trichosanthis Fructus	15 g.
chuān bèi mǔ	Sichuan fritillaria [bulb]	Fritillariae Cirrhosae Bulbus	9 g.
fǎ bàn xià	pinellia [tuber] (processed)	Pinelliae Tuber Praeparatum	9 g.
tiān nán xīng	arisaema [root]	Arisaematis Rhizoma	9 g.
mǔ lì	oyster [shell]	Ostreae Concha (extended decoction)	30 g.
shān cí gū	shancigu [bulb]	Shancigu Bulbus	6 g.

ACUPUNCTURE AND MOXIBUSTION

Main Points: Needle with draining.

PC-06	*nèi guān*
CV-17	*tǎn zhōng*
ST-40	*fēng lóng*
ST-36	*zú sān lǐ*
LR-03	*tài chōng*
GB-21	*jiān jǐng*

Auxiliary points:

For difficult menstruation, add:

SP-06	*sān yīn jiāo*
CV-04	*guān yuán*

2. LIVER AND KIDNEY VACUITY WITH ACCUMULATION OF PHLEGM

Clinical Manifestations: Lumps or masses in the breasts accompanied by irregular menstruation, weakness of the lower back and knees, scanty pale-colored menstrual discharge and (in some cases) amenorrhea.

Tongue: Pale with white coating.

Pulse: Wiry, thready or deep, thready.

Treatment Method: Supplement the liver and kidney, regulate the *chōng* and *rèn*, transform phlegm, dissipate binds.

PRESCRIPTION

Combine Two Immortals Decoction *(èr xiān tāng)* with Four Agents Decoction *(sì wù tāng)*.

Two Immortals Decoction *èr xiān tāng*

xiān máo	curculigo [root]	Curculiginis Rhizoma	9 g.
yín yáng huò	epimedium	Epimedii Herba	9 g.
dāng guī	tangkuei	Angelicae Sinensis Radix	9 g.
bā jǐ tiān	morinda [root]	Morindae Radix	9 g.
huáng bǎi	phellodendron [bark]	Phellodendri Cortex	6 g.
zhī mǔ	anemarrhena [root]	Anemarrhenae Rhizoma	6 g.

with:

Four Agents Decoction *sì wù tāng*

shú dì huáng	cooked rehmannia [root]	Rehmanniae Radix Conquita	9 g.
dāng guī	tangkuei	Angelicae Sinensis Radix	9 g.
bái sháo yào	white peony [root]	Paeoniae Radix Alba	9 g.
chuān xiōng	ligusticum [root]	Ligustici Rhizoma	9 g.

MODIFICATIONS

In cases where there is vacuity of both qi and blood, the prescription is changed to supplement qi and blood and to regulate and rectify the *chōng* and *rèn*. Combine Two Immortals Decoction *(èr xiān tāng)* with Perfect Major Supplementation Decoction *(shí quán dà bǔ tāng)*.

Two Immortals Decoction *èr xiān tāng*

xiān máo	curculigo [root]	Curculiginis Rhizoma	9 g.
yín yáng huò	epimedium	Epimedii Herba	9 g.
dāng guī	tangkuei	Angelicae Sinensis Radix	9 g.
bā jǐ tiān	morinda [root]	Morindae Radix	9 g.
huáng bǎi	phellodendron [bark]	Phellodendri Cortex	6 g.
zhī mǔ	anemarrhena [root]	Anemarrhenae Rhizoma	6 g.

with:

Perfect Major Supplementation Decoction *shí quán dà bǔ tāng*

huáng qí	astragalus [root]	Astragali (seu Hedysari) Radix	9 g.
ròu guì	cinnamon [bark] (abbreviated decoction)	Cinnamomi Cortex	3 g.
rén shēn	ginseng	Ginseng Radix	9 g.
bái zhú	ovate atractylodes [root]	Atractylodis Ovatae Rhizoma	9 g.
fú líng	poria	Poria	9 g.
gān cǎo	licorice [root]	Glycyrrhizae Radix	6 g.
shú dì huáng	cooked rehmannia [root]	Rehmanniae Radix Conquita	9 g.
dāng guī	tangkuei	Angelicae Sinensis Radix	9 g.
bái sháo yào	white peony [root]	Paeoniae Radix Alba	6 g.
chuān xiōng	ligusticum [root]	Ligustici Rhizoma	6 g.

ACUPUNCTURE AND MOXIBUSTION

Main Points: Needle with even supplementation, even draining.

PC-06	*nèi guān*
ST-36	*zú sān lǐ*
SP-06	*sān yīn jiāo*
BL-23	*shèn shū*
CV-04	*guān yuán*
BL-18	*gān shū*

Auxiliary points:

In cases presenting symptoms of afternoon tidal fever, red cheeks, dizziness and vertigo, tinnitus and rapid thready pulse, add:

KI-05	*shuǐ quán*
LR-05	*lǐ gōu*

ALTERNATE THERAPEUTIC METHODS

1. Ear Acupuncture

Main Points: Endocrine, Mammary Gland.

Method: Needle to elicit a moderate sensation; retain needles for fifteen to thirty minutes.

REMARKS

In a small number of patients suffering from *rŭ pì*, mammary nodules can become malignant and necessitate surgical treatment.

FEMALE INFERTILITY

Bú Yùn

1. Kidney Yang Vacuity - 2. Kidney Yin Vacuity - 3. Liver Qi Stagnation - 4. Obstruction of Phlegm-Dampness - 5. Static Blood

Patterns of female infertility are categorized as either primary or secondary. Primary infertility applies to cases where conception has not occurred in two years, where no contraceptive measures have been taken and where the reproductive function of the male partner is normal. Secondary infertility includes cases of mothers who have taken no contraceptive measures but have not conceived again in two years. Infertility from congenital abnormalities are not effectively treated with either medicinal or acumoxa therapy, and are not covered in the this chapter.

ETIOLOGY AND PATHOGENESIS

Since the kidney controls reproduction, infertility is most closely related to the kidney, although the liver, spleen and the *chōng* and *rèn* may also be involved.

Infertility may be the result of the following: 1) constitutional insufficiencies that create kidney yang vacuity and cold in the womb; 2) depletion of essence and blood that creates kidney yin vacuity and lack of nourishment to the *chōng* and *rèn*; 3) emotional disruption leading to liver qi stagnation and disharmony between qi and blood; 4) indulgence in rich fatty foods leading to overweight and spleen vacuity that causes accumulation of phlegm and dampness; or 5) obstruction of the uterine network vessels by the coagulation of cold and static blood.

1. KIDNEY YANG VACUITY

Clinical Manifestations: Inability to conceive, prolonged menstrual cycles, small volume of pale menstrual discharge (or amenorrhea in some cases), accompanied by dull complexion, lassitude, physical cold, lower backache, weakness of the legs, poor libido, copious clear urine, unformed stools.

Tongue: Pale with white coating.

Pulse: Deep, thready, or slow, deep.

Treatment Method: Warm the kidney, invigorate yang, nourish the blood, regulate and rectify the *chōng* and *rèn*.

PRESCRIPTION

Unicorn-Rearing Pill *yù lín zhū*

rén shēn	ginseng	Ginseng Radix	9 g.
bái zhú	ovate atractylodes [root]	Atractylodis Ovatae Rhizoma	9 g.
fú líng	poria	Poria	9 g.
zhì gān cǎo	licorice [root] (honey-fried)	Glycyrrhizae Radix	6 g.
shú dì huáng	cooked rehmannia [root]	Rehmanniae Radix Conquita	12 g.
dāng guī	tangkuei	Angelicae Sinensis Radix	12 g.
bái sháo yào	white peony [root]	Paeoniae Radix Alba	9 g.
chuān xiōng	ligusticum [root]	Ligustici Rhizoma	9 g.
tù sī zǐ	cuscuta [seed]	Cuscutae Semen	12 g.
dù zhòng	eucommia [bark]	Eucommiae Cortex	12 g.
lù jiǎo shuāng	degelatinated deer antler	Cervi Cornu Degelatinum	15 g.
huā jiāo	zanthoxylum [husk]	Zanthoxyli Pericarpium	3 g.

<u>MODIFICATIONS</u>

In cases of severe lower backache, severe lower abdominal coldness and slow deep pulse, the prescription is modified to warm the kidney and invigorate yang. Add:

bā jǐ tiān	morinda [root]	Morindae Radix	12 g.
bǔ gǔ zhī	psoralea [seed]	Psoraleae Semen	9 g.
xiān máo	curculigo [root]	Curculiginis Rhizoma	9 g.
yín yáng huò	epimedium	Epimedii Herba	9 g.

ACUPUNCTURE AND MOXIBUSTION

Main points: Needle with supplementation; add moxibustion.

BL-23	*shèn shū*
CV-04	*guān yuán*
GV-04	*mìng mén*
ST-36	*zú sān lǐ*
SP-06	*sān yīn jiāo*
M-CA-18	*zǐ gōng* (Infant's Palace)

Auxiliary points:

For prolonged menstrual cycle, add:

ST-25	*tiān shū*
ST-29	*guī lái*

2. KIDNEY YIN VACUITY

Clinical Manifestations: Inability to conceive, shortened menstrual cycles, a scanty menstrual discharge that is red in color and contains no blood clots, emaciation, weak aching lower back and legs, dizziness and vertigo, blurred vision, palpitations, insomnia, dry mouth, afternoon fever and (in some cases) vexing heat in the five hearts.

Tongue: Red with little coating.

Pulse: Rapid, thready.

Treatment Method: Moisten kidney yin, nourish the blood, regulate and rectify the *chōng* and *rèn*.

PRESCRIPTION

Essence-Nourishing Jade-Planting Decoction *yǎng jīng zhòng yù tāng*

dāng guī	tangkuei	Angelicae Sinensis Radix	12 g.
bái sháo yào	white peony [root]	Paeoniae Radix Alba	12 g.
shú dì huáng	cooked rehmannia [root]	Rehmanniae Radix Conquita	24 g.
shān zhū yú	cornus [fruit]	Corni Fructus	12 g.

MODIFICATIONS

To further moisten and supplement kidney yin, add:

hàn lián cǎo	eclipta	Ecliptae Herba	12 g.
nǚ zhēn zǐ	ligustrum [fruit]	Ligustri Fructus	12 g.

In cases presenting emaciation, vexing heat in the five hearts and afternoon tidal fever, yin vacuity has given rise to fire. The prescription is modified to moisten yin and clear heat. Add:

guī bǎn	tortoise plastron (extended decoction)	Testudinis Plastrum	30 g.
mǔ dān pí	moutan [root bark]	Moutan Radicis Cortex	9 g.
dì gǔ pí	lycium [root bark]	Lycii Radicis Cortex	12 g.
huáng bǎi	phellodendron [bark]	Phellodendri Cortex	9 g.

ACUPUNCTURE AND MOXIBUSTION

Main points: Needle with supplementation.

BL-23	*shèn shū*
KI-02	*rán gǔ*
KI-13	*qì xué*
KI-03	*tài xī*
SP-06	*sān yīn jiāo*
M-CA-18	*zǐ gōng* (Infant's Palace)

Auxiliary points:

For dizziness and vertigo, add:

GV-20   *bǎi huì*

For blood vacuity with heat, add:

SP-10   *xuè hǎi*

For palpitations and insomnia, add:

HT-07   *shén mén*

3. LIVER QI STAGNATION

Clinical Manifestations: Inability to conceive, irregular menstrual cycles, menstrual cramps, difficult menstrual flow, scanty dark-colored menstrual discharge containing blood clots, premenstrual breast or abdominal distention, emotional depression, irritability.

Tongue: Dark red with thin white coating.

Pulse: Wiry.

Treatment Method: Soothe the liver, move qi, nourish the blood, regulate menstruation.

PRESCRIPTION

Depression-Opening Jade-Planting Decoction *kāi yù zhòng yù tāng*

dāng guī	tangkuei	Angelicae Sinensis Radix	12 g.
bái sháo yào	white peony [root]	Paeoniae Radix Alba	12 g.
bái zhú	ovate atractylodes [root]	Atractylodis Ovatae Rhizoma	9 g.
fú líng	poria	Poria	9 g.
mǔ dān pí	moutan [root bark]	Moutan Radicis Cortex	9 g.
xiāng fù zǐ	cyperus [root]	Cyperi Rhizoma	9 g.
tiān huā fěn	trichosanthes [root]	Trichosanthis Radix	9 g.

MODIFICATIONS

In cases presenting severe fullness and distention of the chest and costal regions, the prescription is modified to soothe the liver and move qi.

Delete:

bái zhú	ovate atractylodes [root]	Atractylodis Ovatae Rhizoma

Add:

qīng pí	unripe tangerine [peel]	Citri Exocarpium Immaturum	9 g.
méi guī huā	rose [flower]	Rosae Flos	6 g.
bái méi huā	white mume [flower]	Mume Flos Albusa	6 g.

In cases of dream-troubled sleep, the prescription is modified to benefit the liver and quiet the spirit. Add:

suān zǎo rén	spiny jujube [kernel]	Ziziphi Spinosi Semen	15 g.
yè jiāo téng	flowery knotweed [stem]	Polygoni Multiflori Caulis	15 g.

In cases manifesting lumps in the breast, the prescription is modified to move qi, invigorate blood and disperse lumps. Add:

wáng bù liú xíng	vaccaria [seed]	Vaccariae Semen	9 g.
jú yè	tangerine [leaf]	Citri Folium	6 g.
jú hé	tangerine [pip]	Citri Semen	9 g.
lù lù tōng	liquidambar [fruit]	Liquidambaris Fructus	6 g.

In cases of distention and burning sensation of the breasts sometimes accompanied by pain upon palpation, the prescription is modified to aid dispersal of the liver, clear heat and resolve toxins. Add:

chuān liàn zǐ	toosendan [fruit]	Toosendan Fructus	9 g.
pú gōng yīng	dandelion	Taraxaci Herba cum Radice	15 g.

ACUPUNCTURE AND MOXIBUSTION

Main points: Needle with draining:

BL-18	*gān shū*
LR-03	*tài chōng*
SP-08	*dì jī*
SP-06	*sān yīn jiāo*
CV-06	*qì hǎi*
M-CA-18	*zǐ gōng* (Infant's Palace)

Auxiliary points:

For distention and pain of the chest and costal regions, add:

PC-06	*nèi guān*
LR-14	*qī mén*

4. OBSTRUCTION BY PHLEGM-DAMPNESS

Clinical Manifestations: Inability to conceive, overweight, prolonged menstrual cycles, amenorrhea in severe cases, copious thick sticky vaginal discharge, pale complexion, dizziness and vertigo, palpitations, thoracic congestion, nausea.

Tongue: White greasy coating.

Pulse: Slippery.

Treatment Method: Dry dampness, dissolve phlegm, move qi, regulate menstruation.

PRESCRIPTION

Uterus-Opening Pill *qí gōng wán*

fǎ bàn xià	pinellia [tuber] (processed)	Pinelliae Tuber Praeparatum	9 g.
cāng zhú	atractylodes [root]	Atractylodis Rhizoma	9 g.
xiāng fù	cyperus [root]	Cyperi Rhizoma	9 g.
fú líng	poria	Poria	12 g.
shén qū	medicated leaven	Massa Fermentata	9 g.
chén pí	tangerine [peel]	Citri Exocarpium	9 g.
chuān xiōng	ligusticum [root]	Ligustici Rhizoma	6 g.

MODIFICATIONS

In cases of heavy menstrual discharge, the prescription is modified to benefit qi and secure the kidney. Delete:

chuān xiōng	ligusticum [root]	Ligustici Rhizoma

Add:

huáng qí	astragalus [root]	Astragali seu Hedysari Radix	12 g.
xù duàn	dipsacus [root]	Dipsaci Radix	12 g.

In cases of palpitations, the prescription is modified to nourish the heart and quiet the spirit. Add:

yuǎn zhì	polygala [root]	Polygalae Radix	9 g.

ACUPUNCTURE AND MOXIBUSTION

Main points: Needle with even supplementation, even draining; add moxibustion.

CV-03	*zhōng jí*
SP-06	*sān yīn jiāo*
ST-40	*fēng lóng*
BL-20	*zú sān lǐ*
M-CA-18	*zǐ gōng* (Infant's Palace)

Auxiliary points:

For vaginal discharge, add:

BL-32	*cì liáo*

For dizziness and vertigo and palpitations, add:

GV-20	*bǎi huì*
HT-07	*shén mén*

5. STATIC BLOOD

Clinical Manifestations: Inability to conceive, prolonged menstrual cycles, scanty blackish-purple menstrual discharge with blood clots, menstrual cramps, lower abdominal pain aggravated on palpation.

Tongue: Dark purplish, sometimes presenting stasis macules on the tongue.

Pulse: Rough, wiry, thready.

Treatment Method: Quicken the blood, expel blood stasis, regulate menstruation.

PRESCRIPTION

Lesser Abdomen Stasis-Expelling Decoction *shào fù zhú yū tāng*

dāng guī	tangkuei	Angelicae Sinensis Radix	9 g.
chì sháo yào	red peony [root]	Paeoniae Radix Rubra	6 g.
pú huáng	typha pollen (wrapped)	Typhae Pollen	9 g.
mò yào	myrrh	Myrrha	6 g.
chuān xiōng	ligusticum [root]	Ligustici Rhizoma	3 g.
wǔ líng zhī	flying squirrel droppings (wrapped)	Trogopteri seu Pteromydis Excrementum	6 g.
yán hú suǒ	corydalis [tuber]	Corydalis Tuber	3 g.
gān jiāng	dried ginger [root]	Zingiberis Rhizoma Exsiccatum	3 g.
ròu guì	cinnamon [bark] (abbreviated decoction)	Cinnamomi Cortex	3 g.
xiǎo huí xiāng	fennel [fruit]	Foeniculi Fructus	3 g.

<u>MODIFICATIONS</u>

Delete:

gān jiāng	dried ginger [root]	Zingiberis Rhizoma Exsiccatum
ròu guì	cinnamon [bark]	Cinnamomi Cortex

Add:

dān shēn	salvia [root]	Salviae Miltiorrhizae Radix	9 g.
xiāng fù zǐ	cyperus [root]	Cyperi Rhizoma	9 g.
guì zhī	cinnamon [twig]	Cinnamomi Ramulus	6 g.

ACUPUNCTURE AND MOXIBUSTION

Main points: Needle with draining; add moxibustion.

CV-03	*zhōng jí*
SP-06	*sān yīn jiāo*
SP-10	*xuè hǎi*
SP-08	*dì jī*
ST-30	*qì chōng*
M-CA-18	*zǐ gōng* (Infant's Palace)

Auxiliary points:

For severe menstrual cramps, add:

BL-32	*cì liáo*
ST-29	*guī lái*

ALTERNATE THERAPEUTIC METHODS

1. Ear Acupuncture

Main points: Endocrine, Kidney, Uterus, Subcortex, Ovary.

Method: Select two to three points each session, and needle to elicit a moderate sensation. Treat once daily, ten sessions per therapeutic course. Auricular needle embedding therapy may also be used.

REMARKS

The inability to conceive involves both the male and female partners; therefore, a thorough examination of the patient's medical history must be made, especially regarding menstruation, childbearing, vaginal discharge and sexual activity. Appropriate gynecological examinations, including salpingography and ovarian function, as well as a spermatographic assay of the male partner, should be undertaken to ensure accurate diagnosis.

PART V

OBSTETRICS

MAMMARY ABSCESS
Rŭ Yōng

1. Initial Stage: Coagulation of Milk - 2. Purulent Stage: Formation of Pus - 3. Rupture Stage: Discharge of Pus

Mammary abscess refers to acute purulent disease of the breast, which is most often observed in first-time mothers during the third or fourth week of postpartum breastfeeding. Mammary abscess corresponds to acute mastitis in Western medicine, which recognizes staphylococcal bacteria as its causative pathogenic agent.

ETIOLOGY AND PATHOGENESIS

The etiology of mammary abscess includes stagnation of liver qi from emotional stress or the binding of heat in the stomach channel from overindulgence in rich food. Both these factors lead to obstruction of the channels and connections, stagnation of qi and stasis of blood, all of which hinder the secretion of milk. Mammary abscess can also be the result of poor hygiene of the nipples and a cracking of the skin that allows invasion by external toxin that coagulates the accumulated milk to form abscesses.

1. INITIAL STAGE: COAGULATION OF MILK

Clinical Manifestations: Swelling, distention, pain and formation of masses in the breast and hindrance of the secretion of milk, often accompanied by aversion to cold, fever, headache, oppression in the chest, nausea, irritability, thirst.

Tongue: Thin yellow or yellow slimy coating.

Pulse: Rapid, wiry or rapid, floating.

Treatment Method: Soothe the liver, clear the stomach, promote lactation, dissipate binds.

PRESCRIPTION
Trichosanthes and Arctium Decoction *guā lóu niú bàng tāng*

guā lóu	trichosanthes [fruit]	Trichosanthis Fructus	15 g.
niú bàng zǐ	arctium [seed]	Arctii Fructus	12 g.
jīn yín huā	lonicera [flower]	Lonicerae Flos	12 g.
lián qiào	forsythia [fruit]	Forsythiae Fructus	12 g.
tiān huā fěn	trichosanthes [root]	Trichosanthis Radix	9 g.
huáng qín	scutellaria [root]	Scutellariae Radix	9 g.
shān zhī zǐ	gardenia [fruit]	Gardeniae Fructus	9 g.
chái hú	bupleurum [root]	Bupleuri Radix	9 g.
qīng pí	unripe tangerine [peel]	Citri Exocarpium Immaturum	9 g.
chén pí	tangerine [peel]	Citri Exocarpium	6 g.
zào jiǎo cì	gleditsia [thorn]	Gleditsiae Spina	6 g.
gān cǎo	licorice [root]	Glycyrrhizae Radix	6 g.

MODIFICATIONS

In cases of severe redness, swelling and pain of the breast, the prescription is modified to quicken the blood, disperse swelling and relieve pain. Add:

chuān shān jiǎ	pangolin scales	Manitis Squama	9 g.
	(or, powdered and stirred in, each time 1.5 g.)		
wáng bù liú xíng	vaccaria [seed]	Vaccariae Semen	9 g.
dān shēn	salvia [root]	Salviae Miltiorrhizae Radix	12 g.

In cases of high fever, the prescription is modified to clear heat. Add:

| shí gāo | gypsum (extended decoction) | Gypsum | 30 g. |
| zhī mǔ | anemarrhena [root] | Anemarrhenae Rhizoma | 9 g. |

In cases of marked qi stagnation, the prescription is modified to soothe the liver and regulate qi. Add:

| jú yè | tangerine [leaf] | Citri Folium | 6 g. |
| chuān liàn zǐ | toosendan [fruit] | Toosendan Fructus | 9 g. |

In cases of distention of the breasts after cessation of breastfeeding, the prescription is modified to return the milk. Add:

| shān zā | crataegus [fruit] | Crataegi Fructus | 12 g. |
| mài yá | barley sprout | Hordei Fructus Germinatus | 30 g. |

In cases of retention of lochia, the prescription is modified to quicken the blood and dispel stasis. Add:

dāng guī	tangkuei	Angelicae Sinensis Radix	9 g.
chuān xiōng	ligusticum [root]	Ligustici Rhizoma	9 g.
yì mǔ cǎo	leonurus	Leonuri Herba	12 g.

In cases where breast masses fail to disperse after treatment, the overuse of cold medicinals has led to stagnation of qi and blood. Symptoms include slight pain in the breast, disappearance of fever, wiry tardy pulse and thin white tongue coating. Treatment should include regulation of liver qi, warming of yang and draining swelling. Use:

Counterflow Cold Powder *sì nì sǎn*

chái hú	bupleurum [root]	Bupleuri Radix	6 g.
bái sháo yào	white peony [root]	Paeoniae Radix Alba	9 g.
zhǐ shí	unripe bitter orange [fruit]	Aurantii Fructus Immaturus	6 g.
zhì gān cǎo	licorice [root] (honey-fried)	Glycyrrhizae Radix	6 g.

Add:

lù jiǎo jiāo	deerhorn glue	Cervi Gelatinum Cornu	9 g.
chuān shān jiǎ	pangolin [scales]	Manitis Squama	9 g.
	(or, powdered and stirred in, each time 1.5 g.)		

ACUPUNCTURE AND MOXIBUSTION

Main points: Needle with draining.

GB-21	jiān jǐng
CV-17	tǎn zhōng
ST-36	zú sān lǐ
ST-34	liáng qiū
ST-18	rǔ gēn
LR-14	qī mén
PC-06	nèi guān

Auxiliary points:

For fever and aversion to cold, add:
> LI-04   *hé gǔ*
> LI-11   *qū chí*

For headache, add:
> GB-20   *fēng chí*

For inability to secrete milk, add:
> SI-01 -   *shào zé*

For marked stagnation of qi, add:
> LR-03   *tài chōng*

For severe swelling and pain of the breast, add:
> GB-41   *zú lín qì*

2. PURULENT STAGE: FORMATION OF PUS

Clinical Manifestations: Enlargement of the mammary masses and an increase in breast swelling, redness of the skin of the breast, continuous high fever, thirst and an increase in the severity of breast pain, which has become constant and throbbing. A softening of the center of the masses that elicits a sensation of wave-like motion on palpation is a definitive sign of purulence.

In cases where masses are deeply situated, a mammary biopsy may be necessary to make a definite diagnosis.

Tongue: Yellow coating.

Pulse: Wiry, rapid.

Treatment Method: Clear heat-toxin, quicken the blood, promote lactation, discharge pus.

PRESCRIPTION

Trichosanthes and Arctium Decoction *guā lóu niú bàng tāng*

guā lóu	trichosanthes [fruit]	Trichosanthis Fructus	15 g.
niú bàng zǐ	arctium [seed]	Arctii Fructus	12 g.
jīn yín huā	lonicera [flower]	Lonicerae Flos	12 g.
lián qiào	forsythia [fruit]	Forsythiae Fructus	12 g.
tiān huā fěn	trichosanthes [root]	Trichosanthis Radix	9 g.
huáng qín	scutellaria [root]	Scutellariae Radix	9 g.
shān zhī zǐ	gardenia [fruit]	Gardeniae Fructus	9 g.
chái hú	bupleurum [root]	Bupleuri Radix	9 g.
qīng pí	unripe tangerine [peel]	Citri Exocarpium Immaturum	9 g.
chén pí	tangerine [peel]	Citri Exocarpium	6 g.
zào jiǎo cì	gleditsia [thorn]	Gleditsiae Spina	6 g.
gān cǎo	licorice [root]	Glycyrrhizae Radix	6 g.

MODIFICATIONS

To increase the strength of the prescription to quicken the blood, disperse swelling and discharge pus, add:

chuān shān jiǎ	pangolin [scales]	Manitis Squama	9 g.
	(or, powdered and stirred in, each time 1.5 g.)		
dāng guī wěi	tangkuei tail	Angelicae Sinensis Radicis Extremitas	6 g.
chì sháo yào	red peony [root]	Paeoniae Radix Rubra	9 g.

In cases of poor constitutions where the pus is not easily discharged, the prescription is modified to relieve inflammation and discharge pus.

Add:

huáng qí	astragalus [root]	Astragali (seu Hedysari) Radix	15 g.
dǎng shēn	codonopsis [root]	Codonopsitis Radix	9 g.
chuān xiōng	ligusticum [root]	Ligustici Rhizoma	6 g.

3. RUPTURE STAGE: DISCHARGE OF PUS

Clinical Manifestations: Discharge of pus from the breast, gradual return of normal body temperature, disappearance of swelling and pain and gradual healing of the superficial lesions.

Tongue: Thin yellow coating.

Pulse: Slight rapid or weak.

Treatment Method: Regulate qi and blood, clear remaining evils.

PRESCRIPTION

Mysterious Four Decoction *sì miào tāng*

huáng qí	astragalus [root]	Astragali (seu Hedysari) Radix	15 g.
dāng guī	tangkuei	Angelicae Sinensis Radix	9 g.
jīn yín huā	lonicera [flower]	Lonicerae Flos	12 g.
zhì gān cǎo	licorice [root] (honey-fried)	Glycyrrhizae Radix	6 g.

MODIFICATIONS

In cases where discharge of pus is poor, where the swelling and pain have not diminished and where the fever has not subsided, it is possible that pus has invaded other lobules of the mammary gland. In such cases, evils have not been completely dispelled and treatment of the initial and purulent stages of mammary abscess should be continued.

When milk is observed to escape through the lesion after the rupture of a carbuncle, the condition is known in traditional Chinese medicine as mammary fistula *(rǔ lòu)*. Treatment should include supplementation of qi and blood to assist in discharging pus.

Use:

Internal Expulsion Toxin-Dispersing Powder *tuō lǐ xiāo dú sǎn*

huáng qí	astragalus [root]	Astragali (seu Hedysari) Radix	12 g.
jīn yín huā	lonicera [flower]	Lonicerae Flos	15 g.
chuān xiōng	ligusticum [root]	Ligustici Rhizoma	9 g.
dāng guī	tangkuei	Angelicae Sinensis Radix	6 g.
bái sháo yào	white peony [root]	Paeoniae Radix Alba	6 g.
bái zhú	ovate atractylodes [root]	Atractylodis Ovatae Rhizoma	6 g.
rén shēn	ginseng	Ginseng Radix	6 g.
fú líng	poria	Poria	9 g.
bái zhǐ	angelica [root]	Angelicae Dahuricae Radix	6 g.
zào jiǎo cì	gleditsia [thorn]	Gleditsiae Spina	6 g.
jié gěng	platycodon [root]	Platycodonis Radix	6 g.
gān cǎo	licorice [root]	Glycyrrhizae Radix	6 g.

ALTERNATE THERAPEUTIC METHODS

1. Ear Acupuncture

Main points: Mammary Gland, Endocrine, Adrenal Gland, Thorax.

Method: Needle to elicit a strong sensation and retain the needles for twenty to thirty minutes.

2. Cupping Therapy

Method: Select appropriately-sized glass fire cups and suction over the site of lesions to draw out the accumulated pus. This treatment is appropriate during the purulent stage of mammary abscess.

3. External Treatments

During the early stage of mammary abscess, the prepared medicine GOLDEN YELLOW POWDER *(jīn huáng sǎn)* mixed with water can be used for external application, or a fifty percent solution of mirabilite *(máng xiāo)* can be applied to the affected area three to four times daily.

During the purulent stage, lancing can aid the drainage of pus. When the masses are small and superficial, pus can be removed with a syringe, after which GOLDEN YELLOW PASTE *(jīn huáng gāo)* can be applied.

During the rupture stage, medicated thread with the prepared medicine EIGHT-TO-TWO POWDER *(bā èr dān)* or the prepared medicine NINE-TO-ONE ELIXIR *(jiǔ yī dān)* can be inserted into the lesions and GOLDEN YELLOW PASTE applied to the area. After completely draining the pus, apply the prepared medicine FLESH-ENGENDERING POWDER *(shēng jī sǎn)* to promote the granulation and healing of the lesions.

REMARKS

Acumoxa therapy is effective in the treatment of mammary abscess during the initial stage prior to the formation of pus. With acumoxa therapy and medicinal therapy, greater therapeutic results can be achieved by applying warm compresses and massage.

While breastfeeding, mothers should follow a feeding schedule and pay attention to the nipple hygiene. When the milk supply exceeds the infant's demand, excessive milk should be expressed by hand or removed with a breast pump after each feeding. This prevents milk stasis. The prompt treatment of abrasions or cracking of the nipples and purulent infections elsewhere on the body is also important to prevent mammary abscess.

Morning Sickness

Rèn Shēn È Zǔ

1. Spleen and Stomach Vacuity - 2. Liver and Stomach Disharmony

Morning sickness refers to patterns of nausea and vomiting during the first trimester of pregnancy, especially during the morning hours. Other symptoms may include dizziness, aversion to food or vomiting upon ingestion of food. Morning sickness is the most commonly observed disorder during the early months of pregnancy. The presentation of mild nausea and vomiting and preference for sour acid foods is a common reaction during early pregnancy and such cases usually do not require treatment; symptoms usually subside naturally in the third month. Treatments offered in this chapter are suitable for more pronounced cases.

Severe cases of morning sickness, observed in Western medicine, can lead to dehydration, electrolyte imbalance and acidosis.

ETIOLOGY AND PATHOGENESIS

The major etiological factor in morning sickness is the failure of stomach qi to descend. The most common pathogenesis is spleen and stomach vacuity or liver and stomach disharmony. With the onset of pregnancy and the termination of menstruation, a relative repletion of qi develops in the *chōng*. When coupled with a constitutional spleen and stomach vacuity, this results in counterflow qi in the stomach channel, the course of which communicates with the *chōng* vessel. This reversal, where stomach qi is ascending, manifests as nausea and vomiting.

Similarly, morning sickness can be caused by liver and stomach disharmony from either constitutional liver repletion or injury to the liver by depression or anger. In both cases yin and blood are redirected to nourish the growing fetus, resulting in a loss of blood to the liver and thus a relative repletion of liver qi. Since the pathway of the liver channel passes through the stomach, the replete liver qi flowing upward disturbs the stomach, causing nausea and vomiting.

1. Spleen and Stomach Vacuity

Clinical Manifestations: Nausea and vomiting, or vomiting upon ingestion of food during the first trimester of pregnancy; vomiting of clear mucus, bland sense of taste, fullness and distention of the epigastrium and abdomen, tiredness, drowsiness.

Tongue: Pale with moist white coating.

Pulse: Slippery, forceless.

Treatment Method: Fortify the spleen, harmonize the stomach, downbear qi, relieve vomiting.

PRESCRIPTION

Saussurea and Amomum Six Gentlemen Decoction
xiāng shā liù jūn zǐ tāng

rén shēn	ginseng	Ginseng Radix	9 g.
bái zhú	ovate atractylodes [root]	Atractylodis Ovatae Rhizoma	9 g.
fú líng	poria	Poria	9 g.
mù xiāng	saussurea [root]	Saussureae (seu Vladimiriae) Radix	6 g.
shā rén	amomum [fruit] (abbreviated decoction)	Amomi Semen seu Fructus	6 g.
zhì gān cǎo	licorice [root] (honey-fried)	Glycyrrhizae Radix	6 g.
chén pí	tangerine [peel]	Citri Exocarpium	9 g.
jiāng bàn xià	pinellia [tuber] (ginger-processed)	Pinelliae Tuber Praeparatum	12 g.

<u>MODIFICATIONS</u>

In cases accompanied by phlegm-rheum, with symptoms of congestion and fullness of the chest and epigastrium and vomiting of phlegm and mucus, the prescription is changed to fortify the spleen, transform phlegm, harmonize the stomach and relieve vomiting.

Use:

Minor Pinellia Poria Decoction *xiǎo bàn xià fú líng tāng*

zhì bàn xià	pinellia [tuber] (processed)	Pinelliae Tuber Praeparatum	9 g.
shēng jiāng	fresh ginger	Zingiberis Rhizoma Recens	9 g.
fú líng	poria	Poria	12 g.

Add:

bái zhú	ovate atractylodes {root}	Atractylodis Ovatae Rhizoma	9 g.
shā rén	amomum [fruit] (abbreviated decoction)	Amomi Semen seu Fructus	6 g.
chén pí	tangerine [peel]	Citri Exocarpium	9 g.
fú lóng gān	oven earth (wrapped; extended decoction)	Terra Flava Usta	30 g.

ACUPUNCTURE AND MOXIBUSTION

Main points: Needle with supplementation.

ST-36	*zú sān lǐ*
CV-13	*shàng wǎn*
CV-12	*zhōng wǎn*
SP-04	*gōng sūn*
PC-06	*nèi guān*

Auxiliary points: Needle with even supplementation, even draining.

For fullness and distention of the epigastria and abdomen, add:

CV-10	*xià wǎn*

In cases accompanied by phlegm-rheum, add:

SP-09	*yīn líng quán*
ST-40	*fēng lóng*

2. LIVER AND STOMACH DISHARMONY

Clinical Manifestations: Vomiting of acid or bitter fluids during early pregnancy, fullness of the chest, costal pain, belching, frequent sighing, distended sensation of the head, dizziness and vertigo, mental depression, thirst, bitter taste in the mouth.

Tongue: Slightly yellow coating.

Pulse: Slippery, wiry.

Treatment Method: Soothe the liver, harmonize the stomach, downbear qi, relieve vomiting.

PRESCRIPTION

Perilla Leaf and Coptis Decoction *sū yè huáng lián tāng*

zǐ sū yè	perilla [leaf] (abbreviated decoction)	Perillae Folium	9 g.
huáng lián	coptis [root]	Coptidis Rhizoma	9 g.

MODIFICATIONS

To further assist in calming the stomach and relieving vomiting, add:

jiāng bàn xià	pinellia [tuber] (ginger-processed)	Pinelliae Tuber Praeparatum	9 g.
chén pí	tangerine [peel]	Citri Exocarpium	9 g.
zhú rú	bamboo shavings	Bambusae Caulis in Taeniam	9 g.
wū méi	mume [fruit]	Mume Fructus	9 g.
huáng qín	scutellaria [root]	Scutellariae Radix	9 g.

In cases of severe vomiting with injury to bodily fluids, accompanied by a red tongue and dry mouth, the prescription is modified to nourish stomach yin.
Add:

lú gēn	phragmites [root]	Phragmititis Rhizoma	15 g.
běi shā shēn	glehnia [root]	Glehniae Radix	12 g.
shí hú	dendrobium [stem] (extended decoction)	Dendrobii Caulis	12 g.

In cases of frequent vomiting and decreased food intake leading to depletion of both qi and yin, with symptoms of emaciation, listlessness, weakness of limbs, dry lips and mouth, decreased urine, dry stools, red tongue with thin dry yellow coating or peeled coating and slippery rapid thready forceless pulse, combine Pulse-Engendering Beverage *(shēng mài yǐn)* with Humor-Increasing Decoction *(zēng yè tāng)*.

Pulse-Engendering Beverage *shēng mài yǐn*

rén shēn	ginseng	Ginseng Radix	9 g.
mài mén dōng	ophiopogon [tuber]	Ophiopogonis Tuber	15 g.
wǔ wèi zǐ	schisandra [berry]	Schisandrae Fructus	6 g.

with:

Humor-Increasing Decoction *zēng yè tāng*

xuán shēn	scrophularia [root]	Scrophulariae Radix	30 g.
mài mén dōng	ophiopogon [tuber]	Ophiopogonis Tuber	15 g.
shēng dì huáng	rehmannia [root] dried/fresh	Rehmanniae Radix Exsiccata seu Recens	24 g.

Add:

chén pí	tangerine [peel]	Citri Exocarpium	6 g.
zhú rú	bamboo shavings	Bambusae Caulis in Taeniam	6 g.
tiān huā fěn	trichosanthes [root]	Trichosanthis Radix	12 g.

ACUPUNCTURE AND MOXIBUSTION

Main points: Needle with draining.

PC-06	*nèi guān*
LR-03	*tài chōng*
ST-36	*zú sān lǐ*
CV-12	*zhōng wǎn*

Auxiliary points:

For oppression in the chest and costal pain, add:

    CV-17   *tǎn zhōng*

For vomiting of bitter fluids, add:

    GB-34   *yáng líng quán*

For distended sensation of the head and dizziness, add:

    GV-20   *bǎi huì*
    M-HN-3   *yìn táng* (Hall of Impression)

ALTERNATE THERAPEUTIC METHODS

1. Ear Acupuncture

Main points: Stomach, Spleen, Liver, *Sān Jiāo*, *Shén Mén*.

Treatment Method: Puncture lightly with needles. Treat once daily, ten sessions per therapeutic course. Auricular needle embedding therapy can also be used.

REMARKS

Use qi-consuming, blood-dissolving herbal medicines prudently in the early months of pregnancy when the developing fetus is as yet unconsolidated. The number of acupoints used should be minimal and the stimulation relatively mild to ensure that no harm comes to the fetus. Patients should remain calm, get plenty of bed rest and abstain from raw cold or rich slimy foods. It is best to eat a greater number of smaller meals to nourish and regulate stomach qi.

In severe cases, traditional and modern therapeutic methods can be used simultaneously. Intravenous infusion may be necessary to correct acidosis and electrolyte imbalance.

POSTPARTUM ABDOMINAL PAIN

Chăn Hòu Fù Tòng

1. Blood Vacuity · 2. Blood Stasis

Patterns of postpartum lower abdominal pain (in common parlance, after-pains) are most frequently observed in first-time mothers.

ETIOLOGY AND PATHOGENESIS

Major etiological factors in the development of postpartum abdominal pain are the restriction of qi and blood flow, which will manifest either as blood vacuity or blood stasis. Patterns of blood vacuity arise following childbirth when blood loss has depleted the *chōng* and *rèn*. This can cause a lack of nourishment of the uterine network vessels, or simply weaken the force of qi and blood circulation.

Postpartum abdominal pain caused by blood stasis can occur when loss of qi during childbirth allows cold evil to invade the uterine network vessels and coagulate the blood, or when the passing of lochia is coupled with an emotional disturbance that leads to a stasis of qi and blood.

1. BLOOD VACUITY

Clinical Manifestations: Dull postpartum lower abdominal pain, softness of the abdomen, pain relieved by external pressure, discharge of a small amount of light-colored lochia, dizziness and vertigo, tinnitus, hard dry stools.

Tongue: Pale with thin coating.

Pulse: Thready, forceless.

Treatment Method: Supplement the blood, boost qi, regulate and rectify the *chōng* and *rèn*, relieve pain.

PRESCRIPTION

Abdomen-Quieting Decoction *cháng níng tāng*

dāng guī	tangkuei	Angelicae Sinensis Radix	12 g.
shú dì huáng	cooked rehmannia [root]	Rehmanniae Radix Conquita	12 g.
rén shēn	ginseng	Ginseng Radix	9 g.
shān yào	dioscorea [root]	Dioscoreae Rhizoma	12 g.
ē jiāo	ass hide glue (dissolved and stirred in)	Asini Corii Gelatinum	9 g.
xù duàn	dipsacus [root]	Dipsaci Radix	9 g.
mài mén dōng	ophiopogon [tuber]	Ophiopogonis Tuber	9 g.
zhì gān cǎo	licorice [root] (honey-fried)	Glycyrrhizae Radix	6 g.
ròu guì	cinnamon [bark] (abbreviated decoction)	Cinnamomi Cortex	3 g.

<u>**MODIFICATIONS**</u>

In cases of severe depletion of bodily fluids with dry stools, the prescription is modified to warm the kidney and moisten the intestines.

Delete:

| *ròu guì* | cinnamon [bark] | Cinnamomi Cortex | |

Add:

| *ròu cōng róng* | cistanche [stem] | Cistanches Caulis | 15 g. |

In cases of vacuous blood accompanied by cold, manifesting as pale greenish complexion, lower abdominal pain that is relieved when heat is applied, cold extremities and slow thready pulse, treatment should nourish the blood and dissipate cold. The prescription is changed to warm and supplement qi and blood and relieve pain. Use:

Tangkuei Center-Fortifying Decoction *dāng guī jiàn zhōng tāng*

dāng guī	tangkuei	Angelicae Sinensis Radix	12 g.
guì zhī	cinnamon [twig]	Cinnamomi Ramulus	9 g.
bái sháo yào	white peony [root]	Paeoniae Radix Alba	18 g.
zhì gān cǎo	licorice [root] (honey-fried)	Glycyrrhizae Radix	6 g.
sheng jiāng	fresh ginger [root]	Zingiberis Rhizoma Recens	9 g.
dà zǎo	jujube	Ziziphi Fructus	4 pc.
yí táng	malt sugar (stirred in)	Granorum Saccharon	30 g.

ACUPUNCTURE AND MOXIBUSTION

Main points: Needle with supplementation; add moxibustion.

CV-04	*guān yuán*
CV-06	*qì hǎi*
BL-17	*gé shū*
ST-36	*zú sān lǐ*
SP-06	*sān yīn jiāo*

Auxiliary points:

For dizziness and vertigo, add:

| GV-20 | *bǎi huì* |
| M-HN-1 | *sì shén cōng* (Alert Spirit Quartet) |

For hard, dry stools, add:

| KI-06 | *zhào hǎi* |
| TB-06 | *zhī gōu* |

2. BLOOD STASIS

Clinical Manifestations: Postpartum lower abdominal pain aggravated by external pressure that is sometimes slightly relieved by the application of heat, discharge of a small volume of dark purple lochia containing blood clots, distention and pain of the chest and hypochondria.

Tongue: Dark-colored with white coating.

Pulse: Deep, tight or rough, wiry.

Treatment Method: Quicken the blood, dispel stasis, dissipate cold, relieve pain.

PRESCRIPTION

Engendering Transformation Decoction *shēng huà tāng*

dāng guī	tangkuei	Angelicae Sinensis Radix	24 g.
chuān xiōng	ligusticum [root]	Ligustici Rhizoma	9 g.
táo rén	peach [kernel]	Persicae Semen	6 g.
gān jiāng	dried ginger [root]	Zingiberis Rhizoma Exsiccatum	3 g.
zhì gān cǎo	licorice [root] (honey-fried)	Glycyrrhizae Cortex	3 g

MODIFICATIONS

When cold is predominant, with symptoms including lower abdominal cold and pain, pale greenish complexion and cold extremities, the prescription is modified to warm the vessels and dissipate cold.
Add:

wú zhū yú	evodia [fruit]	Evodiae Fructus	6 g.
ròu guì	cinnamon [bark] (abbreviated decoction)	Cinnamomi Cortex	6 g.

In cases of lochia containing many blood clots and severe lower abdominal pain, the prescription is modified to quicken the blood and dispel stasis.
Add:

yán hú suǒ	corydalis [tuber]	Corydalis Tuber	9 g.
pú huáng	typha pollen (wrapped)	Typhae Pollen	9 g.
wǔ líng zhī	flying squirrel droppings (wrapped)	Trogopteri seu Pteromydis Excrementum	9 g.

Where lower abdominal distention is more severe than the pain and involves the chest and hypochondrium, the prescription is modified to regulate qi and disperse distention.
Add:

xiāng fù zǐ	cyperus [root]	Cyperi Rhizoma	9 g.
wū yào	lindera [root]	Linderae Radix	9 g.
zhǐ ké	bitter orange [fruit]	Aurantii Fructus	9 g.

ACUPUNCTURE AND MOXIBUSTION

Main points: Needle with draining; add moxibustion.

BL-17	*gé shū*
SP-10	*xuè hǎi*
SP-06	*sān yīn jiāo*
CV-03	*zhōng jí*
LR-03	*tài chōng*

Auxiliary points:

For predominant signs of cold, add:

BL-23	*shèn shū*
CV-04	*guān yuán*

For distention of the chest and hypochondrium, add:

LR-14	*qī mén*
CV-17	*tǎn zhōng*

For inability to pass lochia, add:

CV-06	*qì hǎi*
CV-07	*yīn jiāo*

ALTERNATE THERAPEUTIC METHODS

1. Ear Acupuncture

Main points: Uterus, Liver, Kidney, *Shén Mén*, Endocrine, Adrenal Gland.

Method: Needle to elicit a moderate sensation; retain needles for twenty minutes. Treat once daily. Auricular needle embedding therapy can also be used.

REMARKS

Patients suffering from postpartum abdominal pain should follow a regular daily schedule, abstain from cold raw foods, protect against invasion by wind and cold and avoid situations that can cause anxiety, depression or anger.

THREATENED MISCARRIAGE

Xiān Zhào Liú Chǎn

1. Kidney Qi Depletion - 2. Qi and Blood Vacuity - 3. Blood Heat - 4. Traumatic Injury

SUPPLEMENT: HABITUAL MISCARRIAGE

Huá Tāi

In traditional Chinese medicine, threatened miscarriage refers to two different conditions, namely, leaking fetus *(tāi lòu)*, or uterine bleeding during pregnancy, and stirring fetus *(tāi dòng bù ān)*. Leaking fetus is characterized by slight and intermittent vaginal bleeding without lower backache or abdominal pain. Stirring fetus refers to frequent fetal movement, abdominal pain, bearing-down sensation in the lower abdomen and (in some cases) slight vaginal bleeding. Both conditions warn of possible miscarriage.

As the differential diagnosis and treatment of leaking fetus and stirring fetus are basically equivalent, this chapter discusses the two simultaneously. Habitual miscarriage *(huá tāi)* is discussed in the supplemental section at the end of the chapter.

ETIOLOGY AND PATHOGENESIS

The etiology of threatened miscarriage involves numerous factors. Often there is kidney vacuity, either because of a weak constitution, depleted kidney essence from overindulgent sexual activity or to a history of frequent miscarriages. Other important factors include impairment of the spleen and stomach leading to qi and blood vacuity and internal heat disturbing the fetus, often resulting from stagnation because of emotional stress. Fetal qi can also be adversely affected by the development of another illness during pregnancy. In addition, the effects of traumatic injury, surgery and herbal and pharmaceutical medicines can threaten miscarriage.

1. KIDNEY QI DEPLETION

Clinical Manifestations: Slight vaginal bleeding during pregnancy, dark discharge, lower backache and, in some cases, a bearing down sensation and pain in the abdomen; accompanied by dizziness, vertigo, tinnitus, frequent urination, polyuria at night or urinary incontinence in severe cases. In some cases, there is a history of frequent miscarriage.

Tongue: Pale with white coating.

Pulse: Deep, weak, slippery.

Treatment Method: Secure the kidney, boost qi, calm the fetus.

PRESCRIPTION

Fetal Longevity Pill *shòu tāi wán*

tù sī zǐ	cuscuta [seed]	Cuscutae Semen	12 g.
sāng jì shēng	mistletoe	Loranthi seu Visci Ramus	12 g.
xù duàn	dipsacus [root]	Dipsaci Radix	12 g.
ē jiāo	ass hide glue (dissolved and stirred in)	Asini Corii Gelatinum	9 g.

MODIFICATIONS

To fortify the spleen and boost qi, add:

dǎng shēn	codonopsis [root]	Codonopsitis Radix	9 g.
bái zhú	ovate atractylodes [root]	Atractylodis Ovatae Rhizoma	12 g.

In cases of urinary incontinence, the prescription is modified to warm the kidney and restrain urination. Add:

yì zhì rén	alpinia [fruit]	Alpiniae Oxyphyllae Fructus	6 g.
fù pén zǐ	rubus [berry]	Rubi Fructus	9 g.

2. QI AND BLOOD VACUITY

Clinical Manifestations: Slight vaginal bleeding during pregnancy, discharge that is thin and pale red, and, in some cases, pain and bearing down sensation of the lower back and abdomen, with tiredness, fatigue, pale complexion, palpitations and shortness of breath.

Tongue: Pale with thin white coating.

Pulse: Thready, slippery.

Treatment Method: Supplement qi, nourish the blood, secure the kidney, quiet the fetus.

PRESCRIPTION

Fetal Origin Beverage *tāi yuán yǐn*

rén shēn	ginseng	Ginseng Radix	9 g.
shú dì huáng	cooked rehmannia [root]	Rehmanniae Radix Conquita	12 g.
bái zhǐ	angelica [root]	Angelicae Dahuricae Radix	12 g.
dù zhòng	eucommia [bark]	Eucommiae Cortex	12 g.
bái sháo yào	white peony [root]	Paeoniae Radix Alba	12 g.
chén pí	tangerine [peel]	Citri Exocarpium	6 g.
zhì gān cǎo	licorice [root] (honey-fried)	Glycyrrhizae Radix	6 g.
dāng guī	tangkuei	Angelicae Sinensis Radix	6 g.

MODIFICATIONS

The preceding prescription is usually adjusted to boost qi, nourish the blood and relieve bleeding.

Delete:

dāng guī	tangkuei	Angelicae Sinensis Radix	

Add:

huáng qí	astragalus [root]	Astragali (seu Hedysari) Radix	12 g
ē jiāo	ass hide glue (dissolved and stirred in)	Asini Corii Gelatinum	9 g.

3. BLOOD HEAT

Clinical Manifestations: Vaginal bleeding during pregnancy, discharge that is bright red in color; pain, distention and bearing down sensation of the lower back and abdomen, accompanied by irritability, dry mouth and throat, dark scanty urine and constipation.

Tongue: Red with dry yellow coating.

Pulse: Rapid, slippery or wiry, slippery.

Treatment Principle: Nourish yin, cool the blood, clear heat, quiet the fetus.

PRESCRIPTION

Yin-Safeguarding Brew *bǎo yīn jiān*

shēng dì huáng	rehmannia [root] dried/fresh	Rehmanniae Radix Exsiccata seu Recens	12 g.
shú dì huáng	cooked rehmannia [root]	Rehmanniae Radix Conquita	12 g.
huáng qín	scutellaria [root]	Scutellariae Radix	9 g.
huáng bǎi	phellodendron [bark]	Phellodendri Cortex	9 g.
bái sháo yào	white peony [root]	Paeoniae Radix Alba	12 g.
shān yào	dioscorea [root]	Dioscoreae Rhizoma	12 g.
xù duàn	dipsacus [root]	Dipsaci Radix	9 g.
gān cǎo	licorice [root]	Glycyrrhizae Radix	6 g.

MODIFICATIONS

To cool the blood, relieve bleeding and quiet the fetus, add:

zhù má gēn	ramie	Boehmeriae Radix	30 g.

In cases of heavy vaginal bleeding, the prescription is modified to nourish yin and relieve bleeding.

Add:

ē jiāo	ass hide glue (dissolved and stirred in)	Asini Corii Gelatinum	9 g.
hàn lián cǎo	eclipta	Ecliptae Herba	12 g.

In cases presenting lower backache, the prescription is modified to secure the kidney and quiet the fetus.

Add:

tù sī zǐ	cuscuta [seed]	Cuscutae Semen	12 g.
sāng jì shēng	mistletoe	Loranthi seu Visci Ramus	12 g.

4. TRAUMATIC INJURY

Clinical Manifestations: History of falling, twisting the back or overstrain during pregnancy, resulting in vaginal bleeding; or lower backache and abdominal distention and bearing down sensation.

Tongue: Normal; in some cases dark.

Pulse: Slippery, forceless.

Treatment Method: Supplement qi, regulate blood, quiet the fetus.

PRESCRIPTION

Sagely Cure Decoction *shèng yù tāng*

huáng qí	astragalus [root]	Astragali (seu Hedysari) Radix	12 g.
rén shēn	ginseng	Ginseng Radix	9 g.
dāng guī	tangkuei	Angelicae Sinensis Radix	9 g.
chuān xiōng	ligusticum [root]	Ligustici Rhizoma	6 g.
shú dì huáng	cooked rehmannia [root]	Rehmanniae Radix Conquita	12 g.
shēng dì huáng	rehmannia [root] dried/fresh	Rehmanniae Radix Exsiccata seu Recens	12 g.

MODIFICATIONS

To secure the kidney and quiet the fetus, add:

tù sī zǐ	cuscuta [seed]	Cuscutae Semen	12 g.
sāng jì shēng	mistletoe	Loranthi seu Visci Ramus	12 g.
xù duàn	dipsacus [root]	Dipsaci Radix	12 g.

In cases of heavy vaginal bleeding, the prescription is modified to nourish the blood, relieve bleeding and quiet the fetus.

Delete:

dāng guī	tangkuei	Angelicae Sinensis Radix
chuān xiōng	ligusticum [root]	Ligustici Rhizoma

Add:

ài yè	mugwort [leaf] (charred)	Artemisiae Argyi Folium	9 g.
ē jiāo	ass hide glue (dissolved and stirred in)	Asini Corii Gelatinum	9 g.

REMARKS

Herbal treatment is the main therapeutic modality for threatened miscarriage. Acumoxa therapy is generally not used. Preventative measures include moderating sexual intercourse, regulating the diet and psychological state, avoiding emotional and physical stress and minimizing any circumstances liable to result in falls. When vaginal bleeding and abdominal pain have been alleviated through treatment, pregnancy generally continues normally. Appropriate measures should be undertaken immediately when signs of miscarriage or premature delivery develop. These include increased discharge of blood that may contain blood clots, severe lower backache and abdominal pain.

SUPPLEMENT:

HABITUAL MISCARRIAGE

Huá Tāi

Spontaneous loss of the fetus before the twelfth week of pregnancy is known as *duò tāi,* literally "fetal discharge." Loss between twelve and twenty eight weeks, after the fetus is fully formed, is known as *xiǎo chǎn,* premature labor or miscarriage. Fetal discharge or premature labor that occurs three or more times in succession is termed *huá tāi,* literally, "fetal slippage," and corresponds to habitual miscarriage.

The etiology of habitual miscarriage is complicated, but the pathogenesis mainly involves spleen and kidney vacuity and weakening of the *chōng* and *rèn*.

Clinical Manifestations: Miscarriage following each conception, or miscarriage at a fixed number of weeks, frail physical constitution, lassitude, fatigue, weak aching lower back and knees, palpitations, shortness of breath, frequent night-time urination, loss of appetite, irregular menstruation.

Tongue: Tender and pale with thin white coating.

Pulse: Deep, weak.

Treatment Method: Supplement the kidney, benefit the spleen, regulate and rectify the *chōng* and *rèn*.

PRESCRIPTION

Kidney-Supplementing Penetrating Vessel-Securing Pill
bǔ shèn gù chōng wán

tù sī zǐ	cuscuta [seed]	Cuscutae Semen	240 g.
xù duàn	dipsacus [root]	Dipsaci Radix	90 g.
bā jǐ tiān	morinda [root]	Morindae Radix	90 g.
dù zhòng	eucommia [bark]	Eucommiae Cortex	90 g.
dāng guī	tangkuei	Angelicae Sinensis Radix	90 g.
shú dì huáng	cooked rehmannia [root]	Rehmanniae Radix Conquita	150 g.
lù jiǎo jiāo	deerhorn glue	Cervi Gelatinum Cornu	90 g.
gǒu qǐ zǐ	lycium [berry]	Lycii Fructus	90 g.
ē jiāo	ass hide glue	Asini Corii Gelatinum	120 g.
dǎng shēn	codonopsis [root]	Codonopsitis Radix	120 g.
bái zhú	ovate atractylodes [root]	Atractylodis Ovatae Rhizoma	90 g.
shā rén	amomum [fruit]	Amomi Semen seu Fructus	15 g.
dà zǎo	jujube (pitted)	Ziziphi Fructus	50 pc.

Prepare by grinding the ingredients given into powder, adding honey and forming into small pills. A dose of 6 g. is taken three times a day, or a decoction can be made by using approximately 1/10th the amounts given. This prescription is used in cases of habitual miscarriage where there are no organic pathological changes. It is taken prior to conception and not during menstrual periods.

MODIFICATIONS

Accompanying symptoms of insomnia, dream-troubled sleep, irritability, dry throat, hard dry stools and thin yellow tongue coating are often presented in patients with constitutions tending toward yin vacuity. During pregnancy, yin becomes further depleted, allowing the rise of internal heat to harm the fetus. Treatment should nourish yin and blood and clear vacuity heat. Use:

Yin-Safeguarding Brew *bǎo yīn jiān*

shēng dì huáng	rehmannia [root] dried/fresh	Rehmanniae Radix Exsiccata seu Recens	12 g.
shú dì huáng	cooked rehmannia [root]	Rehmanniae Radix Conquita	12 g.
huáng qín	scutellaria [root]	Scutellariae Radix	9 g.
huáng bǎi	phellodendron [bark]	Phellodendri Cortex	9 g.
bái sháo yào	white peony [root]	Paeoniae Radix Alba	12 g.
shān yào	dioscorea [root]	Dioscoreae Rhizoma	12 g.
xù duàn	dipsacus [root]	Dipsaci Radix	9 g.
gān cǎo	licorice [root]	Glycyrrhizae Radix	6 g.

Kidney-Supplementing Penetrating Vessel-Securing Pill *(bǔ shèn gù chōng wán)* can be used following the clearing of vacuity heat to quiet the fetus.

ECLAMPSIA

Zǐ Xián

1. Liver Wind Stirring Internally - 2. Disruption of the Upper Burner by Phlegm-Fire

Eclampsia may present either during the third trimester of pregnancy, during delivery or following childbirth. It is characterized by the sudden onset of vertigo followed by loss of consciousness, twitching of the limbs, trismus (jaw tetany), staring of the eyes and opisthotonos in severe cases. Patients gradually regain full consciousness and then another attack follows. Prenatal eclampsia is more often observed clinically. The three characteristic features of eclampsia as diagnosed by Western medicine – high blood pressure, edema and albuminuria – may supplement diagnosis.

ETIOLOGY AND PATHOGENESIS

Physical constitutions tending toward vacuity of liver and kidney yin and profusion of liver yang are the major etiology of epilepsy of pregnacy. During pregnancy, essence and blood collect to nourish the growing fetus. Thus less blood is available to the liver. This results in decreased nourishment of the liver and liver wind stirring internally, manifesting as eclampsia. The combination of phlegm and fire that rises and obstructs the orifices may also lead to eclampsia.

1. LIVER WIND STIRRING INTERNALLY

Clinical Manifestations: Dizziness, vertigo, flushed complexion, bitter taste in the mouth, dry throat, palpitations, restlessness and edema of the lower limbs during later pregnancy. The onset of eclampsia is marked by sudden loss of consciousness, twitching of the limbs, staring of the eyes and opisthotonos in severe cases.

Tongue: Red.

Pulse: Slippery, wiry or rapid, wiry.

Treatment Method: Foster yin, quell yang, calm the liver, extinguish wind.

PRESCRIPTION

Antelope Horn and Uncaria Decoction *líng jiǎo gōu téng tāng*

líng yáng jiǎo	antelope horn (powdered and stirred in, each time 0.5 g.)	Antelopis Cornu	3 g.
gōu téng	uncaria [stem and thorn] (abbreviated decoction)	Uncariae Ramulus cum Unco	9 g.
sāng yè	mulberry [leaf]	Mori Folium	6 g.
jú huā	chrysanthemum [flower]	Chrysanthemi Flos	9 g.
chuān bèi mǔ	Sichuan fritillaria [bulb]	Fritillariae Cirrhosae Bulbus	12 g.
zhú rú	bamboo shavings	Bambusae Caulis in Taeniam	9 g.
shēng dì huáng	rehmannia [root] dried/fresh	Rehmanniae Radix Exsiccata seu Recens	15 g.
bái sháo yào	white peony [root]	Paeoniae Radix Alba	9 g.
fú shén	root poria	Poria cum Pini Radice	9 g.
gān cǎo	licorice [root]	Glycyrrhizae Radix	3 g.

ACUPUNCTURE AND MOXIBUSTION

Main points: Needle with even supplementation, even draining.

GV-20	*bǎi huì*
GB-20	*fēng chí*
LR-03	*tài chōng*
PC-06	*nèi guān*
KI-03	*tài xī*

Auxiliary points:

For loss of consciousness, add:

GV-26	*shuǐ gōu*
KI-01	*yǒng quán*

For trismus, add:

ST-07	*xià guān*
ST-06	*jiá chē*

For dizziness and vertigo, add:

M-HN-1	*sì shén cōng* (Alert Spirit Quartet)
M-HN-3	*yìn táng* (Hall of Impression)

For prolonged spasms, add:

GB-34	*yáng líng quán*
LR-08	*qū quán*

2. DISRUPTION OF THE UPPER BURNER BY PHLEGM-FIRE

Clinical Manifestations: Onset of eclampsia during late pregnancy, during delivery or immediately postpartum, with symptoms of sudden loss of consciousness, twitching of the limbs, heavy breathing and whistling respiration.

Tongue: Red with yellow slimy coating.

Pulse: Slippery, wiry.

Treatment Method: Clear heat, expel phlegm, open the orifices.

PRESCRIPTION

Use the prepared medicine BOVINE BEZOAR HEART-CLEARING PILL *(niú-huáng qīng xīn wán)*.

<u>MODIFICATIONS</u>

To reinforce the effects of heat-clearing, phlegm-dissolving and orifice-opening, add:

| *zhú lì* | dried bamboo sap | Bambusae Succus Exsiccatus | 40 g. |

ACUPUNCTURE AND MOXIBUSTION

Main points: Needle with draining.

GV-26	*shuǐ gōu*
GV-20	*bǎi huì*
GV-14	*dà zhuī*
ST-40	*fēng lóng*
LR-03	*tài chōng*
PC-08	*láo gōng*

Auxiliary points:

For trismus (jaw tetany), add:

| LI-04 | *hé gǔ* |
| ST-06 | *jiá chē* |

For yin vacuity, add:

| KI-03 | *tài xī* |

ALTERNATE THERAPEUTIC METHODS

1. Ear Acupuncture

Main points: Liver, Kidney, *Shén Mén*, Subcortex, Occipital.

Method: Needle one to three times daily to elicit a moderate sensation. Auricular needle embedding therapy also may be used.

REMARKS

Eclampsia, a critical condition, often begins as either edema or hypertension during pregnancy. A strict schedule of prenatal examinations should be maintained to detect and treat epilepsy of pregnancy during its developmental stages.

DIFFICULT DELIVERY

Nán Chǎn

1. Vacuity of Qi and Blood - 2. Stagnation of Qi and Stasis of Blood

SUPPLEMENT: MALPOSITION OF THE FETUS

Tāi Wèi Bú Zhèng

Difficult delivery refers to full-term pregnancies where difficulties arise after labor has begun and the delivery of the child is complicated. Labor that exceeds 24 hours in length is termed "protracted labor" *(zhì chǎn).* Irregularities in the force of labor (including irregular uterine contractions as well as poor abdominal pressure), irregularities of the birth canal or irregularities of the fetus or fetal position are often involved in difficult deliveries. The emphasis of the present chapter is on difficult deliveries that are related to irregularities in the force of labor.

ETIOLOGY AND PATHOGENESIS

The pathogenic mechanism of difficult delivery may involve either vacuity of qi and blood or stagnation of qi and stasis of blood. Insufficient qi and blood and the resultant difficult labor may be caused by weak constitutions where both qi and blood are vacuous; bearing down prior to complete dilation of the cervix causing depletion of qi and loss of strength; early breaking of water; or excessive loss of blood during delivery. Stress and anxiety, invasion by cold evil prior to delivery or lack of adequate exercise during pregnancy may all result in the repletion patterns of stagnation of qi, stasis of blood and difficult delivery.

1. VACUITY of Qi AND BLOOD

Clinical Manifestations: Weak labor pains, short contractions followed by long intervals, slow progression of labor, a large volume of light-colored bloody discharge (in some cases), pale complexion, lassitude, palpitations, shortness of breath.

Tongue: Pale with thin coating.

Pulse: Empty or weak.

Treatment Method: Supplement qi, boost the blood, promote the progression of labor.

PRESCRIPTION

Difficult Delivery Formula *nán chǎn fāng*

huáng qí	astragalus [root]	Astragali (seu Hedysari) Radix	30 g.
dǎng shēn	codonopsis [root]	Codonopsitis Radix	12 g.
dāng guī	tangkuei	Angelicae Sinensis Radix	12 g.
fú shén	root poria	Poria cum Pini Radice	9 g.
bái sháo yào	white peony [root]	Paeoniae Radix Alba	9 g.
chuān xiōng	ligusticum [root]	Ligustici Rhizoma	9 g.
gǒu qǐ zǐ	lycium [berry]	Lycii Fructus	12 g.
guī bǎn	tortoise plastron (extended decoction)	Testudinis Plastrum	30 g.

ACUPUNCTURE AND MOXIBUSTION

Main points: Needle with supplementation; add moxibustion.

ST-36	*zú sān lǐ*
SP-06	*sān yīn jiāo*
KI-07	*fù liū*
BL-67	*zhì yīn*

Auxiliary points:

For lassitude, add moxibustion to:

CV-04	*guān yuán*
CV-06	*qì hǎi*

For palpitations and shortness of breath, add:

PC-06	*nèi guān*
KI-03	*tài xī*

2. STAGNATION OF QI AND STASIS OF BLOOD

Clinical Manifestations: Severe lower back pain and abdominal pain during labor, strong contractions at irregular intervals, slow progression of labor, small volume of deep red bloody discharge (in some cases), dark greyish complexion, depressed emotional state, distention and oppression in the chest and epigastrium, periodic nausea and retching.

Tongue: Dark red with normal or slimy coating.

Pulse: Deep, replete.

Treatment Method: Regulate qi, invigorate the blood, dissolve stasis, promote the progression of labor.

PRESCRIPTION

Birth-Hastening Beverage *cuī shēng yǐn*

dāng guī	tangkuei	Angelicae Sinensis Radix	12 g.
chuān xiōng	ligusticum [root]	Ligustici Rhizoma	9 g.
zhǐ ké	bitter orange [fruit]	Aurantii Fructus	9 g.
bái zhǐ	angelica [root]	Angelicae Dahuricae Radix	9 g.
dà fù pí	areca [husk]	Arecae Pericarpium	9 g.

<u>MODIFICATIONS</u>

To quicken the blood and remove stasis, add:

yì mǔ cǎo	leonurus	Leonuri Herba	15 g.

ACUPUNCTURE AND MOXIBUSTION

Main points: Needle with draining.

    LI-04   *hé gǔ*
    SP-06   *sān yīn jiāo*
    M-LE-18a *dú yīn* (Solitary Yin)

Auxiliary points:

For severe abdominal pain, add:

    LR-03   *tài chōng*

For distention and fullness of the chest and costal regions, add:

    PC-06   *nèi guān*
    GB-21   *jǐng*

ALTERNATE THERAPEUTIC METHODS

1. Ear Acupuncture

Main points: Uterus, Subcortex, Endocrine, Kidney, Urinary Bladder.

Method: Needle to elicit a moderate sensation, and manipulate at three to five minute intervals.

REMARKS

The expectant mother should stay calm through her pregnancy, quieting any anxieties and unnecessary tension. She must eat well and follow a schedule that allows adequate rest and physical exercise. Also, she should maintain a fully-aware mental state during labor to insure a normal, uncomplicated birth.

If labor continues to progress at an abnormally slow rate after herbal and acupuncture treatment, it may be necessary to perform a Cesarean section, the decision being made according to the patient's condition.

SUPPLEMENT:

MALPOSITION OF THE FETUS

Tāi Wèi Bú Zhèng

The following treatments may be employed in all cases where prenatal examination reveals the fetus to be in breech, transverse or occipito-posterior position. Treatment generally begins after the 28th week of pregnancy. Abnormal fetal position caused by a narrow pelvic cavity or uterine deformity is best treated by other methods and may require a cesarean section.

ACUPUNCTURE AND MOXIBUSTION

Main point:

    BL-67   *zhì yīn*

Method: During treatment, have the patient loosen restrictive clothing and assume a supine position or recline on a high-backed chair. Apply moxibustion bilaterally for fifteen to twenty minutes with moxa rolls to BL-67 *(zhì yīn)*. Treat once or twice daily, seven days per therapeutic course until the fetus has turned to a cephalic position.

PRESCRIPTION

Carefree Pregnancy Formula *bǎo chǎn wú yōu fāng*

dāng guī	tangkuei	Angelicae Sinensis Radix	4.5 g.
chuān xiōng	ligusticum [root]	Ligustici Rhizoma	4.5 g.
bái sháo yào	white peony [root]	Paeoniae Radix Alba	3.6 g.
huáng qí	astragalus [root]	Astragali (seu Hedysari) Radix	2.4 g.
hòu pò	magnolia [bark]	Magnoliae Cortex	2.1 g.
qiāng huó	notopterygium [root]	Notopterygii Rhizoma	1.5 g.
tù sī zǐ	cuscuta [seed]	Cuscutae Semen	3 g.
chuān bèi mǔ	Sichuan fritillaria [bulb]	Fritillariae Cirrhosae Bulbus	3 g.
zhǐ ké	bitter orange [fruit]	Aurantii Fructus	1.8 g.
ài yè	mugwort [leaf]	Artemisiae Argyi Folium	2.1 g.
shēng jiāng	fresh ginger [root]	Zingiberis Rhizoma Recens	3 pc.
jīng jiè suì	schizonepeta [spike]	Schizonepetae Flos	2.4 g.

MODIFICATIONS

In cases of severe vacuity, the prescription is reinforced to supplement qi. Add:

rén shēn	ginseng	Ginseng Radix	6 g.

Method: Administer one prescription daily or one every two days, ten prescriptions per therapeutic course.

POSTPARTUM SYNCOPE

Chǎn Hòu Xuè Yūn

1. Blood Depletion and Qi Desertion - 2. Blood Stasis and Qi Blockage

In traditional Chinese medicine postpartum syncope *(chǎn hòu xuè yūn)* is a condition manifesting as the sudden onset of vertigo and blurred vision, the inability to sit or stand upright, nausea, vomiting, discomfort or congestion in the chest or loss of consciousness following childbirth.

ETIOLOGY AND PATHOGENESIS

The etiology and pathogenesis of postpartum syncope are differentiated as vacuity and repletion types. Vacuity patterns generally arise in women with pre-existing constitutional qi and blood vacuity, coupled with excessive blood loss during delivery. With excessive blood loss, qi deserts with the blood, failing to nourish the heart and resulting in syncope. Repletion patterns, in contrast, are because of an invasion of cold during delivery. Consequent coagulation of blood leads to blood stasis and internal blockage of qi, which rises, disturbs the heart and causes syncope.

1. DEPLETION OF BLOOD AND ESCAPE OF QI

Clinical Manifestations: Excessive postpartum blood loss, acute onset, vertigo, palpitations, sudden paling of the complexion followed by gradual loss of consciousness with closed eyes, open mouth, cold extremities and cold copious perspiration in severe cases.

Tongue: Pale.

Pulse: Barely perceptible; empty.

Treatment Method: Supplement qi, secure yang qi desertion.

PRESCRIPTION

Pure Ginseng Decoction *dú shēn tāng*

rén shēn	ginseng	Ginseng Radix	30 g.

Decoct with a slow boil and take as a single dose.

<u>MODIFICATIONS</u>

In cases of excessive perspiration and cold extremities, the prescription is modified to revitalize depleted yang, stem counterflow and return the yang.
Use:

Ginseng and Aconite Decoction *shēn fù tāng*

rén shēn	ginseng	Ginseng Radix	30 g.
zhì fù zǐ	aconite [accessory tuber] (processed)	Aconiti Tuber Laterale Praeparatum	15 g.

In cases accompanied by continued vaginal bleeding, the prescription is modified to relieve bleeding.
Add:

fú lóng gān	oven earth (wrapped) (extended decoction)	Terra Flava Usta	30 g.
pào jiāng	blast-fried ginger [root]	Zingiberis Rhizoma Tostum	6 g.
ài yè tàn	mugwort [leaf] (charred)	Artemisiae Argyi Folium	9 g.
xiān hè cǎo	agrimony	Agrimoniae Herba	12 g.

ACUPUNCTURE AND MOXIBUSTION

Main points: Needle with supplementation; add moxibustion.

CV-04	*guān yuán*
CV-06	*qì hǎi*
SP-06	*sān yīn jiāo*
ST-36	*zú sān lǐ*

Auxiliary points:

For vaginal bleeding, add:

SP-01	*yǐn bái*
LR-01	*dà dūn*

For palpitations, add:

HT-07	*shén mén*
PC-04	*xī mén*

2. BLOOD STASIS AND QI BLOCKAGE

Clinical Manifestations: Retention of lochia or passage of a small amount of lochia after childbirth, periodic lower abdominal pain aggravated upon external pressure, discomfort and congestion in the chest, rapid breathing; or loss of consciousness with hands clenched into fists, trismus (jaw tetany), dark purplish complexion, purple lips.

Tongue: Purple.

Pulse: Rough.

Treatment Method: Move qi, quicken the blood, dispel blood stasis.

PRESCRIPTION

Life-Clutching Powder *duó mìng sǎn*

mò yào	myrrh	Myrrha	9 g.
xuè jié	dragon's blood (powdered and stirred in)	Daemonoropis Draconis Resina	1 g.

MODIFICATIONS

To quicken the blood and move qi, add:

dāng guī	tangkuei	Angelicae Sinensis Radix	12 g.
chuān xiōng	ligusticum [root]	Ligustici Rhizoma	9 g.

In cases accompanied by oppression in the chest, nausea or vomiting, the prescription is modified downbear qi.

Add:

jiāng bàn xià	pinellia [tuber] (ginger-processed)	Pinelliae Tuber Praeparatum	9 g.

ACUPUNCTURE AND MOXIBUSTION

Main points: Needle with draining; add moxibustion.

CV-03	*zhōng jí*
CV-07	*yīn jiāo*
SP-06	*sān yīn jiāo*
TB-06	*zhī gōu*
SP-04	*gōng sūn*

Auxiliary points:

For syncope, add:

GV-26	*rén zhōng*
GV-20	*bǎi huì*
KI-01	*yǒng quán*

For lower abdominal pain aggravated by pressure, add:

ST-29	*guī lái*

For hands clenched into fists with trismus (jaw tetany), add:

LR-03	*tài chōng*
LI-04	*hé gǔ*
ST-06	*jiá chē*

ALTERNATE THERAPEUTIC METHODS

1. Ear Acupuncture

Main points: *Shén Mén*, Sympathetic, Liver, Uterus.

Method: Needle to elicit a strong sensation and retain needles one to two hours, manipulating at intervals.

REMARKS

Postpartum syncope may be classified as either repletion or vacuity. Vacuity will manifest as a desertion pattern following excessive blood loss from delivery. Excess will manifest as a tension pattern from coagulation by cold and blood stasis. Regardless of repletion or vacuity, postpartum blood dizziness is an acute condition requiring immediate emergency care. When necessary, traditional Chinese treatment should be combined with Western medicine to ensure prompt relief of pressing symptoms.

LOCHIORRHEA
È Lù Bù Jué

1. Vacuous Qi Failing to Contain Blood · 2. Blood-Heat · 3. Uterine Static Blood Obstruction

Lochiorrhea refers to postpartum patterns where the vaginal discharge of lochia continues for a period of more than twenty days after delivery. When prompt treatment is not undertaken, excessive blood loss can lead to depletion of yin and blood or the invasion of an opportunistic infection that gives rise to a secondary pattern.

ETIOLOGY AND PATHOGENESIS

The major factor in the development of lochiorrhea is pathological change of the *chōng* and *rèn* causing a disruption of the harmonious flow of qi and blood. The *chōng mài* is the sea of blood and the *rèn mài* regulates the uterus and grows the fetus. Blood originates in the viscera and bowels then flows into the *chōng* and *rèn* before being transformed to lochia. Pathological changes of the viscera and bowels that lead to a weakening of these functions may therefore bring about the prolonged discharge of lochia.

Etiological factors include first the weakening of qi of the *chōng* and *rèn*. This may be from a pre-existing qi vacuity in the mother, a loss of blood and consumption of qi during childbirth; or the lack of sufficient postnatal rest and recuperation.

Second, the *chōng* and *rèn* may be damaged by heat, causing blood to escape the vessels. This may be from excessive blood loss during childbirth in patients with a pre-existing yin vacuity; the formation of internal heat; stagnation of liver qi with resultant heat; invasion of external heat evil; or excessive consumption of warm dry herbal medicines in the postpartum period.

Finally, following childbirth, the uterine network vessels are subject to blood stasis and internal obstruction. This may be from invasion by cold evil into the depleted *chōng* and *rèn*, or from retention of a fragment of the placenta. In either case, blood flowing outside the vessels may lead to a continuous discharge of lochia for a protracted period.

1. VACUOUS QI FAILING TO CONTAIN BLOOD

Clinical Manifestations: Continuous discharge of a large volume of light red thin odorless lochia, bearing down sensation in the lower abdomen, tiredness, fatigue, disinclination to speak and a pale complexion.

Tongue: Pale.

Pulse: Weak, tardy.

Treatment Method: Supplement qi, contain the blood.

PRESCRIPTION
Center-Supplementing Qi-Boosting Decoction *bǔ zhōng yì qì tāng*

huáng qí	astragalus [root]	Astragali (seu Hedysari) Radix	15 g.
rén shēn	ginseng	Ginseng Radix	9 g.
bái zhú	ovate atractylodes [root]	Atractylodis Ovatae Rhizoma	9 g.
dāng guī	tangkuei	Angelicae Sinensis Radix	9 g.
chén pí	tangerine [peel]	Citri Exocarpium	6 g.
shēng mā	cimicifuga [root]	Cimicifugae Rhizoma	3 g.
chái hú	bupleurum [root]	Bupleuri Radix	3 g.
zhì gān cǎo	licorice [root] (honey-fried)	Glycyrrhizae Radix	6 g.

MODIFICATIONS

To warm yang, boost qi and contain the blood, the prescription is enhanced by adding:

lù jiǎo jiāo	deerhorn glue (dissolved and stirred-in)	Cervi Gelatinum Cornu	9 g.
ài yè tàn	mugwort [leaf] (charred)	Artemisiae Argyi Folium	9 g.

ACUPUNCTURE AND MOXIBUSTION

Main points: Needle with supplementation; add moxibustion.

CV-04	*guān yuán*
ST-36	*zú sān lǐ*
SP-06	*sān yīn jiāo*
CV-06	*qì hǎi*

Auxiliary points:

For bearing down sensation in the lower abdomen, add:

GV-20	*bǎi huì*
CV-12	*zhōng wǎn*

2. BLOOD-HEAT

Clinical Manifestations: Discharge of a large volume of red thick foul-smelling lochia, flushed complexion, dry mouth and throat.

Tongue: Red.

Pulse: Rapid or rapid, thready.

Treatment Method: Clear heat, nourish yin, relieve bleeding.

PRESCRIPTION
Yin-Safeguarding Brew *bǎo yīn jiān*

shēng dì huáng	rehmannia [root] dried/fresh	Rehmanniae Radix Exsiccata seu Recens	12 g.
shú dì huáng	cooked rehmannia [root]	Rehmanniae Radix Conquita	12 g.
huáng qín	scutellaria [root]	Scutellariae Radix	9 g.
huáng bǎi	phellodendron [bark]	Phellodendri Cortex	9 g.
bái sháo yào	white peony [root]	Paeoniae Radix Alba	12 g.
shān yào	dioscorea [root]	Dioscoreae Rhizoma	12 g.
xù duàn	dipsacus [root]	Dipsaci Radix	9 g.
gān cǎo	licorice [root]	Glycyrrhizae Radix	6 g.

MODIFICATIONS

To help to clear heat, nourish yin and stopp bleeding, the prescription is modified by adding:

ē jiāo	ass hide glue (dissolved and stirred-in)	Asini Corii Gelatinum	9 g.
hàn lián cǎo	eclipta	Ecliptae Herba	12 g.
hǎi piāo xiāo	cuttlefish [bone]	Sepiae seu Sepiellae Os	9 g.

In cases accompanied by liver qi stagnation, with symptoms of distention and pain of the costal regions, irritability, yellow tongue coating and rapid wiry pulse, the prescription is changed to soothe the liver, clear heat and relieve bleeding. Use:

Moutan and Gardenia Free Wanderer Powder *dān zhī xiāo yáo sǎn*

chái hú	bupleurum [root]	Bupleuri Radix	9 g.
bái sháo yào	white peony [root]	Paeoniae Radix Alba	12 g.
dāng guī	tangkuei	Angelicae Sinensis Radix	9 g.
bái zhú	ovate atractylodes [root]	Atractylodis Ovatae Rhizoma	9 g.
fú líng	poria	Poria	9 g.
mǔ dān pí	moutan [root bark]	Moutan Radicis Cortex	9 g.
shān zhī zǐ	gardenia [fruit]	Gardeniae Fructus	9 g.
zhì gān cǎo	licorice [root] (honey-fried)	Glycyrrhizae Radix	6 g.
shēng jiāng	fresh ginger [root]	Zingiberis Rhizoma Recens	3 g.
bò hé	mint (abbreviated decoction)	Menthae Herba	3 g.

plus:

shēng dì huáng	rehmannia [root] dried/fresh	Rehmanniae Radix Exsiccata seu Recens	15 g.
hàn lián cǎo	eclipta	Ecliptae Herba	12 g.
qiàn cǎo gēn	madder [root] (abbreviated decoction)	Rubiae Radix	12 g.

ACUPUNCTURE AND MOXIBUSTION

Main points: Needle with even supplementation, even draining.

CV-03	*zhōng jí*
SP-10	*xuè hǎi*
LR-06	*zhōng dū*
KI-10	*yīn gǔ*

Auxiliary points:
For stagnation of liver qi, add:

LR-02	*xíng jiān*
LR-14	*qī mén*

3. UTERINE STATIC BLOOD OBSTRUCTION

Clinical Manifestations: Dribbling discharge of a small volume of dark purplish lochia containing blood clots, spasmodic pains in the lower abdomen, pain increased with external pressure.

Tongue: Dark purplish, sometimes presenting stasis macules on the tongue.

Pulse: Wiry or deep and rough.

Treatment Method: Quicken the blood, dispel stasis.

PRESCRIPTION

Engendering Transformation Decoction *shēng huà tāng*

dāng guī	tangkuei	Angelicae Sinensis Radix	24 g.
chuān xiōng	ligusticum [root]	Ligustici Rhizoma	9 g.
táo rén	peach [kernel]	Persicae Semen	6 g.
pào jiāng	blast-fried ginger [root]	Zingiberis Rhizoma Tostum	3 g.
zhì gān cǎo	licorice [root] (honey-fried)	Glycyrrhizae Radix	3 g.

MODIFICATIONS

To reinforce removal of stasis and arresting bleeding, add:

yì mǔ cǎo	leonurus	Leonuri Herba	15 g.
pú huáng	typha pollen (wrapped)	Typhae Pollen	9 g.

In cases accompanied by qi vacuity with empty bearing down sensation in the lower abdomen, the prescription is modified to supplement qi and remove stasis. Add:

dǎng shēn	codonopsis [root]	Codonopsitis Radix	12 g.
huáng qí	astragalus [root]	Astragali (seu Hedysari) Radix	12 g.

In cases of prolonged blood stasis that has given rise to heat and foul-smelling lochia, the prescription is modified to clear heat and resolve toxin. Add:

zǎo xiū	paris [root]	Paridis Rhizoma	9 g.
pú gōng yīng	dandelion	Taraxaci Herba cum Radice	12 g.

ACUPUNCTURE AND MOXIBUSTION

Main points: Needle with draining; add moxibustion.

CV-03	*zhōng jí*
CV-06	*qì hǎi*
ST-29	*guī lái*
SP-08	*dì jī*

Auxiliary points:

For cold and pain in the umbilical region, add moxibustion to:

CV-08	*shén què*
CV-07	*yīn jiāo*

ALTERNATE THERAPEUTIC METHODS

1. Ear Acupuncture

Main points: Uterus, *Shén Mén,* Sympathetic, Endocrine, Spleen, Liver, Kidney, Subcortex.

Method: Select two to three points each session, needle to elicit a moderate sensation, and retain needles fifteen to twenty minutes. Treat once daily. Auricular needle embedding therapy may also be used.

REMARKS

During postpartum recuperation, attention must be paid to the mother's psychological state, avoiding circumstances that may generate anger, anxiety or pensiveness. Raw or cold foods should be avoided, as should overwork. Abstaining from sexual activity is wise.

INSUFFICIENT LACTATION
Rŭ Shăo
1. Qi and Blood Vacuity - 2. Liver Qi Stagnation

SUPPLEMENT: TERMINATION OF LACTATION
Huí Rŭ

Insufficient lactation (diminished lactation or scant breast milk) refers to patterns manifesting as decreased secretion of milk after childbirth resulting in an inability to satisfy the infant's need. Severe cases involve complete cessation of milk production, hence the term *rŭ zhī bù xíng* (absence of breast milk) in traditional Chinese medicine. In Western medicine this includes the conditions labeled oligogalactia, galactostasis and agalactia.

ETIOLOGY AND PATHOGENESIS

Two etiological factors are involved in insufficient lactation. The first is vacuity of qi and blood from either the weakened constitution of the mother or from excessive blood loss during childbirth, both of which affect milk production and lead to vacuity patterns.

The second factor is postpartum emotional disturbances causing liver qi stagnation and obstruction of the channels. This affects the normal flow of milk, giving rise to a repletion pattern of diminished lactation.

1. QI AND BLOOD VACUITY

Clinical Manifestations: Decreased or complete cessation of milk secretion, thin clear milk, soft flaccid breasts with no sensation of distention, lusterless complexion, tiredness, fatigue, loss of appetite, loose stools.

Tongue: Pale.

Pulse: Weak, thready.

Treatment Method: Boost qi, supplement blood, free the milk.

PRESCRIPTION
Lactation Elixir *tōng rŭ dān*

huáng qí	astragalus [root]	Astragali (seu Hedysari) Radix	30 g.
rén shēn	ginseng	Ginseng Radix	9 g.
dāng guī	tangkuei	Angelicae Sinensis Radix	12 g.
mài mén dōng	ophiopogon [tuber]	Ophiopogonis Tuber	9 g.
mù tōng	mutong [stem]	Mutong Caulis	6 g.
jié gĕng	platycodon [root]	Platycodonis Radix	6 g.

The above herbs are traditionally decocted in pig's feet soup.

MODIFICATIONS

The following substitutions are frequently made:

Delete:

| *mù tōng* | mutong [stem] | Mutong Caulis | |

Add:

| *tōng cǎo* | rice-paper plant pith | Tetrapanacis Medulla | 6 g. |

ACUPUNCTURE AND MOXIBUSTION

Main points: Needle with supplementation; add moxibustion.

CV-17	*tǎn zhōng*
ST-18	*rǔ gēn*
BL-20	*pí shū*
ST-36	*zú sān lǐ*
SI-01	*shào zé*

Auxiliary points:

For loss of appetite and loose stools, add:

| CV-12 | *zhōng wǎn* |
| ST-25 | *tiān shū* |

For excessive blood loss, add:

| BL-17 | *gé shū* |
| BL-18 | *gān shū* |

2. LIVER QI STAGNATION

Clinical Manifestations: Diminution or complete cessation of milk secretion; distention and pain of the breasts; fullness and discomfort of the chest, hypochondrium and epigastrium; psychological depression or irritability; dizziness and vertigo and loss of appetite.

Tongue: Thin, or thin yellow coating.

Pulse: Wiry.

Treatment Method: Soothe the liver, resolve depression, free the connections, promote lactation.

PRESCRIPTION

Lactation-Promoting Gushing Spring Powder *xià rǔ yǒng quán sǎn*

dāng guī	tangkuei	Angelicae Sinensis Radix	9 g.
bái sháo yào	white peony [root]	Paeoniae Radix Alba	9 g.
shēng dì huáng	rehmannia [root] dried/fresh	Rehmanniae Radix Exsiccata seu Recens	9 g.
chái hú	bupleurum [root]	Bupleuri Radix	6 g.
qīng pí	unripe tangerine [peel]	Citri Exocarpium Immaturum	9 g.
tiān huā fěn	trichosanthes [root]	Trichosanthis Radix	9 g.
lòu lú	rhaponticum-echinops [root]	Rhapontici seu Echinopis Radix	9 g.
tōng cǎo	rice-paper [plant pith]	Tetrapanacis Medulla	6 g.
jié gěng	platycodon [root]	Platycodonis Radix	6 g.
bái zhǐ	angelica [root]	Angelicae Dahuricae Radix	6 g.
chuān shān jiǎ	pangolin [scales]	Manitis Squama	9 g.
	(or, powdered and administered separately, each time 1.5 g.)		
wáng bù liú xíng	vaccaria [seed]	Vaccariae Semen	9 g.
gān cǎo	licorice [root]	Glycyrrhizae Radix	3 g.
chuān xiōng	ligusticum [root]	Ligustici Rhizoma	9 g.

MODIFICATIONS

In cases manifesting fever, the prescription is modified to clear heat. Add:

huáng qín	scutellaria [root]	Scutellariae Radix	9 g.
pú gōng yīng	dandelion	Taraxaci Herba cum Radice	9 g.

In cases where breasts are hard, distended, feverish and painful, with palpable lumps, the prescription is modified to free the connections and disperse lumps. Add:

sī guā luò	loofah	Luffae Fasciculus Vascularis	12 g.
lù lù tōng	liquidambar [fruit]	Liquidambaris Fructus	12 g.
xià kū cǎo	prunella [spike]	Prunellae Spica	12 g.

Apply externally over swollen areas:

pú gōng yīng	dandelion	Taraxaci Herba cum Radice	60 g.

(Mash fresh dandelions into a poultice or make a paste with the powder of the dried herb.)

ACUPUNCTURE AND MOXIBUSTION

Main points: Needle with draining.

CV-17	*tăn zhōng*
ST-18	*rŭ gēn*
SI-01	*shào zé*
PC-06	*nèi guān*
LR-03	*tài chōng*

Auxiliary points:

For distention and fullness of the chest and hypochondrium, add:

LR-14	*qī mén*

For epigastric fullness and distention, add:

CV-12	*zhōng wăn*
ST-36	*zú sān lĭ*

ALTERNATE THERAPEUTIC METHODS

1. Ear Acupuncture

Main points: Thorax, Endocrine, Liver, Kidney.

Method: Needle to elicit a moderate sensation and retain the needles fifteen to twenty minutes. Treat once daily.

REMARKS

The therapeutic efficacy of Chinese herbal medicine and acumoxa therapy in the treatment of diminished lactation is relatively high. During treatment, the patient's diet should include nutritious foods such as pig's feet soup and fresh carp soup, which are especially beneficial in cases of qi and blood vacuity. During the breastfeeding months, mothers should avoid emotional stress. Attention should be paid to the method of breastfeeding to ensure that proper techniques are adopted before difficulties arise.

SUPPLEMENT:

TERMINATION OF LACTATION

Huí Rŭ

For mothers who do not wish to breastfeed, one or more of the following methods of decreasing milk production can be used.

PRESCRIPTION

| *mài yá* | barley sprout | Hordei Fructus Germinatus | 200 g. |
| *chán tuì* | cicada molting | Cicadae Periostracum | 5 g. |

Decoct the given amounts in water to serve as a daily dose.

| *máng xiāo* | mirabilite | Mirabilitum | 120 g. |
| | (uncooked and crushed into dry powder.) | | |

Place the powder in a cloth bag and, after manually evacuating the breast, hold the bag firmly over the breast. After this first bag has become saturated with milk, repeat with a second bag.

ACUPUNCTURE AND MOXIBUSTION

Main Points: Needle with draining and follow with ten minutes of moxibustion.

GB-41   *zú lín qì*
GB-37   *guāng míng*

Treat once daily for a total of three to five days.

PART VI

PEDIATRICS

WHOOPING COUGH

Dùn Ké

1A. Initial Coughing Stage: External Wind-Cold - 1B. Initial Coughing Stage: External Wind-Heat - 2. Spasmodic Coughing Stage - 3A. Recovery Stage: Lung Yin Vacuity - 3B. Recovery Stage: Spleen and Stomach Qi Vacuity

Whooping cough is a common pediatric infectious respiratory disease. It is characterized by a recurring spasmodic cough marked by the sound made during inspiration which resembles a rooster's crow. Since this cough often alleviates spontaneously then begins again, it is called "paroxysmal cough." Because of its long course, averaging five to twelve weeks, paroxysmal cough is also known as the "hundred days cough." In Western medicine, it is known as pertussis.

Paroxysmal coughs may occur during any season, but are most prevalent during winter and spring. Children under the age of five are most likely to be infected.

ETIOLOGY AND PATHOGENESIS

The major cause of whooping cough is attack by seasonal external evils resulting in phlegm-turbidity, dysfunction of the ability of the lung to downbear and the upward counterflow ascent of lung qi.

Paroxysmal cough is clinically categorized into three stages. During the initial coughing stage, it presents as an external pattern of the defense aspect *(wèi)* and is similar to the common cold. With continued development, the coughing gradually becomes more severe as seasonal evils accumulate and are transformed into phlegm-heat. This second development is the spasmodic coughing stage. Although the lung is most affected during this stage, other internal organs may also become involved, leading to various secondary patterns. In the final recovery stage, evils have been dispelled for the most part, but the qi is still depleted. Pathological changes at this stage are mainly in the lung and spleen.

1A. INITIAL COUGHING STAGE: EXTERNAL WIND COLD

Clinical Manifestations: Coughing with thin white foamy phlegm, fever, sneezing, runny nose.

Tongue: Thin white coating.

Pulse: Floating, with a light red index vessel.

Treatment Method: Dispel wind, dissipate cold, diffuse the lung, relieve coughing.

PRESCRIPTION

Apricot Kernel and Perilla Powder *xìng sū sǎn*

xìng rén	apricot [kernel] (abbreviated decoction)	Armeniacae Semen	*6 g.	(1.5-3 g.)
zǐ sū yè	perilla [leaf]	Perillae Folium	6 g.	(1.5-3 g.)
zhǐ ké	bitter orange [fruit]	Aurantii Fructus	6 g.	(1.5-3 g.)
qián hú	peucedanum [root]	Peucedani Radix	6 g.	(1.5-3 g.)
jié gěng	platycodon [root]	Platycodonis Radix	6 g.	(1.5-3 g.)
zhì bàn xià	(processed) pinellia	Pinelliae Tuber Praeparatum	6 g.	(1.5-3 g.)
fú líng	poria	Poria	6 g.	(1.5-3 g.)
chén pí	tangerine [peel]	Citri Exocarpium	6 g.	(1.5-3 g.)
shēng jiāng	fresh ginger [root]	Zingiberis Rhizoma Recens	6 g.	(1.5-3 g.)
gān cǎo	licorice [root]	Glycyrrhizae Radix	6 g.	(1.5-3 g.)
dà zǎo	jujube	Ziziphi Fructus	2 pc.	(1-2 pc.)

*(Note: Generally speaking, the dose of each ingredient of a decoction for a child at or over five years of age is half of that for an adult. For a child under five it is one quarter of the adult dose. The doses given in parenthesis are for reference only.)

MODIFICATIONS

In cases where cold evil is predominant, the prescription is changed to dissipate cold, diffuse the lung, transform phlegm and relieve coughing.
Use:

Florid Canopy Powder *huá gài sǎn*

má huáng	ephedra	Ephedrae Herba	6 g.	(1.5-3 g.)
xìng rén	apricot [kernel] (abbreviated decoction)	Armeniacae Semen	9 g.	(3-4.5 g.)
zǐ sū zǐ	perilla [fruit]	Perillae Fructus	9 g.	(3-4.5 g.)
sāng bái pí	mulberry [root bark]	Mori Radicis Cortex	9 g.	(3-4.5 g.)
fú líng	poria	Poria	6 g.	(1.5-3 g.)
chén pí	tangerine [peel]	Citri Exocarpium	6 g.	(1.5-3 g.)
zhì gān cǎo	licorice [root]	Glycyrrhizae Radix	6 g.	(1.5-3 g.)
plus:				
bǎi bù	stemona [root]	Stemonae Radix	9 g.	(3-4.5 g.)
fǎ bàn xià	pinellia [tuber] (processed)	Pinelliae Tuber Praeparatum	9 g.	(3-4.5 g.)

ACUPUNCTURE AND MOXIBUSTION

Main Points: Needle with draining; add moxibustion.

BL-12	fēng mén
LU-07	liè quē
LI-04	hé gǔ
TB-05	wài guān

1B. INITIAL COUGHING STAGE: EXTERNAL WIND-HEAT

Clinical Manifestations: Coughing with thick sticky yellow phlegm that is difficult to expectorate, chills and fever, sore red throat

Tongue: Thin yellow coating.

Pulse: Floating; with a light red index vessel.

Treatment Method: Dispel wind, clear heat, diffuse the lung, relieve coughing.

PRESCRIPTION

Mulberry Leaf and Chrysanthemum Beverage *sāng jú yǐn*

sāng yè	mulberry [leaf]	Mori Folium	9 g.	(3-4.5 g.)
jú huā	chrysanthemum [flower]	Chrysanthemi Flos	9 g.	(3-4.5 g.)
lián qiào	forsythia [fruit]	Forsythiae Fructus	9 g.	(3-4.5 g.)
lú gēn	phragmites [root]	Phragmititis Rhizoma	9 g.	(3-4.5 g.)
xìng rén	apricot [kernel] (abbreviated decoction)	Armeniacae Semen	9 g.	(3-4.5 g.)
jié gěng	platycodon [root]	Platycodonis Radix	9 g.	(3-4.5 g.)
bò hé	mint (abbreviated decoction)	Menthae Herba	6 g	(1.5-3 g.)
gān cǎo	licorice [root]	Glycyrrhizae Radix	6 g.	(1.5-3 g.)

<u>MODIFICATIONS</u>

In cases where heat evil is predominant, the prescription is changed to clear heat, diffuse the lung, transform phlegm and relieve coughing. Use:

Ephedra, Apricot Kernel, Gypsum and Licorice Decoction *má xìng shí gān tāng*

má huáng	ephedra	Ephedrae Herba	6 g.	(1.5-3 g.)
xìng rén	apricot [kernel] (abbreviated decoction)	Armeniacae Semen	9 g.	(3-4.5 g.)
shí gāo	gypsum (extended decoction)	Gypsum	30 g.	(9-15 g.)
zhì gān cǎo plus:	licorice [root] (honey-fried)	Glycyrrhizae Radix	6 g.	(1.5-3 g.)
bǎi bù	stemona [root]	Stemonae Radix		3-4.5 g.

When phlegm is thick, yellow and difficult to expectorate, further additions may be required to clear heat and transform phlegm. Combine with:

Indigo and Clamshell Powder *dài gé sǎn*

qīng dài	indigo (stirred in)	Indigo Pulverata Levis	3 g.	(1-1.5 g.)
hǎi gé ké	clamshell (powdered and wrapped)	Cyclinae (seu Meretricis) Concha	12 g.	(3-6 g.)
guā lóu plus:	trichosanthes [fruit]	Trichosanthis Fructus	6–9 g.	(1.5-3 g.)

ACUPUNCTURE AND MOXIBUSTION

Main Points: Needle with draining.

BL-12	*fēng mén*
LU-07	*liè quē*
LU-05	*chǐ zé*
GV-14	*dà zhuī*

Auxiliary points:

For itchy and inflamed throat, bleed:

LU-11	*shào shāng*

2. SPASMODIC COUGHING STAGE

Clinical Manifestations: A recurring spasmodic cough manifesting in extended bouts of continuous coughing. The sound of the cough during deep inhalation is similar to a rooster's crow. Temporary relief from coughing is seen only after the expectoration of phlegm or the vomiting of food matter. During the night the coughing becomes more severe. Accompanying symptoms include fever, dry mouth, constipation, concentrated urine, blood-streaked phlegm, epistaxis or (in some cases) subconjunctival hemorrhage.

Pulse: Rapid, slippery, with a purplish-red index vessel.

Tongue: Red with yellow coating.

Treatment Method: Clear heat, drain the lung, transform phlegm, relieve coughing.

PRESCRIPTION

Mulberry Root Bark Decoction *sāng bái pí tāng*

sāng bái pí	mulberry [root bark]	Mori Radicis Cortex	12 g.	(3-6.0 g.)
fǎ bàn xià	pinellia [tuber] (processed)	Pinelliae Tuber Praeparatum	9 g.	(3-4.5 g.)
zǐ sū zǐ	perilla [fruit]	Perillae Fructus	9 g.	(3-4.5 g.)
xìng rén	apricot [kernel] (abbreviated decoction)	Armeniacae Semen	9 g.	(3-4.5 g.)
zhè bèi mǔ	Zhejiang fritillaria [bulb]	Fritillariae Verticillatae Bulbus	9 g.	(3-4.5 g.)
huáng qín	scutellaria [root]	Scutellariae Radix	9 g.	(3-4.5 g.)
huáng lián	coptis [root]	Coptidis Rhizoma	6 g.	(1.5-3 g.)
shān zhī zǐ	gardenia [fruit]	Gardeniae Fructus	9 g.	(3-4.5 g.)

MODIFICATIONS

In cases of continuous spasmodic coughing, the prescription is modified to relax spasms and suppress coughing. Add:

bái jiāng cán	silkworm	Bombyx Batryticatus	3-6.0 g.
wú gōng	centipede	Scolopendra	0.5-1.5 g.

In cases of coughing with repeated vomiting affecting food intake, the prescription is modified to harmonize the stomach and downbear lung qi. Add:

dài zhě shí	hematite (extended decoction)	Haematitum	6-12 g.
pí pá yè	loquat [leaf]	Eriobotryae Folium	3-6 g.

In cases of hacking cough with scanty phlegm and red tongue with little coating, the prescription is modified to moisten the lung and relieve coughing.

Delete:

huáng qín	scutellaria [root]	Scutellariae Radix
huáng lián	coptis [root]	Coptidis Rhizoma

Add:

běi shā shēn	glehnia [root]	Glehniae Radix	3-6 g.
tiān mén dōng	asparagus [tuber]	Asparagi Tuber	3-6 g.
mài mén dōng	ophiopogon [tuber]	Ophiopogonis Tuber	3-6 g

In cases with coughing up of blood, epistaxis and subconjunctival hemorrhage, the prescription is modified to cool the blood and relieve bleeding. Add:

bái máo gēn	imperata [root]	Imperatae Rhizoma	6-12 g.
cè bǎi yè	biota [leaf]	Biotae Folium	3-6 g.
sān qī	notoginseng [root]	Notoginseng Radix	3-4.5 g.

In cases of red swollen eyes, the prescription is modified to clear liver fire. Add:

lóng dǎn cǎo	gentian [root]	Gentianae Radix	1.5-3 g.

ACUPUNCTURE AND MOXIBUSTION

Main Points: Needle with draining.

GV-14	*dà zhuī*
GV-12	*shēn zhù*
LU-05	*chǐ zé*
ST-40	*fēng lóng*

Auxiliary points:

For fever, add:

LI-11	*qū chí*

For coughing blood and epistaxis, add:

LU-06	*kǒng zuì*
GV-23	*shàng xīng*

3A. RECOVERY STAGE: LUNG YIN VACUITY

Clinical Manifestations: A decrease in frequency and severity of coughing; dry cough with little phlegm, dry throat and thirst.

Pulse: Rapid, thready, with a pale greenish index vessel.

Tongue: Red with peeled coating.

Treatment Method: Supplement yin, moisten the lung, relieve coughing.

PRESCRIPTION

Adenophora/Glehnia and Ophiopogon Decoction *shā shēn mài dōng tāng*

běi shā shēn	glehnia [root]	Glehniae Radix	9 g	(3-4.5 g)
mài mén dōng	ophiopogon [tuber]	Ophiopogonis Tuber	9 g.	(3-4.5 g.)
tiān huā fěn	trichosanthes [root]	Trichosanthis Radix	12 g	(3-6 g.)
yù zhú	Solomon's seal [root]	Polygonati Yuzhu Rhizoma	9 g.	(3-4.5 g.)
biǎn dòu	lablab [bean]	Lablab Semen	12 g.	(3-6 g.)
sāng yè	mulberry [leaf]	Mori Folium	6 g.	(3-4.5 g.)
gān cǎo	licorice [root]	Glycyrrhizae Radix	6 g	(3-4.5 g.)

MODIFICATIONS

The prescription is often reinforced to transform phlegm and relieve coughing. Add:

jié gěng	platycodon [root]	Platycodonis Radix	3-4.5 g.
xìng rén	apricot [kernel] (abbreviated decoction)	Armeniacae Semen	3-4.5 g.

In cases where phlegm is difficult to expectorate with dry stools, the prescription is modified to transform phlegm and free the stool. Add:

guā lóu	trichosanthes [fruit]	Trichosanthis Fructus	6-9 g.

ACUPUNCTURE AND MOXIBUSTION

Main Points: Needle with supplementation.

BL-13	*fèi shū*
LU-09	*tài yuān*
ST-36	*zú sān lǐ*
BL-43 (38)	*gāo huāng shū*
KI-03	*tài xī*

3B. RECOVERY STAGE: SPLEEN AND STOMACH QI VACUITY

Clinical Manifestations: Forceless coughing with thin phlegm, shortness of breath, tiredness, fatigue, loss of appetite, spontaneous perspiration.

Tongue: Pale with white coating.

Pulse: Thready, weak, with a pale-greenish index vessel.

Treatment Method: Strengthen spleen and stomach qi, relieve coughing.

PRESCRIPTION

Ginseng and Schisandra Decoction *rén shēn wǔ wèi zǐ tāng*

rén shēn	ginseng	Ginseng Radix	6 g.	(1.5-3 g.)
bái zhú	ovate atractylodes [root]	Atractylodis Ovatae Rhizoma	6 g.	(1.5-3 g.)
fú líng	poria	Poria	6 g.	(1.5-3 g.)
wǔ wèi zǐ	schisandra [berry]	Schisandrae Fructus	3 g.	(1-1.5 g.)
mài mén dōng	ophiopogon [tuber]	Ophiopogonis Tuber	6 g.	(1.5-3 g.)
zhì gān cǎo	licorice [root] (honey-fried)	Glycyrrhizae Radix	6 g.	(1.5-3 g.)
shēng jiāng	fresh ginger [root]	Zingiberis Rhizoma Recens	2 g.	(0.5-1 g.)
dà zǎo	jujube	Ziziphi Fructus	2 pc.	(1-2 pc.)

MODIFICATIONS

In cases with spontaneous perspiration and a tendency to catch colds, the prescription is modified to boost qi and consolidate the surface.

Add:

huáng qí	astragalus [root]	Astragali (seu Hedysari) Radix	6-9 g.
fáng fēng	ledebouriella [root]	Ledebouriellae Radix	3-4.5 g.

ACUPUNCTURE AND MOXIBUSTION

Main Points: Needle with supplementation.

BL-13	fèi shū
BL-20	pí shū
LU-09	tài yuān
ST-36	zú sān lǐ

Auxiliary points:

For poor appetite and loose stools, add:

CV-12	zhōng wǎn
ST-25	tiān shū
CV-06	qì hǎi

For lack of warmth in the extremities, add:

CV-04	guān yuán

ALTERNATE THERAPEUTIC METHODS

1. Ear Acupuncture

Main Points: Trachea, Lung, *Shén Mén*, Sympathetic.

Method: Select two or three points each session and needle to elicit a moderate sensation. Needle ears alternately once daily.

2. Plum-Blossom Needle Therapy

Main Points: Needle once daily to elicit a moderate sensation:

Governor Vessel channel: along the channel over back and nape of neck

GV-14	*dà zhuī*
CV-12	*zhōng wǎn*
PC-06	*nèi guān*
LU-09	*tài yuān*
ST-40	*fēng lóng*

REMARKS

During treatment patients should get ample bed-rest in a well-ventilated room exposed to plenty of sunlight. Hot spicy foods, smoke and other irritating substances should be avoided.

INFANTILE DIARRHEA

Xiǎo Ér Fù Xiè

1. Food Stagnation - 2. Damp-Heat - 3. Wind-Cold - 4. Spleen Qi Vacuity - 5. Spleen and Kidney Yang Vacuity

Infantile diarrhea is characterized by an increase in frequency of bowel movements and a loose, runny or even watery consistency of stools. A commonly observed pediatric illnesses, it is especially prevalent in children under two years of age. In general, the younger the age, the higher the occurrence of diarrhea. Infantile diarrhea may occur in any of the four seasons, although it is most prevalent during summer and autumn.

ETIOLOGY AND PATHOGENESIS

During the early years of life, the viscera and bowels are tender and the transporting and transforming functions of the spleen and stomach are frail. Hence, diarrhea easily develops as a result of external evils, internal injury from dietary imbalance, weakening of the spleen and stomach during extended illness or depletion of spleen and kidney yang. If treatment is not adequate, diarrhea may give rise to more critical patterns such as injury to yin, injury to yang or injury to both yin and yang.

1. FOOD STAGNATION

Clinical Manifestations: Abdominal distention, borborygmus, intermittent abdominal pain followed by the passage of runny foul-smelling stools, alleviation of pain after moving the bowels, frequent belching, vomiting of undigested food (in some cases), loss of appetite, restless sleep.

Tongue: Thick slimy coating.

Pulse: Slippery.

Treatment Method: Disperse food, abduct stagnation.

PRESCRIPTION

Harmony-Preserving Pill bǎo hé wán

shān zhā	crataegus [fruit]	Crataegi Fructus	18 g.	(4.5-9 g.)
shén qū	medicated leaven	Massa Medicata Fermentata	9 g.	(3-4.5 g.)
zhì bàn xià	pinellia [tuber] (processed)	Pinelliae Tuber Praeparatum	9 g.	(3-4.5 g.)
fú líng	poria	Poria	9 g.	(3-4.5 g.)
chén pí	tangerine [peel]	Citri Exocarpium	6 g.	(1.5-3 g.)
lián qiáo	forsythia [fruit]	Forsythiae Fructus	6 g.	(1.5-3 g.)
lái fú zǐ	radish [seed]	Raphani Semen	6 g.	(1.5-3 g.)

MODIFICATIONS

In cases of severe abdominal pain and distention, the prescription is modified to regulate qi, disperse distention and relieve pain. Add:

mù xiāng	saussurea [root]	Saussureae (seu Vladimiriae) Radix	3-4.5 g.
hòu pò	magnolia [bark]	Magnoliae Cortex	3-4.5 g.

In cases of severe vomiting, add:

huò xiāng	agastache-patchouli	Agastaches seu Pogostemi Herba	3-4.5 g.
shēng jiāng	fresh ginger [root]	Zingiberis Rhizoma Recens	3-4.5 g.

ACUPUNCTURE AND MOXIBUSTION

Main Points: Needle with draining.

CV-12	*zhōng wǎn*
CV-11	*jiàn lǐ*
ST-25	*tiān shū*
CV-06	*qì hǎi*
ST-36	*zú sān lǐ*
M-LE-1	*lǐ nèi tíng* (Li Inner Court)

Auxiliary points:

For vomiting, add:

PC-06	*nèi guān*
CV-13	*shàng wǎn*

For abdominal pain and distention, add:

CV-10	*xià wǎn*
LI-04	*hé gǔ*

2. DAMP-HEAT

Cinical Manifestations: Runny yellow foul-smelling stools often containing small amounts of mucus; abdominal pain, fever, thirst, burning sensation of the anus, dark scanty urine.

Tongue: Yellow slimy coating.

Pulse: Rapid, slippery.

Treatment Method: Clear heat, disinhibit dampness.

PRESCRIPTION

Pueraria, Scutellaria and Coptis Decoction
gé gēn huáng qín huáng lián tāng

gé gēn	pueraria [root]	Puerariae Radix	15 g.	(4.5-9 g.)
huáng lián	coptis [root]	Coptidis Rhizoma	9 g.	(3-4.5 g.)
huáng qín	scutellaria [root]	Scutellariae Radix	6 g.	(1.5-3 g.)
zhì gān cǎo	licorice [root] (honey-fried)	Glycyrrhizae Radix	6 g	(1.5-3 g.)

MODIFICATIONS

In cases where urine is dark and scanty, the prescription is modified to reinforce heat clearing and dampness draining. Add:

huá shí	talcum (wrapped)	Talcum	3-6 g.
gān cǎo	licorice [root]	Glycyrrhizae Radix	0.5-1 g.

In cases of severe abdominal pain, the prescription is modified to regulate qi and relieve pain.
Add:

bái sháo yào	white peony [root]	Paeoniae Radix Alba	3-4.5 g.
mù xiāng	saussurea [root]	Saussureae (seu Vladimiriae) Radix	3-4.5 g.

In cases of frequent vomiting, the prescription is modified to downbear qi and relieve vomiting.
Add:

jiāng bàn xià	pinellia [tuber]	Pinelliae Tuber Praeparatum (ginger-processed)	3-4.5 g.
shēng jiāng	fresh ginger	Zingiberis Rhizoma Recens	1.5-3 g.

In cases where damp evil is predominant, with thick slimy tongue coating and mild thirst, the prescription is modified to dry dampness.
Add:

hòu pò	magnolia bark	Magnoliae Cortex	3-4.5 g.
cāng zhú	atractylodes [root]	Atractylodis Rhizoma	3-4.5 g.

In cases where heat evil is prevalent, with symptoms including high fever, irritability, and excessive thirst, the prescription is modified to clear heat.
Add:

shí gāo	gypsum (extended decoction)	Gypsum	9-15 g.

ACUPUNCTURE AND MOXIBUSTION

Main Points: Needle with draining.

CV-12	*zhōng wǎn*
ST-25	*tiān shū*
LI-11	*qū chí*
ST-36	*zú sān lǐ*
ST-44	*nèi tíng*

Auxiliary points:

For high fever, add:

LI-04	*hé gǔ*
GV-14	*dà zhuī*

For predominant dampness, add:

SP-09	*yīn líng quán*

3. WIND-COLD

Clinical Manifestations: Thin clear often foamy stools without marked foul odor, borborygmus, abdominal pain, fever and in some cases aversion to cold.

Tongue: White slimy coating.

Pulse: Slippery or floating.

Treatment Method: Dispel wind, dissipate cold.

PRESCRIPTION

Agastache/Patchouli Qi-Righting Powder *huò xiāng zhèng qì sǎn*

huò xiāng	agastache/patchouli	Agastaches seu Pogostemi Herba	6 g.	(1.5-3 g.)
zǐ sū yè	perilla [leaf] (abbreviated decoction)	Perillae Folium	4.5 g.	(1-3 g.)
bái zhǐ	angelica [root]	Angelicae Dahuricae Radix	3 g.	(1-1.5 g.)
dà fù pí	areca [husk]	Arecae Pericarpium	3 g.	(1-1.5 g.)
fú líng	poria	Poria	9 g.	(3-4.5 g.)
bái zhú	ovate atractylodes [root]	Atractylodis Ovatae Rhizoma	6 g.	(1.5-3 g.)
chén pí	tangerine [peel]	Citri Exocarpium	6 g.	(1.5-3 g.)
jiāng bàn xià	pinellia [tuber] (ginger-processed)	Pinelliae Tuber Praeparatum	6 g.	(1.5-3 g.)
hòu pò	magnolia [bark]	Magnoliae Cortex	3 g.	(1-1.5 g.)
jié gěng	platycodon [root]	Platycodonis Radix	4.5 g.	(1-3 g.)
zhì gān cǎo	licorice [root] (honey-fried)	Glycyrrhizae Radix	3 g.	(1-1.5 g.)
shēng jiāng	fresh ginger root]	Zingiberis Rhizoma Recens	3 g.	(1-1.5 g.)
dà zǎo	jujube	Ziziphi Fructus	2 pc.	(1-2 pc.)

MODIFICATIONS

In cases of severe abdominal pain, the prescription is modified to regulate qi and relieve pain.

Add:

mù xiāng	saussurea [root]	Saussureae (seu Vladimiriae) Radix	3-4.5 g.
shā rén	amomum [fruit] (abbreviated decoction)	Amomi Semen seu Fructus	1.5-3 g.

In cases accompanied by food accumulation and stagnation, the prescription is modified to disperse food and abduct stagnation.

Add:

shān zhā	crataegus [fruit]	Crataegi Fructus	3-6 g.
shén qū	medicated leaven	Massa Medicata Fermentata	3-6 g.

In cases with dark scanty urine, the prescription is modified to disinhibit dampness and free and disinhibit urine.

Add:

zé xiè	alisma [tuber]	Alismatis Rhizoma	3-6 g.
zhū líng	polyporus	Polyporus	3-6 g.

ACUPUNCTURE AND MOXIBUSTION

Main Points: Needle with draining; add moxibustion.

CV-12	*zhōng wǎn*
ST-25	*tiān shū*
LI-04	*hé gǔ*
ST-37	*shàng jù xū*
SP-09	*yīn líng quán*

Auxiliary points:

For severe abdominal pain and diarrhea, add moxibustion.

CV-08	*shén què*

For vomiting and abdominal distention, add:

PC-06	*nèi guān*
SP-04	*gōng sūn*

4. SPLEEN QI VACUITY

Cinical Manifestations: Pale-colored liquid stools without marked foul odor, bowel movements often occurring directly after meals, variation in severity of diarrhea, sallow complexion, poor appetite, emaciation, lassitude, fatigue.

Tongue: Pale with white coating.

Pulse: Tardy, thready.

Treatment Method: Fortify the spleen, boost qi.

PRESCRIPTION

Ginseng, Poria and Ovate Atractylodes Powder *shēn líng bái-zhú sǎn*

rén shēn	ginseng	Ginseng Radix	12 g.	(3-6 g.)
bái zhú	ovate atractylodes [root]	Atractylodis Ovatae Rhizoma	12 g.	(3-6 g.)
fú líng	poria	Poria	12 g.	(3-6 g.)
shān yào	dioscorea [root]	Dioscoreae Rhizoma	12 g.	(3-6 g.)
bái biǎn dòu	lablab [bean]	Lablab Semen	9 g.	(3-4.5 g.)
lián zǐ	lotus [fruit-seed]	Nelumbinis Fructus seu Semen	6 g.	(1.5-3 g.)
yì yǐ rén	coix [seed]	Coicis Semen	6 g.	(1.5-3 g.)
shā rén	amomum [fruit] (abbreviated decoction)	Amomi Semen seu Fructus	6 g.	(1.5-3 g.)
jié gěng	platycodon [root]	Platycodonis Radix	6 g.	(1.5-3 g.)
zhì gān cǎo	licorice [root] (honey-fried)	Glycyrrhizae Radix	12 g.	(3-6 g.)

MODIFICATIONS

In cases of abdominal distention and pain, the prescription is modified to regulate qi and relieve pain.
Add:

mù xiāng	saussurea [root]	Saussureae (seu Vladimiriae) Radix	3-4.5 g.

In cases of prolonged diarrhea without signs of food accumulation and stagnation, the prescription is modified to consolidate retention and relieve diarrhea.
Add:

hē zǐ	chebule [fruit]	Chebulae Fructus	1.5-3 g.
chì shí zhī	halloysite (wrapped)	Halloysitum Rubrum	3-6 g.

In cases where stools are watery with undigested food, the prescription is modified to warm the middle burner and dissipate cold.
Add:

gān jiāng	dried ginger [root]	Zingiberis Rhizoma Exsiccatum	3-6 g.

ACUPUNCTURE AND MOXIBUSTION

Main Points: Needle with supplementation; add moxibustion.

BL-20	*pí shū*
CV-12	*zhōng wǎn*
ST-25	*tiān shū*
ST-36	*zú sān lǐ*
LR-13	*zhāng mén*

Auxiliary points:

For abdominal distention and pain, add:

CV-06	*qì hǎi*
SP-04	*gōng sūn*

5. SPLEEN AND KIDNEY YANG VACUITY

Cinical Manifestations: Prolonged diarrhea, bowel movements directly following meals, thin clear stools containing undigested food matter, physical cold, cold extremities, pale complexion, listlessness and in some cases anal prolapse.

Tongue: Pale with white coating.

Pulse: Weak, thready.

Treatment Method: Supplement the spleen, warm the kidney.

PRESCRIPTION

Combine Aconite Center-Rectifying Decoction *(fù-zǐ lǐ zhōng tāng)* with Four Spirits Pill *(sì shén wán)*.

Aconite Center-Rectifying Decoction *fù zǐ lǐ zhōng tāng*

zhì fù zǐ	aconite accessory tuber (processed) (extended decoction)	Processed Aconiti Tuber Laterale	6 g.	(1.5-3 g.)
rén shēn	ginseng	Ginseng Radix	9 g.	(3-4.5 g.)
bái zhú	ovate atractylodes [root]	Atractylodis Ovatae Rhizoma	9 g.	(3-4.5 g.)
pào jiāng	blast-fried ginger [root]	Zingiberis Rhizoma Tostum	6 g.	(1.5-3 g.)
zhì gān cǎo	licorice [root] (honey-fried)	Glycyrrhizae Radix	6 g.	(1.5-3 g.)

with:

Four Spirits Pill *sì shén wán*

bǔ gǔ zhī	psoralea [seed]	Psoraleae Semen	12 g.	(3-6 g.)
ròu dòu kòu	nutmeg	Myristicae Semen	6 g.	(1.5-3 g.)
wǔ wèi zǐ	schisandra [berry]	Schisandrae Fructus	6 g.	(1.5-3 g.)
wú zhū yú	evodia [fruit]	Evodiae Fructus	3 g.	(1-1.5 g.)

MODIFICATIONS

In cases of anal prolapse, the prescription is modified to upraise center qi.
Add:

huáng qí	astragalus [root]	Astragali (seu Hedysari) Radix	3-6 g.
zhì shēng má	cimicifuga [root] (honey-fried)	Cimicifugae Rhizoma	1-1.5 g.

In cases of prolonged diarrhea, the prescription is modified to consolidate retention with astringent medicines.
Add:

hē zǐ	chebule	Chebulae Fructus	1.5-3 g.
chì shí zhī	halloysite (wrapped)	Halloysitum Rubrum	3-6 g.

ACUPUNCTURE AND MOXIBUSTION

Main Points: Needle with supplementation; add moxibustion.

BL-20	*pí shū*
BL-23	*shèn shū*
ST-36	*zú sān lǐ*
ST-25	*tiān shū*
CV-06	*qì hǎi*

Auxiliary points:

For cold extremities, add moxibustion to:

    CV-04   *guān yuán*

For anal prolapse, add:

    GV-01   *cháng qiáng*
    BL-25   *dà cháng shū*
    BL-57   *chéng shān*
    GV-20   *bǎi huì* (with moxibustion)

ALTERNATE THERAPEUTIC METHODS

1. Moxibustion Therapy

Method: Locate the point at the intersection of the vertical line of the tip of the external malleolus and the line separating the lighter skin of the soles from the darker skin of the back of the feet. Apply moxibustion bilaterally with a moxa roll for ten to fifteen minutes, two to three times daily. Applicable in all types of infantile diarrhea.

2. Cupping Therapy

Main Point: BL-25 - *dà cháng shū*

Method: Apply cupping bilaterally for five to ten minutes, once daily. Applicable for all types of infantile diarrhea.

3. Umbilical Plaster Treatment

Method: Grind the following into a fine powder:

wú zhū yú	evodia [fruit]	Evodiae Fructus	30 g.
dīng xiāng	clove	Caryophylli Flos	2 g.
hú jiāo	pepper	Piperis Fructus	30 pc.

At each treatment, add aged vinegar or vegetable oil to 1.5 g. of this medicinal powder; mix to the consistency of a smooth paste. Spread the paste over the umbilical region and cover with gauze. Apply once daily. Umbilical plaster treatment is applicable in infantile diarrhea from dietary imbalance, wind cold and spleen vacuity.

REMARKS

During the treatment of infantile diarrhea, particular attention must be paid to the patient's diet. In milder cases, it is best to decrease the milk intake of the child, both by shortening the length of nursing sessions and by increasing the interval between them. In more severe cases, intake of foodstuffs is initially terminated for eight to twelve hours. Following amelioration of the patient's condition, small amounts of breast milk or other easily digested foods may be given, gradually increasing the servings.

Regulation of the diet is also important after recovery of the patient. In addition, the skin of the child's buttocks must be kept clean and dry. After each bowel movement the area must be cleaned well with warm water and talcum powder or ointment should be applied to prevent diaper rash.

INFANTILE MALNUTRITION

Xiǎo Ér Gān Jī

1. Spleen and Stomach Vacuity - 2. Infection by Parasitic Worms

Infantile malnutrition *(xiǎo ér gān jī)* is a chronic condition marked by emaciation, sallow complexion, poor hair growth, marked abdominal distention, protrusion of the superficial abdominal veins, irregular eating habits and listlessness.

The Chinese character *gān* has two meanings. The first is "sweet," which refers to the etiology of the condition, namely, injury of the spleen and stomach by excessive consumption of rich sweet foods. The second meaning is "dry" or "polelike," describing the clinical manifestations, which include extreme thinness with depletion of qi, blood and fluids.

Termed infantile malnutrition in Western terminology, this condition is most often observed in children under five years of age.

ETIOLOGY AND PATHOGENESIS

The transportation and transformation functions of the spleen and stomach are delicate during the early years of life. The major cause of infantile malnutrition involves dysfunction of the spleen and stomach and is directly related to this delicacy. Of the numerous factors harmful to the transportation and transformation function of the spleen and stomach, those most often involved in the development of infantile malnutrition include an improper diet that lacks essential nutrients, injury to the spleen and stomach from excessive breastfeeding, infection by parasitic worms that consume qi and blood, and spleen and stomach vacuity from prolonged illness.

While the major pathological changes take place in the spleen and stomach, prolongation of the condition with concurrent depletion of qi and blood can also damage other viscera and bowels, causing various secondary patterns.

1. SPLEEN AND STOMACH VACUITY

Clinical Manifestations:
Early stage: Gradual onset, loss of weight, sallow lusterless complexion, thinning of the hair, refusal of food or poor appetite, lack of alertness, restlessness, frequent crying and loose stools.

With further pathological development: Internal food accumulation and stagnation, emaciation, marked abdominal distention with protrusion of the navel and superficial abdominal veins, scaly skin, dry brittle hair, listlessness, dry lips and mouth, periodic low-grade fever and restless sleep with the eyes often left unclosed.

Tongue: Slimy, scummy or completely peeled coating.

Pulse: Thready, weak.

Treatment Method: Fortify the spleen and stomach, disperse food accumulation and stasis, transform stagnation.

PRESCRIPTION

Use Life-Promoting Spleen-Fortifying Pill *(zī shēng jiàn pí wán)* or Gan Accumulation Powder *(gān jī sǎn)*.

Life-Promoting Spleen-Fortifying Pill* *zī shēng jiàn pí wán*

dǎng shēn	codonopsis [root]	Codonopsitis Radix	3-6 g.
bái zhú	ovate atractylodes [root]	Atractylodis Ovatae Rhizoma	3-6 g.
fú líng	poria	Poria	3-6 g.
shān yào	dioscorea [root]	Dioscoreae Rhizoma	6-9 g.
biǎn dòu	lablab [bean]	Lablab Semen	3-6 g.
yì yǐ rén	coix [seed]	Coicis Semen	6-9 g.
lián zǐ	lotus [fruit-seed]	Nelumbinis Fructus seu Semen	3-6 g.
huáng lián	coptis [root]	Coptidis Rhizoma	1-3 g.
huò xiāng	agastache/patchouli	Agastaches seu Pogostemi Herba	1-3 g.
bái dòu kòu	cardamom	Amomi Cardamomi Fructus	1-3 g.
	(abbreviated decoction)		
zhǐ shí	unripe bitter orange [fruit]	Aurantii Fructus Immaturus	1-3 g.
zhǐ ké	bitter orange	Aurantii Fructus	1-3 g.
zé xiè	alisma [tuber]	Alismatis Rhizoma	1-3 g.
jié gěng	platycodon [root]	Platycodonis Radix	1-3 g.
mài yá	barley sprout	Hordei Fructus Germinatus	3-6 g.
shén qū	medicated leaven	Massa Medicata Fermentata	3-6 g.
shān zhā	crataegus [fruit]	Crataegi Fructus	3-6 g.
zhì gān cǎo	licorice [root] (honey-fried)	Glycyrrhizae Radix	3-6 g.

*This formula is only for children.

or:

Gan Accumulation Powder* *gān jī sǎn*

jī nèi jīn	gizzard lining	Galli Gigerii Endothelium	3-6 g.
cāng zhú	atractylodes [root]	Atractylodis Rhizoma	3-6 g.
ròu dòu kòu	nutmeg	Myristicae Semen	3-6 g.
xiāng fù zǐ	cyperus [root]	Cyperi Rhizoma	1.5-3 g.
hú huáng lián	picrorhiza [root]	Picrorhizae Rhizoma	3-6 g.
shén qū	medicated leaven	Massa Medicata Fermentata	3-6 g.
shā rén	amomum [fruit]	Amomi Semen seu Fructus	1-3 g.
	(abbreviated decoction)		
mài yá	barley sprout	Hordei Fructus Germinatus	3-6 g.

*This formula is only for children.

MODIFICATIONS

Where food accumulation and statis is severe, with marked abdominal distention, belching, refusal of food and thick slimy tongue coating, Life-Promoting Spleen-Fortifying Pill *(zī shēng jiàn pí wán)* is modified to promote splenic transportation and disperse food accumulation and stagnation.

Delete:

dǎng shēn	codonopsis [root]	Codonopsitis Radix
bái zhú	ovate atractylodes [root]	Atractylodis Ovatae Rhizoma
shān yào	dioscorea [root]	Dioscoreae Rhizoma

Add:

jī nèi jīn	gizzard lining	Galli Gigerii Endothelium	1.5-4.5 g.

In cases with loose stools, the prescription is modified to warm spleen yang. Add a small dose of:

pào jiāng	(blast-fried) ginger [root]	Zingiberis Rhizoma Tostum	1-1.5 g.

In the later stages of malnutrition with the presentation of extreme emaciation, Eight-Gem Decoction *(bā zhēn tāng)* is used instead of the preceding prescriptions to simultaneously supplement qi and blood.

Eight-Gem Decoction *bā zhēn tāng*

shú dì huáng	cooked rehmannia [root]	Rehmanniae Radix Conquita	12 g.	(3-6 g.)
dāng guī	tangkuei	Angelicae Sinensis Radix	9 g.	(3-4.5 g.)
bái sháo yào	white peony [root]	Paeoniae Radix Alba	9 g.	(3-4.5 g.)
chuān xiōng	ligusticum [root]	Ligustici Rhizoma	6 g.	(1.5-3 g.)
rén shēn	ginseng	Ginseng Radix	9 g.	(3-4.5 g.)
bái zhú	ovate atractylodes [root]	Atractylodis Ovatae Rhizoma	9 g.	(3-4.5 g.)
fú líng	poria	Poria	9 g.	(3-4.5 g.)
zhì gān cǎo	licorice [root] (honey-fried)	Glycyrrhizae Radix	6 g.	(1.5-3 g.)
shēng jiāng	fresh ginger [root]	Zingiberis Rhizoma Recens	3 g.	(1-1.5 g.)
dà zǎo	jujube	Ziziphi Fructus	3 pc.	(1-2 pc.)

MODIFICATIONS

In cases of spleen yang vacuity, with symptoms of pale complexion and tongue, Eight-Gem Decoction *(bā zhēn tang),* is modified to warm yang and move the spleen.

Delete:

bái sháo yào	white peony [root]	Paeoniae Radix Alba

Add:

pào jiāng	blast-fried ginger [root]	Zingiberis Rhizoma Tostum	1-3 g.
zhì fù zǐ	aconite [accessory tuber] (processed) (extended decoction)	Aconiti Tuber Laterale Praeparatum	1.5-6 g.

Where the tongue is red with little coating and the mouth is dry, Eight-Gem Decoction *(bā zhēn tāng)* is modified to nourish yin. Add:

wū méi	mume [fruit]	Mume Fructus	3-6 g.
shí hú	dendrobium [stem] (extended decoction)	Dendrobii Caulis	3-6 g.

ACUPUNCTURE AND MOXIBUSTION

Main Points:

1)

	CV-12	*zhōng wǎn*
	BL-21	*wèi shū*
	M-UE-9	*sì fèng* (Four Seams)
	LR-13	*zhāng mén*
	ST-36	*zú sān lǐ*
	BL-20	*pí shū*
	SP-04	*gōng sūn*

2) Use a three-edged or a thick filiform needle to pierce the *sì fèng* (Four Seams) points to a depth of 0.3 cm. Withdraw the needle immediately and squeeze a drop of yellowish-white fluid from the lesion. Follow the above procedure once daily.

Needle the auxillary points with supplementation at a superficial depth followed by immediate needle withdrawal.

Auxiliary points:

For food accumulation and stagnation, add:

    CV-11　　　*jiàn lǐ*

For abdominal distention and/or loose stools, add:

    CV-10　　　*xià wǎn*
    ST-25　　　*tiān shū*
    CV-06　　　*qì hǎi*

For restless sleep, add:

    PC-05　　　*jiān shǐ*

2. INFECTION BY PARASITIC WORMS

Clinical Manifestations: In addition to the above symptoms, patients may be prone to overeating or the ingestion of inedible matter, abdominal distention with protrusion of superficial abdominal veins, frequent abdominal pain and grinding of the teeth during sleep.

Tongue: Pale.

Pulse: Wiry, thready.

Treatment Method: Digest food accumulation and stagnation, expel worms.

PRESCRIPTION

Chubby Child Pill* *féi ér wān*

shén qū	medicated leaven	Massa Medicata Fermentata	300 g.
huáng lián	coptis [root]	Coptidis Rhizoma	300 g.
ròu dòu kòu	nutmeg	Myristicae Semen	150 g.
shǐ jūn zǐ	quisqualis [fruit]	Quisqualis Fructus	150 g.
mài yá	barley sprout	Hordei Fructus Germinatus	150 g.
bīng láng	areca [nut]	Arecae Semen	120 g.
mù xiāng	saussurea [root]	Saussureae (seu Vladimiriae) Radix	60 g.

*This formula is only for children.

Grind the above constituents into a fine powder, add fresh pig's bile and form into small 3 g. balls. Administer one ball dissolved in boiling water. The medication should be taken once daily, in the morning on an empty stomach. Reduce the dosage for infants younger than one year.

ACUPUNCTURE AND MOXIBUSTION

Main Points: Needle first with draining, then with supplementation. Needle superficially and withdraw immediately without retention.

    CV-14　　　*jù què*
    CV-12　　　*zhōng wǎn*
    ST-25　　　*tiān shū*
    ST-36　　　*zú sān lǐ*
    M-UE-9　　*sì fèng* (Four Seams)
    M-LE-34　*bǎi chóng wō* (Hundred Worm Nest)

Auxiliary points:

For severe abdominal distention, add:

    LR-13　　　*zhāng mén*
    CV-06　　　*qì hǎi*

ALTERNATE THERAPEUTIC METHODS

1. Plum-Blossom Needle Therapy

Main points:

BL-21	*wèi shū*
BL-20	*pí shū*
M-UE-9	*sì fèng* (Four Seams)
BL-22	*sān jiāo shū*
ST-36	*zú sān lǐ*
M-BW-35	*huá tuó jiā jǐ* (Hua Tuo's Paravertebrals)

Method: Use a plum-blossom needle to tap lightly over the above acupoints once every two days.

REMARKS

Infants must be fed fixed portions at regular intervals to avoid the detrimental effects of excessive hunger or overeating. Do not permit indulgence in rich oily foods. During treatment of infantile malnutrition, the fundamental principle is protection of the spleen and stomach. When food intake is possible, stomach qi is still substantial and the prognosis fair. When food intake is not possible, the prognosis is poor. To increase therapeutic effectiveness, diet therapy and tuina spinal massage may be used.

INFANTILE CONVULSIONS
Xiǎo Ér Jīng Fēng

**1A. Acute Fright Wind – External Wind - 1B. Acute Fright Wind –
Internal Phlegm-Heat - 1C. Acute Fright Wind – Sudden Fright or Fear -
2A. Chronic Fright Wind – Spleen Vacuity and Liver Exuberance -
2B. Chronic Fright Wind – Liver and Kidney Yin Vacuity**

Convulsions or fright wind (*jīng fēng*) refers to patterns presenting the following major symptoms: muscular spasms of the limbs, jaw tetany, opisthotonos and clouding of the consciousness. Infantile convulsions are most frequently seen in children under five years old, as children become less vulnerable with age. Convulsions can be abrupt or gradual with replete or vacuous clinical manifestations and are classified as either acute or chronic.

Fright wind can be present in numerous Western diseases, including high fever and acute infectious diseases of the central nervous system, such as epidemic cerebrospinal meningitis, encephalitis B, toxic bacillary dysentery and toxic pneumonia. Chronic convulsions, on the other hand, can appear with prolonged diarrhea or vomiting, metabolic or nutritional disturbances and chronic infectious diseases of the central nervous system, such as tubercular meningitis. Refer to this chapter for the differential diagnosis and treatment of infantile convulsions from any of these conditions.

ETIOLOGY AND PATHOGENESIS

Infantile convulsions can result from a variety of different factors. Acute infantile convulsions can be instigated by external evils that can transform into heat. In the extreme, heat gives rise to internal wind, causing convulsions. Improper diet and eating habits can lead to food stasis and the production of phlegm-heat, which eventually results in acute convulsions. Surprise or fear, both of which can disrupt the flow of qi and blood, can also bring on acute convulsions. These are repletion patterns with major pathological changes occurring in the liver and heart.

Chronic infantile convulsions are usually the result of vacuity, and may be brought about by prolonged vomiting, diarrhea or extended illness. Excessive restraint of a weakened spleen by the liver, or a dual liver and kidney yin vacuity, both can lead to the production of wind and convulsions. Chronic convulsions can also develop following acute convulsions.

1A. ACUTE FRIGHT WIND – EXTERNAL WIND

Clinical Manifestations: Abrupt onset, high fever, thirst, headache, inflamed throat, mental disturbance, irritability, limb spasms, jaw tetany, neck rigidity, rolling back of the eyes and, in severe cases, opisthotonos.

Tongue: Red with yellow coating.

Pulse: Rapid, wiry; greenish-purple index vessel.

Treatment Method: Clear heat, dispel evil, open the orifices, extinguish wind.

PRESCRIPTION

Scourge-Clearing Toxin-Vanquishing Beverage *qīng wēn bài dú yǐn*

shí gāo	gypsum (extended decoction)	Gypsum	30 g.	(9-15 g.)
shēng dì huáng	rehmannia [root] dried/fresh	Rehmanniae Radix Exsiccata seu Recens	15 g.	(4.5-9 g.)
xī jiǎo	rhinoceros horn (powdered and stirred in)	Rhinocerotis Cornu	6 g.	(1.5-3 g.)
huáng lián	coptis [root]	Coptidis Rhizoma	6 g.	(1.5-3 g.)
shān zhī zǐ	gardenia [fruit]	Gardeniae Fructus	6 g.	(1.5-3 g.)
huáng qín	scutellaria [root]	Scutellariae Radix	6 g.	(1.5-3 g.)
zhī mǔ	anemarrhena [root]	Anemarrhenae Rhizoma	6 g.	(1.5-3 g.)
chì sháo yào	red peony [root]	Paeoniae Radix Rubra	6 g.	(1.5-3 g.)
xuán shēn	scrophularia [root]	Scrophulariae Radix	6 g.	(1.5-3 g.)
lián qiào	forsythia [fruit]	Forsythiae Fructus	6 g.	(1.5-3 g.)
mǔ dān pí	moutan [root bark]	Moutan Radicis Cortex	6 g.	(1.5-3 g.)
jié gěng	platycodon [root]	Platycodonis Radix	3 g.	(1-1.5 g.)
zhú yè	black bamboo [leaf]	Bambusae Folium	3 g.	(1-1.5 g.)
gān cǎo	licorice [root]	Glycyrrhizae Radix	3 g.	(1-1.5 g.)

*Use of *xī jiǎo* (rhinoceros horn) is prohibited in North America by the endangered species laws. Water Buffalo Horn *(shuǐ niú jiǎo)* may be substituted. Increase the dose to 15 g., extended decoction.)

MODIFICATIONS

To reinforce clearing heat, eradicating wind and relieving convulsions, add:

líng yáng jiǎo	antelope horn (or, powdered and stirred in, each time 0.1-0.2 g.)	Antelopis Cornu	1-1.5 g.
gōu téng	uncaria [stem and thorn] (abbreviated decoction)	Uncariae Ramulus cum Unco	3-6 g.
shí jué míng	abalone shell (extended decoction)	Haliotidis Concha	9-15 g.

In more severe cases of high fever, convulsions and coma, the prescription is modified to clear heat, open the orifices and relieve convulsions. Combine with the given prescription any one of the following prepared medicines: PEACEFUL PALACE BOVINE BEZOAR PILL *(ān gōng niú huáng wán)*, PURPLE SNOW ELIXIR *(zǐ xuě dān)*, or SUPREME JEWEL ELIXIR *(zhì bǎo dān)*.

In cases accompanied by phlegm-dampness, with a thick yellow slimy tongue coating, the prescription is modified to expel phlegm, dispel dampness and open the orifices. Add:

shí chāng pú	acorus [root]	Acori Rhizoma	3-4.5 g.
yù jīn	curcuma [tuber]	Curcumae Tuber	3-4.5 g.
dǎn xīng	(bile-processed) arisaema [root]	Arisaematis Rhizoma cum Felle Bovis	1.5-3 g.
fǎ bàn xià	pinellia [tuber] (processed)	Pinelliae Tuber Praeparatum	3-4.5 g.

With repeated vomiting, the prescription is changed to expel phlegm-turbidity and relieve vomiting. Add the prepared medicine, JADE AXIS ELIXIR *(yù shū dān)*.

In cases presenting constipation, the prescription is modified for offensive precipitation.

Add:

dà huáng	rhubarb (abbreviated decoction)	Rhei Rhizoma	3-4.5 g.
máng xiāo	mirabilite (stirred in)	Mirabilitum	3-4.5 g.

In cases with abdominal pain where the stools contain pus and blood, the prescription is modified for offensive precipitation to stop dysentery.

Add:

Pulsatilla Decoction *bái tóu wēng tāng*

bái tóu wēng	pulsatilla [root]	Pulsatillae Radix	15 g.	(4.5-9 g.)
huáng bǎi	phellodendron [bark]	Phellodendri Cortex	12 g.	(3-6 g.)
qín pí	ash [bark]	Fraxini Cortex	12 g.	(3-6 g.)
huáng lián	coptis [root]	Coptidis Rhizoma	6 g.	(1.5-3 g.)

ACUPUNCTURE AND MOXIBUSTION

Main points: Needle with draining; bleed at the jing points.

LU-11	*shào shāng*
LI-01	*shāng yáng*
HT-09	*shào chōng*
SI-01	*shào zé*
PC-09	*zhōng chōng*
TB-01	*guān chōng*
GV-14	*dà zhuī*
LI-04	*hé gǔ*
LR-03	*tài chōng*
GB-34	*yáng líng quán*

Auxiliary points:

For severe heat, add:

LI-11   *qū chí*

For loss of consciousness, add:

GV-26   *rén zhōng*

For vomiting, add:

CV-12	*zhōng wǎn*
PC-06	*nèi guān*

1B. ACUTE FRIGHT WIND - INTERNAL PHLEGM-HEAT

Clinical Manifestations: Initial symptoms include loss of appetite, vomiting, fever, abdominal pain and constipation or stools containing pus and blood, followed by sudden loss of consciousness, convulsions, wheezing respiration, abdominal fullness and distention, heavy breathing.

Tongue: Thick yellow slimy coating.

Pulse: Wiry, slippery.

Treatment Method: Clear heat, transform phlegm, open the orifices, relieve convulsions.

PRESCRIPTION

Use the prepared medicine CHILDREN'S RETURN-OF-SPRING ELIXIR *(xiǎo ér huí chūn dān)*.

MODIFICATIONS

In cases of vomiting, the prescription is modified to relieve vomiting. Add the prepared medicine, JADE AXIS ELIXIR *(yù shū dān)*.

In cases accompanied by food stagnation, the prescription is modified to disperse food stagnation. Add:

Harmony-Preserving Pill *bǎo hé wán*

shān zhā	crataegus [fruit]	Crataegi Fructus	18 g.	(4.5-9 g.)
shén qū	medicated leaven	Massa Medicata Fermentata	9 g.	(3-4.5 g.)
zhì bàn xià	pinellia [tuber] (processed)	Pinelliae Tuber Praeparatum	9 g.	(3-4.5 g.)
fú líng	poria	Poria	9 g.	(3-4.5 g.)
chén pí	tangerine [peel]	Citri Exocarpium	6 g.	(1.5-3 g.)
lián qiào	forsythia [fruit]	Forsythiae Fructus	6 g.	(1.5-3 g.)
lái fú zǐ	radish [seed]	Raphani Semen	6 g.	(1.5-3 g.)

ACUPUNCTURE AND MOXIBUSTION

Main points: Needle with draining.

GV-26	*rén zhōng*
TB-19	*lú xí*
CV-12	*zhōng wǎn*
ST-40	*fēng lóng*
HT-07	*shén mén*
LR-03	*tài chōng*

Auxiliary points:

For rolling back of the eyes, add:

GV-24	*shén tíng*
GV-22	*xìn huì*
GV-08	*jīn suō*

For jaw tetany, add:

ST-06	*jiá chē*
LI-04	*hé gǔ*

For abdominal distention, add:

ST-25	*tiān shū*
CV-06	*qì hǎi*

1C. ACUTE FRIGHT WIND - SUDDEN FRIGHT OR FEAR

Clinical Manifestations: No fever, lack of warmth in the limbs, restless sleep followed by crying or wailing and jumpiness after awakening, greenish complexion, intermittent convulsions.

Tongue: Thin coating.

Pulse: Deep; greenish-purple index vessel.

Treatment Method: Relieve convulsions, quiet the spirit.

PRESCRIPTION

Combine the prepared medicines AMBER DRAGON-EMBRACING PILL *(hǔ pò bào lóng wán)* and CINNABAR SPIRIT-QUIETING PILL *(zhū shā ān shén wán).*

ACUPUNCTURE AND MOXIBUSTION

Main points: Needle with draining.

GV-21	*qián dǐng*
M-HN-3	*yìn táng* (Hall of Impression)
HT-07	*shén mén*
KI-01	*yǒng quán*

Auxiliary points:

For prolonged convulsions, add:

TB-19	*lú xí*
GV-22	*xìn huì*

For lethargic stupor, add:

GV-26	*rén zhōng*

2A. CHRONIC FRIGHT WIND - SPLEEN VACUITY AND LIVER EXUBERANCE

Clinical Manifestations: Emaciation, sallow complexion, tiredness, fatigue, heavy sleep with exposure of the eyeballs, intermittent convulsions, incomplete closure of fontanels, lack of warmth in the limbs, loose runny greenish stools, slight edema of the face and back of feet.

Tongue: Pale with white coating.

Pulse: Deep, weak.

Treatment Method: Strengthen the spleen, calm the liver, relieve convulsions.

PRESCRIPTION

Liver-Relaxing Spleen-Rectifying Decoction* *huǎn gān lì pí tāng*

rén shēn	ginseng	Ginseng Radix	3–6 g.
fú líng	poria	Poria	3–6 g.
bái zhú	ovate atractylodes [root]	Atractylodis Ovatae Rhizoma	3–6 g.
guì zhī	cinnamon [twig]	Cinnamomi Ramulus	3–6 g.
bái sháo yào	white peony [root]	Paeoniae Radix Alba	4.5–9 g.
chén pí	tangerine [peel]	Citri Exocarpium	3–6 g.
shān yào	dioscorea [root]	Dioscoreae Rhizoma	4.5–9 g.
biǎn dòu	lablab [bean]	Lablab Semen	3–6 g.
shēng jiāng	fresh ginger [root] (roasted in hot ashes)	Zingiberis Rhizoma Recens	3–6 g.
zhì gān cǎo	licorice [root]	Glycyrrhizae Radix	3–6 g.
dà zǎo	jujube	Ziziphi Fructus	3–5 pc.

*This formula is only for children.

MODIFICATIONS

To reinforce the effects of soothing the liver and relieving convulsions, add:

gōu téng	uncaria [stem and thorn] (abbreviated decoction)	Uncariae Ramulus cum Unco	3–6 g.
tiān má	gastrodia [root]	Gastrodiae Rhizoma	3–4.5 g.
jú huā	chrysanthemum [flower]	Chrysanthemi Flos	3-4.5 g.

In cases of prolonged illness leading to vacuity of spleen and kidney yang, with lack of warmth in the limbs, pale complexion, stools containing undigested food, lack of vitality and a slow deep pulse, the prescription is changed to warm and supplement the spleen and kidney, relieve convulsions and quiet the spirit. Combine True-Securing Decoction *(gù zhēn tāng)* with Cold-Dispelling Fright-Assuaging Decoction *(zhú hán dàng jīng tāng).*

True-Securing Decoction *gù zhēn tāng*

huáng qí	astragalus [root]	Astragali (seu Hedysari) Radix	9 g.	(3-4.5 g.)
rén shēn	ginseng	Ginseng Radix	6 g.	(1.5-3 g.)
bái zhú	ovate atractylodes [root]	Atractylodis Ovatae Rhizoma	6 g.	(1.5-3 g.)
fú líng	poria	Poria	6 g.	(1.5-3 g.)
shān yào	dioscorea [root]	Dioscoreae Rhizoma	9 g.	(3-4.5 g.)
zhì gān cǎo	licorice [root] (honey-fried)	Glycyrrhizae Radix	6 g.	(1.5-3 g.)
zhì fù zǐ	aconite [accessory tuber]	Aconiti Tuber Laterale	6 g.	(1.5-3 g.)
ròu guì	cinnamon [bark] (abbreviated decoction)	Cinnamomi Cortex	3 g.	(1-1.5 g.)

with:

Cold-Dispelling Fright-Assuaging Decoction* *zhú hán dàng jīng tāng*

hú jiāo	pepper	Piperis Fructus	1-3 g.
pào jiāng	blast-fried ginger [root]	Zingiberis Rhizoma Tostum	3 4.5 g.
ròu guì	cinnamon [bark] (abbreviated decoction)	Cinnamomi Cortex	1.5-3 g.
dīng xiāng	clove	Caryophylli Flos	1.5-3 g.
fú lóng gān	oven earth	Terra Flava Usta	30-60 g.
	(decoct in water first, then decoct the other herbs in this decoction)		

*This formula is only for children.

Add:

lóng gǔ	dragon bone (extended decoction)	Mastodi Ossis Fossilia	4.5-9 g.
mǔ lì	oyster shell (extended decoction)	Ostreae Concha	4.5-9 g.
cí shí	loadstone (extended decoction)	Magnetitum	4.5-9 g.

ACUPUNCTURE AND MOXIBUSTION

Main points: Needle with supplementation; add moxibustion.

BL-20	*pí shū*
BL-21	*wèi shū*
ST-36	*zú sān lǐ*
GV-20	*bǎi huì*
M-HN-3	*yìn táng* (Hall of Impression)
LR-03	*tài chōng*

Auxiliary points:

For vacuity of spleen and kidney yang, add:

BL-23	*shèn shū*
CV-04	*guān yuán*

2B. CHRONIC FRIGHT WIND – LIVER AND KIDNEY YIN VACUITY

Clinical Manifestations: Restlessness, red cheeks, emaciation, feverish palms and soles, intermittent convulsions, hard, dry stools.

Tongue: Red with little or no coating.

Pulse: Rapid, thready.

Treatment Method: Supplement and boost liver and kidney yin, relieve convulsions.

PRESCRIPTION

Use Major Wind-Stabilizing Pill *(dà dìng fēng zhū)* or Triple-Armored Pulse-Restorative Decoction *(sān jiǎ fù mài tāng)*.

Major Wind-Stabilizing Pill *dà dìng fēng zhū*

bái sháo yào	white peony [root]	Paeoniae Radix Alba	18 g. (4.5-9 g.)
ē jiāo	ass hide glue (dissolved and stirred in)	Asini Corii Gelatinum	9 g. (3-4.5 g.)
guī bǎn	tortoise plastron (extended decoction)	Testudinis Plastrum	12 g. (3-6 g.)
shēng dì huáng	rehmannia [root] dried/fresh	Rehmanniae Radix Exsiccatum seu Recens	18 g. (4.5-9 g.)
huǒ má rén	hemp [seed]	Cannabis Semen	6 g. (1.5-3 g.)
wǔ wèi zǐ	schisandra [berry]	Schisandrae Fructus	6 g. (1.5-3 g.)
mǔ lì	oyster shell (extended decoction)	Ostreae Concha	12 g. (3-6 g.)
mài mén dōng	ophiopogon [tuber]	Ophiopogonis Tuber	18 g. (4.5-9 g.)
biē jiǎ	turtle shell (extended decoction)	Amydae Carapax	12 g. (3-6 g.)
jī zǐ huáng	egg yolk (stirred in while the decoction cools)	Galli Vitellus	2 pc. (1-2 pc.)
zhì gān cǎo	licorice [root] (honey-fried)	Glycyrrhizae Radix	12 g. (4.5-9 g.)

or:

Triple-Armored Pulse-Restorative Decoction *sān jiǎ fù mài tāng*

zhì gān cǎo	licorice [root] (honey-fried)	Glycyrrhizae Radix	18 g. (4.5-9 g.)
shú dì huáng	rehmannia [root] (cooked)	Rehmanniae Radix Conquita	18 g. (4.5-9 g.)
bái sháo yào	white peony [root]	Paeoniae Radix Alba	18 g. (4.5-9 g.)
mài mén dōng	ophiopogon [tuber]	Ophiopogonis Tuber	15 g. (4.5-9 g.)
ē jiāo	ass hide glue (dissolved and stirred in)	Asini Corii Gelatinum	9 g. (3-4.5 g.)
mǔ lì	oyster shell (extended decoction)	Ostreae Concha	15 g. (4.5-9 g.)
biē jiǎ	turtle shell (extended decoction))	Amydae Carapax	24 g. (6-12 g.)
guī bǎn	tortoise plastron (extended decoction)	Testudinis Plastrum	30 g. (9-15 g.)

MODIFICATIONS

In cases of tidal fever caused by vacuity of yin, the prescription is modified to clear vacuity-heat. Add:

yín chái hú	lanceolate stellaria [root]	Stellariae Lanceolatae Radix	3-4.5 g.
dì gǔ pí	lycium [root bark]	Lycii Radicis Cortex	3-4.5 g.
qīng hāo	sweet wormwood (abbreviated decoction)	Artemisiae Apiaceae seu Annuae Herba	3-4.5 g.

ACUPUNCTURE AND MOXIBUSTION

Main points: Needle with supplementation.

BL-18	*gān shū*
BL-23	*shèn shū*
GV-24	*shén tíng*

GV-20   *băi huì*
KI-02   *rán gŭ*
LR-03   *tài chōng*

Auxiliary points:

For tidal fever, add:

BL-43 (38)   *gāo huāng shū*

ALTERNATE THERAPEUTIC METHODS

1. Ear Acupuncture

Main Points: Sympathetic, *Shén Mén*, Subcortex, Brain, Heart.

Method: Needle to elicit a strong sensation. Manipulate every ten minutes and retain the needles for sixty minutes.

REMARKS

During convulsions, the child should be placed on their side, with a tongue depressor wrapped in several layers of gauze between the teeth to prevent biting the tongue. When there is threat of suffocation, phlegm and other secretions should be aspirated from the throat at regular intervals. Following convulsions, the child is usually very fatigued and should be allowed ample rest, and the room kept quiet at all times. The child's diet should be modified to include fruits, vegetables and ample liquids, and to restrict greasy or rich foods.

INFANTILE PALSY

Xiǎo Ér Má Bì

1. Evils Entering the Lung and Stomach - 2. Evils Entering the Channels and Connections - 3. Qi Vacuity with Blood Stasis - 4. Liver and Kidney Depletion

Infantile palsy is a contagious disease caused by toxic, seasonal and epidemic evils. During the initial stages, the clinical manifestations are similar to those of the common cold, and may include fever, coughing, inflamed throat, general aches and pains and sometimes vomiting and diarrhea. Paralysis of the limbs can manifest with continued development and, eventually, muscular atrophy and deformity of the joints.

Infantile palsy generally affects children under five years of age, especially those between six months and two years. School-age children and adults have also been known to contract the disease. Although epidemics are most common during the summer and autumn, infantile palsy may occur in any of the four seasons. In Western medicine, infantile palsy is known as polio or poliomyelitis.

ETIOLOGY AND PATHOGENESIS

The etiology of infantile palsy primarily involves toxic wind, heat and dampness evils. These seasonal epidemic evils enter through the nose and mouth, invade the lung and stomach, and cause, during the initial stages, symptoms very similar to those of the common cold. Epidemic toxins spread internally along the channels and connections, which they eventually obstruct, hindering the flow of qi and blood and thereby denying nutrients to the sinews, ultimately causing flaccid paralysis of the limbs. In extended cases lacking adequate treatment, qi becomes depleted and blood stagnates, giving rise to patterns of repletion in the midst of vacuity. In cases of long-term paralysis, the liver and kidney are affected, leading to an insufficiency of essence and blood, muscular atrophy and deformity of the bones and joints. In such cases, recovery is very difficult.

1. EVILS ENTERING THE LUNG AND STOMACH

Clinical Manifestations: Fever, perspiration, coughing, runny nose, sore inflamed throat, general malaise, headache, vomiting, abdominal pain and diarrhea in some cases.

Tongue: Red with thin yellow sometimes slimy coating.

Pulse: Rapid or soft, rapid.

Treatment Method: Course wind, clear heat, disinhibit dampness, resolve the exterior.

PRESCRIPTION

Pueraria, Scutellaria and Coptis Decoction
gé gēn huáng qín huáng lián tāng

gé gēn	pueraria [root]	Puerariae Radix	*15 g.	(4.5-9 g.)
huáng qín	scutellaria [root]	Scutellariae Radix	9 g.	(3-4.5 g.)
huáng lián	coptis [root]	Coptidis Rhizoma	6 g.	(3-4.5 g.)
zhì gān cǎo	licorice [root] (honey-fried)	Glycyrrhizae Radix	6 g.	(3-4.5 g.)

MODIFICATIONS

In cases where dampness evil predominates, the prescription is modified to harmonize the stomach and transform dampness.

Add:

huò xiāng	agastache/patchouli	Agastaches seu Pogostemi Herba	(3-4.5 g.)
yì yǐ rén	coix [seed]	Coicis Semen	(9-15 g.)
zhì bàn xià	pinellia [tuber] (processed)	Pinelliae Tuber Praeparatum	(3-4.5 g.)

In cases of irritability and restlessness, the prescription is modified to settle and quiet the spirit.

Add:

dēng xīn cǎo	juncus [pith]	Junci Medulla	(1-1.5 g.)
dì lóng	earthworm	Lumbricus	(3-4.5 g.)

In cases of sleepiness with slimy tongue coating, the prescription is modified to transform phlegm-turbidity.

Add:

dǎn xīng	arisaema [root] (bile-processed)	Arisaematis Rhizoma cum Felle Bovis	(1.5-3 g.)
fú líng	poria	Poria	(3-6 g.)
shí chāng pú	acorus [root]	Acori Rhizoma	(3-4.5 g.)

In cases presenting frequent nausea and vomiting with a yellow slimy tongue coating, the prescription is modified to relieve vomiting.

Add:

jiāng bàn xià	(ginger-processed) pinellia [tuber]	Pinelliae Tuber Praeparatum	(3-4.5 g.)
zhú rú	bamboo shavings	Bambusae Caulis in Taeniam	(3-4.5 g.)

In cases with constipation the prescription is modified to clear heat and moisten the intestines.

Add:

quán guā lóu	whole trichosanthes [fruit]	Trichosanthis Fructus Integer	(3-6 g.)
jué míng zǐ	fetid cassia [seed]	Cassiae Torae Semen	(3-6 g.)

ACUPUNCTURE AND MOXIBUSTION

Main points: Needle with draining.

LI-04	*hé gǔ*
LU-07	*liè quē*
GB-20	*fēng chí*
LI-11	*qū chí*
SP-09	*yīn líng quán*
SP-06	*sān yīn jiāo*

Auxiliary points:

For fever, add:

GV-14	*dà zhuī*
LU-11	*shào shāng*
LI-01	*shāng yáng*

For vomiting and diarrhea, add:

CV-12	*zhōng wǎn*
ST-36	*zú sān lǐ*

2. EVILS ENTERING THE CHANNELS AND CONNECTIONS

Clinical Manifestations: In general, three to four days after the symptoms from invasion of the stomach and lung subside, the following will appear: fever, perspiration, pains in the limbs, difficulty rotating the torso, crying, restlessness and eventual paralysis. Paralysis can occur in any part of the body, although the lower limbs are most commonly affected, either unilaterally or bilaterally. Unilateral facial paralysis may also be observed. The temperature of the skin of the affected side will be somewhat cooler than that of the unaffected side. In cases where the abdominal muscles have been affected, marked protrusion of the abdomen will be noted when the child cries. When the bladder has been affected, there may be either urinary retention or incontinence.

Tongue: Yellow slimy coating.

Pulse: Soft, rapid.

Treatment Method: Clear heat, transform dampness, course and free the channels and connections.

PRESCRIPTION

Notopterygium Dampness-Overcoming Decoction *qiāng huó shèng shī tāng*

qiāng huó	notopterygium [root]	Notopterygii Rhizoma	6 g.	(1.5-3 g.)
dú huó	tuhuo [angelica root]	Angelicae Duhuo Radix	6 g.	(1.5-3 g.)
gǎo běn	Chinese lovage [root]	Ligustici Sinensis Rhizoma et Radix	6 g.	(1.5-3 g.) (1.5-3 g.)
fáng fēng	ledebouriella [root]	Ledebouriellae Radix	6 g.	(1.5-3 g.)
màn jīng zǐ	vitex [fruit]	Viticis Fructus	6 g.	(1.5-3 g.)
chuān xiōng	ligusticum [root]	Ligustici Rhizoma	6 g.	(1.5-3 g.)
zhì gān cǎo	licorice [root] (honey-fried)	Glycyrrhizae Radix	3 g.	(1-1.5 g.)

MODIFICATIONS

To clear heat and dispel dampness, add:

cāng zhú	atractylodes [root]	Atractylodis Rhizoma	1.5-3 g.
huáng bǎi	phellodendron [bark]	Phellodendri Cortex	1.5-3 g.
fáng jǐ	fangji [root]	Fangji Radix	1.5-3 g.
yì yǐ rén	coix [seed]	Coicis Semen	3-6 g.

In cases of facial paralysis or general muscular aches and pains, the prescription is modified to dispel wind and transform phlegm.
Add:

Pull Aright Powder *qiān zhèng sǎn*

zhì bái fù zǐ	aconite/typhonium [tuber] (processed)	Aconiti Coreani seu Typhonii Gigantei Tuber Praeparatum	6 g.
bài jiàng cǎo	baijiang	Baijiang Herba cum Radice	6 g.
quán xiē	scorpion	Buthus	6 g.

Grind equal proportions of these ingredients into a powder. Take a 1-1.5 g. dose with warm water or alcohol.

Because of the warm drying characteristics of this prescription, it is to be used cautiously for blood vacuity with internal heat. To counter the drying effects, add:

shēng dì huáng	rehmannia [root] dried/fresh	Rehmanniae Radix Exsiccata seu Recens	3-4.5 g.
mài mén dōng	ophiopogon [tuber]	Ophiopogonis Tuber	3-4.5 g.

ACUPUNCTURE AND MOXIBUSTION

Main points: Needle with draining.

LI-11	*qū chí*
ST-36	*zú sān lǐ*
SP-09	*yīn líng quán*
SP-06	*sān yīn jiāo*

Auxiliary points:

For facial paralysis, add:

LI-20	*yíng xiāng*
LI-04	*hé gǔ*
ST-06	*jiá chē*
ST-04	*dì cāng*
GB-14	*yáng bái*

For paralysis of the abdominal muscles, add:

CV-12	*zhōng wǎn*
ST-25	*tiān shū*

For pain and paralysis of the upper limbs, add:

LI-15	*jiān yú*
LI-04	*hé gǔ*
TB-05	*wài guān*

For paralysis and pain of the lower limbs, add:

GB-30	*huán tiào*
GB-34	*yáng líng quán*

For retention or incontinence of urine, add:

CV-03	*zhōng jí*
BL-28	*páng guāng shū*
CV-04	*guān yuán*
GV-20	*bǎi huì*

3. QI VACUITY WITH BLOOD STASIS

Clinical Manifestations: After the fever subsides, the limbs become numb, flaccid and weak. This pattern usually presents in patients who have not recovered after six months of illness. Accompanying symptoms include sallow complexion and a tendency to perspire. Apart from symptoms of local paralysis, other clinical manifestations are not apparent.

Tongue: Pale, or dark with white coating.

Pulse: Tardy or weak.

Treatment Method: Supplement qi, quicken the blood, clear channels and connections.

PRESCRIPTION

Yang-Supplementing Five-Returning Decoction *bǔ yáng huán wǔ tāng*

huáng qí	astragalus [root]	Astragali (seu Hedysari) Radix	30–120 g. (9-60 g.)
	(Use 30 g. at the beginning and increase dosage gradually)		
dāng guī	tangkuei	Angelicae Sinensis Radix	6 g. (1.5-3 g.)
chì sháo yào	red peony [root]	Paeoniae Radix Rubra	6 g. (1.5-3 g.)
dì lóng	earthworm	Lumbricus	3 g. (1-1.5 g.)
chuān xiōng	ligusticum [root]	Ligustici Rhizoma	3 g (1-1.5 g.)
hóng huā	carthamus [flower]	Carthami Flos	3 g. (1-1.5 g.)
táo rén	peach [kernel]	Persicae Semen	3 g. (1-1.5 g.)

MODIFICATIONS

In cases of paralysis of the upper limbs, the prescription is modified to dispel wind and clear the channels and connections.
Add:

sāng zhī	mulberry [twig]	Mori Ramulus	4.5-9 g.
guì zhī	cinnamon [twig]	Cinnamomi Ramulus	3-4.5 g.

In cases of paralysis of the lower limbs, the prescription is modified to supplement the kidney and strengthen sinew and bone.
Add:

sāng jì shēng	mistletoe	Loranthi seu Visci Ramus	3-6 g.
niú xī	achyranthes [root]	Achyranthis Bidentatae Radix	3-6 g.
xù duàn	dipsacus [root]	Dipsaci Radix	3-6 g.
dù zhòng	eucommia [bark]	Eucommiae Cortex	3-6 g.

In cases where damp-heat has not been completely dispelled, the prescription is modified to clear heat and disinhibit dampness.
Add:

Mysterious Three Pill *sān miào wán*

cāng zhú	atractylodes [root]	Atractylodis Rhizoma	9 g.	(3-4.5 g.)
huáng bǎi	phellodendron [bark]	Phellodendri Cortex	9 g.	(3-4.5 g.)
chuān niú xī	cyathula [root]	Cyathulae Radix	9 g.	(3-4.5 g.)

ACUPUNCTURE AND MOXIBUSTION

Main points: Needle with even supplementation, even draining; add moxibustion.

CV-04	guān yuán
CV-06	qì hǎi
ST-36	zú sān lǐ
SP-10	xuè hǎi
SP-06	sān yīn jiāo

Auxiliary points:

For paralysis of the upper limbs, add:

LI-15	jiān yú
TB-14	jiān liáo
LI-11	qū chí
TB-05	wài guān
LI-04	hé gǔ
GV-14	dà zhuī
SI-14	jiān wài shū
SI-03	hòu xī

For paralysis of the lower limbs, add:

GB-30	*huán tiào*
GB-31	*fēng shì*
GB-34	*yáng líng quán*
GB-39	*xuán zhōng*
ST-32	*fú tù*
BL-60	*kūn lún*
SP-09	*yīn líng quán*
KI-03	*tài xī*
GV-03	*yāo yáng guān*
BL-30	*bái huán shū*

4. LIVER AND KIDNEY DEPLETION

Clinical Manifestations: Over time there is evident muscular atrophy of the paralyzed limb, which is markedly shorter and thinner than the unaffected limb. There may also be deformity of the bones and joints of the area paralyzed, including anterior or lateral curvature of the spine; or plantar, inverted or everted club foot.

Tongue: Pale.

Pulse: Thready, deep.

Treatment Method: Supplement the liver and kidney, warm and clear channels and connections.

PRESCRIPTION

Hidden Tiger Pill *hŭ qián wán*

shú dì huáng	cooked rehmannia [root]	Rehmanniae Radix Conquita	24 g.	(6-12 g.)
zhī mŭ	anemarrhena [root]	Anemarrhenae Rhizoma	12 g.	(3-6 g.)
guī băn	tortoise plastron (extended decoction)	Testudinis Plastrum	30 g.	(9-15 g.)
huáng băi	phellodendron [bark]	Phellodendri Cortex	9 g.	(3-4.5 g.)
bái sháo yào	white peony [root]	Paeoniae Radix Alba	9 g.	(3-4.5 g.)
hŭ gŭ	tiger bone*	Tigris Os	6 g.	(1.5-3 g.)
chén pí	tangerine peel	Citri Exocarpium	6 g.	(1.5-3 g.)
suŏ yáng	cynomorium [stem]	Cynomorii Caulis	6 g.	(1.5-3 g.)
gān jiāng	dried ginger [root]	Zingiberis Rhizoma Exsiccatum	3 g.	(1-1.5 g.)

*(Editor's note: *hŭ gŭ* (tiger bone) is prohibited in North America by endangered species laws. Leg bone of pig or dog may be substituted.)

MODIFICATIONS

In cases of cold extremities and a thready pulse, the prescription is modified to supplement qi, quicken the blood, warm and clear the channels and connections. Add:

huáng qí	astragalus [root]	Astragali (seu Hedysari) Radix	4.5-9 g.
guì zhī	cinnamon twig	Cinnamomi Ramulus	3-4.5 g.
dāng guī	tangkuei	Angelicae Sinensis Radix	3-6 g.

ACUPUNCTURE AND MOXIBUSTION

Main points: Needle with supplementation; add moxibustion.

BL-18	*gān shū*
BL-23	*shèn shū*
GV-03	*yāo yáng guān*
GB-34	*yáng líng quán*

GB-39	xuán zhōng
KI-03	tài xī
LI-11	qū chí
ST-36	zú sān lǐ

Auxiliary points:

For difficulty in raising the shoulder, add:

GB-21	jiān jǐng
LI-15	jiān yú
TB-14	jiàn liáo
LI-16	jù gǔ
SI-11	tiān zōng
LI-14	bì nào

For difficulty in flexion and extension of the elbow, add:

LU-03	tiān fǔ
PC-02	tiān quán
LU-05	chǐ zé
PC-03	qū zé
PC-06	nèi guān

For difficulty in inward or outward rotation of the hand, add:

LI-10	shǒu sān lǐ
TB-04	yáng chí
LI-05	yáng xī
SI-03	hòu xī
TB-09	sì dú
HT-03	shào hǎi

For flaccid wrist drop, add:

TB-05	wài guān
SI-05	yáng gǔ
M-UE-33	zhōng quán (Central Spring)
	(in the depression between LI-05 *(yáng xī)* and TB-04 *(yáng chí)*

For difficulty in lifting the leg, add:

ST-31	bì guān
GB-30	huán tiào
ST-32	fú tù
M-BW-35	huá tuó jiā jí (Hua Tuo's Paravertebrals) (Lower back L1–L5)

For difficulty in flexion and extension of the knee, add:

ST-33	yīn shì
ST-34	liáng qiū
ST-37	shàng jù xū
ST-35	dú bí

For back of the knee, add:

BL-36 (50)	chéng fú
BL-40 (54)	wěi zhōng
BL-57	chéng shān

For flaccid drop foot, add:

ST-39	xià jù xū
ST-41	jiě xī

For inverted club foot, add:

GB-39	xuán zhōng
BL-58	fēi yáng
BL-63	jīn mén
GB-40	qiū xū
BL-62	shēn mài

For everted club foot, add:

SP-06	sān yīn jiāo
KI-03	tài xī
KI-06	zhào hǎi

For dorsiflected club foot, add:

BL-57   *chéng shān*
BL-60   *kūn lún*
KI-03   *tài xī*

ALTERNATE THERAPEUTIC METHODS

1. Ear Acupuncture

Main points: Lung, *Shén Mén*, Subcortex, Cervical Vertebrae, Thoracic Vertebrae, Lumbo-Sacral Vertebrae.

Method: Select three to four points each session, needle to elicit a moderate sensation and retain needles for thirty minutes. Treat once daily.

2. Plum-Blossom Needle Therapy

Area of Treatment:

In cases of paralysis of the upper limbs, select these points on the affected side:

Governing Vessel (cervical and T1–T4 portion)
Large Intestine Channel
Small Intestine Channel
LI-11   *qū chí*
LI-04   *hé gǔ*
TB-05   *wài guān*

In cases of paralysis of the lower limbs, select lumbo-sacral portions of the following channels on the affected side:

Governing Vessel
Bladder Channel
Stomach Channel
Spleen Channel
Liver Channel
Gallbladder Channel

In cases of paralysis of the abdominal muscles, add the abdominal portions of:

Stomach Channel
Spleen Channel
Gallbladder Channel

Method: Treat once daily.

REMARKS

During the initial stages, infantile palsy is usually a repletion pattern. In later stages it becomes vacuous, or replete in the midst of vacuity. Generally speaking, treatment during the early stages corresponds to treatment for attacks by external evils or stomach and intestinal disorders. During the later stages, treatment is based on the length of illness as well as the pattern and includes methods to boost qi and quicken the blood, supplement the liver and kidney or course and clear the channels and connections.

Acumoxa therapy has good therapeutic benefits in treating sequelae of infantile palsy. Acupoints of the affected side are generally selected, although, given that treatment is quite protracted, contralateral needling can also be used, first to the unaffected, then the affected side. Apart from herbal and acumoxa therapy treatment, the use of physical therapy or tuina massage is a definite aid to recovery. In cases of severe deformation of bones and joints, orthopedic surgery may be required.

ENURESIS

Yí Niào

1. Vacuity of Kidney Yang - 2. Vacuity of Lung and Spleen Qi - 3. Damp-Heat of the Liver Channel

Patterns of enuresis are characterized by the involuntary passage of urine during sleep. Enuresis is considered a pathological condition in children over three years of age and particularly so in children five years of age or older. In milder cases, bed-wetting can occur once in several nights, while in more severe cases, bed-wetting occurs once every night or even several times each night. Enuresis can also be present in adults, although rarely.

ETIOLOGY AND PATHOGENESIS

The etiology of enuresis most often involves vacuity. In children with frail constitutions, kidney yang may be insufficient, leading to weakening of the urinary bladder's holding function. Vacuity of lung and spleen qi can also lead to loss of control over the water passage of the lower burner, resulting in enuresis. There is also a repletion pattern that is caused by damp-heat of the liver channel.

1. VACUITY OF KIDNEY YANG

Clinical Manifestations: Frequent bed-wetting, up to several times each night, accompanied by a pale complexion, tiredness, fatigue, copious clear urine, frequent urination, cold extremities, physical cold, weak aching lower back and legs.

Tongue: Pale.

Pulse: Slow, deep, forceless.

Treatment Method: Warm and supplement kidney yang, secure and astringe the urine.

PRESCRIPTION

MILD CASES:

Stream-Reducing Pill *suō quán wán*

wū yào	lindera [root]	Linderae Radix	9 g.	(3-4.5 g.)
yì zhì rén	alpinia [fruit]	Alpiniae Oxyphyllae Fructus	9 g.	(3-4.5 g.)
shān yào	dioscorea [root]	Dioscoreae Rhizoma	12 g.	(3-6 g.)

SEVERE CASES:
Cuscuta Seed Pill *tù sī zǐ wán*

tù sī zǐ	cuscuta [seed]	Cuscutae Semen	12 g.	(3-6 g.)
ròu cōng róng	cistanche [stem]	Cistanches Caulis	12 g.	(3-6 g.)
jī nèi jīn	gizzard lining	Galli Gigerii Endothelium	9 g.	(3-4.5 g.)
wǔ wèi zǐ	schisandra [berry]	Schisandrae Fructus	6 g.	(1.5-3 g.)
zhì fù zǐ	aconite [accessory tuber] (processed) (extended decoction)	Aconiti Tuber Laterale Praeparatum	6 g.	(1.5-3 g.)
duàn mǔ lì	oyster shell (calcined) (extended decoction)	Ostreae Concha Calcinatum	15 g.	(4.5-9 g.)

MODIFICATIONS

In cases accompanied by phlegm-dampness where patients are difficult to rouse from sleep, the prescription is modified to transform phlegm-dampness, open the orifices, and awaken the spirit.
Add:

dǎn xīng	arisaema [root] [bile-processed]	Arisaematis Rhizoma cum Felle Bovis	1.5-3 g.
fǎ bàn xià	pinellia [tuber] (processed)	Pinelliae Tuber Praeparatum	3-4.5 g.
shí chāng pú	acorus [root]	Acori Rhizoma	3-4.5 g.
yuǎn zhì	polygala [root]	Polygalae Radix	3-4.5 g.

In cases presenting with poor appetite and loose stools, the prescription is modified to fortify the spleen and regulate the stomach.
Add:

dǎng shēn	codonopsis [root]	Codonopsitis Radix	3-6 g.
bái zhú	ovate atractylodes [root]	Atractylodis Ovatae Rhizoma	3-4.5 g.
fú líng	poria	Poria	3-6 g.
shān zhā	crataegus [fruit]	Crataegi Fructus	3-6 g.

ACUPUNCTURE AND MOXIBUSTION

Main points: Needle with supplementation; add moxibustion.

CV-04	*guān yuán*
CV-03	*zhōng jí*
BL-23	*shèn shū*
BL-28	*páng guāng shū*
KI-03	*tài xī*
SP-06	*sān yīn jiāo*

Auxiliary points:

For excessive deep sleep, add:

GV-20	*bǎi huì*
HT-07	*shén mén*

For several bed-wettings each night, add moxibustion to:

LR-01	*dà dūn*

2. VACUITY OF LUNG AND SPLEEN QI

Clinical Manifestations: Enuresis with frequent short urinations, often seen when the constitution is weak during recovery from illness. Accompanying symptoms include shortness of breath, disinclination to speak, tiredness, fatigue, sallow complexion, loss of appetite, loose stools and spontaneous perspiration.

Tongue: Pale with white coating.

Pulse: Tardy or deep, thready.

Treatment Method: Supplement spleen and lung qi, consolidate the urine-holding function of the urinary bladder.

PRESCRIPTION

Combine Center-Supplementing Qi-Boosting Decoction *(bŭ zhōng yì qì tāng)* with Stream-Reducing Pill *(suō quán wán)*.

Center-Supplementing Qi-Boosting Decoction *bŭ zhōng yì qì tāng*

huáng qí	astragalus [root]	Astragali (seu Hedysari) Radix	15 g.	(4.5-9 g.)
rén shēn	ginseng	Ginseng Radix	9 g.	(3-4.5 g.)
bái zhú	ovate atractylodes [root]	Atractylodis Ovatae Rhizoma	9 g.	(3-4.5 g.)
dāng guī	tangkuei	Angelicae Sinensis Radix	9 g.	(3-4.5 g.)
chén pí	tangerine [peel]	Citri Exocarpium	6 g.	(1.5-3 g.)
shēng má	cimicifuga [root]	Cimicifugae Rhizoma	3 g.	(1-1.5 g.)
chái hú	bupleurum [root]	Bupleuri Radix	3 g.	(1-1.5 g.)
zhì gān căo	licorice [root] (honey-fried)	Glycyrrhizae Radix	6 g.	(1.5-3 g.)

MODIFICATIONS

In cases of excessively deep sleep, the prescription is modified to clear the heart and awaken the spirit.

Add:

shí chāng pú	acorus [root]	Acori Rhizoma	3-4.5 g.

In cases of loose stools, the prescription is modified to warm the spleen and dispel cold.

Add:

pào jiāng	blast-fried ginger (root)	Zingiberis Rhizoma Exsiccatum	1.5-3 g.

ACUPUNCTURE AND MOXIBUSTION

Main points: Needle with supplementation; add moxibustion.

BL-20	*pí shū*
CV-06	*qì hăi*
SP-06	*sān yīn jiāo*
LU-09	*tài yuān*
ST-36	*zú sān lĭ*

Auxiliary points:

For frequent urination, add:

GV-20	*băi huì*
BL-32	*cì liáo*

3. DAMP-HEAT OF THE LIVER CHANNEL

Clinical Manifestations: Bed-wetting, decreased urinary volume that is fishy in odor and yellow in color; restlessness and agitation, talking in the sleep, grinding of teeth during sleep, red lips.

Tongue: Yellow slimy coating.

Pulse: Rapid, slippery.

Treatment Method: Drain the liver, clear heat, disinhibit dampness.

PRESCRIPTION

Gentian Liver-Draining Decoction *lóng dǎn xiè gān tāng*

lóng dǎn cǎo	gentian [root]	Gentianae Radix	6 g.	(1.5-3 g.)
huáng qín	scutellaria [root]	Scutellariae Radix	9 g.	(3-4.5 g.)
shān zhī zǐ	gardenia [fruit]	Gardeniae Fructus	9 g.	(3-4.5 g.)
zé xiè	alisma [tuber]	Alismatis Rhizoma	12 g.	(3-6 g.)
mù tōng	mutong [stem]	Mutong Caulis	9 g.	(3-4.5 g.)
dāng guī	tangkuei	Angelicae Sinensis Radix	3 g.	(1.5-3 g.)
chē qián zǐ	plantago [seed] (wrapped)	Plantaginis Semen	9 g.	(3-4.5 g.)
shēng dì huáng	rehmannia [root] dried/fresh	Rehmanniae Radix Exsiccata seu Recens	9 g.	(3-4.5 g.)
chái hú	bupleurum [root]	Bupleuri Radix	6 g.	(1.5-3 g.)
gān cǎo	licorice [root]	Glycyrrhizae Radix	6 g.	(1.5-3 g.)

MODIFICATIONS

In cases of prolonged damp-heat that shows signs of red tongue with little coating, injury has been done to kidney yin. The prescription is modified to nourish yin and downbear fire.

Add:

Anemarrhena, Phellodendron and Rehmannia Pill *zhī bǎi dì huáng wán*

shú dì huáng	cooked rehmannia [root]	Rehmanniae Radix Conquita	24 g.	(6-12 g.)
shān zhū yú	cornus [fruit]	Corni Fructus	12 g.	(3-6 g.)
shān yào	dioscorea [root]	Dioscoreae Rhizoma	12 g.	(3-6 g.)
zé xiè	alisma [tuber]	Alismatis Rhizoma	9 g.	(3-4.5 g.)
fú líng	poria	Poria	9 g.	(3-4.5 g.)
mǔ dān pí	moutan [root bark]	Moutan Radicis Cortex	9 g.	(3-4.5 g.)
zhī mǔ	anemarrhena [root]	Anemarrhenae Rhizoma	9 g.	(3-4.5 g.)
huáng bǎi	phellodendron [bark]	Phellodendri Cortex	9 g.	(3-4.5 g.)

ACUPUNCTURE AND MOXIBUSTION

Main points: Needle with draining.

BL-28	*páng guāng shū*
CV-03	*zhōng jí*
SP-09	*yīn líng quán*
SP-06	*sān yīn jiāo*
LR-02	*xíng jiān*

Auxiliary points:

For frequent dreaming, add:

HT-07	*shén mén*

For depletion of kidney yin, add:

KI-03	*tài xī*

ALTERNATE THERAPEUTIC METHODS

1. Ear Acupuncture

Main points: Kidney, Urinary Bladder, Brain, Subcortex, and *Ā Shì* points.

Method: Select two to three points each session, needle to elicit a moderate sensation and retain the needles for twenty minutes. Treat once daily. Auricular needle-embedding therapy can also be used.

REMARKS

Because toilet habits are not fully established, enuresis is not considered a pathological condition in infants under three years of age. Enuresis because of organic pathological changes, such as spina bifida, deformities of the urinary tract, or organic cerebral pathological changes, as well as enterobiasis, should be treated according to the primary cause.

The entire family should cooperate in aiding the child, including moderate fluid intake after the nighttime meal, reminding the child to empty his or her bladder before going to bed, waking him or her once or twice at set intervals during the night to urinate and helping to form the habit of awakening during the night to urinate. Whole-hearted efforts should also be made to help the child overcome any sense of inferiority or timidity, and establish the confidence to eliminate the bed-wetting problem.

MUMPS

Zhà Sāi

1. External Epidemic Warm-Toxin - 2. Internal Epidemic Heat-Toxin

Zhà sāi, or mumps, is an acute contagious disease that presents with fever, swelling and tenderness of the parotid glands as its distinguishing characteristics. Mumps may be contracted in any of the four seasons, although it is more prevalent during winter and spring. School-age children are most commonly affected and the prognosis is generally favorable. In older children, mumps can be accompanied by pain and swelling of the testicles and, in severe cases, loss of consciousness and convulsions.

ETIOLOGY AND PATHOGENESIS

Wind-heat seasonal epidemic evils are the major etiological factor in the development of mumps. Such toxins invade the body through the nose and mouth, after which they combine with phlegm-fire to congest the shaoyang channels and obstruct the flow of qi and blood, with the result of swelling, hardness and pain in the area just under the ears above the parotid glands. Since the gallbladder channel and the liver channel are externally and internally related, and the liver channel encircles the external genitalia, severe seasonal heat-toxin can invade the liver channel, causing redness, swelling and pain of the testicles. If toxins move inward to affect the heart and liver, convulsions and loss of consciousness can result.

1. EXTERNAL EPIDEMIC WARM-TOXIN

Clinical Manifestations: Mild fever and aversion to cold, unilateral or bilateral swelling over the parotid glands, unclear swelling boundary, no apparent redness in the swollen area, pain and springy sensation on palpation, some difficulty in chewing, redness and pain of the throat.

Tongue: Red with thin yellow coating.

Pulse: Rapid, floating.

Treatment Method: Dispel wind, clear heat, resolve toxins, relieve swelling.

PRESCRIPTION

Lonicera and Forsythia Powder *yín qiào sǎn*

jīn yín huā	lonicera [flower]	Lonicerae Flos	9 g.	(3-4.5 g.)
lián qiào	forsythia [fruit]	Forsythiae Fructus	9 g.	(3-4.5 g.)
dàn dòu chǐ	fermented soybean	Glycines Semen Fermentatum Insulsum	6 g.	(1.5-3 g.)

niú bàng zǐ	arctium [seed]	Arctii Fructus	9 g. (3-4.5 g.)
bò hé	mint (abbreviated decoction)	Menthae Herba	6 g. (1.5-3 g.)
jīng jiè suì	schizonepeta [spike] (abbreviated decoction)	Schizonepetae Flos	6 g. (1.5-3 g.)
jié gěng	platycodon [root]	Platycodonis Radix	6 g. (1.5-3 g.)
gān cǎo	licorice [root]	Glycyrrhizae Radix	6 g. (1.5-3 g.)
lú gēn	phragmites [root]	Phragmititis Rhizoma	9 g. (3-4.5 g.)

MODIFICATIONS

In cases of redness, swelling and pain of the throat, the prescription is modified to reinforce resolving toxins and easing the throat.

Delete:

jīng jiè	schizonepeta	Schizonepetae Herba et Flos	

Add:

mǎ bó	puffball	Lasiosphaera seu Calvatia	1.5-3 g.
bǎn lán gēn	isatis [root]	Isatidis Radix	3-6 g.

In cases of severe swelling and pain of the parotid area, the prescription is modified to clear the liver, dissipate binds and disperse swelling. Add:

xià kū cǎo	prunella [spike]	Prunellae Spica	3-6 g.

ACUPUNCTURE AND MOXIBUSTION

Main points: Needle with draining.

ST-06	jiá chē
TB-17	yì fēng
TB-05	wài guān
LI-04	hé gǔ

Auxiliary points:

For fever and aversion to cold, add:

LU-07	liè quē

For high fever, add:

LI-11	qū chí
GV-14	dà zhuī
LU-11	shào shāng (Bleed)

2. INTERNAL EPIDEMIC HEAT-TOXIN

Clinical Manifestations: Heat, pain, redness and swelling of the area over the parotid glands; difficulty chewing; high fever, headache, irritability; thirst, redness, pain and swelling of the throat; dark scanty urine; dry hard stools; vomiting. In severe cases, there is redness and swelling of the testes, loss of consciousness or convulsions.

Tongue: Red with yellow coating.

Pulse: Rapid, slippery.

Treatment Method: Clear heat, resolve toxin, soften hardness, dissipate binds.

PRESCRIPTION

Universal Salvation Toxin-Dispersing Beverage *pǔ jì xiāo dú yǐn*

bǎn lán gēn	isatis [root]	Isatidis Radix	12 g. (3-6 g.)
huáng qín	scutellaria [root]	Scutellariae Radix	9 g. (3-4.5 g.)
huáng lián	coptis [root]	Coptidis Rhizoma	9 g. (3-4.5 g.)
xuán shēn	scrophularia [root]	Scrophulariae Radix	9 g. (3-4.5 g.)
lián qiào	forsythia [fruit]	Forsythiae Fructus	9 g. (3-4.5 g.)
chái hú	bupleurum [root]	Bupleuri Radix	6 g. (1.5-3 g.)
niú bàng zǐ	arctium [seed]	Arctii Fructus	9 g. (3-4.5 g.)
bái jiāng cán	silkworm	Bombyx Batryticatus	6 g. (1.5-3 g.)
jié gěng	platycodon [root]	Platycodonis Radix	6 g. (1.5-3 g.)
shēng mā	cimicifuga [root]	Cimicifugae Rhizoma	6 g. (1.5-3 g.)
bò hé	mint (abbreviated decoction)	Menthae Herba	3 g. (1-1.5 g.)
mǎ bó	puffball	Lasiosphaera seu Calvatia	3 g. (1-1.5 g.)
chén pí	tangerine [peel]	Citri Exocarpium	6 g. (1.5-3 g.)
gān cǎo	licorice [root]	Glycyrrhizae Radix	3 g. (1-1.5 g.)

MODIFICATIONS

In cases of swollen parotid glands with hard masses that are not easily dispersed, the prescription is modified to soften hardness and dissipate binds.

Delete:

gān cǎo	licorice [root]	Glycyrrhizae Radix

Add:

xià kū cǎo	prunella [spike]	Prunellae Spica	3-6 g.
hǎi zǎo	sargassum	Sargassi Herba	3-6 g.
kūn bù	kelp	Algae Thallus	3-6 g.

In cases of congestion of heat-toxin with constipation, the prescription is modified to drain heat and free the stool.

Add:

dà huáng	rhubarb (abbreviated decoction)	Rhei Rhizoma	3-4.5 g.
máng xiāo	mirabilite (stirred in)	Mirabilitum	3-4.5 g.

In cases accompanied by pain and swelling of the testes, the prescription is changed to clear and purge liver fire, quicken the blood and relieve pain.

Use:

Gentian Liver-Draining Decoction *lóng dǎn xiè gān tāng*

lóng dǎn cǎo	gentian [root]	Gentianae Radix	6 g. (1.5-3 g.)
huáng qín	scutellaria [root]	Scutellariae Radix	9 g. (3-4.5 g.)
shān zhī zǐ	gardenia [fruit]	Gardeniae Fructus	9 g. (3-4.5 g.)
zé xiè	alisma [tuber]	Alismatis Rhizoma	12 g. (3-6 g.)
mù tōng	mutong [stem]	Mutong Caulis	9 g (3-4.5 g.)
dāng guī	tangkuei	Angelicae Sinensis Radix	3 g. (1-1.5 g.)
chē qián zǐ	plantago [seed] (wrapped)	Plantaginis Semen	9 g. (3-4.5 g)
shēng dì huáng	rehmannia [root] dried/fresh	Rehmanniae Radix Exsiccata seu Recens	9 g. (3-4.5 g.)
chái hú	bupleurum [root]	Bupleuri Radix	6 g. (1.5-3 g.)
gān cǎo	licorice [root]	Glycyrrhizae Radix	6 g. (1.5-3 g.)

Delete:

shēng dì huáng	rehmannia [root] dried/fresh	Rehmanniae Radix Exsiccata seu Recens
chē qián zǐ	plantago [seed]	Plantaginis Semen
zé xiè	alisma [tuber]	Alismatis Rhizoma
gān cǎo	licorice [root]	Glycyrrhizae Radix

Add:

chì sháo yào	red peony [root]	Paeoniae Radix Rubra	3-4.5 g.
táo rén	peach [kernel]	Persicae Semen	3-4.5 g.
yán hú suǒ	corydalis [tuber]	Corydalis Tuber	3-4.5 g.
chuān liàn zǐ	toosendan [fruit]	Toosendan Fructus	3-4.5 g.

In cases accompanied by convulsions, loss of consciousness and a crimson tongue, Universal Salvation Toxin-Dispersing Beverage *(pǔ jì xiāo dú yǐn)* is modified to clear heat-toxin, extinguish wind and suppress convulsions.

Delete:

jié gěng	platycodon [root]	Platycodonis Radix
niú bàng zǐ	arctium [seed]	Arctii Fructus
bò hé	mint	Menthae Herba
chái hú	bupleurum [root]	Bupleuri Radix
shēng mā	cimicifuga [root]	Cimicifugae Rhizoma
mǎ bó	puffball	Lasiosphaera seu Calvatia
gān cǎo	licorice [root]	Glycyrrhizae Radix

Add:

xià kū cǎo	prunella [spike]	Prunellae Spica	3-6 g.
pú gōng yīng	dandelion	Taraxaci Herba cum Radice	3-6 g.
gōu téng	uncaria [stem and thorn] (abbreviated decoction	Uncariae Ramulus cum Unco	3-6 g.
chán tuì	cicada molting	Cicadae Periostracum	3-4.5 g.
quán xiē	scorpion	Buthus	1.5-3 g.

In addition, use the prepared formulas PURPLE SNOW ELIXIR *(zǐ xuě dān)* or SUPREME JEWEL ELIXIR *(zhì bǎo dān)*, to increase the heat clearing, wind eradicating and orifice opening.

ACUPUNCTURE AND MOXIBUSTION

Main points: Needle with draining.

TB-22	*hé liáo*
TB-05	*wài guān*
LI-04	*hé gǔ*
LI-11	*qū chí*
LU-11	*shào shāng*
TB-01	*guān chōng*
ST-40	*fēng lóng*

Auxiliary points:

For high fever, add:

GV-14	*dà zhuī*

Bleed the twelve jing points:

LU-11	*shào shāng*
LI-01	*shāng yáng*
PC-09	*zhōng chōng*
TB-01	*guān chōng*
HT-09	*shào chōng*
SI-01	*shào zé*

For pain and swelling of the testes, add:

LR-03	*tài chōng*
LR-08	*qū quán*

For headache, add:

GB-20	*fēng chí*
GB-43	*xiá xī*

For convulsions and loss of consciousness, add:

GV-26	*shuǐ gōu*

ALTERNATE THERAPEUTIC METHODS

1. Ear Acupuncture

Main points: Parotid Gland, Cheek, *Shén Mén*, Helix 4, 5, 6.

Method: Select two to three points each session, and needle to elicit a strong sensation. Treat once or twice daily, three days per therapeutic course.

2. External Treatment

Grind the ingredients in the following prescription into a fine powder and mix with an enough vinegar to form a smooth paste. Spread the plaster over the parotid area three to four times daily.

Indigo Powder *qīng dài sǎn*

qīng dài	indigo	Indigo Pulverata Levis	60 g.
huáng bǎi	phellodendron [bark]	Phellodendri Cortex	60 g.
shí gāo	gypsum	Gypsum	120 g.
huá shí	talcum	Talcum	120 g.

REMARKS

Mumps is a communicable respiratory illness. Patients should be quarantined during treatment, generally until five days after the swelling completely subsides. During the period of high fever, patients should be given plenty of bed rest and a liquid or semi-liquid diet, restricting rich, slimy and fibrous foods.

As a preventative for children who have been exposed to the illness administer a daily decoction of 15–30 g. isatis root *(bǎn lán gēn)* for three to five days.

MEASLES

Má Zhěn

1. Uncomplicated Patterns: - 1A. Febrile Stage - 1B. Eruption Stage - 1C. Recovery Stage - 2. Complicated Patterns: - 2A. Oppression of the Lung by Heat Evil - 2B. Invasion of the Throat by Heat Evil - 2C. Accumulation of Heat-Toxin in the Heart and Liver

Measles is a common communicable pediatric respiratory illness. Its distinguishing characteristics include fever, coughing, stuffy nose, runny nose, tearing of the eyes and a red rash covering the entire body. Measles can occur at any time throughout the year, although it is more prevalent during the winter and spring. Measles is a highly contagious illness most common in children between the ages of six months and five years. One attack of measles generally gives lifetime immunity to the illness.

ETIOLOGY AND PATHOGENESIS

The etiology of measles involves attack by seasonal heat-toxin. Under ordinary circumstances, the development of measles can be thought of as an initial febrile stage, eruption stage and recovery stage. During the initial febrile stage, one finds defense aspect patterns resembling the common cold, with symptoms of fever, coughing, sneezing and runny nose. As the toxins invade the qi aspect, a red rash develops over the entire body. The appearance of the rash marks the beginning of the eruption stage and is the result an effort by correct qi to disperse toxins through the body surface. Evils are expelled with the rash and the fever diminishes, with some injury to fluids. The illness then moves into the recovery stage. This represents the uncomplicated course of measles.

Following the appearance of the rash over the entire body, there may be further internal invasion of evils. These can create various complications and are considered unfavorable. If correct qi is insufficient, further invasion of the body by internal evils may occur, or if seasonal heat-toxin is severe and cannot be overcome, the outward expulsion of toxins does not take place, resulting in secondary patterns. Complicated patterns can occur at any stage during the development of measles; however, complications most often occur during the eruption stage.

1A. UNCOMPLICATED PATTERNS – FEBRILE STAGE

Clinical Manifestations: Fever, aversion to cold or drafts, stuffy runny nose, sneezing, coughing, frontal headache, red eyelids, tearing of the eyes, fatigue and sleepiness. After two to three days of fever, the mucous membranes on the inside of the cheeks become red and the mucous patches characteristic of measles gradually appear. They begin next to the molars and consist of a small white dot surrounded by a ring of redness, known in Western medicine as Koplik's spots. Urine is concentrated and scanty, stools sometimes loose or runny. This stage, from the first signs of fever to the appearance of the rash, lasts approximately three days.

Tongue: Thin, white or slightly yellow coating.

Pulse: Rapid, floating.

Treatment Method: Clear and diffuse the lung, outthrust the exterior with cool pungent herbs.

PRESCRIPTION

Toxin-Diffusing Exterior-Effusing Decoction* *xuān dú fā biǎo tāng*

gé gēn	pueraria [root]	Puerariae Radix	3-6 g.
shēng mā	cimicifuga [root]	Cimicifugae Rhizoma	1.5-3 g.
niú bàng zǐ	arctium [seed]	Arctii Fructus	3-6 g.
lián qiào	forsythia [fruit]	Forsythiae Fructus	3-6 g.
zhú yè	black bamboo [leaf]	Bambusae Folium	1.5-3 g.
qián hú	peucedanum [root]	Peucedani Radix	3-6 g.
jīng jiè	schizonepeta (abbreviated decoction)	Schizonepetae Herba et Flos	1.5-3 g.
fáng fēng	ledebouriella [root]	Ledebouriellae Radix	1.5-3 g.
zhǐ ké	bitter orange [fruit]	Aurantii Fructus	1.5-3 g.
mù tōng	mutong [stem]	Mutong Caulis	1.5-3 g.
jié gěng	platycodon [root]	Platycodonis Radix	1.5-3 g.
gān cǎo	licorice [root]	Glycyrrhizae Radix	1.5-3 g.
bò hé	mint (abbreviated decoction)	Menthae Herba	1.5-3 g.
yán suī	coriander	Coriandi Herba cum Radice	1.5-3 g.

*This formula is only for children.

MODIFICATIONS

In cases of high fever without perspiration, the prescription is modified to aid eruption of rash and dispersion of evils.
Add:

xiān fú píng	fresh duckweed	Lemnae Herba Recens	3-4.5 g.

In cases of marked soreness of the throat, the prescription is modified to course wind heat, clear the lung, and disinhibit the pharynx.
Add:

mǎ bó	puffball	Lasiosphaera seu Calvatia	1.5-3 g.
shè gān	belamcanda [root]	Belamcandae Rhizoma	3-4.5 g.

In cases of high fever with injury to yin where eruption of the rash is hindered, the prescription is modified to nourish yin and promote eruption of the rash.
Add:

shēng dì huáng	rehmannia [root] (dried/fresh)	Rehmanniae Radix Exsiccata seu Recens	3-4.5 g.
xuán shēn	scrophularia [root]	Scrophulariae Radix	3-4.5 g.
tiān huā fěn	trichosanthes root	Trichosanthis Radix	3-6 g.

In cases of poor physical constitution, with lack of strength necessary to erupt the rash and dispel evils, accompanied by pale complexion and pale tongue, the prescription is modified to assist correct qi and effuse the rash.

Add:

rén shēn	ginseng	Ginseng Radix	3-4.5 g.
huáng qí	astragalus [root]	Astragali (seu Hedysari) Radix	3-6 g.
huáng jīng	polygonatum [root]	Polygonati Huangjing Rhizoma	3-6 g.

In cases where wind-cold has invaded the body surface, preventing the unhindered eruption of the rash, the prescription is modified to promote eruption of the rash with warm pungent herbs.

Add:

má huáng	ephedra	Ephedrae Herba	1.5-3 g.
xì xīn	asarum	Asiasari Herba cum Radice	1-1.5 g.

In cases where evils have invaded the construction aspect, with symptoms of hindered eruption of the rash, high fever, irritability, thirst and deep red tongue, the prescription is modified to cool construction and promote eruption of the rash.

Add:

shí hú	dendrobium [stem]	Dendrobii Caulis	3-6 g.
shēng dì huáng	rehmannia [root] dried/fresh	Rehmanniae Radix Exsiccata seu Recens	3-6 g.
dàn dòu chǐ	fermented soybean (unsalted)	Glycines Semen Fermentatum Insulsum	3-6 g.

1B. UNCOMPLICATED PATTERNS – ERUPTION STAGE

Clinical Manifestations: Continued fever with simultaneous eruption of rash. The rash begins along the hairline behind the ears, gradually spreading over the forehead, cheeks, neck, chest, abdomen, four limbs and, when fully erupted, to the palms, soles and top of the nose. The rash begins as small separate spots that gradually become denser – bright red at first, dark red later – and slightly raised above the surface of the skin. Accompanying symptoms include excessive thirst, bloodshot eyes with increased discharge, more severe coughing, irritability or sleepiness. This stage, from the first signs of rash to full eruption of the rash, lasts approximately three days.

Tongue: Red with yellow coating.

Pulse: Rapid.

Treatment Method: Clear heat, resolve toxin, promote eruption of rash.

PRESCRIPTION

Clearing and Resolving Exterior-Outthrusting Decoction*
qīng jiě tòu biǎo tāng

sāng yè	mulberry [leaf]	Mori Folium	3-6 g.
jú huā	chrysanthemum [flower]	Chrysanthemi Flos	3-6 g.
jīn yín huā	lonicera [flower]	Lonicerae Flos	3-6 g.
lián qiào	forsythia [fruit]	Forsythiae Fructus	3-6 g.
chán tuì	cicada molting	Cicadae Periostracum	3-4.5 g.
niú bàng zǐ	arctium [seed]	Arctii Fructus	3-6 g.
xī hé liǔ	tamarisk [twig and leaf]	Tamaricis Ramulus et Folium	3-6 g.
gé gēn	pueraria [root]	Puerariae Radix	3-6 g.
shēng má	cimicifuga [root]	Cimicifugae Rhizoma	3-6 g.
zǐ cǎo	puccoon [root]	Lithospermi, Macrotomiae, seu Onosmatis Radix	3-6 g.
gān cǎo	licorice [root]	Glycyrrhizae Radix	3-4.5 g.

*This formula is only for children.

MODIFICATIONS

In cases where rash is bright red or dark purplish, manifesting in large patches, the prescription is modified to clear heat and cool the blood.
Add:

shēng dì huáng	rehmannia [root] dried/fresh	Rehmanniae Radix Exsiccata seu Recens	3-6 g.
mǔ dān pí	moutan [root bark]	Moutan Radicis Cortex	3-6 g.

In cases of severe coughing, the prescription is modified to clear the lung and transform phlegm.
Add:

jié gěng	platycodon [root]	Platycodonis Radix	3-4.5 g.
sāng bái pí	mulberry [root bark]	Mori Radicis Cortex	3-4.5 g.
xìng rén	apricot [kernel] (abbreviated decoction)	Armeniacae Semen	3-4.5 g.

In cases of high fever, with flushed complexion and irritability, the prescription is modified to clear heat and drain fire.
Add:

shān zhī zǐ	gardenia [fruit]	Gardeniae Fructus	3-4.5 g.
huáng lián	coptis [root]	Coptidis Rhizoma	1.5-3 g.
shí gāo	gypsum (extended decoction)	Gypsum	9-15 g.

In cases of bleeding gums or epistaxis, the prescription is modified to cool the blood and relieve bleeding.
Add:

ǒu jié tàn	lotus root node (charred)	Nelumbinis Rhizomatis Nodus Carbonisatus	3-6 g.
bái máo gēn	imperata [root]	Imperatae Rhizoma	6-12 g.

1C. UNCOMPLICATED PATTERNS – RECOVERY STAGE

Clinical Manifestations: After complete eruption of the rash, the fever begins to subside and the voice is slightly hoarse with dry coughing and thirst. The rash gradually disappears in the same sequence as that of eruption and the skin becomes darker and flakes off. Appetite improves, and vitality returns.

Tongue: Red with dry coating.

Pulse: Thready, slightly rapid.

Treatment Method: Nourish yin, boost qi, clear remaining evils.

PRESCRIPTION

Adenophora-Glehnia and Ophiopogon Decoction *shā shēn mài dōng tāng*

běi shā shēn	glehnia [root]	Glehniae Radix	9 g. (3-4.5 g.)
mài mén dōng	ophiopogon [tuber]	Ophiopogonis Tuber	9 g. (3-4.5 g.)
tiān huā fěn	trichosanthes [root]	Trichosanthis Radix	12 g. (3-6 g.)
yù zhú	Solomon's seal [root]	Polygonati Yuzhu Rhizoma	9 g. (3-4.5 g.)
biǎn dòu	lablab [bean]	Lablab Semen	12 g. (3-6 g.)
sāng yè	mulberry [leaf]	Mori Folium	6 g. (1.5-3 g.)
gān cǎo	licorice [root]	Glycyrrhizae Radix	6 g. (1.5-3 g.)

MODIFICATIONS

In cases where heat is not completely cleared, the prescription is modified to clear the lung and clear vacuity heat.

Add:

dì gŭ pí	lycium [root bark]	Lycii Radicis Cortex	3-4.5 g.
yín chái hú	lanceolate stellaria [root]	Stellariae Lanceolatae Radix	3-4.5 g.

In cases of poor appetite, the prescription is modified to strengthen the stomach and promote appetite.

Add:

gŭ yá	rice sprout	Oryzae Fructus Germinatus	3-6 g.
mài yá	barley sprout	Hordei Fructus Germinatus	3-6 g.

In cases of hard dry stools, the prescription is modified to moisten and free the stool.

Add:

quán guā lóu	whole trichosanthes [fruit]	Trichosanthis Fructus Integer	3-6 g.
huŏ má rén	hemp [seed]	Cannabis Semen	3-6 g.

2A. COMPLICATED PATTERNS – OPPRESSION OF THE LUNG BY HEAT-TOXIN

Clinical Manifestations: Incomplete eruption of rash; premature disappearance of rash; or extensive concentrated purplish rash, unabated high fever, coughing, wheezing, flaring of the nostrils during respiration, thirst, restlessness.

Tongue: Red with dry yellow coating.

Pulse: Rapid.

Treatment Method: Diffuse the lung, open oppression, clear heat, resolve toxin.

PRESCRIPTION

Ephedra, Apricot Kernel, Gypsum and Licorice Decoction
má xìng shí gān tāng

má huáng	ephedra	Ephedrae Herba	6 g. (1.5-3 g.)
xìng rén	apricot kernel	Armeniacae Semen	9 g. (3-4.5 g.)
shí gāo	gypsum (extended decoction)	Gypsum	18 g. (4.5-9 g.)
zhì gān căo	licorice [root] (honey-fried)	Glycyrrhizae Radix	6 g. (1.5-3 g.)

MODIFICATIONS

In cases of extreme fever, the prescription is modified to clear lung heat.

Add:

huáng qín	scutellaria [root]	Scutellariae Radix	3-4.5 g.
yú xīng căo	houttuynia	Houttuyniae Herba cum Radice	4.5-9 g.

In cases of severe coughing and wheezing, the prescription is modified to drain the lung and relieve coughing and wheezing.

Add:

tíng lì zĭ	tingli [seed]	Descurainiae seu Lepidii Semen	3-4.5 g.

In addition, to downbear qi and transform phlegm, add:

qián hú	peucedanum [root]	Peucedani Radix	3-4.5 g.

In cases of dry, hard stools, the prescription is modified to drain fire and free the stool.

Add:

dà huáng	rhubarb (abbreviated decoction)	Rhei Rhizoma	3-4.5 g.
máng xiāo	mirabilite (stirred in)	Mirabilitum	3-4.5 g.

In cases of copious phlegm, the prescription is modified to dissolve and eliminate phlegm.

Add:

tiān zhú huáng	bamboo sugar	Bambusae Concretio Silicea	1.5-3 g.
zhú lì	dried bamboo sap (stirred in)	Bambusae Succus Exsiccatus	9-18 g.
zhè bèi mǔ	Zhejiang fritillaria [bulb]	Fritillariae Verticillatae Bulbus	3-4.5 g.

2B. COMPLICATED PATTERNS – INVASION OF THE THROAT BY HEAT-TOXIN

Clinical Manifestations: Swelling and pain of the throat, hoarse voice, heavy coughing similar to a dog barking.

Tongue: Red with yellow slimy coating.

Pulse: Rapid, slippery.

Treatment Method: Clear heat-toxin, ease the throat, disperse swelling.

PRESCRIPTION

Combine Pharynx-Clearing Phlegm-Precipitating Decoction *(qīng yān xià tán tāng)* with the prepared medicine SIX SPIRITS PILL *(liù shén wán)*.

Pharynx-Clearing Phlegm-Precipitating Decoction *qīng yān xià tán tāng*

xuán shēn	scrophularia [root]	Scrophulariae Radix	12 g. (3-6 g.)
jié gěng	platycodon [root]	Platycodonis Radix	9 g. (3-4.5 g.)
niú bàng zǐ	arctium [seed]	Arctii Fructus	9 g. (3-4.5 g.)
shè gān	belamcanda [root]	Belamcandae Rhizoma	9 g. (3-4.5 g.)
jīng jiè	schizonepeta (abbreviated decoction)	Schizonepetae Herba et Flos	6 g. (1.5-3 g.)
mǎ dōu líng	aristolochia [fruit]	Aristolochiae Fructus	9 g. (3-4.5 g.)
zhè bèi mǔ	Zhejiang fritillaria, bulb	Fritillariae Verticillatae Bulbus	12 g. (3-6 g.)
guā lóu	trichosanthes [fruit]	Trichosanthis Fructus	12 g. (3-6 g.)
gān cǎo	licorice [root]	Glycyrrhizae Radix	9 g. (3-4.5 g.)

MODIFICATIONS

To reinforce clearing heat-toxin, with symptoms of sore throat and lymphatic swelling, add:

bǎn lán gēn	isatis [root]	Isatidis Radix	3-6 g.
jīn yín huā	lonicera [flower]	Lonicerae Flos	3-6 g.
tíng lì zǐ	tingli [seed]	Descurainiae seu Lepidii Semen	3-4.5 g.

In cases of hard, dry stools, the prescription is modified to drain fire and free the stool.

Add:

dà huáng	rhubarb (abbreviated decoction)	Rhei Rhizoma	3-4.5 g.
máng xiāo	mirabilite (stirred in)	Mirabilitum	3-4.5 g.

2c. COMPLICATED PATTERNS – ACCUMULATION OF HEAT-TOXIN IN THE HEART AND LIVER

Clinical Manifestations: High fever, restlessness, delirium, concentrated purplish-red rash manifesting in large patches over the entire body, flaring of the nostrils during respiration, loss of consciousness and convulsions when severe.

Tongue: Deep red.

Pulse: Rapid, wiry.

Treatment Method: Clear the heart, resolve toxin, subdue liver, extinguish wind.

PRESCRIPTION

Antelope Horn and Uncaria Decoction *líng jiǎo gōu téng tāng*

líng yáng jiǎo	antelope horn	Antelopis Cornu	3 g.	(1-1.5 g.)
	(or, powdered and stirred in, each time 0.5 g.)			
gōu téng	uncaria [stem and thorn]	Uncariae Ramulus cum Unco	9 g.	(3-4.5 g.)
	(abbreviated decoction)			
sāng yè	mulberry [leaf]	Mori Folium	6 g.	(1.5-3 g.)
jú huā	chrysanthemum [flower]	Chrysanthemi Flos	9 g.	(3-4.5 g.)
chuān bèi mǔ	Sichuan fritillaria [bulb]	Fritillariae Cirrhosae Bulbus	12 g.	(3-6 g.)
zhú rú	bamboo shavings	Bambusae Caulis in Taeniam	9 g.	(3-4.5 g.)
shēng dì huáng	rehmannia [root] dried/fresh	Rehmanniae Radix Exsiccata seu Recens	15 g.	(4.5-9 g.)
bái sháo yào	white peony [root]	Paeoniae Radix Alba	9 g.	(3-4.5 g.)
fú shén	root poria	Poria cum Pini Radice	9 g.	(3-4.5 g.)
gān cǎo	licorice [root]	Glycyrrhizae Radix	3 g.	(1-1.5 g.)

MODIFICATIONS

In severe cases of loss of consciousness, the prescription is modified to increase the effects of clearing heat, suppressing convulsions, and opening the orifices. Add:

shí chāng pú	acorus [root]	Acori Rhizoma	3-4.5 g.
dǎn xīng	[bile-processed] arisaema [root]	Arisaematis Rhizoma cum Felle Bovis	1.5-3 g.
yù jīn	curcuma [tuber]	Curcumae Tuber	3-4.5 g.

When necessary, add the prepared medicines PURPLE SNOW ELIXIR *(zǐ xuě dān)* or PEACEFUL PALACE BOVINE BEZOAR PILL *(ān gōng niú huáng wán)*.

ALTERNATE THERAPEUTIC METHODS

In cases of incomplete eruption of the measles rash, one of the following external treatments can be adopted in addition to the prescription of internal herbal medicine.

External Prescription One:

má huáng	ephedra	Ephedrae Herba	15 g.
xiān fú píng	fresh duckweed	Lemnae Herba Recens	15 g.
yán suī	coriander	Coriandri Herba cum Radice	15 g.
huáng mǐ jǔ	yellow rice wine	Oryzae Vinum Aureum	60 cc.

Add to an appropriate amount of water and boil, allowing the steam to fill the sickroom, as well as wetting towels with the decoction and applying to the patient's face, chest and back.

External Prescription Two:

xiān fú píng	fresh duckweed	Lemnae Herba Recens	15 g.
xī hé liǔ	tamarisk [twig and leaf]	Tamaricis Ramulus et Folium	30 g.
zǐ sū yè	perilla [leaf]	Perillae Folium	15 g.
yán suī	coriander	Coriandri Herba cum Radice	15 g.

Decoct in water and use the decoction to scrub the patient with a towel.

REMARKS

Whether or not complications are likely is of little importance during the initial development of measles. Herbal medicine constitutes the major treatment, and is recommended in all cases. The treatment method depends on the patient's constitution and the stage of illness development and includes promoting eruption of the rash, clearing heat-toxin or nourishing yin. In general, promoting the eruption of the rash is used during the initial febrile stage, clearing heat-toxin during the eruption stage, and nourishing yin during the recovery stage.

When promoting the eruption of rash, avoid depletion of fluids; when clearing heat-toxin, avoid disruption by cold; when nourishing yin, avoid incomplete expulsion of evils. In cases of severe heat-toxin, regardless of whether or not the rash has erupted completely, clear heat-toxin and promote eruption of rash simultaneously; such cases have a tendency to develop complicated patterns like pneumonia.

Promoting the eruption of the rash can also be accomplished through warm dispersion and supplementation, but this method is called for only in a few cases where the physical constitution is weak and a pattern of vacuity cold presents. It is not to be used imprudently.

Nursing care is also important during the treatment of measles. The sickroom should be well-ventilated without being drafty; overly bright light should be avoided. The patient's mouth, nose and eyes should be regularly cleaned, and the patient be allowed plenty to drink. The diet should be light and bland and consists mainly of easily digested foods, such as liquids and purees. Rich, slimy and spicy foods should be restricted.

PART VII

OPHTHALMOLOGY

SORE, RED AND SWOLLEN EYES

Mù Chì Zhŏng Tòng

1. External Wind-Heat - 2. Exuberant Liver and Gallbladder Fire

Redness, pain, and swelling of the eyes is an acute symptom presented in a variety of eye illnesses. In traditional Chinese medicine, it is also known as red eye *(hóng yăn)*, or fire eye *(huŏ yăn)*. In ancient medical works the etiology, clinical manifestations and communicability of eye illnesses gave basis to such terms as wind-heat eye *(fēng rè yăn)*, epidemic reddening of the eye *(tiān xíng chì mù)* and epidemic reddening of the eye with corneal opacity *(tiān xíng chì mù bào yì)*.

Redness, pain and swelling of the eyes is commonly observed in ophthalmic conditions including acute conjunctivitis, pseudo membranous conjunctivitis and epidemic keratoconjunctivitis.

ETIOLOGY AND PATHOGENESIS

Redness, pain and swelling of the eyes is often the result of invasion by seasonal wind-heat evils; these factors can lodge in the eyes and are not easily dispersed. A second possible pathogenesis involves exuberance of liver and gallbladder fire that follows the course of these channels, rising to disturb the eyes.

1. EXTERNAL WIND-HEAT

Clinical Manifestations: Redness, pain and swelling of the eyes; over-sensitivity to light, excessive tearing, dryness and/or itching of the eyes or eyes with a gummy exudate that are difficult to open. These symptoms are accompanied by sensitivity to draughts, fever, headache, stuffy nose, dry mouth and thirst.

Tongue: Thin yellow coating.

Pulse: Rapid, floating.

Treatment Method: Dispel wind, clear heat, disperse swelling, relieve pain.

PRESCRIPTION

Lung-Clearing Beverage *xiè fèi yĭn*

shí gāo	gypsum (extended decoction)	Gypsum	15 g.
chì sháo yào	red peony [root]	Paeoniae Radix Rubra	9 g.
huáng qín	scutellaria [root]	Scutellariae Radix	9 g.
lián qiào	forsythia [fruit]	Forsythiae Fructus	12 g.
sāng bái pí	mulberry [root bark]	Mori Radicis Cortex	12 g.

shān zhī zǐ	gardenia [fruit]	Gardeniae Fructus	6 g.
mù tōng	mutong [stem]	Mutong Caulis	6 g.
jīng jiè	schizonepeta (abbreviated decoction)	Schizonepetae Herba et Flos	6 g.
fáng fēng	ledebouriella [root]	Ledebouriellae Radix	6 g.
qiāng huó	notopterygium [root]	Notopterygii Rhizoma	3 g.
bái zhǐ	angelica [root]	Angelicae Dahuricae Radix	3 g.
zhǐ ké	bitter orange [fruit]	Aurantii Fructus	3 g.
gān cǎo	licorice [root]	Glycyrrhizae Radix	6 g.

MODIFICATIONS

To reinforce dispersing wind, clearing heat and brightening the eyes, add:

sāng yè	mulberry [leaf]	Mori Folium	9 g.
jú huā	chrysanthemum [flower]	Chrysanthemi Flos	9 g.
chán tuì	cicada molting	Cicadae Periostracum	6 g.

In cases of constipation, the prescription is modified to drain heat and free the stool.
Add:

| dà huáng | rhubarb (abbreviated decoction) | Rhei Rhizoma | 6 g. |
| máng xiāo | mirabilite (stirred in) | Mirabilitum | 6 g. |

ACUPUNCTURE AND MOXIBUSTION

Main points: Needle with draining.

LI-11	qū chí
LI-04	hé gǔ
TB-05	wài guān
BL-01	jīng míng
GB-20	fēng chí
M-HN-9	tài yáng (Greater Yang) (bleed)

Auxiliary points:

For headache, add:

| M-HN-3 | yìn táng (Hall of Impression) |

For irritability, add:

| TB-01 | guān chōng |

2. EXUBERANCE OF LIVER AND GALLBLADDER FIRE

Clinical Manifestations: Symptoms of redness, pain and swelling of the eyes, over-sensitivity to light, tearing, dryness and/or itching of the eyes or eyes with a gummy exudate that are difficult to open; accompanied by symptoms of dry bitter-tasting mouth, dry throat, irritability, tinnitus, headache, constipation and dark urine.

Tongue: Redness of the tip and sides with yellow coating.

Pulse: Rapid, wiry.

Treatment Method: Drain liver and gallbladder fire.

PRESCRIPTION

Gentian Liver-Draining Decoction *lóng dǎn xiè gān tāng*

lóng dǎn cǎo	gentian [root]	Gentianae Radix	6 g.
huáng qín	scutellaria [root]	Scutellariae Radix	9 g.
shān zhī zǐ	gardenia [fruit]	Gardeniae Fructus	9 g.
zé xiè	alisma [tuber]	Alismatis Rhizoma	12 g.
mù tōng	mutong [stem]	Mutong Caulis	9 g.
dāng guī	tangkuei	Angelicae Sinensis Radix	3 g.
chē qián zǐ	plantago [seed] (wrapped)	Plantaginis Semen	9 g.
shēng dì huáng	rehmannia [root] dried/fresh	Rehmanniae Radix Exsiccata seu Recens	9 g.
chái hú	bupleurum [root]	Bupleuri Radix	6 g.
gān cǎo	licorice [root]	Glycyrrhizae Radix	6 g.

MODIFICATIONS

In cases of constipation, the prescription is modified to free the stool and drain heat. Add:

dà huáng	rhubarb (abbreviated decoction)	Rhei Rhizoma	9 g.
máng xiāo	mirabilite (stirred in)	Mirabilitum	9 g.

After the bowels begin moving, the prescription is modified to clear the liver and boost the eyes.

Delete:

dà huáng	rhubarb	Rhei Rhizoma
máng xiāo	mirabilite	Mirabilitum

Add:

jīn yín huā	lonicera [flower]	Lonicerae Flos	9 g.
pú gōng yīng	dandelion	Taraxaci Herba cum Radice	9 g.
cì jí lí	tribulus [fruit]	Tribuli Fructus	9 g.
jué míng zǐ	fetid cassia [seed]	Cassiae Torae Semen	12 g.

ACUPUNCTURE AND MOXIBUSTION

Main points: Needle with draining.

LI-04	*hé gǔ*
BL-01	*jīng míng*
M-HN-9	*tài yáng* (Greater Yang) (bleed)
GB-20	*fēng chí*
LR-03	*tài chōng*
LR-02	*xíng jiān*

Auxiliary points:

For headache and tinnitus, add:

GB-43	*xiá xī*

ALTERNATE THERAPEUTIC METHODS

1. Ear Acupuncture

Main points: Eye, Eye 1, Eye 2, Liver.

Method: Needle to elicit a strong sensation and retain needles for thirty minutes.

The tip of the ear and the small veins on the back of the ear can be pricked with a three-edged needle to let blood.

2. Picking Therapy

Method: Locate painful pressure points between the shoulder blades, or select GV-14 *(dà zhuī)* and two points 0.5 cun to its left and right. Employ a thicker needle to break the skin; then pick up and snap the glistening white fibers from underlying tissues.

REMARKS

In order to prevent infection of the eye and injury to blood vessels, needling of acupoints located within the orbits, such as BL-01 *(jīng míng)* should be preceded by strict sterilization. The insertion of the needles should be slow, with manipulation consisting of delicate rotation without lifting or thrusting. During the course of treatment, patients should control their tempers, avoid overindulgent sexual activity and abstain from spicy foods. Attention should also be paid to eye hygiene, adequate sleep and reduction of activities strenuous to the eyes.

STYE

Zhēn Yǎn

1. External Wind-Heat - 2. Heat Brewing in the Stomach and Spleen

Stye refers to certain inflamed grain-sized swellings appearing along the edge of the eyelid. Known as hordeolum in Western medicine, styes are most commonly found in teenagers.

ETIOLOGY AND PATHOGENESIS

Styes can result from the invasion of external wind-heat or from the over-consumption of spicy or rich foods leading to heat brewing in the stomach and spleen and disturbing the eyes.

1. EXTERNAL WIND-HEAT

Clinical Manifestations: Initial pain and itching of the affected eyelid, followed by localized redness and swelling along the edge of the eyelid; formation of a grain-sized mass that is fixed on palpation. Accompanying symptoms include aversion to drafts, fever, headache, coughing, general malaise.

Tongue: Thin yellow coating.

Pulse: Rapid, floating.

Treatment Method: Course wind, clear heat.

PRESCRIPTION

Lonicera and Forsythia Powder *yín qiào sǎn*

jīn yín huā	lonicera [flower]	Lonicerae Flos	9 g.
lián qiáo	forsythia [fruit]	Forsythiae Fructus	9 g.
dàn dòu chǐ	fermented soybean (unsalted)	Glycines Semen Fermentatum Insulsum	6 g.
niú bàng zǐ	arctium [seed]	Arctii Fructus	9 g.
bò hé	mint (abbreviated decoction)	Menthae Herba	6 g.
jīng jiè suì	schizonepeta [spike] (abbreviated decoction)	Schizonepetae Flos	6 g.
jié gěng	platycodon [root]	Platycodonis Radix	6 g.
gān cǎo	licorice [root]	Glycyrrhizae Radix	6 g.
lú gēn	phragmites [root]	Phragmititis Rhizoma	9 g.

MODIFICATIONS

In cases of severe heat, the prescription is modified to assist clearing heat.

Delete:

jīng jiè	schizonepeta	Schizonepetae Herba et Flos
dàn dòu chǐ	fermented soybean (unsalted)	Glycines Semen Fermentatum Insulsum

Add:

huáng qín	scutellaria [root]	Scutellariae Radix	9 g.
huáng lián	coptis [root]	Coptidis Rhizoma	6 g.

ACUPUNCTURE AND MOXIBUSTION

Main points: Needle with draining.

BL-01	*jīng míng*
BL-02	*zǎn zhú*
LR-02	*xíng jiān*
LI-04	*hé gǔ*
M-HN-9	*tài yáng* (Greater Yang) (bleed)

Auxiliary points:

For fever and aversion to draughts, add:

TB-05	*wài guān*

For headache, add:

GB-20	*fēng chí*

2. HEAT BREWING IN THE STOMACH AND SPLEEN

Clinical Manifestations: Localized redness and swelling on the affected eyelid, with a lesion that is large, hot, painful and aggravated by physical contact. Accompanying symptoms include thirst, irritability, halitosis, constipation and dark urine.

Tongue: Red body with yellow coating.

Pulse: Rapid.

Treatment Method: Clear stomach heat, disperse swelling.

PRESCRIPTION

Combine Yellow-Draining Powder *(xiè huáng sǎn)* with Stomach-Clearing Powder *(qīng wèi sǎn)*.

Yellow-Draining Powder *xiè huáng sǎn*

shí gāo	gypsum (extended decoction)	Gypsum	15 g.
shān zhī zǐ	gardenia [fruit]	Gardeniae Fructus	9 g.
fáng fēng	ledebouriella [root]	Ledebouriellae Radix	9 g.
huò xiāng	agastache/patchouli	Agastaches seu Pogostemi Herba	6 g.
gān cǎo	licorice [root]	Glycyrrhizae Radix	6 g.

with:

Stomach-Clearing Powder *qīng wèi sǎn*

huáng lián	coptis [root]	Coptidis Rhizoma	9 g.
shēng dì huáng	rehmannia [root] dried/fresh	Rehmanniae Radix Exsiccata seu Recens	12 g.
mǔ dān pí	moutan [root bark]	Moutan Radicis Cortex	9 g.
shēng má	cimicifuga [root]	Cimicifugae Rhizoma	6 g.
dāng guī	tangkuei	Angelicae Sinensis Radix	3 g.

<u>MODIFICATIONS</u>

In cases presenting constipation, the prescription is modified to drain heat and free the stool.

Add:

dà huáng	rhubarb (abbreviated decoction)	Rhei Rhizoma	9 g.
máng xiāo	mirabilite (stirred in)	Mirabilitum	9 g.

ACUPUNCTURE AND MOXIBUSTION

Main points: Needle with draining.

LI-04	*hé gǔ*
M-HN-9	*tài yáng* (Greater Yang)
ST-01	*chéng qì*
ST-02	*sì bái*
SP-09	*yīn líng quán*

Auxiliary points:

For constipation, add:

LI-11	*qū chí*
ST-37	*shàng jù xū*

For halitosis, add:

CV-24	*chéng jiāng*

ALTERNATE THERAPEUTIC METHODS

1. Ear Acupuncture

Main points: Eye, Liver, Spleen, Ear Apex.

Method: Needle once daily to elicit a strong sensation. Bleed at the apex and at the small veins on the back of the ear.

2. Cupping Therapy

Method: Use a three-edged needle to bleed GV-14 *(dà zhuī)*. Follow with fire-cupping.

3. Picking Therapy

Method: Locate grain-sized light red papules between the shoulder blades, bilateral from the first to the seventh thoracic vertebrae. Needle such points with a three-edged needle and squeeze out a small amount of blood or fluid. Afterward, wipe clean with a cotton ball. Squeeze points three to five times. Alternately, papules can be broken open with a thicker filiform needle and the underlying white glistening, fibers picked up and snapped.

REMARKS

In cases of recurring styes, the pathogenesis often involves qi and blood vacuity allowing wind evil to enter the body. The incomplete clearing of evils where heat-toxin brewing persists can also result in the recurrence of styes. To prevent recurrence, treatment should address the overall symptoms. In addition, styes should not be squeezed or pressed to avoid spreading infection. In acupuncture treatment of styes, only acupoints outside the locale of inflammation and swelling are selected.

UPPER EYELID DROOP

Shàng Bāo Xià Chuí

1. Kidney Yang Vacuity - 2. Spleen Qi Vacuity - 3. Liver Blood Vacuity with Wind Evil Damaging the Connections

Eyelid ptosis is the biomedical name for a condition characterized by a drooping of the upper eyelid that partially blocks the pupil and impairs vision. Eyelid droop can be congenital or acquired, and can affect either one or both eyes. This chapter considers all cases of eyelid droop caused by paralysis of the oculomotor nerve, myasthenia gravis, traumatic injury or trachoma (infectious conjunctivitis). In Western medicine, eyelid ptosis is also known as blepharoptosis.

ETIOLOGY AND PATHOGENESIS

Cases of congenital eyelid droop are generally the result of kidney yang vacuity leading to spleen yang vacuity. Acquired eyelid droop, on the other hand, can be caused by two conditions: vacuity of spleen qi failing to nourish the muscles; or depletion of liver blood with wind evil lodging in the eyelid, causing obstruction of the channels and connections and hindering the flow of qi and blood.

1. KIDNEY YANG VACUITY

Clinical Manifestations: Congenital eyelid ptosis; inability to raise the upper eyelid when looking at objects.

Tongue: Pale.

Pulse: Deep, weak.

Treatment Method: Warm kidney yang, assist spleen yang.

PRESCRIPTION

Right-Restoring [Kidney Yang] Beverage yòu guī yǐn

shú dì huáng	cooked rehmannia [root]	Rehmanniae Radix Conquita	24 g.
shān yào	dioscorea [root]	Dioscoreae Rhizoma	12 g.
gǒu qǐ zǐ	lycium [berry]	Lycii Fructus	12 g.
shān zhū yú	cornus [fruit]	Corni Fructus	12 g.
dù zhòng	eucommia [bark]	Eucommiae Cortex	9 g.
gān cǎo	licorice [root]	Glycyrrhizae Radix	6 g.
zhì fù zǐ	aconite [accessory tuber] (processed) (extended decoction)	Aconiti Tuber Laterale Praeparatum	9 g.
ròu guì	cinnamon bark (abbreviated decoction)	Cinnamomi Cortex	6 g.

<u>MODIFICATIONS</u>

To supplement spleen yang qi, add:

rén shēn	ginseng	Ginseng Radix	9 g.
bái zhú	ovate atractylodes [root]	Atractylodis Ovatae Rhizoma	9 g.

ACUPUNCTURE AND MOXIBUSTION

Main points: Needle with supplementation.

BL-02	*zǎn zhú*	through to	BL-01	*jīng míng*
M-HN-6	*yú yāo* (Fish's Lumbus)	through to	TB-23	*sī zhú kōng*
M-HN-9	*tài yáng* (Greater Yang)	through to	GB-01	*tóng zǐ liáo*
CV-04	*guān yuán* (add moxibustion)			
ST-36	*zú sān lǐ* (add moxibustion)			
BL-23	*shèn shū* (add moxibustion)			
BL-20	*pí shū* (add moxibustion)			

2. SPLEEN QI VACUITY

Clinical Manifestations: Slow onset of eyelid droop, improvement of the condition in the morning or following rest and aggravation in the afternoon or following strain; accompanied by tiredness, fatigue, dizziness and vertigo, poor appetite, numbness of the affected eyelid and, in severe cases, difficulty in swallowing.

Tongue: Pale with thin white coating.

Pulse: Weak, forceless.

Treatment Method: Boost spleen qi.

PRESCRIPTION

Center-Supplementing Qi-Boosting Decoction *bǔ zhōng yì qì tāng*

huáng qí	astragalus [root]	Astragali (seu Hedysari) Radix	15 g.
rén shēn	ginseng	Ginseng Radix	9 g.
bái zhú	ovate atractylodes [root]	Atractylodis Ovatae Rhizoma	9 g.
dāng guī	tangkuei	Angelicae Sinensis Radix	9 g.
chén pí	tangerine [peel]	Citri Exocarpium	6 g.
shēng má	cimicifuga [root]	Cimicifugae Rhizoma	3 g.
chái hú	bupleurum [root]	Bupleuri Radix	3 g.
zhì gān cǎo	licorice [root] (honey-fried)	Glycyrrhizae Radix	6 g.

ACUPUNCTURE AND MOXIBUSTION

Main points: Needle with supplementation.

BL-02	*zǎn zhú*	through to	BL-01	*jīng míng*
M-HN-6	*yú yāo* (Fish's Lumbus)	through to	TB-23	*sī zhú kōng*
M-HN-9	*tài yáng* (Greater Yang)	through to	GB-01	*tóng zǐ liáo*
ST-36	*zú sān lǐ* (add moxibustion)			
SP-06	*sān yīn jiāo* (add moxibustion)			
CV-06	*qì hǎi* (add moxibustion)			
BL-20	*pí shū* (add moxibustion)			

3. LIVER BLOOD VACUITY WITH WIND EVIL
DAMAGING THE CONNECTIONS

Clinical Manifestations: Abrupt onset of one-sided eyelid ptosis, frequently with outward deviation of the eyeball and double vision. Prior to the emergence of eyelid droop, patients present a lusterless complexion, dizziness, vertigo and tinnitus. After onset, external patterns are often present, with symptoms including aversion to cold, fever and headache.

Tongue: Pale.

Pulse: Thready, wiry.

Treatment Method: Nourish liver blood, dispel wind evil.

PRESCRIPTION

Blood-Nourishing Tangkuei and Rehmannia Decoction
yǎng xuè dāng guī dì huáng tāng

shēng dì huáng	rehmannia [root] dried/fresh	Rehmanniae Radix Exsiccata seu Recens	12 g.
dāng guī	tangkuei	Angelicae Sinensis Radix	9 g.
bái sháo yào	white peony [root]	Paeoniae Radix Alba	9 g.
chuān xiōng	ligusticum [root]	Ligustici Rhizoma	9 g.
gǎo běn	Chinese lovage [root]	Ligustici Sinensis Rhizoma et Radix	9 g.
fáng fēng	ledebouriella [root]	Ledebouriellae Radix	9 g.
bái zhǐ	angelica [root]	Angelicae Dahuricae Radix	9 g.
xì xīn	asarum	Asiasari Herba cum Radice	3 g.

ACUPUNCTURE AND MOXIBUSTION

Main points: Needle with even supplementation, even draining.

BL-02	*zǎn zhú*	through to	BL-01	*jīng míng*
M-HN-6	*yú yāo* (Fish's Lumbus)	through to	TB-23	*sī zhú kōng*
M-HN-9	*tài yáng* (Greater Yang)	through to	GB-01	*tóng zǐ liáo*
GB-20	*fēng chí*			
LI-04	*hé gǔ*			
SP-06	*sān yīn jiāo*			
BL-18	*gān shū*			

ALTERNATE THERAPEUTIC METHODS

1. Plum-Blossom Needle Therapy

Method: On the affected side, tap with a plum-blossom needle over the course of the bladder and gallbladder channels, as well as over the orbicularis oculi muscle. Work from the top downward and from the inside to the outside.

REMARKS

In severe cases of congenital eyelid ptosis, surgical treatment may be considered.

TEARING PATTERNS
Liú Lèi Zhèng
1. Liver and Kidney Vacuity

Tearing of the eyes, or lacrimation, refers to an ophthalmic condition where the tears frequently escape from the lower margins of the eyes. Tearing can be divided into hot tearing and cold tearing.

Hot tearing generally refers to infectious diseases of the eyes, such as wind-heat eye *(fēng rè yǎn)*, epidemic reddening of the eyes *(tiān xíng chì mù)* and epidemic reddening of the eye with corneal opacity *(tiān xíng chì mù bào yì)*. For these conditions, diagnosis and treatment can be made according to the chapter "Sore, Red and Swollen Eyes."

The emphasis of this chapter is on patterns of cold tearing, which are most prevalent during the winter months. These mainly affect the elderly and are characterized by the secretion of clear cool tears that are thin in consistency and unaccompanied by symptoms of redness, pain or corneal opacity.

Cold tearing resembles dacryorrhea, a biomedically-defined condition caused by deviation in the location of the margin of the eyelid, obstruction of the lacrimal passages or incomplete drainage of tears. The secretion of tears as a result of emotional factors is not considered a pathological condition.

ETIOLOGY AND PATHOGENESIS

Cold tearing is most often from liver and kidney vacuity, the weakened functions of retention allowing external wind to evoke tearing.

1. LIVER AND KIDNEY VACUITY

Clinical Manifestations: Frequent clear cool tears that are thin in consistency, increase on exposure to wind but without apparent redness, pain or swelling of the eyes. Accompanying symptoms include dizziness, tinnitus, blurred vision and weak aching lower back and knees.

Tongue: Red body with little coating.

Pulse: Weak, thready.

Treatment Method: Nourish the liver, boost the kidney.

PRESCRIPTION

Left-Restoring [Kidney Yin] Beverage *zuǒ guī yǐn*

shú dì huáng	cooked rehmannia [root]	Rehmanniae Radix Conquita	24 g.
shān yào	dioscorea [root]	Dioscoreae Rhizoma	12 g.
gǒu qǐ zǐ	lycium [berry]	Lycii Fructus	12 g.
shān zhū yú	cornus [fruit]	Corni Fructus	12 g.
fú líng	poria	Poria	9 g.
zhì gān cǎo	licorice [root] (honey-fried)	Glycyrrhizae Radix	6 g.

MODIFICATIONS:

In cases of excessive tearing on exposure to wind, the prescription is modified to expel wind and stop tearing.
Add:

bái zhǐ	angelica [root]	Angelicae Dahuricae Radix	9 g.
fáng fēng	ledebouriella [root]	Ledebouriellae Radix	9 g.

In cases of qi and blood vacuity, manifesting as pale complexion, tiredness, fatigue, poor memory and palpitations, the prescription is modified to boost qi and nourish the blood.
Add:

dǎng shēn	codonopsis [root]	Codonopsitis Radix	12 g.
bái zhú	ovate atractylodes [root]	Atractylodis Ovatae Rhizoma	9 g.
dāng guī	tangkuei	Angelicae Sinensis Radix	9 g.
bái sháo yào	white peony [root]	Paeoniae Radix Alba	9 g.

In cases of kidney yang vacuity with symptoms of physical cold and cold extremities, the prescription is modified to warm and supplement kidney yang.
Add:

bā jǐ tiān	morinda [root]	Morindae Radix	12 g.
ròu cōng róng	cistanche [stem]	Cistanches Caulis	12 g.
sāng piāo xiāo	mantis egg-case	Mantidis Oötheca	6 g.

ACUPUNCTURE AND MOXIBUSTION

Main points: Needle with supplementation.

  BL-01 *jīng míng*
  BL-02 *zǎn zhú*
  GB-20 *fēng chí*
  BL-18 *gān shū* (with moxibustion)
  BL-23 *shèn shū* (with moxibustion)

Auxiliary points:

For blurred vision, add:
  SI-06 *yǎng lǎo*
  ST-01 *chéng qì*
For excessive tearing upon exposure to wind, add:
  LI-04 *hé gǔ*

ALTERNATE THERAPEUTIC METHODS

1. Ear Acupuncture

Main points: Liver, Eye 1, Eye 2.

Method: Needle to elicit a strong sensation. Retain needles for thirty minutes.

REMARKS

Acupuncture has been found to be highly effective in the treatment of tearing when there is no evidence of obstruction in the lacrimal passages. When needling the acupoint BL-01 *(jīng míng),* manipulation should be delicate so as not to cause subcutaneous or conjunctival bleeding. In cases where the lacrimal passages are extremely narrow or obstructed, probing of the passages or surgery may be required.

NEARSIGHTEDNESS
Jìn Shì
1. Depletion of Liver Blood and Kidney Essence

Myopia or nearsightedness is an eye disorder involving abnormal refraction, in which the eyes may be focused clearly on objects nearby, but not on distant objects. Myopia is common during the teenage years.

ETIOLOGY AND PATHOGENESIS

The etiology and pathogenesis of myopia involves insufficiency because of constitutional factors, or depletion of the blood and essence of the liver and kidney. Depletion may be from poor working habits, including poor lighting, improper posture or excessively long periods of reading, writing or close work.

1. DEPLETION OF LIVER BLOOD AND KIDNEY ESSENCE

Clinical Manifestations: Symptoms of weakening of vision, clear image of close objects and a blurred image of distant objects often accompanied by headache, rapid fatigue of the eyes, and sometimes accompanied by dizziness and vertigo, tinnitus, weak aching lower back and knees, insomnia and poor memory.

Pulse: Weak, thready.

Treatment Method: Supplement liver blood and kidney essence, brighten the eyes.

PRESCRIPTION

Lycium Berry, Chrysanthemum and Rehmannia Decoction
qǐ jú dì huáng tāng

shú dì huáng	cooked rehmannia [root]	Rehmanniae Radix Conquita	24 g.
shān zhū yú	cornus [fruit]	Corni Fructus	12 g.
shān yào	dioscorea [root]	Dioscoreae Rhizoma	12 g.
zé xiè	alisma [tuber]	Alismatis Rhizoma	9 g.
mǔ dān pí	moutan [root bark]	Moutan Radicis Cortex	9 g.
fú líng	poria	Poria	9 g.
gǒu qǐ zǐ	lycium [berry]	Lycii [Fructus]	9 g.
jú huā	chrysanthemum [flower]	Chrysanthemi Flos	9 g.

MODIFICATIONS

In cases accompanied by spleen and stomach qi vacuity, the prescription is modified to fortify the spleen and boost the stomach. Add:

dǎng shēn	codonopsis [root]	Codonopsitis Radix	12 g.
bái zhú	ovate atractylodes [root]	Atractylodis Ovatae Rhizoma	9 g.
chén pí	tangerine [peel]	Citri Exocarpium	9 g.
mài yá	barley sprout	Hordei Fructus Germinatus	12 g.

ACUPUNCTURE AND MOXIBUSTION

Main points: Needle with even supplementation, even draining.

BL-01	*jīng míng*
BL-02	*zǎn zhú*
ST-01	*chéng qì*
GB-20	*fēng chí*
GB-37	*guāng míng*
BL-18	*gān shū*
BL-23	*shèn shū*
LI-04	*hé gǔ*
M-HN-13	*yì míng* (Shielding Brightness)

Auxiliary points:

For spleen and stomach vacuity, add:

ST-36	*zú sān lǐ*
SP-06	*sān yīn jiāo*
ST-02	*sì bái*

ALTERNATE THERAPEUTIC METHODS

1. Ear Acupuncture

Main points: Eye, Liver, Kidney.

Method: Needle to elicit a moderate sensation and retain needles for thirty minutes. Treat once every second day, ten sessions per therapeutic course.

2. Plum-Blossom Needle Therapy

1. Tap over the acupoints in the region surrounding the eyes, as well as over bilateral back-shu points and GB-20 *(fēng chí)*. Treat once daily, ten sessions per therapeutic course.

2.**Main point:** *Zhèng guāng* (just below the upper edge of the orbit directly beneath the midpoint of the line connecting BL-02 *(zǎn zhú)* and M-HN-6 *(yú yāo,* Fish's Lumbus).

Auxiliary points: GB-20 *(fēng chí)*, GV-14 *(dà zhuī)*, PC-06 *(nèi guān)*.

Method: Tap with moderate force twenty to fifty times within a radius of 0.4-0.6 cm. of each acupoint. In most cases, only the major acupoint is selected, the auxiliary acupoints being selected only when therapeutic effects have been poor. Treat once daily, fifteen sessions per therapeutic course.

REMARKS

Acupuncture has been found to be quite effective in the treatment of myopia. In needling BL-01 *(jīng míng),* the insertion is slow with a delicate rotation. To prevent bleeding, the point is pressed with a cotton ball for one minute after withdrawing the needle.

When needling GB-20 *(fēng chí)* and M-HN-13 *(yī míng,* Shielding Brightness), the effects are stronger when the needling sensation is felt in the vicinity of the eyes. If the given treatment fails to produce good results, eyeglasses or surgical treatment may be necessary to fully correct the patient's vision.

BLUE-EYE BLINDNESS

Qīng Máng

1. Liver and Kidney Vacuity - 2. Qi and Blood Vacuity - 3. Stagnation of Liver Qi - 4. Stagnation of Qi and Blood

Blue-eye blindness refers to eye diseases where there is a gradual loss of vision and eventual blindness, yet the eyes reveal no external abnormality. Refer to this chapter for all cases of primary optic atrophy as well as disorders of the fundus of the eye resulting in optic atrophy. In Western medicine, these include papillitis, diabetic retinopathy, retinal arterial embolism and pigmentary degeneration of the retina.

ETIOLOGY AND PATHOGENESIS

Blue-eye blindness can be the result of either congenital weakness or depletion of the blood and essence of the liver and kidney. Other factors include vacuity of both qi and blood from an extended illness or an excessive loss of blood, and depression of liver qi from emotional depression. Stagnation of qi and stasis of blood through a traumatic injury to the head or eyes can also cause blue-eye blindness.

1. LIVER AND KIDNEY VACUITY

Clinical Manifestations: Dryness of the eyes, loss of vision or blindness and pathological changes of the fundus of the eyes signalling optic atrophy, accompanied by symptoms of dizziness, vertigo, tinnitus, lower backache, seminal emission.

Tongue: Red with little coating.

Pulse: Thready or rapid, thready.

Treatment Method: Supplement the liver and kidney, brighten the eyes.

PRESCRIPTION

Eye Brightener Rehmannia Pill *míng mù dì huáng wán*

shú dì huáng	cooked rehmannia [root]	Rehmanniae Radix Conquita	12 g.
shēng dì huáng	rehmannia [root] dried/fresh	Rehmanniae Radix Exsiccata seu Recens	12 g.
shān yào	dioscorea [root]	Dioscoreae Rhizoma	12 g.
shān zhū yú	cornus [fruit]	Corni Fructus	12 g.
zé xiè	alisma [tuber]	Alismatis Rhizoma	9 g.
fú líng	poria	Poria	9 g.
mǔ dān pí	moutan [root bark]	Moutan Radicis Cortex	9 g.
chái hú	bupleurum [root]	Bupleuri Radix	6 g.
dāng guī	tangkuei	Angelicae Sinensis Radix	9 g.
wǔ wèi zǐ	schisandra [berry]	Schisandrae Fructus	6 g.

<u>MODIFICATIONS</u>

To free the connections and open the orifices, add:

niú xī	achyranthes [root]	Achyranthis Bidentatae Radix	9 g.
shè xiāng	musk (each time, stirred in)	Moschus	0.1 g.

In cases presenting signs of vacuous kidney yang, such as physical cold, cold extremities, pale tongue and deep pulse, the prescription is modified to warm and supplement kidney yang.
Add:

tù sī zǐ	cuscuta [seed]	Cuscutae Semen	12 g.
ròu guì	cinnamon [bark] (abbreviated decoction)	Cinnamomi Cortex	6 g.
bǔ gǔ zhī	psoralea [seed]	Psoraleae Semen	9 g.
gǒu qǐ zǐ	lycium [berry]	Lycii [Fructus]	12 g.

ACUPUNCTURE AND MOXIBUSTION

Main points: Needle with supplementation.

BL-01	*jīng míng*
M-HN-8	*qiú hòu* (Back of the Ball)
ST-01	*chéng qì*
GB-20	*fēng chí*
GB-37	*guāng míng*
BL-23	*shèn shū* (with moxibustion)
BL-18	*gān shū* (with moxibustion)
KI-03	*tài xī*

Auxiliary points:

For vacuity of kidney yang, add acupuncture and moxibustion to:

CV-04	*guān yuán*
CV-06	*qì hǎi*

2. QI AND BLOOD VACUITY

Clinical Manifestations: Eye symptoms as noted above and accompanied by tiredness, fatigue, shortness of breath, disinclination to speak, dizziness and vertigo, palpitations, insomnia, poor memory, loss of appetite, loose stools.

Tongue: Pale with thin white coating.

Pulse: Weak, thready.

Treatment Method: Benefit qi, nourish the blood, brighten the eyes.

PRESCRIPTION

Ginseng Construction-Nourishing Decoction (Pill)
rén shēn yǎng róng tāng (wán)

rén shēn	ginseng	Ginseng Radix	9 g.
bái zhú	ovate atractylodes [root]	Atractylodis Ovatae Rhizoma	9 g.
fú líng	poria	Poria	9 g.
huáng qí	astragalus [root]	Astragali (seu Hedysari) Radix	12 g.
shú dì huáng	cooked rehmannia [root]	Rehmanniae Radix Conquita	9 g.
dāng guī	tangkuei	Angelicae Sinensis Radix	9 g.
bái sháo yào	white peony [root]	Paeoniae Radix Alba	12 g.
chén pí	tangerine peel	Citri Exocarpium	9 g.

ròu guì	cinnamon bark (abbreviated decoction)	Cinnamomi Cortex	3 g.
wǔ wèi zǐ	schisandra [berry]	Schisandrae Fructus	6 g.
yuǎn zhì	polygala [root]	Polygalae Radix	6 g.
zhì gān cǎo	licorice [root] (honey-fried)	Glycyrrhizae Radix	6 g.
shēng jiāng	fresh ginger [root]	Zingiberis Rhizoma Recens	3 g.
dà zǎo	jujube	Ziziphi Fructus	3 pc.

MODIFICATIONS

To free the connections and open the orifices, add a selection from:

niú xī	achyranthes [root]	Achyranthis Bidentatae Radix	9 g.
chuān xiōng	ligusticum [root]	Ligustici Rhizoma	9 g.
hóng huā	carthamus [flower]	Carthami Flos	6 g.
shè xiāng	musk (each time, stirred in)	Moschus	0.1 g.
shí chāng pú	acorus [root]	Acori Rhizoma	9 g.

ACUPUNCTURE AND MOXIBUSTION

Main points: Needle with supplementation.

BL-01	*jīng míng*
M-HN-8	*qiú hòu* (Back of the Ball)
M-HN-13	*yì míng* (Shielding Brightness)
GB-20	*fēng chí*
ST-36	*zú sān lǐ*
SP-06	*sān yīn jiāo*
GB-37	*guāng míng*

Auxiliary points:

For insomnia and palpitations, add:

| BL-15 | *xīn shū* |
| HT-07 | *shén mén* |

3. STAGNATION OF LIVER QI

Clinical Manifestations: Eye symptoms as noted above, but accompanied by emotional stress, dizziness and vertigo, distending pain of the eyes, bitter taste in the mouth, costal pain.

Pulse: Wiry.

Treatment Method: Soothe the liver, brighten the eyes.

PRESCRIPTION

Free Wanderer Powder *xiāo yáo sǎn*

chái hú	bupleurum [root]	Bupleuri Radix	9 g.
bái sháo yào	white peony [root]	Paeoniae Radix Alba	12 g.
dāng guī	tangkuei	Angelicae Sinensis Radix	9 g.
bái zhú	ovate atractylodes [root]	Atractylodis Ovatae Rhizoma	9 g.
fú líng	poria	Poria	9 g.
zhì gān cǎo	licorice [root] (honey-fried)	Glycyrrhizae Radix	6 g.
bò hé	mint (abbreviated decoction)	Menthae Herba	3 g.
shēng jiāng	fresh ginger [root]	Zingiberis Rhizoma Recens	3 g.

Modifications

To reinforce the blood-quickening and connection-freeing actions of this prescription, add:

xiāng fù zǐ	cyperus [root]	Cyperi Rhizoma	9 g.
yù jīn	curcuma [tuber]	Curcumae Tuber	9 g.
chuān xiōng	ligusticum [root]	Ligustici Rhizoma	9 g.

In cases of stagnation of liver qi transforming into heat, add:

mǔ dān pí	moutan [root bark]	Moutan Radicis Cortex	9 g.
shān zhī zǐ	gardenia [fruit]	Gardeniae Fructus	9 g.

ACUPUNCTURE AND MOXIBUSTION

Main points: Needle with even supplementation, even draining.

BL-01	*jīng míng*
M-HN-8	*qiú hòu* (Back of the Ball)
GB-20	*fēng chí*
GB-37	*guāng míng*
LR-03	*tài chōng*
GB-34	*yáng líng quán*
LR-14	*qī mén*

4. STAGNATION OF QI AND BLOOD

Clinical Manifestations: Eye symptoms as noted above but generally following traumatic injury to the head or eyes, and accompanied by headache and poor memory.

Tongue: Dark-colored.

Pulse: Rough.

Treatment Method: Move qi, quicken the blood, clear the connections, brighten the eyes.

PRESCRIPTION

House of Blood Stasis-Expelling Decoction *xuè fǔ zhú yū tāng*

táo rén	peach [kernel]	Persicae Semen	12 g.
hóng huā	carthamus [flower]	Carthami Flos	9 g.
dāng guī	tangkuei	Angelicae Sinensis Radix	9 g.
shēng dì huáng	rehmannia [root] dried/fresh	Rehmanniae Radix Exsiccata seu Recens	9 g.
chuān xiōng	ligusticum [root]	Ligustici Rhizoma	4.5 g.
chì sháo yào	red peony [root]	Paeoniae Radix Rubra	6 g.
niú xī	achyranthes [root]	Achyranthis Bidentatae Radix	9 g.
jié gěng	platycodon [root]	Platycodonis Radix	4.5 g.
chái hú	bupleurum [root]	Bupleuri Radix	3 g.
zhǐ ké	bitter orange [fruit]	Aurantii Fructus	6 g.
gān cǎo	licorice [root]	Glycyrrhizae Radix	3 g.

Modifications

In cases of extended illness where qi has become vacuous, this prescription is modified to benefit qi.

Delete:

niú xī	achyranthes [root]	Achyranthis Bidentatae Radix	
zhǐ ké	bitter orange [fruit]	Aurantii Fructus	
jié gěng	platycodon [root]	Platycodonis Radix	

Add:

huáng qí	astragalus [root]	Astragali (seu Hedysari) Radix	12 g.
bái zhú	ovate atractylodes [root]	Atractylodis Ovatae Rhizoma	12 g.
chén pí	tangerine [peel]	Citri Exocarpium	9 g.

ACUPUNCTURE AND MOXIBUSTION

Main points: Needle with even supplementation and draining stimulus.

BL-01	*jīng míng*
M-HN-8	*qiú hòu* (Back of the Ball)
GB-20	*fēng chí*
GB-37	*guāng míng*
SP-06	*sān yīn jiāo*
BL-17	*gé shū*
LI-04	*hé gǔ*

Auxiliary points:

For extended illness where qi is vacuous, add:

ST-36	*zú sān lǐ*
CV-06	*qì hǎi*

ALTERNATE THERAPEUTIC METHODS

1. Ear Acupuncture

Main points: Eye 1, Eye 2, Liver, Kidney, Subcortex, Occiput.

Method: Use intradermal needles at above points. Replace once weekly.

2. Scalp Acupuncture

Location: *Shi Qu*: Optic region: Bilateral lines 4 cm in length beginning level with the external occipital protuberance 1 cm to each side of it, and running upward parallel to the anterior-posterior or midline of the head.

Method: Have the patient assume a sitting or lying position. After routine sterilization of the above note region, select a 2.5–3 cun, #26–#28 needle and insert it obliquely into the optic region. The needle is inserted into the subcutaneous tissues, the tip is neither in the skin nor periosteum. After insertion, needle manipulation consists of twisting and rotating at a frequency of approximately two hundred and forty rotations per minute without lifting or thrusting. After eliciting a numb, distending sensation, retain the needle for five to ten minutes before repeating the procedure. Again retain, manipulate, then withdraw the needle, pressing the lesion firmly with a cotton ball to prevent bleeding. Needle once daily or once every second day; ten to fifteen treatments constitute a therapeutic course.

REMARKS

In the treatment of blue-eye blindness, apart from differential diagnosis and treatment, the addition of the following herbs to free the connections and open the orifices enhances the therapeutic effect:

shè xiāng	musk (each time, stirred in)	Moschus	0.1 g.
niú xī	achyranthes [root]	Achyranthis Bidentatae Radix	9 g.
hóng huā	carthamus [flower]	Carthami Flos	9 g.
shí chāng pú	acorus [root]	Acori Rhizoma	9 g.

SUDDEN BLINDNESS

Bào Máng

1. Qi Stagnation and Blood Stasis - 2. Exuberant Liver Fire

In the absence of any ophthalmic disorder, a sudden severe decrease in sight or the complete loss of sight in one or both eyes is known as sudden blindness. Several illnesses known to Western medicine can result in sudden blindness. These include embolism of the central retinal artery and acute optic neuritis.

ETIOLOGY AND PATHOGENESIS

Sudden blindness can result from emotional upset such as sudden anger, fright or fear, or from the invasion of external heat evil into the viscera and bowels, both of which can cause liver fire to rise to the eyes. Stagnation of qi and blood can also result in sudden blindness when essence is not transported to the eyes.

1. QI STAGNATION AND BLOOD STASIS

Clinical Manifestations: Sudden severe decrease or complete loss of sight, with some abnormality found in the fundus of the eye, accompanied by headache, distended sensation of the eyes and irritability.

Tongue: Dark and purplish with stasis macules on the tongue.

Pulse: Rough.

Treatment Method: Rectify qi, quicken the blood, clear the orifices.

PRESCRIPTION

Orifice-Freeing Blood-Quickening Decoction *tōng qiào huó xuè tāng*

chì sháo yào	red peony [root]	Paeoniae Radix Rubra	3 g.
chuān xiōng	ligusticum [root]	Ligustici Rhizoma	3 g.
táo rén	peach kernel	Persicae Semen	9 g.
hóng huā	carthamus [flower]	Carthami Flos	9 g.
cōng bái	scallion white	Allii Fistulosi Bulbus Recens	3 g.
dà zǎo	jujube	Ziziphi Fructus	5 pc.
shè xiāng	musk (each time; stirred in)	Moschus	0.1 g.
huáng jiǔ	yellow wine	Vinum Aureum	50 cc.

MODIFICATIONS:

In cases accompanied by stagnation of liver qi, the prescription is modified to soothe the liver and regulate qi.

Add:

yù jīn	curcuma [tuber]	Curcumae Tuber	9 g.
qīng pí	unripe tangerine [peel]	Citri Exocarpium Immaturum	9 g.

In cases of severe retinal edema, the prescription is modified to quicken the blood, dissolve stasis, disinhibit water and disperse swelling.
Add:

hǔ pò	amber (each time; powdered and stirred in)	Succinum	1.5 g.
zé lán	lycopus	Lycopi Herba	12 g.
yì mǔ cǎo	leonurus	Leonuri Herba	12 g.

In cases of severe bleeding at the fundus of the eye, the prescription is modified to dissolve stasis and relieve bleeding.
Add:

pú huáng	typha pollen (wrapped)	Typhae Pollen	9 g.
qiàn cǎo gēn	madder [root]	Rubiae Radix	12 g.
sān qī	notoginseng [root]	Notoginseng Radix	9 g.
	(or, powdered and administered separately, 1.5 g. each time)		

ACUPUNCTURE AND MOXIBUSTION

Main points: Needle with draining.

BL-01	*jīng míng*
GB-01	*tóng zǐ liáo*
M-HN-8	*qiú hòu* (Back of the Ball)
PC-06	*nèi guān*
BL-17	*gé shū*
SP-06	*sān yīn jiāo*

Auxiliary points:

For distended sensation of the eye, bleed at:

TB-01	*guān chōng*

2. EXUBERANT LIVER FIRE

Clinical Manifestations: Ophthalmic symptoms as above, accompanied by pain of the eyeball upon external pressure and pain behind the eyes during eye movement, as well as headache, tinnitus, irritability, insomnia, profuse dreaming, bitter taste in the mouth, dry throat.

Tongue: Red with yellow coating.

Pulse: Rapid, wiry.

Treatment Method: Clear the liver, drain fire.

PRESCRIPTION
Gentian Liver-Draining Decoction *lóng dǎn xiè gān tāng*

lóng dǎn cǎo	gentian [root]	Gentianae Radix	6 g.
huáng qín	scutellaria [root]	Scutellariae Radix	9 g.
shān zhī zǐ	gardenia [fruit]	Gardeniae Fructus	9 g.
zé xiè	alisma [tuber]	Alismatis Rhizoma	12 g.
mù tōng	mutong [stem]	Mutong Caulis	9 g.
dāng guī	tangkuei	Angelicae Sinensis Radix	3 g.
chē qián zǐ	plantago [seed] (wrapped)	Plantaginis Semen	9 g.
shēng dì huáng	rehmannia [root] dried/fresh	Rehmanniae Radix Exsiccata seu Recens	9 g.
chái hú	bupleurum [root]	Bupleuri Radix	6 g.
gān cǎo	licorice [root]	Glycyrrhizae Radix	6 g.

MODIFICATIONS

In cases of severe edema and congestion of the optic papilla, or exudation and bleeding of the neighboring region of the retina, the prescription is modified to cool and invigorate the blood.

Add:

mǔ dān pí	moutan [root bark]	Moutan Radicis Cortex	9 g.
chì sháo yào	red peony [root]	Paeoniae Radix Rubra	9 g.

ACUPUNCTURE AND MOXIBUSTION

Main points: Needle with draining.

BL-01	*jīng míng*
GB-01	*tóng zǐ liáo*
M-HN-8	*qiú hòu* (Back of the Ball)
GB-20	*fēng chí*
LR-03	*tài chōng*
GB-37	*guāng míng*

REMARKS

Sudden blindness is a severe condition and, in clinical practice, it is usually necessary to confirm the diagnosis with fundoscopy. A comprehensive treatment combining both Chinese and Western medical techniques is recommended.

ROUND CORNEAL NEBULA

Yuán Yì Nèi Zhàng

1. Liver and Kidney Vacuity - 2. Spleen Qi Vacuity - 3. Upper Burner Liver Heat - 4. Yin Depletion and Damp-Heat

Round corneal nebula is a chronic condition where clouding of the eyes leads to gradual vision impairment and, ultimately, blindness. It is most frequently observed in older patients. In the vast majority of cases, both eyes are affected, although one eye often develops a nebula before the other. The Chinese medical term "round corneal nebula" is derived from the characteristic round silvery or brown-colored opacity observed filling the pupil in the later stages of the disease. Round corneal nebula corresponds to the cataract of Western medicine.

ETIOLOGY AND PATHOGENESIS

The etiology and pathogenesis of corneal nebulae can involve either vacuity of the liver and kidney with advancing years and the consequent insufficiency of essence and blood, or weakening of the spleen's ability to transport qi and essence upward to nourish the eyes. In addition, stagnant heat in the liver channel or depletion of yin coupled with the ascent of damp-heat evil can also cause corneal nebulae.

1. LIVER AND KIDNEY VACUITY

Clinical Manifestations: Unclear vision, dizziness, tinnitus, weak aching lower back and knees.

Tongue: Red with little coating.

Pulse: Thready.

Treatment Method: Moisten the liver and kidney, boost essence, nourish the blood, brighten the eyes.

PRESCRIPTION

Lycium Berry, Chrysanthemum and Rehmannia Decoction
qǐ jú dì huáng tāng

shú dì huáng	cooked rehmannia [root]	Rehmanniae Radix Conquita	24 g.
shān zhū yú	cornus [fruit]	Corni Fructus	12 g.
shān yào	dioscorea [root]	Dioscoreae Rhizoma	12 g.
zé xiè	alisma [tuber]	Alismatis Rhizoma	9 g.
mǔ dān pí	moutan [root bark]	Moutan Radicis Cortex	9 g.
fú líng	poria	Poria	9 g.
gǒu qǐ zǐ	lycium [berry]	Lycii [Fructus]	9 g.
jú huā	chrysanthemum [flower]	Chrysanthemi Flos	9 g.

MODIFICATIONS

In cases of severe essence and blood depletion, the prescription is modified to supplement essence, nourish the blood and brighten the eyes.

Add:

tù sī zǐ	cuscuta [seed]	Cuscutae Semen	12 g.
shí hú	dendrobium [stem] (extended decoction)	Dendrobii Caulis	12 g.
dāng guī	tangkuei	Angelicae Sinensis Radix	9 g.
bái sháo yào	white peony [root]	Paeoniae Radix Alba	9 g.

In cases of kidney yang vacuity presenting cold extremities, copious clear urine, pale tongue and deep weak pulse, the prescription is changed to warm and supplement kidney yang while boosting essence, nourishing the blood and brightening the eyes.

Use:

Right-Restoring [Kidney Yang] Pill *yòu guī wán*

shú dì huáng	cooked rehmannia [root]	Rehmanniae Radix Conquita	24 g.
shān yào	dioscorea [root]	Dioscoreae Rhizoma	12 g.
shān zhū yú	cornus [fruit]	Corni Fructus	9 g.
gǒu qǐ zǐ	lycium [berry]	Lycii [Fructus]	9 g.
lù jiǎo jiāo	deerhorn glue (dissolved and stirred in)	Cervi Gelatinum Cornu	12 g.
tù sī zǐ	cuscuta [seed]	Cuscutae Semen	12 g.
dù zhòng	eucommia [bark]	Eucommiae Cortex	12 g.
dāng guī	tangkuei	Angelicae Sinensis Radix	9 g.
ròu guì	cinnamon [bark] (abbreviated decoction)	Cinnamomi Cortex	6 g.
zhì fù zǐ	aconite [accessory tuber] (processed) (extended decoction)	Aconiti Tuber Laterale Praeparatum	6 g.

ACUPUNCTURE AND MOXIBUSTION

Main points: Needle with supplementation; add moxibustion.

BL-01	*jīng míng*
M-HN-8	*qiú hòu* (Back of the Ball)
BL-02	*zǎn zhú*
GB-20	*fēng chí*
BL-18	*gān shū*
BL-23	*shèn shū*
KI-07	*fù liū*
GB-37	*guāng míng*

Auxiliary points:

For vacuity of kidney yang, add:

CV-04	*guān yuán*
GV-04	*mìng mén*

2. SPLEEN QI VACUITY

Clinical Manifestations: Blurred vision, tiredness, fatigue, sallow complexion, poor appetite, loose stools.

Tongue: Pale with white coating.

Pulse: Weak, thready.

Treatment Method: Supplement the spleen, boost qi, brighten the eyes.

PRESCRIPTION

Center-Supplementing Qi-Boosting Decoction *bǔ zhōng yì qì tāng*

huáng qí	astragalus [root]	Astragali (seu Hedysari) Radix	15 g.
rén shēn	ginseng	Ginseng Radix	9 g.
bái zhú	ovate atractylodes [root]	Atractylodis Ovatae Rhizoma	9 g.
dāng guī	tangkuei	Angelicae Sinensis Radix	9 g.
chén pí	tangerine [peel]	Citri Exocarpium	6 g.
shēng má	cimicifuga [root]	Cimicifugae Rhizoma	3 g.
chái hú	bupleurum [root]	Bupleuri Radix	3 g.
zhì gān cǎo	licorice [root] (honey-fried)	Glycyrrhizae Radix	6 g.

MODIFICATIONS

In cases where the weakening of the spleen has allowed damp accumulation, with loose or liquid stools, the prescription is modified to fortify the spleen and disperse dampness.

Delete:

dāng guī	tangkuei	Angelicae Sinensis Radix

Add:

fú líng	poria	Poria	12 g.
biǎn dòu	lablab [bean]	Lablab Semen	12 g.
yì yǐ rén	coix [seed]	Coicis Semen	30 g.

ACUPUNCTURE AND MOXIBUSTION

Main points: Needle with supplementation; add moxibustion.

BL-01	*jīng míng*
M-HN-8	*qiú hòu* (Back of the Ball)
BL-02	*zǎn zhú*
LI-04	*hé gǔ*
ST-36	*zú sān lǐ*
SP-06	*sān yīn jiāo*
BL-20	*pí shū*
ST-02	*sì bái*

3. UPPER BURNER LIVER HEAT

Clinical Manifestations: Headache, discomfort of the eyes, blurred vision, excessive secretion of mucus and tears from the eyes, bitter taste in the mouth, dry throat.

Pulse: Rapid, wiry.

Treatment Method: Clear the liver, brighten the eyes.

PRESCRIPTION

Abalone Shell Powder *shí jué míng sǎn*

shí jué míng	abalone shell (extended decoction)	Haliotidis Concha	30 g.
jué míng zǐ	fetid cassia [seed]	Cassiae Torae Semen	12 g.
shān zhī zǐ	gardenia [fruit]	Gardeniae Fructus	9 g.
chì sháo yào	red peony [root]	Paeoniae Radix Rubra	9 g.
dà huáng	rhubarb	Rhei Rhizoma	6 g.
mài mén dōng	ophiopogon [tuber]	Ophiopogonis Tuber	6 g.
jīng jiè	schizonepeta (abbreviated decoction)	Schizonepetae Herba et Flos	6 g.
qiāng huó	notopterygium [root]	Notopterygii Rhizoma	6 g.
mù zéi	equisetum	Equiseti Herba	9 g.

<u>**MODIFICATIONS**</u>

In cases of exuberance of liver fire, the prescription is reinforced to clear the liver, purge fire and brighten the eyes.

Add:

jú huā	chrysanthemum [flower]	Chrysanthemi Flos	9 g.
xià kū cǎo	prunella [spike]	Prunellae Spica	9 g.

ACUPUNCTURE AND MOXIBUSTION

Main points: Needle with draining.

BL-01	*jīng míng*
M-HN-8	*qiú hòu* (Back of the Ball)
BL-02	*zǎn zhú*
GB-20	*fēng chí*
LR-03	*tài chōng*
GB-37	*guāng míng*
LR-02	*xíng jiān*
GB-43	*xiá xī*

4. YIN DEPLETION AND DAMP-HEAT

Clinical Manifestations: Constitutional yin vacuity, dryness of the eyes, blurred vision, irritability, halitosis, difficult bowel movements.

Tongue: Red with yellow slimy coating.

Pulse: Soft, rapid.

Treatment Method: Nourish yin, clear heat, transform dampness, brighten the eyes.

PRESCRIPTION

Sweet Dew Beverage *gān lù yǐn*

shú dì huáng	cooked rehmannia [root]	Rehmanniae Radix Conquita	9 g.
shēng dì huáng	rehmannia [root] dried/fresh	Rehmanniae Radix Exsiccata seu Recens	9 g.
tiān mén dōng	asparagus [tuber]	Asparagi Tuber	9 g.
mài mén dōng	ophiopogon [tuber]	Ophiopogonis Tuber	9 g.
yīn chén hāo	capillaris	Artemisiae Capillaris Herba	15 g.
shí hú	dendrobium [stem] (extended decoction)	Dendrobii Caulis	9 g.
huáng qín	scutellaria [root]	Scutellariae Radix	9 g.
zhǐ ké	bitter orange [fruit]	Aurantii Fructus	9 g.
pí pá yè	loquat [leaf]	Eriobotryae Folium	9 g.
gān cǎo	licorice [root]	Glycyrrhizae Radix	6 g.

ACUPUNCTURE AND MOXIBUSTION

Main points: Needle with even supplementation, even draining.

BL-01	*jīng míng*
M-HN-8	*qiú hòu* (Back of the Ball)
BL-02	*zǎn zhú*
LI-04	*hé gǔ*
GB-37	*guāng míng*
KI-03	*tài xī*
SP-09	*yīn líng quán*
SP-06	*sān yīn jiāo*

ALTERNATE THERAPEUTIC METHODS

1. Ear Acupuncture

Auricular points: Eye, Eye 1, Eye 2, Liver, Kidney.

Method: Needle to elicit a mild to moderate sensation and retain needles fifteen to thirty minutes. Treat once every two days.

REMARKS

The course of development of round corneal nebula is extended, but once clouding of the lens has occurred, it is difficult to correct. Acupuncture or herbal medicine treatment should therefore be sought during the early stages of disease. Those cases already in the later stages are best referred for surgical treatment.

PART VIII

OTORHINOLARYNGOLOGY

TINNITUS AND DEAFNESS
Ěr Míng, Ěr Lóng

**1. Exuberant Liver and Gallbladder Fire - 2. External Wind-Heat -
3. Binding Depression of Phlegm-Fire - 4. Kidney Essence Depletion -
5. Spleen and Stomach Qi Vacuity**

Tinnitus and deafness are both hearing disorders. *Ěr míng* refers to the subjective sensation of ringing in the ears (tinnitus), while *ěr lóng* refers to a decrease in or complete loss of hearing (deafness). Tinnitus and deafness can occur as symptoms of a variety of disorders or they can occur in isolation. Since deafness often develops from tinnitus, the two are largely equivalent in etiology, pathogenesis and treatment. For this reason, they are generally discussed as a unit in Chinese medicine. Tinnitus and deafness resulting from earwax, foreign objects or purulent ear (otitis media) are not discussed in this chapter.

ETIOLOGY AND PATHOGENESIS

Tinnitus and deafness are generally differentiated according to repletion and vacuity. Patterns of repletion can result from the following: emotional stress stirring liver and gallbladder fire which then rises to disturb the ears, invasion of the ear by external wind-heat or excessive consumption of alcohol and rich foods leading to stagnation of phlegm-fire. Vacuity patterns are a result of either the depletion of kidney essence from poor physical constitution, extended illness, overindulgent sexual activity or an inability of spleen and stomach qi to rise and nourish the ears which is rooted in poor diet and excessive work.

1. EXUBERANT LIVER AND GALLBLADDER FIRE

Clinical Manifestations: Sudden onset of tinnitus or deafness with the tinnitus resembling ocean waves or claps of thunder, onset of symptoms or increase in severity of symptoms with anger or frustration; headache, dizziness and vertigo, earache, distending sensation of the ears, flushed complexion, dry mouth, irritability, restless sleep, distention and pain of the chest and hypochondrium, constipation, dark urine.

Tongue: Red with yellow coating.

Pulse: Rapid, wiry, forceful.

Treatment Method: Clear liver and gallbladder fire.

PRESCRIPTION

Gentian Liver-Draining Decoction *lóng dǎn xiè gān tāng*

lóng dǎn cǎo	gentian [root]	Gentianae Radix	6 g.
huáng qín	scutellaria [root]	Scutellariae Radix	9 g.
shān zhī zǐ	gardenia [fruit]	Gardeniae Fructus	9 g.
zé xiè	alisma [tuber]	Alismatis Rhizoma	12 g.
mù tōng	mutong [stem]	Mutong Caulis	9 g.
dāng guī	tangkuei	Angelicae Sinensis Radix	3 g.
chē qián zǐ	plantago seed (wrapped)	Plantaginis Semen	9 g.
shēng dì huáng	rehmannia [root] dried/fresh	Rehmanniae Radix Exsiccata seu Recens	9 g.
chái hú	bupleurum [root]	Bupleuri Radix	6 g.
gān cǎo	licorice [root]	Glycyrrhizae Radix	6 g.

MODIFICATIONS

To open the orifices, add:

shí chāng pú	acorus [root]	Acori Rhizoma	9 g.

In cases of constipation, the prescription is modified to free the stool and drain heat.

Add:

dà huáng	rhubarb (abbreviated decoction)	Rhei Rhizoma	9 g.

In cases of liver qi stagnation where fire is not marked, the prescription is changed to soothe the liver, move qi and open the orifices.

Use:

Free Wanderer Powder *xiāo yáo sǎn*

chái hú	bupleurum [root]	Bupleuri Radix	9 g.
bái sháo yào	white peony [root]	Paeoniae Radix Alba	12 g.
dāng guī	tangkuei	Angelicae Sinensis Radix	9 g.
bái zhú	ovate atractylodes [root]	Atractylodis Ovatae Rhizoma	9 g.
fú líng	poria	Poria	9 g.
zhì gān cǎo	licorice [root] (honey-fried)	Glycyrrhizae Radix	6 g.
bò hé	mint (abbreviated decoction)	Menthae Herba	3 g.
shēng jiāng	fresh ginger [root]	Zingiberis Rhizoma Recens	3 g.

Add:

shí chāng pú	acorus [root]	Acori Rhizoma	9 g.
màn jīng zǐ	vitex [fruit]	Viticis Fructus	9 g.
xiāng fù zǐ	cyperus [root]	Cyperi Rhizoma	9 g.

ACUPUNCTURE AND MOXIBUSTION

Main points: Needle with draining.

TB-17	*yì fēng*
GB-02	*tīng huì*
TB-03	*zhōng zhǔ*
GB-43	*xiá xī*
LR-03	*tài chōng*
GB-40	*qiū xū*

2. EXTERNAL WIND-HEAT

Clinical Manifestations: Symptoms are initially those of the common cold but develop to include the subjective sensation of distention and obstruction within the ears, tinnitus and impairment of hearing, often accompanied by headache, aversion to wind, fever and dry mouth.

Tongue: Thin yellow coating.

Pulse: Rapid, floating.

Treatment Method: Course wind, clear heat.

PRESCRIPTION

Lonicera and Forsythia Powder *yín qiào săn*

jīn yín huā	lonicera [flower]	Lonicerae Flos	9 g.
lián qiào	forsythia [fruit]	Forsythiae Fructus	9 g.
dàn dòu chǐ	fermented soybean (unsalted)	Glycines Semen Fermentatum Insulsum	6 g.
niú bàng zǐ	arctium [seed]	Arctii Fructus	9 g.
bò hé	mint (abbreviated decoction)	Menthae Herba	6 g.
jīng jiè suì	schizonepeta [spike] (abbreviated decoction)	Schizonepetae Flos	6 g.
jié gěng	platycodon [root]	Platycodonis Radix	6 g.
gān cǎo	licorice [root]	Glycyrrhizae Radix	6 g.
lú gēn	phragmites [root]	Phragmititis Rhizoma	9 g.

MODIFICATIONS

The prescription is reinforced to increase wind heat-dispersing and orifice-clearing actions.

Add:

màn jīng zǐ	vitex [fruit]	Viticis Fructus	9 g.
shēng mā	cimicifuga [root]	Cimicifugae Rhizoma	9 g.
jú huā	chrysanthemum [flower]	Chrysanthemi Flos	9 g.

To move qi and open the orifices, add:

shí chāng pú	acorus [root]	Acori Rhizoma	9 g.
lù lù tōng	liquidambar [fruit]	Liquidambaris Fructus	6 g.

ACUPUNCTURE AND MOXIBUSTION

Main points: Needle with draining.

TB-17	*yì fēng*
GB-02	*tīng huì*
TB-03	*zhōng zhù*
GB-43	*xiá xī*
TB-05	*wài guān*
LI-04	*hé gǔ*

3. BINDING DEPRESSION OF PHLEGM-FIRE

Clinical Manifestations: Tinnitus and deafness accompanied by dizzy spells, sensation of heaviness of the head, oppression in the chest, profuse phlegm, bitter taste in the mouth and irregularity of urination and bowel movements.

Tongue: Red with yellow slimy coating.

Pulse: Slippery, wiry or rapid, slippery.

Treatment Method: Clear fire, transform phlegm.

PRESCRIPTION

Supplemented Two Matured Ingredients Decoction *jiā wèi èr chén tāng*

fǎ bàn xià	pinellia [tuber] (processed)	Pinelliae Tuber Praeparatum	12 g.
chén pí	tangerine [peel]	Citri Exocarpium	12 g.
fú líng	poria	Poria	9 g.
huáng qín	scutellaria [root]	Scutellariae Radix	9 g.
huáng lián	coptis [root]	Coptidis Rhizoma	9 g.
gān cǎo	licorice [root]	Glycyrrhizae Radix	6 g.
shēng jiāng	fresh ginger [root]	Zingiberis Rhizoma Recens	3 g.
bò hé	mint (abbreviated decoction)	Menthae Herba	6 g.

MODIFICATIONS

To reinforce the clearing heat and dissolving phlegm, add:

xìng rén	apricot [kernel] (abbreviated decoction)	Armeniacae Semen	9 g.
guā lóu rén	trichosanthes [seed]	Trichosanthis Semen	12 g.
dǎn xīng	bile-processed arisaema [root]	Arisaematis Rhizoma cum Felle Bovis	6 g.

ACUPUNCTURE AND MOXIBUSTION

Main points: Needle with draining.

TB-17	*yì fēng*
GB-02	*tīng huì*
TB-03	*zhōng zhù*
GB-43	*xiá xī*
ST-40	*fēng lóng*
PC-08	*láo gōng*

4. KIDNEY ESSENCE DEPLETION

Clinical Manifestations: Tinnitus resembling the buzzing of cicadas, intermittent spells of tinnitus, worsening of symptoms at night, extended course of illness and gradual loss of hearing, accompanied by dizziness and vertigo, insomnia, weak aching lower back and knees and seminal emission.

Tongue: Red with little coating.

Pulse: Thready, or rapid, thready.

Treatment Method: Supplement the kidney, secure essence.

PRESCRIPTION

Deafness Left-Benefiting Loadstone Pill *ěr lóng zuǒ cí wán*

shú dì huáng	cooked rehmannia [root]	Rehmanniae Radix Conquita	24 g.
shān zhū yú	cornus [fruit]	Corni Fructus	12 g.
shān yào	dioscorea [root]	Dioscoreae Rhizoma	12 g.
mǔ dān pí	moutan [root bark]	Moutan Radicis Cortex	9 g.
zé xiè	alisma [tuber]	Alismatis Rhizoma	9 g.
fú líng	poria	Poria	9 g.
shí chāng pú	acorus [root]	Acori Rhizoma	6 g.
wǔ wèi zǐ	schisandra [berry]	Schisandrae Fructus	6 g.
cí shí	loadstone (extended decoction)	Magnetitum	30 g.

<u>MODIFICATIONS</u>

In cases presenting symptoms of vacuity of kidney yang, including cold extremities, impotence, pale tongue and weak pulse, the prescription is modified to warm and supplement kidney yang.

Add:

zhì fù zǐ	aconite [accessory tuber] (processed) (extended decoction)	Aconiti Tuber Laterale Praeparatum	9 g.
ròu guì	cinnamon [bark] (abbreviated decoction)	Cinnamomi Cortex	6 g.
bǔ gǔ zhī	psoralea [seed]	Psoraleae Semen	9 g.
tù sī zǐ	cuscuta [seed]	Cuscutae Semen	12 g.

ACUPUNCTURE AND MOXIBUSTION

Main points: Needle with supplementation; may apply moxibustion.

TB-17	*yì fēng*
GB-02	*tīng huì*
BL-23	*shèn shū*
KI-03	*tài xī*
CV-04	*guān yuán*
GV-04	*mìng mén*

5. SPLEEN AND STOMACH QI VACUITY

Clinical Manifestations: Tinnitus and deafness aggravated by overwork, and a sensation of emptiness and coolness within the ears, accompanied by tiredness, fatigue, poor appetite, loose stools, epigastric distention after eating and a sallow withered complexion.

Tongue: Pale with white coating.

Pulse: Weak.

Treatment Method: Strengthen the spleen and stomach, boost qi.

PRESCRIPTION

Center-Supplementing Qi-Boosting Decoction *bǔ zhōng yì qì tāng*

huáng qí	astragalus [root]	Astragali (seu Hedysari) Radix	15 g.
rén shēn	ginseng	Ginseng Radix	9 g.
bái zhú	ovate atractylodes [root]	Atractylodis Ovatae Rhizoma	9 g.
dāng guī	tangkuei	Angelicae Sinensis Radix	9 g.
chén pí	tangerine peel	Citri Exocarpium	6 g.
shēng mā	cimicifuga [root]	Cimicifugae Rhizoma	3 g.
chái hú	bupleurum [root]	Bupleuri Radix	3 g.
zhì gān cǎo	licorice [root] (honey-fried)	Glycyrrhizae Radix	6 g.

<u>MODIFICATIONS</u>

The prescription may be reinforced to open the orifices.

Add:

shí chāng pú	acorus [root]	Acori Rhizoma	9 g.
màn jīng zǐ	vitex [fruit]	Viticis Fructus	9 g.
gé gēn	pueraria [root]	Puerariae Radix	12 g.

ACUPUNCTURE AND MOXIBUSTION

Main points: Needle with supplementation; add moxibustion

TB-17	*yì fēng*
GB-02	*tīng huì*
BL-20	*pí shū*
BL-21	*wèi shū*
ST-36	*zú sān lǐ*
CV-06	*qì hǎi*

ALTERNATE THERAPEUTIC METHODS

1. Ear Acupuncture

Main points: Subcortex, Endocrine, Liver, Kidney, Inner Ear, *Shén Mén*.

Method: Needle to elicit a moderate sensation and retain needles for thirty minutes. Treat once daily or once every second day, fifteen to twenty sessions per course.

2. Scalp Acupuncture

Main points: *Yùn Tīng Qū* (Vertigo and Hearing Region)

Method: Retain needles for twenty minutes, manipulating needles periodically. Treat once daily or once every second day.

REMARKS

During the treatment of tinnitus and deafness, patients should make every attempt to regulate their diet, emotional state and sleeping schedule. Also, they should avoid strong tea, coffee, chocolate, alcohol and other stimulants.

Tuina self-massage is beneficial in the treatment of tinnitus and deafness. First cover the ears with the palms of the hands and then beat the areas over the occipital bone and mastoid processes with the fingers. Next, rhythmically lift and press the palms of the hands, opening and closing the orifice of the ear. Repeat this process morning and night, maintaining the rhythm for several minutes.

Acupuncture has been found to be highly effective in the treatment of neural tinnitus and deafness.

Purulent Ear

Tíng Ěr

1. External Wind-Heat - 2. Exuberant Liver and Gallbladder Fire - 3. Damp-Encumbered Vacuous Spleen - 4. Kidney Yin Vacuity with Toxin Accumulation

Purulent ear is an ear disease resembling the acute and chronic otitis media of Western medicine. Major clinical manifestations include perforation or rupture of the tympanic membrane and drainage of a purulent discharge into the external ear. Purulent ear is most often seen in children.

ETIOLOGY AND PATHOGENESIS

The development of purulent ear may be caused by the following: invasion of external wind-heat evils into the orifices of the ears, exuberant liver and gallbladder fire that penetrates the channels and disturbs the ears, dampness resulting from weakened spleen function rising to the ears or depletion of kidney yin with accumulation of toxins.

Cases may be either acute or chronic, and the course of illness brief or long. In general, acute cases where suppuration has just begun are classified as repletion patterns, and chronic cases where suppuration is prolonged are classified either as vacuity patterns or patterns of repletion in the midst of vacuity.

1. EXTERNAL WIND-HEAT

Clinical Manifestations: Acute onset, pain within the ear, sensations of distention or blockage, tinnitus and impairment of hearing, followed by a gradual increase in the severity of the ear pain, which spreads to involve the head. After a bout of excruciating pain, there is often a perforation of the eardrum and drainage of a purulent discharge. This is followed by a decrease in pain and other accompanying symptoms and may be concurrent with fever, aversion to cold, headache, stuffy nose and runny nose.

Tongue: Thin yellow coating

Pulse: Rapid, floating.

Treatment Method: Course wind-heat, resolve toxins, promote suppuration.

PRESCRIPTION

Vitex Fruit Powder *màn jīng zǐ sǎn*

màn jīng zǐ	vitex [fruit]	Viticis Fructus	12 g.
jú huā	chrysanthemum [flower]	Chrysanthemi Flos	12 g.
shēng mā	cimicifuga [root]	Cimicifugae Rhizoma	9 g.
shēng dì huáng	rehmannia [root] dried/fresh	Rehmanniae Radix Exsiccata seu Recens	12 g.
chì sháo yào	red peony [root]	Paeoniae Radix Rubra	9 g.
mài mén dōng	ophiopogon [tuber]	Ophiopogonis Tuber	12 g.
fú líng	poria	Poria	12 g.
mù tōng	mutong [stem]	Mutong Caulis	6 g.
sāng bái pí	mulberry [root bark]	Mori Radicis Cortex	12 g.
qián hú	peucedanum [root]	Peucedani Radix	9 g.
zhì gān cǎo	licorice [root] (honey-fried)	Glycyrrhizae Radix	6 g.

MODIFICATIONS

In cases of severe heat where there is danger of convulsions, the prescription is modified to calm the liver and extinguish wind.
Add:

gōu téng	uncaria [stem and thorn] (abbreviated decoction)	Uncariae Ramulus cum Unco	12 g.
chán tuì	cicada molting	Cicadae Periostracum	9 g.

After perforation of the eardrum and drainage of pus, the prescription is changed to dispel dampness, resolve toxins, quicken the blood and promote suppuration.
Use:

Immortal Formula Life-Giving Beverage *xiān fāng huó mìng yǐn*

jīn yín huā	lonicera [flower]	Lonicerae Flos	12 g.
zhè bèi mǔ	Zhejiang fritillaria [bulb]	Fritillariae Verticillatae Bulbus	9 g.
tiān huā fěn	trichosanthes [root]	Trichosanthis Radix	9 g.
chuān shān jiǎ	pangolin scales	Manitis Squama	6 g.
zào jiǎo cì	gleditsia [thorn]	Gleditsiae Spina	6 g.
bái zhǐ	angelica [root]	Angelicae Dahuricae Radix	6 g.
chén pí	tangerine [peel]	Citri Exocarpium	6 g.
chì sháo yào	red peony [root]	Paeoniae Radix Rubra	9 g.
dāng guī wěi	tangkuei tail	Angelicae Sinensis Radicis Extremitas	6 g.
rǔ xiāng	frankincense	Olibanum	6 g.
mò yào	myrrh	Myrrha	6 g.
fáng fēng	ledebouriella [root]	Ledebouriellae Radix	6 g.

Add:

chē qián zǐ	plantago [seed] (wrapped)	Plantaginis Semen	9 g.
dì fū zǐ	kochia [fruit]	Kochiae Fructus	9 g.
kǔ shēn	flavescent sophora [root]	Sophorae Flavescentis Radix	9 g.

ACUPUNCTURE AND MOXIBUSTION

Main points: Needle with draining.

TB-17	*yì fēng*
GB-20	*fēng chí*
SI-19	*tīng gōng*
LI-04	*hé gǔ*
TB-05	*wài guān*

Auxiliary points:

For severe heat, add:

      GV-14   *dà zhuī*
      LI-11   *qū chí*

For headache, add:

      M-HN-9   *tài yáng* (Greater Yang)
      GV-23   *shàng xīng*

2. EXUBERANT LIVER AND GALLBLADDER FIRE

Clinical Manifestations: Ear symptoms as described above with exudation of a thick yellow pus, or pus mixed with blood in severe cases, accompanied by bitter taste in the mouth, dry throat, constipation and dark urine.

Tongue: Red with yellow coating.

Pulse: Rapid, wiry.

Treatment Method: Drain the liver and gallbladder, resolve toxins, promote suppuration.

PRESCRIPTION

Gentian Liver-Draining Decoction *lóng-dǎn xiè gān tāng*

lóng dǎn cǎo	gentian [root]	Gentianae Radix	6 g.
huáng qín	scutellaria [root]	Scutellariae Radix	9 g.
shān zhī zǐ	gardenia [fruit]	Gardeniae Fructus	9 g.
zé xiè	alisma [tuber]	Alismatis Rhizoma	12 g.
mù tōng	mutong [stem]	Mutong Caulis	9 g.
dāng guī	tangkuei	Angelicae Sinensis Radix	3 g.
chē qián zǐ	plantago [seed] (wrapped)	Plantaginis Semen	9 g.
shēng dì huáng	rehmannia [root] dried/fresh	Rehmanniae Radix Exsiccata seu Recens	9 g.
chái hú	bupleurum [root]	Bupleuri Radix	6 g.
gān cǎo	licorice [root]	Glycyrrhizae Radix	6 g.

MODIFICATIONS

In cases with constipation, the prescription is modified to drain heat and free the stool.

Add:

dà huáng	rhubarb (abbreviated decoction)	Rhei Rhizoma	9 g.
máng xiāo	mirabilite (stirred in)	Mirabilitum	9 g.

After perforation of the eardrum and drainage of pus, the prescription is modified to dispel dampness, resolve toxins, quicken the blood and promote suppuration. Use:

Immortal Formula Life-Giving Beverage *xiān fāng huó mìng yǐn*

jīn yín huā	lonicera [flower]	Lonicerae Flos	12 g.
zhè bèi mǔ	Zhejiang fritillaria [bulb]	Fritillariae Verticillatae Bulbus	9 g.
tiān huā fěn	trichosanthes [root]	Trichosanthis Radix	9 g.
chuān shān jiǎ	pangolin scales	Manitis Squama	6 g.
zào jiǎo cì	gleditsia [thorn]	Gleditsiae Spina	6 g.
bái zhǐ	angelica [root]	Angelicae Dahuricae Radix	6 g.
chén pí	tangerine peel	Citri Exocarpium	6 g.
chì sháo yào	red peony [root]	Paeoniae Radix Rubra	9 g.
dāng guī wěi	tangkuei tail	Angelicae Sinensis Radicis Extremitas	6 g.
rǔ xiāng	frankincense	Olibanum	6 g.
mò yào	myrrh	Myrrha	6 g.
fáng fēng	ledebouriella [root]	Ledebouriellae Radix	6 g.

Add:

chē qián zǐ	plantago [seed] (wrapped)	Plantaginis Semen	9 g.
dì fū zǐ	kochia [fruit]	Kochiae Fructus	9 g.
kǔ shēn	flavescent sophora [root]	Sophorae Flavescentis Radix	9 g.

ACUPUNCTURE AND MOXIBUSTION

Main points: Needle with draining.

TB-17	*yì fēng*
GB-20	*fēng chí*
GB-02	*tīng huì*
GB-41	*zú lín qì*
LR-02	*xíng jiān*

Auxiliary points:

For severe heat, add:

GV-14	*dà zhuī*
LI-11	*qū chí*

For headache, add:

M-HN-9	*tài yáng* (Greater Yang)
GV-23	*shàng xīng*

3. DAMP-ENCUMBERED VACUOUS SPLEEN

Clinical Manifestations: Drainage of a large quantity of clear thin pus into the external auditory canal, fluctuations of the quantity drained and poor response to treatment. Accompanying symptoms include dizziness and vertigo, sensation of heaviness of the head, fatigue, sallow withered complexion, poor appetite and loose stools.

Tongue: Pale with moist white coating.

Pulse: Soft, weak.

Treatment Method: Strengthen the spleen, dispel dampness, promote suppuration.

PRESCRIPTION

Internal Expulsion Toxin-Dispersing Powder *tuō lǐ xiāo dú sǎn*

huáng qí	astragalus [root]	Astragali (seu Hedysari) Radix	12 g.
jīn yín huā	lonicera [flower]	Lonicerae Flos	15 g.
chuān xiōng	ligusticum [root]	Ligustici Rhizoma	9 g.
dāng guī	tangkuei	Angelicae Sinensis Radix	6 g.
bái sháo yào	white peony [root]	Paeoniae Radix Alba	6 g.
bái zhú	ovate atractylodes [root]	Atractylodis Ovatae Rhizoma	6 g.
rén shēn	ginseng	Ginseng Radix	6 g.
fú líng	poria	Poria	9 g.
bái zhǐ	angelica [root]	Angelicae Dahuricae Radix	6 g.
zào jiǎo cì	gleditsia [thorn]	Gleditsiae Spina	6 g.
jié gěng	platycodon [root]	Platycodonis Radix	6 g.
gān cǎo	licorice [root]	Glycyrrhizae Radix	6 g.

MODIFICATIONS

In cases where there is evidence of dampness transforming into heat, the prescription is modified to clear heat, disinhibit dampness, and resolve toxins.

Add:

chē qián zǐ	plantago [seed] (wrapped)	Plantaginis Semen	9 g.
dì fū zǐ	kochia [fruit]	Kochiae Fructus	9 g.
pú gōng yīng	dandelion	Taraxaci Herba cum Radice	12 g.
yú xīng cǎo	houttuynia	Houttuyniae Herba cum Radice	12 g.

ACUPUNCTURE AND MOXIBUSTION

Main points: Needle with supplementation; add moxibustion.

TB-17	*yì fēng*
ST-36	*zú sān lǐ*
SP-09	*yīn líng quán*
BL-20	*pí shū*
SP-03	*tài bái*

4. KIDNEY YIN VACUITY WITH TOXIN ACCUMULATION

Clinical Manifestations: Discharge of a small amount of thin pus into the external auditory canal, extended course of illness and marked hearing impairment, accompanied by dizziness and vertigo, tinnitus, tiredness, fatigue, weak aching lower back and knees, seminal emission and premature ejaculation.

Pulse: Weak, thready.

Treatment Method: Supplement kidney yin, resolve toxins, promote suppuration.

PRESCRIPTION
Anemarrhena, Phellodendron and Rehmannia Pill *zhī bǎi dì huáng wán*

shú dì huáng	cooked rehmannia [root]	Rehmanniae Radix Conquita	24 g.
shān zhū yú	cornus [fruit]	Corni Fructus	12 g.
shān yào	dioscorea [root]	Dioscoreae Rhizoma	12 g.
zé xiè	alisma [tuber]	Alismatis Rhizoma	9 g.
fú líng	poria	Poria	9 g.
mǔ dān pí	moutan [root bark]	Moutan Radicis Cortex	9 g.
zhī mǔ	anemarrhena [root]	Anemarrhenae Rhizoma	9 g.
huáng bǎi	phellodendron [bark]	Phellodendri Cortex	9 g.

MODIFICATIONS

To resolve toxins and promote suppuration, add:

mù tōng	mutong [stem]	Mutong Caulis	6 g.
xià kū cǎo	prunella [spike]	Prunellae Spica	9 g.
jié gěng	platycodon [root]	Platycodonis Radix	9 g.

In cases accompanied by damp-heat, where the pus is turbid and foul smelling, the prescription is modified to quicken the blood, clear heat, dispel dampness and promote suppuration.

Add:

chuān shān jiǎ	pangolin scales	Manitis Squama	9 g.
	(or, powdered and administered separately, each time 1.5 g.)		
zào jiǎo cì	gleditsia [thorn]	Gleditsiae Spina	9 g.
yú xīng cǎo	houttuynia	Houttuyniae Herba cum Radice	12 g.
zé lán	lycopus	Lycopi Herba	12 g.

In cases of vacuity of kidney yang, the prescription is modified to warm and supplement kidney yang, quicken the blood and promote suppuration.

Use:

Kidney Qi Pill *shèn qì wán*

shú dì huáng	cooked rehmannia [root]	Rehmanniae Radix Conquita	24 g.
shān yào	dioscorea [root]	Dioscoreae Rhizoma	12 g.
shān zhū yú	cornus [fruit]	Corni Fructus	12 g.
zé xiè	alisma [tuber]	Alismatis Rhizoma	9 g.
fú líng	poria	Poria	9 g.
mǔ dān pí	moutan [root bark]	Moutan Radicis Cortex	9 g.
zhì fù zǐ	aconite [accessory tuber] (processed) (extended decoction)	Aconiti Tuber Laterale Praeparatum	3 g.
ròu guì	cinnamon [bark] (abbreviated decoction)	Cinnamomi Cortex	3 g.

Add:

zào jiǎo cì	gleditsia [thorn]	Gleditsiae Spina	9 g.
jié gěng	platycodon [root]	Platycodonis Radix	9 g.
táo rén	peach [kernel]	Persicae Semen	6 g.
hóng huā	carthamus [flower]	Carthami Flos	6 g.

ACUPUNCTURE & MOXIBUSTION

Main points: Needle with supplementation.

TB-17	*yì fēng*
GB-02	*tīng huì*
BL-23	*shèn shū*
KI-03	*tài xī*
SP-09	*yīn líng quán*

Auxiliary points:

For kidney yang vacuity, add acupuncture and moxibustion at:

CV-04	*guān yuán*
GV-04	*mìng mén*

ALTERNATE THERAPEUTIC METHODS

1. Ear Acupuncture

Main points: Kidney, Inner Ear, Endocrine, Occiput, External Ear.

Method: Needle once daily to elicit a moderate sensation. Retain needles for twenty to thirty minutes. Blood may be let at the small veins on the back of the ear.

REMARKS

During treatment, patients should minimize the consumption of eggs, seafood and legumes. Where there is perforation of the eardrum, patients need to refrain from swimming, or else take appropriate measures before swimming.

NOSEBLEED

Bí Nǜ

1. Exuberance of Lung Heat - 2. Exuberance of Stomach Heat - 3. Effulgent Liver Fire - 4. Vacuity of Liver and Kidney Yin - 5. Spleen Failing to Manage the Blood

Nosebleed, or epistaxis, is commonly observed in a variety of conditions. This chapter focuses on nosebleed that results from a dysfunction of the viscera and bowels, and does not include those caused by traumatic injury.

ETIOLOGY AND PATHOGENESIS

The etiology of nosebleeds is closely linked to the functioning of the lung, stomach, liver and spleen. Nosebleed is most commonly caused by the invasion of external wind-heat or dryness-heat causing exuberant heat in the lungs or consumption of strong alcoholic beverages or spicy foods resulting in an exuberance of stomach heat. Other factors include exuberant liver fire following anger or frustration, effulgent fire caused by liver and kidney yin vacuity that follows prolonged illnesses, overindulgent sexual activity or failure of vacuous spleen qi to secure the blood due to anxiety and worry, overwork or poor dietary habits.

1. EXUBERANCE OF LUNG HEAT

Clinical Manifestations: Nosebleed with a moderate amount of bright red blood, dryness and feverish sensation of the nasal cavity accompanied by fever, cough with little phlegm and dry mouth.

Tongue: Red tip with thin white dry coating.

Pulse: Rapid or rapid, floating.

Treatment Method: Course wind, clear heat, cool the blood, relieve bleeding.

PRESCRIPTION

Mulberry Leaf and Chrysanthemum Beverage *sāng jú yǐn*

sāng yè	mulberry [leaf]	Mori Folium	9 g.
jú huā	chrysanthemum [flower]	Chrysanthemi Flos	9 g.
lián qiào	forsythia [fruit]	Forsythiae Fructus	9 g.
lú gēn	phragmites [root]	Phragmitis Rhizoma	9 g.
xìng rén	apricot [kernel] (abbreviated decoction)	Armeniacae Semen	9 g.
jié gěng	platycodon [root]	Platycodonis Radix	9 g.
bò hé	mint (abbreviated decoction)	Menthae Herba	6 g.
gān cǎo	licorice [root]	Glycyrrhizae Radix	6 g.

MODIFICATIONS

To cool the blood and relieve bleeding, add:

mǔ dān pí	moutan [root bark]	Moutan Radicis Cortex	9 g.
bái máo gēn	imperata [root]	Imperatae Rhizoma	15 g.
shān zhī zǐ	gardenia [fruit] (charred)	Gardeniae Fructus Carbonisatus	9 g.

ACUPUNCTURE AND MOXIBUSTION

Main points: Needle with draining.

GB-20   *fēng chí*
LI-20   *yíng xiāng*
LI-04   *hé gǔ*
LI-11   *qū chí*

Auxiliary points:

For severe heat, add:

TB-5   *wài guān*
LI-01   *shāng yáng*

2. EXUBERANCE OF STOMACH HEAT

Clinical Manifestations: Nosebleed with a large amount of bright red or dark red blood, dry nasal cavity, dry mouth, halitosis, excessive thirst, hard dry stools and dark scanty urine.

Tongue: Red with dry yellow coating.

Pulse: Surging, rapid.

Treatment Method: Clear the stomach, drain fire, cool the blood, relieve bleeding.

PRESCRIPTION

Rhinoceros Horn and Rehmannia Decoction *xī jiǎo dì huáng tāng*

xī jiǎo	rhinoceros horn* (powdered and stirred in)	Rhinocerotis Cornu	3 g.
shēng dì huáng	rehmannia [root] dried/fresh	Rehmanniae Radix Exsiccata seu Recens	30 g.
bái sháo yào	white peony [root]	Paeoniae Radix Alba	12 g.
mǔ dān pí	moutan [root bark]	Moutan Radicis Cortex	9 g.

*Use of *xī jiǎo* (rhinoceros horn) is prohibited in North America by the endangered species law. Water Buffalo Horn *(shuǐ niú jiǎo)* may be substituted. Increase the dose to 15 g., extended decoction.)

MODIFICATIONS

To clear stomach heat, add:

shí gāo	gypsum (extended decoction)	Gypsum	30 g.
zhī mǔ	anemarrhena [root]	Anemarrhenae Rhizoma	9 g.

In cases of hard dry stools, the prescription is modified to free the stool and clear heat.

Add:

dà huáng	rhubarb (abbreviated decoction)	Rhei Rhizoma	9 g.
guā lóu rén	trichosanthes [seed]	Trichosanthis Semen	12 g.

ACUPUNCTURE AND MOXIBUSTION

Main points: Needle with draining.

ST-44	*nèi tíng*
SP-01	*yǐn bái*
GV-23	*shàng xīng*
LI-02	*èr jiān*

3. EFFULGENT LIVER FIRE

Clinical Manifestations: Nosebleed, discharge of large amounts of dark red blood, headache, dizziness and vertigo, bitter taste in the mouth, dry throat, discomfort and fullness of the chest and hypochondria, flushed complexion, bloodshot eyes, restlessness, irritability.

Tongue: Red with yellow coating.

Pulse: Rapid, wiry.

Treatment Method: Clear the liver, drain fire, cool the blood, relieve bleeding.

PRESCRIPTION

Gentian Liver-Draining Decoction *lóng dǎn xiè gān tāng*

lóng dǎn cǎo	gentian [root]	Gentianae Radix	6 g.
huáng qín	scutellaria [root]	Scutellariae Radix	9 g.
shān zhī zǐ	gardenia [fruit]	Gardeniae Fructus	9 g.
zé xiè	alisma [tuber]	Alismatis Rhizoma	12 g.
mù tōng	mutong [stem]	Mutong Caulis	9 g.
dāng guī	tangkuei	Angelicae Sinensis Radix	3 g.
chē qián zǐ	plantago [seed] (wrapped)	Plantaginis Semen	9 g.
shēng dì huáng	rehmannia [root] dried/fresh	Rehmanniae Radix Exsiccata seu Recens	9 g.
chái hú	bupleurum [root]	Bupleuri Radix	6 g.
gān cǎo	licorice [root]	Glycyrrhizae Radix	6 g.

MODIFICATIONS

To clear and soothe the liver, drain fire and regulate the blood, add:

méi guī huā	rose	Rosae Flos	6 g.
líng yáng jiǎo	antelope [horn]	Antelopis Cornu	3 g.

(decocted separately, or ground into powder and administered separately, each time 0.5 g.)

The prescription may be modified to clear rising fire. According to the patient's condition, select from and add:

xī jiǎo	rhinoceros horn (powdered and stirred in)*	Rhinocerotis Cornu	3 g.
shí gāo	gypsum (extended decoction)	Gypsum	30 g.
huáng lián	coptis [root]	Coptidis Rhizoma	6 g.
zhú rú	bamboo shavings	Bambusae Caulis in Taeniam	9 g.
qīng hāo	sweet wormwood (abbreviated decoction)	Artemisiae Apiaceae seu Annuae Herba	9 g.

---

*Use of *xī jiǎo* (rhinoceros horn) is prohibited in North America by the endangered species law. Water Buffalo Horn *(shuǐ niú jiǎo)* may be substituted. Increase the dose to 15 g., extended decoction.)

ACUPUNCTURE AND MOXIBUSTION

Main points: Needle with draining.

LR-02	*xíng jiān*
BL-40 (54)	*wěi zhōng*
GV-27	*duì duān*
LR-08	*qū quán*
BL-45 (40)	*yī xǐ*

4. VACUITY OF LIVER AND KIDNEY YIN

Clinical Manifestations: Intermittently recurring nosebleed, discharge of small amount of blood, dry mouth with little saliva, tidal fever, night sweating, dizziness and vertigo, blurred vision, palpitations, insomnia, tinnitus, vexing heat in the five hearts.

Tongue: Red with little coating.

Pulse: Rapid, thready.

Treatment Method: Nourish yin, drain fire, cool the blood, relieve bleeding.

PRESCRIPTION

Anemarrhena, Phellodendron and Rehmannia Decoction
zhī bǎi dì huáng tāng

shú dì huáng	cooked rehmannia [root]	Rehmanniae Radix Conquita	24 g.
shān zhū yú	cornus [fruit]	Corni Fructus	12 g.
shān yào	dioscorea [root]	Dioscoreae Rhizoma	12 g.
zé xiè	alisma [tuber]	Alismatis Rhizoma	9 g.
fú líng	poria	Poria	9 g.
mǔ dān pí	moutan [root bark]	Moutan Radicis Cortex	9 g.
zhī mǔ	anemarrhena [root]	Anemarrhenae Rhizoma	9 g.
huáng bǎi	phellodendron [bark]	Phellodendri Cortex	9 g.

MODIFICATIONS

To cool the blood and relieve bleeding, add:

hàn lián cǎo	eclipta	Ecliptae Herba	12 g.
ǒu jié	lotus [root node]	Nelumbinis Rhizomatis Nodus	12 g.
ē jiāo	ass hide glue (dissolved and stirred in)	Asini Corii Gelatinum	9 g.

In cases of severe depletion of blood, the prescription is changed to supplement the blood and relieve bleeding.

Combine with the given prescription:

Ass Hide Glue and Mugwort Four Agents Decoction *jiāo ài sì wù tāng*

ē jiāo	ass hide glue (dissolved and stirred in)	Asini Corii Gelatinum	9 g.
ài yè	mugwort [leaf]	Artemisiae Argyi Folium	9 g.
shēng dì huáng	rehmannia [root] dried/fresh	Rehmanniae Radix Exsiccata seu Recens	12 g.
dāng guī	tangkuei	Angelicae Sinensis Radix	9 g.
bái sháo yào	white peony [root]	Paeoniae Radix Alba	12 g.
chuān xiōng	ligusticum [root]	Ligustici Rhizoma	6 g.
gān cǎo	licorice [root]	Glycyrrhizae Radix	6 g.

ACUPUNCTURE AND MOXIBUSTION

Main points: Needle with even supplementation, even drainage.

BL-23	*shèn shū*
KI-03	*tài xī*
KI-01	*yǒng quán*
LR-03	*tài chōng*
BL-07	*tōng tiān*

5. SPLEEN FAILING TO MANAGE THE BLOOD

Clinical Manifestations: Nosebleed, discharge of a varying amount of light red blood, lusterless complexion, poor appetite, tiredness, fatigue, disinclination to speak.

Tongue: Pale with thin coating.

Pulse: Weak, tardy.

Treatment Method: Fortify the spleen, boost qi, secure the blood, relieve bleeding.

PRESCRIPTION

Spleen-Returning Decoction *guī pí tāng*

huáng qí	astragalus [root]	Astragali (seu Hedysari) Radix	9 g.
rén shēn	ginseng	Ginseng Radix	9 g.
bái zhú	ovate atractylodes [root]	Atractylodis Ovatae Rhizoma	9 g.
fú shén	root poria	Poria cum Pini Radice	9 g.
lóng yǎn ròu	longan [flesh]	Longanae Arillus	9 g.
suān zǎo rén	spiny jujube [kernel]	Ziziphi Spinosi Semen	9 g.
mù xiāng	saussurea [root]	Saussureae (seu Vladimiriae) Radix	6 g.
dāng guī	tangkuei	Angelicae Sinensis Radix	6 g.
yuǎn zhì	polygala [root]	Polygalae Radix	3 g.
zhì gān cǎo	licorice [root] (honey-fried)	Glycyrrhizae Radix	6 g.
shēng jiāng	fresh ginger [root]	Zingiberis Rhizoma Recens	3 g.
dà zǎo	jujube [fruit]	Ziziphi Fructus	5 pc.

MODIFICATIONS

The prescription is modified to ameliorate the spleen's failure to contain the blood and relieve bleeding.

Delete:

shēng jiāng	fresh ginger [root]	Zingiberis Rhizoma Recens

Add:

cè bǎi yè	biota [leaf]	Biotae Folium	12 g.
dì yú	sanguisorba [root]	Sanguisorbae Radix	12 g.

ACUPUNCTURE AND MOXIBUSTION

Main points: Needle with supplementation; add moxibustion.

CV-12	*zhōng wǎn*
BL-20	*pí shū*
ST-36	*zú sān lǐ*
SP-01	*yǐn bái*

ALTERNATE THERAPEUTIC METHODS

1. Ear Acupuncture

Main points: Inner Nose, Lung, Adrenal, Forehead.

Method: Manipulate one to two minutes to elicit a moderate sensation. Retain needles twenty to thirty minutes. Treat once daily.

REMARKS

Nosebleed should be treated according to the principle, "when acute, treat the branch." During nosebleeds, patients should assume a semi-supine position. Cold compresses, external pressure and nasal packing can be used when necessary. Avoiding spicy or stimulating foods helps to minimize aggravation of the condition.

DEEP-SOURCE NASAL CONGESTION

Bí Yuān

1. Lung Wind-Heat - 2. Gallbladder Heat - 3. Spleen and Stomach Damp-Heat - 4. Lung Vacuity Cold - 5. Spleen Qi Vacuity

Deep-source nasal congestion *(bí yuān)*, also known as *nǎo lòu* (brain leak) in Chinese, is a commonly observed rhinological disease characterized by turbid fishy-smelling nasal discharge, stuffy nose and impairment or complete loss of the sense of smell. Deep-source nasal congestion is generally presented in Western medical conditions such as acute and chronic sinusitis and chronic rhinitis.

ETIOLOGY AND PATHOGENESIS

Deep-source nasal congestion and discharge is categorized according to repletion and vacuity. Repletion patterns are usually caused by the invasion of external wind-heat or external wind-cold that transforms to heat. These evils can enter the lung, ultimately obstructing the orifice of the nose. Other repletion etiologies include stagnation of qi following emotional upset, which transforms into heat that accumulates in the gallbladder; and internal damp-heat of the spleen and stomach caused by improper diet and eating habits. Repletion patterns are usually acute and of short duration.

Vacuity patterns are either due to lung vacuity cold or to spleen qi vacuity. Vacuity patterns are of long duration and respond poorly to treatment.

1. LUNG WIND-HEAT

Clinical Manifestations: Fever, aversion to cold, headache, stuffy nose, turbid yellow fishy-smelling nasal discharge, coughing in some cases.

Tongue: Red tip with thin yellow coating.

Pulse: Rapid, floating.

Treatment Method: Dispel wind, clear heat, diffuse the lung, free the orifice.

PRESCRIPTION

Xanthium Powder *cāng ěr zǐ sǎn*

cāng ěr zǐ	xanthium [fruit]	Xanthii Fructus	9 g.
xīn yí	magnolia [flower] (wrapped)	Magnoliae Flos	6 g.
bái zhǐ	angelica [root]	Angelicae Dahuricae Radix	6 g.
bò hé	mint (abbreviated decoction)	Menthae Herba	6 g.

MODIFICATIONS

To reinforce dispersing wind and clearing heat, add:

huáng qín	scutellaria [root]	Scutellariae Radix	6 g.
jú huā	chrysanthemum [flower]	Chrysanthemi Flos	9 g.
gé gēn	pueraria [root]	Puerariae Radix	9 g.
lián qiào	forsythia [fruit]	Forsythiae Fructus	9 g.

ACUPUNCTURE AND MOXIBUSTION

Main points: Needle with draining.

LU-07	*liè què*
LI-04	*hé gǔ*
M-HN-14	*bí tōng* (Clear Nose)
LI-20	*yíng xiāng*
M-HN-3	*yìn táng* (Hall of Impression)
GB-20	*fēng chí*

Auxiliary points:

For pain of the superciliary arch, add:

BL-02	*zǎn zhú*

2. GALLBLADDER HEAT

Clinical Manifestations: Heavy discharge of thick turbid yellow foul-smelling mucus from the nose, with severe headache and marked pain on external pressure in the area between the eyebrows or in the zygomatic region, accompanied by symptoms of fever, bitter taste in the mouth, dry throat, tinnitus, deafness, insomnia, dream-troubled sleep, restlessness, irascibility.

Tongue: Red with yellow coating.

Pulse: Rapid, wiry.

Treatment Method: Drain gallbladder heat, dispel turbidity, free the orifice.

PRESCRIPTION

Gentian Liver-Draining Decoction *lóng dǎn xiè gān tāng*

lóng dǎn cǎo	gentian [root]	Gentianae Radix	6 g.
huáng qín	scutellaria [root]	Scutellariae Radix	9 g.
shān zhī zǐ	gardenia [fruit]	Gardeniae Fructus	9 g.
zé xiè	alisma [tuber]	Alismatis Rhizoma	12 g.
mù tōng	mutong [stem]	Mutong Caulis	9 g.
dāng guī	tangkuei	Angelicae Sinensis Radix	3 g.
chē qián zǐ	plantago [seed] (wrapped)	Plantaginis Semen	9 g.
shēng dì huáng	rehmannia [root] dried/fresh	Rehmanniae Radix Exsiccata seu Recens	9 g.
chái hú	bupleurum [root]	Bupleuri Radix	6 g.
gān cǎo	licorice [root]	Glycyrrhizae Radix	6 g.

MODIFICATIONS

To dispel turbidity and clear the orifice, add:

cāng ěr zǐ	xanthium [fruit]	Xanthii Fructus	9 g.
xīn yí	magnolia [flower] (wrapped)	Magnoliae Flos	6 g.
bái zhǐ	angelica [root]	Angelicae Dahuricae Radix	6 g.
huò xiāng	agastache/patchouli	Agastaches seu Pogostemi Herba	6 g.

In cases with constipation, the prescription is modified to free the stool and drain heat.

Add:

dà huáng	rhubarb (abbreviated decoction)	Rhei Rhizoma	6 g.
máng xiāo	mirabilite (stirred in)	Mirabilitum	6 g.

ACUPUNCTURE AND MOXIBUSTION

Main points: Needle with draining.

GB-20	*fēng chí*
GB-43	*xiá xī*
M-HN-3	*yìn táng* (Hall of Impression)
LI-20	*yíng xiāng*
M-HN-14	*bí tōng* (Clear Nose)
GV-23	*shàng xīng*

Auxiliary points:

For headache, add:

GV-20	*bǎi huì*
M-HN-9	*tài yáng* (Greater Yang)

3. SPLEEN AND STOMACH DAMP-HEAT

Clinical Manifestations: Heavy turbid yellow nasal discharge, severe continuous nasal congestion, loss of the sense of smell, redness and swelling within the nasal cavity and distending pain within the nose (swelling and distention being especially marked). Accompanying general symptoms include heaviness and aching of the head, fatigue, epigastric discomfort and fullness, loss of appetite, dark yellow urine.

Tongue: Red with slimy yellow coating.

Pulse: Rapid, slippery or soft, rapid.

Treatment Method: Clear heat, drain dampness, dispel turbidity, open the orifice.

PRESCRIPTION

Combine Scutellaria and Talcum Decoction *(huáng-qín huá-shí tāng)* with Xanthium Powder *(cāng ěr zǐ sǎn)*.

Scutellaria and Talcum Decoction *huáng qín huá shí tāng*

huáng qín	scutellaria [root]	Scutellariae Radix	9 g.
huá shí	talcum (wrapped)	Talcum	12 g.
fú líng	poria	Poria	12 g.
zhū líng	polyporus	Polyporus	9 g.
tōng cǎo	rice-paper plant pith	Tetrapanacis Medulla	6 g.
dà fù pí	areca [husk]	Arecae Pericarpium	9 g.
bái dòu kòu	cardamom (abbreviated decoction)	Amomi Cardamomi Fructus	6 g.

with:

Xanthium Powder *cāng ěr zǐ sǎn*

cāng ěr zǐ	xanthium [fruit]	Xanthii Fructus	9 g.
xīn yí	magnolia [flower]	Magnoliae Flos	6 g.
bái zhǐ	angelica [root]	Angelicae Dahuricae Radix	6 g.
bò hé	mint (abbreviated decoction)	Menthae Herba	6 g.

MODIFICATIONS

In cases of severe heat, the prescription is modified to aid in purging spleen and stomach heat. Add:

shí gāo	gypsum (extended decoction)	Gypsum	15 g.
huáng lián	coptis [root]	Coptidis Rhizoma	6 g.
dà huáng	rhubarb (abbreviated decoction)	Rhei Rhizoma	6 g.

ACUPUNCTURE AND MOXIBUSTION

Main points: Needle with draining.

LI-20	*yíng xiāng*
M-HN-14	*bí tōng* (Clear Nose)
GV-23	*shàng xīng*
SP-09	*yīn líng quán*
SP-06	*sān yīn jiāo*
ST-36	*zú sān lǐ*

Auxiliary points:

For headache, add:

LI-04	*hé gǔ*
M-HN-3	*yìn táng* (Hall of Impression)

4. LUNG VACUITY COLD

Clinical Manifestations: Clear sticky nasal discharge, nasal congestion that is intermittently mild or severe, impairment of the sense of smell with increase in severity of nasal discharge and congestion upon exposure to wind or cold; with accompanying symptoms including shortness of breath, loss of strength, sluggish speech, weak voice, spontaneous perspiration, aversion to draughts and coughing with expectoration of phlegm (in some cases).

Tongue: Pale with thin white coating.

Pulse: Weak.

Treatment Method: Warm and supplement lung qi, dissipate cold, clear the orifice.

PRESCRIPTION

Lung-Warming Decoction *wēn fèi tāng*

huáng qí	astragalus [root]	Astragali (seu Hedysari) Radix	12 g.
qiāng huó	notopterygium [root]	Notopterygii Rhizoma	9 g.
fáng fēng	ledebouriella [root]	Ledebouriellae Radix	9 g.
dīng xiāng	clove	Caryophylli Flos	3 g.
má huáng	ephedra	Ephedrae Herba	6 g.
gé gēn	pueraria [root]	Puerariae Radix	9 g.
cōng bái	scallion white	Allii Fistulosi Bulbus Recens	6 g.
shēng mā	cimicifuga [root]	Cimicifugae Rhizoma	6 g.
gān cǎo	licorice [root]	Glycyrrhizae Radix	6 g.

MODIFICATIONS

To clear the orifice, add:

cāng ěr zǐ	xanthium [fruit]	Xanthii Fructus	9 g.
bái zhǐ	angelica [root]	Angelicae Dahuricae Radix	9 g.
xīn yí	magnolia flower	Magnoliae Flos	6 g.
xì xīn	asarum	Asiasari Herba cum Radice	3 g.

In cases of cold and pain of the forehead, the prescription is modified to dissipate cold and relieve pain.

Add:

gǎo běn	Chinese lovage [root]	Ligustici Sinensis Rhizoma et Radix	9 g.
chuān xiōng	ligusticum [root]	Ligustici Rhizoma	9 g.

ACUPUNCTURE AND MOXIBUSTION

Main points: Needle with supplementation; add moxibustion.

LI-20	*yíng xiāng*
GV-23	*shàng xīng*
GB-20	*fēng chí*
LI-04	*hé gǔ*
GV-20	*bǎi huì*
ST-36	*zú sān lǐ*

Auxiliary points:

For marked vacuity of lung qi, add:

BL-13	*fèi shū*
CV-06	*qì hǎi*

5. SPLEEN QI VACUITY

Clinical Manifestations: Heavy thick milky sticky nasal discharge without foul odor, severe nasal congestion and impairment or complete loss of the sense of smell, accompanied by heaviness of the limbs, loss of strength, poor appetite, loose stools, sallow withered complexion, heavy sensation of the head, dizziness and vertigo.

Tongue: Pale with white coating.

Pulse: Weak, tardy.

Treatment Method: Supplement spleen qi, drain dampness, clear the orifice.

PRESCRIPTION

Ginseng, Poria and Ovate Atractylodes Powder *shēn líng bái zhú sǎn*

rén shēn	ginseng	Ginseng Radix	12 g.
fú líng	poria	Poria	12 g.
bái zhú	ovate atractylodes [root]	Atractylodis Ovatae Rhizoma	12 g.
shān yào	dioscorea [root]	Dioscoreae Rhizoma	12 g.
biǎn dòu	lablab [bean]	Lablab Semen	9 g.
lián zǐ	lotus fruit-seed	Nelumbinis Fructus seu Semen	6 g.
yì yǐ rén	coix [seed]	Coicis Semen	6 g.
jié gěng	platycodon [root]	Platycodonis Radix	6 g.
shā rén	amomum [fruit] (abbreviated decoction)	Amomi Semen seu Fructus	6 g.
zhì gān cǎo	licorice [root] (honey-fried)	Glycyrrhizae Radix	12 g.

MODIFICATIONS

To reinforce the spleen-strengthening and damp-draining, add:

huáng qí	astragalus [root]	Astragali (seu Hedysari) Radix	12 g.
zé xiè	alisma [tuber]	Alismatis Rhizoma	9 g.

To dispel turbidity and clear the orifice, add:

bái zhǐ	angelica [root]	Angelicae Dahuricae Radix	9 g.
xīn yí	magnolia [flower] (wrapped)	Magnoliae Flos	6 g.
cāng ěr zǐ	xanthium [fruit]	Xanthii Fructus	9 g.

In cases where dampness transforms into heat, the prescription is modified to clear heat and drain dampness.
Add:

huáng lián	coptis [root]	Coptidis Rhizoma	6 g.
chē qián zǐ	plantago [seed] (wrapped)	Plantaginis Semen	9 g.
mù tōng	mutong [stem]	Mutong Caulis	6 g.

ACUPUNCTURE AND MOXIBUSTION

Main points: Needle with supplementation; add moxibustion.

GV-20	*bǎi huì*
LI-20	*yíng xiāng*
M-HN-14	*bí tōng* (Clear Nose)
GV-23	*shàng xīng*
ST-36	*zú sān lǐ*
SP-09	*yīn líng quán*

Auxiliary points:

For severe vacuity of spleen qi, add:

CV-04	*guān yuán*
BL-20	*pí shū*

For headache, add:

BL-02	*zǎn zhú*
M-HN-3	*yìn táng* (Hall of Impression)

ALTERNATE THERAPEUTIC METHODS

1. Ear Acupuncture

Auricular points: Inner Nose, Adrenal, Lung, Forehead. In cases of allergic rhinitis, add: Anti-asthma, Endocrine.

Method: Needle to elicit a strong sensation and retain needles for twenty to thirty minutes. Alternately, embed needles for five to seven days.

REMARKS

During the treatment of deep-source nasal congestion, patients should avoid spicy foods and abstain from smoking and ingesting alcohol beverages.

SORE SWOLLEN THROAT

Yān Hóu Zhŏng Tòng

1. Lung Wind-Heat - 2. Exuberant Lung and Stomach Heat - 3. Depletion of Lung and Kidney Yin

Soreness and swelling of the throat is a commonly observed disorder when there are pathological changes in the throat. In traditional Chinese medicine it is often seen in cases of *rŭ é* (baby moth), which corresponds to tonsillitis, and *hóu bì* (throat block), which corresponds to inflammation of the throat. This chapter also refers to cases of acute and chronic tonsillitis as well as acute and chronic pharyngitis as diagnosed by Western medicine.

ETIOLOGY AND PATHOGENESIS

Patterns of sore swollen throat are classified according to repletion and vacuity, and relate to the channel pathways of the lung, stomach and kidney. Repletion patterns result from the invasion of the lung by wind-heat or from an overconsumption of spicy foods that has caused exuberant stomach and lung heat to rise into the throat. Vacuity patterns are generally the result of lung and kidney yin depletion with frenetic vacuity fire rising to the throat.

1. LUNG WIND-HEAT

Clinical Manifestations: Redness, swelling and pain of the throat, acute onset of symptoms, increased pain upon swallowing or coughing, sensation of dryness and burning of the throat accompanied by fever, aversion to cold and cough with thick sticky phlegm that may be yellow.

Tongue: Red tip with thin yellow coating.

Pulse: Rapid, floating.

Treatment Method: Course wind, clear heat, disperse swelling, disinhibit the pharynx.

PRESCRIPTION

Wind-Coursing Heat-Clearing Decoction *shū fēng qīng rè tāng*

jīng jiè	schizonepeta (abbreviated decoction)	Schizonepetae Herba et Flos	6 g.
fáng fēng	ledebouriella [root]	Ledebouriellae Radix	6 g.
niú bàng zǐ	arctium [seed]	Arctii Fructus	9 g.
jīn yín huā	lonicera [flower]	Lonicerae Flos	9 g.
lián qiào	forsythia [fruit]	Forsythiae Fructus	9 g.
sāng bái pí	mulberry [root bark]	Mori Radicis Cortex	9 g.
huáng qín	scutellaria [root]	Scutellariae Radix	6 g.

chì sháo yào	red peony [root]	Paeoniae Radix Rubra	6 g.
xuán shēn	scrophularia [root]	Scrophulariae Radix	6 g.
zhè bèi mǔ	Zhejiang fritillaria [bulb]	Fritillariae Verticillatae Bulbus	6 g.
jié gěng	platycodon [root]	Platycodonis Radix	6 g.
tiān huā fěn	trichosanthes [root]	Trichosanthis Radix	9 g.
gān cǎo	licorice [root]	Glycyrrhizae Radix	6 g.

ACUPUNCTURE AND MOXIBUSTION

Main points: Needle with draining.

LU-11	*shào shāng* (bleed)
LU-05	*chǐ zé*
LI-04	*hé gǔ*
LI-11	*qū chí*

Auxiliary points:

For hoarseness of the voice, add:

| LU-07 | *liè quē* |
| LI-18 | *fú tú* |

2. EXUBERANT LUNG AND STOMACH HEAT

Clinical Manifestations: Severe pain with redness and swelling of the throat, pain often radiating to the base of the ear and beneath the jaw, difficulty swallowing, sensation of throat obstruction with hoarseness in some cases; accompanied by symptoms of high fever, excessive thirst, headache, halitosis, thick sticky yellow phlegm, constipation, dark scanty urine.

Tongue: Red with thick yellow coating.

Pulse: Surging.

Treatment Method: Clear heat, resolve toxins, disperse swelling, disinhibit the pharynx.

PRESCRIPTION

Pharynx-Clearing Diaphragm-Disinhibiting Decoction *qīng yān lì gé tāng*

jīn yín huā	lonicera [flower]	Lonicerae Flos	12 g.
lián qiào	forsythia [fruit]	Forsythiae Fructus	12 g.
huáng qín	scutellaria [root]	Scutellariae Radix	9 g.
shān zhī zǐ	gardenia [fruit]	Gardeniae Fructus	9 g.
jīng jiè	schizonepeta (abbreviated decoction)	Schizonepetae Herba et Flos	6 g.
fáng fēng	ledebouriella [root]	Ledebouriellae Radix	6 g.
niú bàng zǐ	arctium [seed]	Arctii Fructus	9 g.
xuán shēn	scrophularia [root]	Scrophulariae Radix	9 g.
bò hé	mint (abbreviated decoction)	Menthae Herba	6 g.
dà huáng	rhubarb (abbreviated decoction)	Rhei Rhizoma	9 g.
máng xiāo	mirabilite (stirred in)	Mirabilitum	9 g.

MODIFICATIONS

In cases of coughing with expectoration of large amounts of thick yellow phlegm, the prescription is modified to clear heat and transform phlegm.

Select from and add:

shè gān	belamcanda [root]	Belamcandae Rhizoma	9 g.
guā lóu	trichosanthes [fruit]	Trichosanthis Fructus	9 g.
zhè bèi mǔ	Zhejiang fritillaria [bulb]	Fritillariae Verticillatae Bulbus	9 g.

| *tiān zhú huáng* | bamboo sugar | Bambusae Concretio Silicea | 6 g. |
| *zhú rú* | bamboo shavings | Bambusae Caulis in Taeniam | 6 g. |

In cases presenting persistent high fever, the prescription is modified to clear heat and drain fire.

Add:

| *shí gāo* | gypsum (extended decoction) | Gypsum | 30 g. |
| *zhī mǔ* | anemarrhena [root] | Anemarrhenae Rhizoma | 9 g. |

In cases of severe pain and swelling of the throat, the prescription is reinforced to further clear heat, resolve toxins, disperse swelling and relieve pain. Use the preceding prescription with the prepared formula, SIX SPIRITS PILL (*liù shén wán*).

ACUPUNCTURE AND MOXIBUSTION

Main points: Needle with draining.

LI-01	*shāng yáng* (bleed)
ST-44	*nèi tíng*
CV-22	*tiān tú*
ST-40	*fēng lóng*

Auxiliary points:

For high fever, add:

| GV-14 | *dà zhuī* |
| LI-11 | *qū chí* |

For constipation, add:

| ST-37 | *shàng jù xū* |

3. DEPLETION OF LUNG AND KIDNEY YIN

Clinical Manifestations: Slow onset or extended course of illness, slight redness, swelling and pain of the throat with dryness, itching or possible burning sensation of the throat, symptoms milder in the morning and more severe in the afternoon and at night. There may be dry cough with scanty sticky phlegm or no phlegm. Accompanying symptoms include dizziness and vertigo, blurred vision, weak aching lower back and knees, irritability, insomnia and vexing heat in the five hearts.

Tongue: Red with little coating.

Pulse: Rapid, thready.

Treatment Method: Nourish yin, downbear fire, disinhibit the pharynx.

PRESCRIPTION

Combine Yin-Nourishing Lung-Clearing Decoction (*yǎng yīn qīng fèi tāng*) with Anemarrhena, Phellodendron and Rehmannia Decoction (Pill) (*zhī bǎi dì-huáng tāng [wán]*).

Yin-Nourishing Lung-Clearing Decoction *yǎng yīn qīng fèi tāng*

shēng dì huáng	rehmannia [root] dried/fresh	Rehmanniae Radix Exsiccata seu Recens	12 g.
mài mén dōng	ophiopogon [tuber]	Ophiopogonis Tuber	12 g.
xuán shēn	scrophularia [root]	Scrophulariae Radix	12 g.
chuān bèi mǔ	Sichuan fritillaria [bulb]	Fritillariae Cirrhosae Bulbus	9 g.
mǔ dān pí	moutan [root bark]	Moutan Radicis Cortex	9 g.
bái sháo yào	white peony [root]	Paeoniae Radix Alba	9 g.
bò hé	mint (abbreviated decoction)	Menthae Herba	6 g.
gān cǎo	licorice [root]	Glycyrrhizae Radix	6 g.

with:

Anemarrhena, Phellodendron and Rehmannia Decoction (Pill)
zhī bǎi dì huáng tāng (wán)

shú dì huáng	cooked rehmannia [root]	Rehmanniae Radix Conquita	24 g.
shān zhū yú	cornus [fruit]	Corni Fructus	12 g.
shān yào	dioscorea [root]	Dioscoreae Rhizoma	12 g.
zé xiè	alisma [tuber]	Alismatis Rhizoma	9 g.
fú líng	poria	Poria	9 g.
mǔ dān pí	moutan [root bark]	Moutan Radicis Cortex	9 g.
zhī mǔ	anemarrhena [root]	Anemarrhenae Rhizoma	9 g.
huáng bǎi	phellodendron [bark]	Phellodendri Cortex	9 g.

MODIFICATIONS

In cases of vacuity of both qi and yin with accompanying symptoms of poor appetite, fatigue, shortness of breath and disinclination to speak, the prescription is modified to supplement both qi and yin.
Add:

huáng qí	astragalus [root]	Astragali (seu Hedysari) Radix	12 g.
dǎng shēn	codonopsis [root]	Codonopsitis Radix	9 g.
huáng jīng	polygonatum [root]	Polygonati Huangjing Rhizoma	9 g.

ACUPUNCTURE AND MOXIBUSTION

Main points: Needle with even supplementation, even draining.

CV-23	lián quán
KI-03	tài xī
LU-07	liè quē
KI-06	zhào hǎi
LU-10	yú jì

Auxiliary points:

For vexing heat in the five hearts add:

HT-08	shào fǔ

For vacuity of both qi and yin, add:

CV-06	qì hǎi
ST-36	zú sān lǐ

ALTERNATE THERAPEUTIC METHODS

1. Ear Acupuncture

Auricular points: Throat, Tonsils, Lungs, Helix 1-6.

Method: Manipulate for two to three minutes to elicit a moderate to strong sensation and retain the needles for thirty to sixty minutes once daily. In cases of severe redness, swelling and pain of the throat, one to five drops of blood can be let at Helix 1-6 or at the small veins on the back of the ear.

REMARKS

During treatment patients should not smoke, drink alcohol or consume spicy foods.

LOSS OF VOICE

Shī Yīn

1. Acute Loss of Voice - 1A. Wind-Heat Invasion - 1B. Wind-Cold Invasion - 1C. Stagnation of Liver Qi - 2. Chronic Loss of Voice - 2A. Lung and Kidney Yin Vacuity - 2B. Spleen and Lung Qi Vacuity - 2C. Qi Stagnation, Blood Stasis and Congealed Phlegm

In its milder stages, loss of voice refers to hoarseness of the voice. When it is severe, it refers to aphonia. Clinically, loss of voice is divided into acute and chronic types. Acute loss of voice, known in Chinese as *bào yīn* (sudden loss of voice) is characterized by sudden onset and a short course of illness. Chronic loss of voice, termed *jiǔ yīn* (enduring loss of voice), is slow in onset and longer in duration. Refer to this chapter for all conditions of acute or chronic laryngitis, strain or nodulation of the vocal cords and loss of voice from hysteria.

ETIOLOGY AND PATHOGENESIS

Patterns of acute loss of voice are repletion types caused by invasion of external wind-heat or wind-cold, or following bouts of rage or depression. Chronic loss of voice is a vacuity type, from weakening of the lung, spleen or kidney; vacuity of lung and kidney yin is commonly observed. Vacuity patterns, or patterns complicated by both vacuity and repletion, can be caused by various etiologies, including vacuity of lung and spleen qi, qi stagnation, blood stasis and congealed phlegm.

1A. ACUTE LOSS OF VOICE – WIND-HEAT INVASION

Clinical Manifestations: Sudden hoarseness of the voice accompanied by sore throat, dry nose, fever, thirst, coughing and expectoration of yellow phlegm.

Tongue: Thin yellow coating.

Pulse: Rapid, floating.

Treatment Method: Course wind, clear heat, ease the throat, open the voice.

PRESCRIPTION

Wind-Coursing Heat-Clearing Decoction *shū fēng qīng rè tāng*

jīng jiè	schizonepeta (abbreviated decoction)	Schizonepetae Herba et Flos	9 g.
fáng fēng	ledebouriella [root]	Ledebouriellae Radix	9 g.
niú bàng zǐ	arctium [seed]	Arctii Fructus	9 g.
jīn yín huā	lonicera [flower]	Lonicerae Flos	9 g.
lián qiào	forsythia [fruit]	Forsythiae Fructus	9 g.
sāng bái pí	mulberry [root bark]	Mori Radicis Cortex	9 g.

huáng qín	scutellaria [root]	Scutellariae Radix	6 g.
chì sháo yào	red peony [root]	Paeoniae Radix Rubra	6 g.
xuán shēn	scrophularia [root]	Scrophulariae Radix	6 g.
zhè bèi mǔ	Zhejiang fritillaria [bulb]	Fritillariae Verticillatae Bulbus	6 g.
jié gěng	platycodon [root]	Platycodonis Radix	6 g.
tiān huā fěn	trichosanthes [root]	Trichosanthis Radix	9 g.
gān cǎo	licorice [root]	Glycyrrhizae Radix	6 g.

MODIFICATIONS

The prescription can be reinforced by adding:

| *chán tuì* | cicada molding | Cicadae Periostracum | 9 g. |
| *pàng dà hài* | sterculia | Sterculiae Semen | 9 g. |

In cases of internal invasion of heat evil, with more severe symptoms including constipation, the prescription is changed to clear heat, resolve toxins, disinhibit the pharynx and open the voice.
Use:

Pharynx-Clearing Diaphragm-Disinhibiting Decoction *qīng yān lì gé tāng*

jīn yín huā	lonicera [flower]	Lonicerae Flos	12 g.
lián qiào	forsythia [fruit]	Forsythiae Fructus	12 g.
huáng qín	scutellaria [root]	Scutellariae Radix	9 g.
shān zhī zǐ	gardenia [fruit]	Gardeniae Fructus	9 g.
jīng jiè	schizonepeta (abbreviated decoction)	Schizonepetae Herba et Flos	6 g.
fáng fēng	ledebouriella [root]	Ledebouriellae Radix	6 g.
niú bàng zǐ	arctium [seed]	Arctii Fructus	9 g.
xuán shēn	scrophularia [root]	Scrophulariae Radix	9 g.
bò hé	mint (abbreviated decoction)	Menthae Herba	6 g.
dà huáng	rhubarb (abbreviated decoction)	Rhei Rhizoma	9 g.
máng xiāo	mirabilite (stirred in)	Mirabilitum	9 g.

Add:

| *chán tuì* | cicada molding | Cicadae Periostracum | 9 g. |
| *pàng dà hài* | sterculia | Sterculiae Semen | 9 g. |

In cases where phlegm is yellow and copious, the prescription is modified to clear heat and transform phlegm.
Add:

zhè bèi mǔ	Zhejiang fritillaria [bulb]	Fritillariae Verticillatae Bulbus	9 g.
tiān zhú huáng	bamboo sugar	Bambusae Concretio Silicea	6 g.
guā lóu	trichosanthes [fruit]	Trichosanthis Fructus	9 g.

ACUPUNCTURE AND MOXIBUSTION

Main points: Needle with draining.

LI-04	*hé gǔ*
LU-05	*chǐ zé*
CV-23	*lián quán*
LI-17	*tiān dǐng*
HT-05	*tōng lǐ*

Auxiliary points:

For severe sore throat, add:

| LI-02 | *èr jiān* |

1B. ACUTE LOSS OF VOICE – WIND-COLD INVASION

Clinical Manifestations: Sudden hoarseness of the voice accompanied by aversion to cold, fever, stuffy nose, secretion of thin clear mucus from the nose, itchy throat, coughing, expectoration of thin phlegm, no apparent thirst.

Tongue: Thin white coating.

Pulse: Tight, floating.

Treatment Method: Course wind, dispel cold, ventilate the lung, open the voice.

PRESCRIPTION

Six-Ingredient Decoction *liù wèi tāng*

jīng jiè suì	schizonepeta [spike] (abbreviated decoction)	Schizonepetae Flos	9 g.
fáng fēng	ledebouriella [root]	Ledebouriellae Radix	9 g.
bái jiāng cán	silkworm	Bombyx Batryticatus	9 g.
bò hé	mint (abbreviated decoction)	Menthae Herba	6 g.
jié gěng	platycodon [root]	Platycodonis Radix	6 g.
gān cǎo	licorice [root]	Glycyrrhizae Radix	6 g.

MODIFICATIONS

To reinforce dispersing wind, dispelling cold, ventilating the lung and easing the throat, add:

zǐ sū zǐ	perilla [fruit] (abbreviated decoction)	Perillae Fructus	9 g.
xìng rén	apricot [kernel] (abbreviated decoction)	Armeniacae Semen	9 g.
chán tuì	cicada molting	Cicadae Periostracum	9 g.

In cases of coughing with expectoration of large amounts of phlegm, the prescription is modified to transform phlegm and relieve coughing.
Add:

fǎ bàn xià	pinellia [tuber] (processed)	Pinelliae Tuber Praeparatum	9 g.
bái qián	cynanchum [root]	Cynanchi Baiqian Radix et Rhizoma	9 g.

ACUPUNCTURE AND MOXIBUSTION

Main points: Needle with draining; add moxibustion.

LI-04	*hé gǔ*
TB-05	*wài guān*
CV-23	*lián quán*
LI-17	*tiān dǐng*
HT-05	*tōng lǐ*

Auxiliary points:

For coughing with copious phlegm, add:

LU-07	*liè quē*

1C. ACUTE LOSS OF VOICE – STAGNATION OF LIVER QI

Clinical Manifestations: Sudden hoarseness of the voice or aphonia accompanied by irritability, dizziness, tinnitus, fullness and distention of the chest and hypochondrium, frequent sighing.

Tongue: Thin, white or slimy coating.

Pulse: Wiry.

Treatment Method: Course the liver, regulate qi, open the voice.

PRESCRIPTION

Pinellia and Magnolia Bark Decoction *bàn xià hòu pò tāng*

zhì bàn xià	(processed) pinellia [tuber	Pinelliae Tuber Praeparatum	12 g.
hòu pò	magnolia [bark]	Magnoliae Cortex	9 g.
fú líng	poria	Poria	12 g.
shēng jiāng	fresh ginger [root]	Zingiberis Rhizoma Recens	9 g.
zǐ sū yè	perilla [leaf]	Perillae Folium	6 g.

MODIFICATIONS

In cases of severe emotional depression, the prescription is reinforced to rectify qi and relieve depression. Combine the preceding prescription with the prepared medicine, DEPRESSION-OVERCOMING PILL *(yuè jú wán)*.

ACUPUNCTURE AND MOXIBUSTION

Main points: Needle with draining.

LI-04	*hé gǔ*
LR-03	*tài chōng*
CV-23	*lián quán*
LI-17	*tiān dǐng*
HT-05	*tōng lǐ*

2A. CHRONIC LOSS OF VOICE – LUNG AND KIDNEY YIN VACUITY

Clinical Manifestations: Progressive hoarseness of the voice, often aggravated by stress and overstrain or following long periods of speaking. Accompanying symptoms include dryness of the throat and mouth, dry cough with little phlegm, weak aching lower back and knees, tidal fever, night sweating, dizziness, tinnitus.

Tongue: Red with little coating.

Pulse: Rapid, thready.

Treatment Method: Nourish lung and kidney yin, downbear fire, ease the throat, open the voice.

PRESCRIPTION

Lily Bulb Metal-Securing Decoction *bǎi hé gù jīn tāng*

shēng dì huáng	rehmannia [root] dried/fresh	Rehmanniae Radix Exsiccata seu Recens	9 g.
shú dì huáng	cooked rehmannia [root]	Rehmanniae Radix Conquita	9 g.
mài mén dōng	ophiopogon [tuber]	Ophiopogonis Tuber	9 g.
bǎi hé	lily [bulb]	Lilii Bulbus	9 g.
bái sháo yào	white peony [root]	Paeoniae Radix Alba	9 g.
dāng guī	tangkuei	Angelicae Sinensis Radix	6 g.
chuān bèi mǔ	Sichuan fritillaria [bulb]	Fritillariae Cirrhosae Bulbus	9 g.
xuán shēn	scrophularia [root]	Scrophulariae Radix	9 g.
jié gěng	platycodon [root]	Platycodonis Radix	6 g.
gān cǎo	licorice [root]	Glycyrrhizae Radix	6 g.

MODIFICATIONS

The prescription can be reinforced by adding:

chán tuì	cicada molting	Cicadae Periostracum	6 g.
mù hú dié	oroxylum [seed]	Oroxyli Semen	6 g.
shí hú	dendrobium [stem] (extended decoction)	Dendrobii Caulis	9 g.

In cases of frenetic vacuity fire, the prescription is modified to nourish yin and diminish vacuity fire.
Add:

huáng bǎi	phellodendron [bark]	Phellodendri Cortex	9 g.
zhī mǔ	anemarrhena [root]	Anemarrhenae Rhizoma	9 g.

ACUPUNCTURE AND MOXIBUSTION

Main points: Needle with even supplementation, even draining.

LU-10	*yú jì*
KI-03	*tài xī*
CV-23	*lián quán*
LI-17	*tiān dǐng*
KI-06	*zhào hǎi*

2B. CHRONIC LOSS OF VOICE – SPLEEN AND LUNG QI VACUITY

Clinical Manifestations: Prolonged hoarseness of the voice, aggravated by overwork, and often more marked in the morning. The voice is faint, speaking requires a tremendous effort and cannot be sustained. Accompanying symptoms include shortness of breath, slow speech, tiredness, fatigue, poor appetite, loose stools.

Tongue: Pale with white coating.

Pulse: Weak, forceless.

Treatment Method: Supplement the lung and spleen, boost qi, open the voice.

PRESCRIPTION

Center-Supplementing Qi-Boosting Decoction *bǔ zhōng yì qì tāng*

huáng qí	astragalus [root]	Astragali (seu Hedysari) Radix	15 g
rén shēn	ginseng	Ginseng Radix	9 g.
bái zhú	ovate atractylodes [root]	Atractylodis Ovatae Rhizoma	9 g.
dāng guī	tangkuei	Angelicae Sinensis Radix	9 g.
chén pí	tangerine peel	Citri Exocarpium	6 g.
shēng mā	cimicifuga [root]	Cimicifugae Rhizoma	3 g.
chái hú	bupleurum [root]	Bupleuri Radix	3 g.
zhì gān cǎo	licorice [root] (honey-fried)	Glycyrrhizae Radix	6 g.

MODIFICATIONS

The prescription can be reinforced to benefit the throat by adding:

hē zǐ	chebule	Chebulae Fructus	9 g.
shí chāng pú	acorus [root]	Acori Rhizoma	9 g.

In cases where dampness and phlegm are prevalent, the prescription is modified to expel phlegm and dampness.

Add:

fǎ bàn xià	pinellia [tuber] (processed)	Pinelliae Tuber Praeparatum	9 g.
fú líng	poria	Poria	12 g.
biǎn dòu	lablab [bean]	Lablab Semen	12 g.

ACUPUNCTURE AND MOXIBUSTION

Main points: Needle with supplementation; add moxibustion.

LU-09	*tài yuān*
ST-36	*zú sān lǐ*
SP-06	*sān yīn jiāo*
CV-23	*lián quán*
LI-17	*tiān dǐng*

2C. CHRONIC LOSS OF VOICE – QI STAGNATION, BLOOD STASIS AND CONGEALED PHLEGM

Clinical Manifestations: Prolonged loss of voice where tremendous effort is required to speak; an uncomfortable sensation of a foreign object lodged in the throat. Accompanying symptoms include oppression in the chest and expectoration of phlegm. Laryngoscopic examination often reveals nodules or polyps of the vocal cords.

Tongue: Dark, purplish.

Pulse: Rough.

Treatment Method: Move qi, quicken the blood, transform phlegm, open the voice.

PRESCRIPTION

Epiglottis Stasis-Expelling Decoction *huì yàn zhú yū tāng*

táo rén	peach [kernel]	Persicae Semen	9 g.
hóng huā	carthamus [flower]	Carthami Flos	9 g.
shēng dì huáng	rehmannia [root] dried/fresh	Rehmanniae Radix Exsiccata seu Recens	9 g.
dāng guī	tangkuei	Angelicae Sinensis Radix	9 g.
chì sháo yào	red peony [root]	Paeoniae Radix Rubra	9 g.
xuán shēn	scrophularia [root]	Scrophulariae Radix	9 g.
chái hú	bupleurum [root]	Bupleuri Radix	6 g.
zhǐ ké	bitter orange [fruit]	Aurantii Fructus	6 g.
jié gěng	platycodon [root]	Platycodonis Radix	6 g.
gān cǎo	licorice [root]	Glycyrrhizae Radix	6 g.

MODIFICATIONS

In cases of vacuous lung and kidney yin, combine the preceding prescription with:

Lily Bulb Metal-Securing Decoction *bǎi hé gù jīn tāng*

shēng dì huáng	rehmannia [root] dried/fresh	Rehmanniae Radix Exsiccata seu Recens	9 g.
shú dì huáng	cooked rehmannia [root]	Rehmanniae Radix Conquita	9 g.
mài mén dōng	ophiopogon [tuber]	Ophiopogonis Tuber	9 g.
bǎi hé	lily [bulb]	Lilii Bulbus	9 g.
bái sháo yào	white peony [root]	Paeoniae Radix Alba	9 g.
dāng guī	tangkuei	Angelicae Sinensis Radix	6 g.
chuān bèi mǔ	Sichuan fritillaria [bulb]	Fritillariae Cirrhosae Bulbus	9 g.
xuán shēn	scrophularia [root]	Scrophulariae Radix	9 g.
jié gěng	platycodon [root]	Platycodonis Radix	6 g.
shēng gān cǎo	licorice [root] (raw)	Glycyrrhizae Radix Cruda	6 g.

Where lung and spleen qi are vacuous, combine the preceding prescription with:

Center-Supplementing Qi-Boosting Decoction *bŭ zhōng yì qì tāng*

huáng qí	astragalus [root]	Astragali (seu Hedysari) Radix	15 g.
rén shēn	ginseng	Ginseng Radix	9 g.
bái zhú	ovate atractylodes [root]	Atractylodis Ovatae Rhizoma	9 g.
dāng guī	tangkuei	Angelicae Sinensis Radix	9 g.
chén pí	tangerine [peel]	Citri Exocarpium	6 g.
shēng má	cimicifuga [root]	Cimicifugae Rhizoma	3 g.
chái hú	bupleurum [root]	Bupleuri Radix	3 g.
zhì gān căo	licorice [root] (honey-fried)	Glycyrrhizae Radix	6 g.

In cases with copious phlegm, the prescription is modified to transform phlegm. Add:

chuān bèi mŭ	Sichuan fritillaria [bulb]	Fritillariae Cirrhosae Bulbus	9 g.
guā lóu zĭ	trichosanthes [seed]	Trichosanthis Semen	9 g.
hăi fú shí	pumice	Pumex	9 g.

ACUPUNCTURE AND MOXIBUSTION

Main points: Needle with even supplementation, even draining.

LI-04	*hé gŭ*
LR-03	*tài chōng*
PC-06	*nèi guān*
CV-23	*lián quán*
LI-17	*tiān dĭng*

Auxiliary points:

For vacuity of lung and kidney yin, add:

KI-03	*tài xī*

For vacuity of lung and spleen qi, add:

ST-36	*zú sān lĭ*
SP-06	*sān yīn jiāo*

For copious phlegm, add:

ST-40	*fēng lóng*

ALTERNATE THERAPEUTIC METHODS

1. Ear Acupuncture

Auricular points: Lung, Throat, Neck, Trachea, Heart, Kidney.

Method: Needle to elicit a strong sensation in acute cases and a mild sensation in chronic cases. Five sessions constitute one course of treatment, although, in prolonged cases, one course can be ten to fifteen sessions.

REMARKS

To prevent aggravation of their condition, patients should minimize speaking, avoid yelling or screaming and abstain from spicy foods, alcohol and tobacco. In cases of enduring loss of voice where herbal medicine and acupuncture have had little effect, examination by a biomedical specialist is recommended.

PART IX

STOMATOLOGY

MOUTH SORES

Kŏu Chuāng

1. Exuberant Heart and Spleen Heat - 2. Vacuity Fire

Mouth sores *(kŏu chuāng)* are commonly called canker sores in the West. These are small superficial yellowish-white ulcerations that appear on the mucous membranes of the oral cavity, specifically the tongue, the gums and the insides of the lips and cheeks. *Kŏu chuāng* are round or oval in shape and have a concave surface surrounded by a red ring. They can appear one or more at a time and are accompanied by a localized burning pain.

Clinically, mouth sores are categorized according to vacuity and repletion. Repletion patterns are the result of exuberant heart and spleen heat. This corresponds to aphthous stomatitis in Western medicine. Vacuity patterns are generally caused by depletion of yin with effulgent fire. These frequently recur. Mouth sores are most common in adults.

ETIOLOGY AND PATHOGENESIS

Repletion patterns involve over-consumption of alcohol or spicy foods or the invasion of external wind, fire or dryness that results in exuberant heart and spleen heat. This heat traverses the corresponding channels and attacks the tissues of the oral cavity.

Vacuity patterns result from yin vacuity constitutions, prolonged illnesses or overwork, all of which can lead to vacuity of heart and kidney yin . This can cause a rise of exuberant vacuity fire into the oral cavity. In prolonged cases, it is possible that injury to yin can also injure yang.

1. EXUBERANT HEART AND SPLEEN HEAT

Clinical Manifestations: Ulceration of the mucous membranes of the oral cavity, sores that are yellowish-white in color with surrounding mucous membranes that are bright red and slightly swollen. In severe cases a large number of sores will merge into patches and localized burning and pain will be aggravated while speaking and eating. Accompanying signs may include fever, thirst, halitosis, constipation and dark urine.

Tongue: Red with yellow coating.

Pulse: Rapid.

Treatment Method: Clear heat, resolve toxins, disperse swelling, relieve pain.

PRESCRIPTION

Diaphragm-Cooling Powder *liáng gé săn*

lián qiáo	forsythia [fruit]	Forsythiae Fructus	12 g.
huáng qín	scutellaria [root]	Scutellariae Radix	9 g.
shān zhī zǐ	gardenia [fruit]	Gardeniae Fructus	9 g.
bò hé	mint (abbreviated decoction)	Menthae Herba	9 g.
zhú yè	black bamboo [leaf]	Bambusae Folium	6 g.
dà huáng	rhubarb (abbreviated decoction)	Rhei Rhizoma	6 g.
gān căo	licorice [root]	Glycyrrhizae Radix	9 g.
máng xiāo	mirabilite (stirred in)	Mirabilitum	9 g.

MODIFICATIONS

In cases where heat evil is profuse with marked pain, the prescription is modified to clear heat and relieve pain.
Add:

huáng lián	coptis [root]	Coptidis Rhizoma	6 g.
huáng băi	phellodendron [bark]	Phellodendri Cortex	6 g.

In cases of vexation in the heart, dark urine and difficult urination, the prescription is modified to clear the heart and promote diuresis.
Combine with:

Red-Abducting Powder *dăo chì săn*

shēng dì huáng	rehmannia [root] dried/fresh	Rehmanniae Radix Exsiccata seu Recens	15 g.
mù tōng	mutong [stem]	Mutong Caulis	6 g.
zhú yè	black bamboo [leaf]	Bambusae Folium	9 g.
gān căo	licorice [root]	Glycyrrhizae Radix	6 g.

ACUPUNCTURE AND MOXIBUSTION

Main points: Needle with draining.

CV-24	*chéng jiāng*
ST-06	*jiá chē*
PC-08	*láo gōng*
LI-04	*hé gŭ*
LI-11	*qū chí*
ST-36	*zú sān lĭ*
GV-27	*duì duān*

2. VACUITY FIRE

Clinical Manifestations: Ulceration of the mucous membranes of the oral cavity; a relatively small number of sores that are grayish-white in color, with the surrounding mucous membranes pale or unchanged in color and no fusion of sores into patches; local pain aggravated during eating and frequent recurrence of sores. Accompanying symptoms include weakness and aching of the lower back and knees and dry throat.

Tongue: Dry with little coating.

Pulse: Rapid, thready.

Treatment Method: Nourish yin, downbear fire, relieve pain.

PRESCRIPTION
Anemarrhena, Phellodendron and Rehmannia Decoction
zhī bǎi dì huáng tāng

shú dì huáng	cooked rehmannia [root]	Rehmanniae Radix Conquita	24 g.
shān zhū yú	cornus [fruit]	Corni Fructus	12 g.
shān yào	dioscorea [root]	Dioscoreae Rhizoma	12 g.
zé xiè	alisma [tuber]	Alismatis Rhizoma	9 g.
fú líng	poria	Poria	9 g.
mǔ dān pí	moutan [root bark]	Moutan Radicis Cortex	9 g.
zhī mǔ	anemarrhena [root]	Anemarrhenae Rhizoma	9 g.
huáng bǎi	phellodendron [bark]	Phellodendri Cortex	9 g.

MODIFICATIONS

In cases accompanied by depletion of stomach yin, the prescription is modified to nourish stomach yin and downbear fire.
Add:

shēng dì huáng	rehmannia [root] dried/fresh	Rehmanniae Radix Exsiccata seu Recens	12 g.
mài mén dōng	ophiopogon [tuber]	Ophiopogonis Tuber	9 g.
shí hú	dendrobium [stem] (extended decoction)	Dendrobii Caulis	9 g.
xuán shēn	scrophularia [root]	Scrophulariae Radix	9 g.

In cases of frequent recurrence where both vacuous qi and blood are preventing a complete recovery, the prescription is modified to supplement both qi and blood. Use the above prescription with:

Eight-Gem Decoction *bā zhēn tāng*

shú dì huáng	cooked rehmannia [root]	Rehmanniae Radix Conquita	12 g.
dāng guī	tangkuei	Angelicae Sinensis Radix	9 g.
bái sháo yào	white peony [root]	Paeoniae Radix Alba	9 g.
chuān xiōng	ligusticum [root]	Ligustici Rhizoma	6 g.
rén shēn	ginseng	Ginseng Radix	9 g.
bái zhú	ovate atractylodes [root]	Atractylodis Ovatae Rhizoma	9 g.
fú líng	poria	Poria	12 g.
zhì gān cǎo	licorice [root] (honey-fried)	Glycyrrhizae Radix	6 g.
shēng jiāng	fresh ginger [root]	Zingiberis Rhizoma Recens	3 g.
dà zǎo	jujube	Ziziphi Fructus	3 pc.

To downbear vacuity fire to the kidney add a small dose of:

| *ròu guì* | cinnamon [bark] (abbreviated decoction) | Cinnamomi Cortex | 1.5 g. |

In cases where injury to yin has led to injury to yang with symptoms of physical cold, cold extremities, pale tongue and deep pulse, the prescription is changed in order to warm and supplement kidney yang.
Use:

Golden Coffer Kidney Qi Pill *jīn guì shèn qì wán*

shú dì huáng	cooked rehmannia [root]	Rehmanniae Radix Conquita	24 g.
shān yào	dioscorea [root]	Dioscoreae Rhizoma	12 g.
shān zhū yú	cornus [fruit]	Corni Fructus	12 g.
zé xiè	alisma [tuber]	Alismatis Rhizoma	9 g.
fú líng	poria	Poria	9 g.
mǔ dān pí	moutan [root bark]	Moutan Radicis Cortex	9 g.
zhì fù zǐ	aconite [accessory tuber] (processed) (extended decoction)	Aconiti Tuber Laterale Praeparatum	3 g.
ròu guì	cinnamon [bark] (abbreviated decoction)	Cinnamomi Cortex	3 g.

ACUPUNCTURE AND MOXIBUSTION

Main points: Needle with even supplementation, even draining.

CV-24	*chéng jiāng*
ST-06	*jiá chē*
PC-08	*láo gōng*
KI-03	*tài xī*
LR-02	*xíng jiān*
CV-23	*lián quán*
ST-36	*zú sān lǐ*
SP-06	*sān yīn jiāo*

ALTERNATE THERAPEUTIC METHODS

1. Ear Acupuncture

Main points: Mouth, Heart, Spleen, Tongue, Kidney, *Shén Mén*, Endocrine.

Method: Choose two to four points. Needle to elicit a moderate sensation, and retain needles for twenty to thirty minutes. Treat once daily.

REMARKS

During treatment, patients should pay attention to oral hygiene, avoid spicy or irritating foods and abstain from alcohol and smoking. In the daily routine, work and relaxation should be balanced, and physical exercise and sexual activity moderated.

TOOTHACHE

Yá Tòng

1. Wind-Fire Toothache - 2. Stomach Fire Toothache - 3. Vacuity Fire Toothache

Patterns presenting tooth pain as the major symptom are grouped under the heading of toothache. Such pain is aggravated by heat, cold or consumption of acid or sweet foods. Patterns of toothache are frequently observed in medical mouth disorders including those Western medicine labels as acute and chronic pulpitis, dental caries and periodontitis.

ETIOLOGY AND PATHOGENESIS

Toothache can be caused by a many factors, and patterns are generally classified according to repletion and vacuity. Repletion patterns usually involve the hand and foot yang ming channels, which pass through the lower and upper gums respectively. Large intestine or stomach heat, as well as invasion of the yang ming channels by external wind, can all accumulate evils in the yang ming channels. This transforms into fire which, following the course of the channels upward, gives rise to repletion type toothache. The kidney controls the bones and the teeth are the "surplus" of the bones. Vacuity of kidney yin with consequent frenetic vacuity fire most often constitutes the etiology and pathogenesis of vacuity-type toothaches.

1. WIND-FIRE TOOTHACHE

Clinical Manifestations: Periodic toothache with redness and swelling of the gums, accompanied by aversion to cold, fever, dry mouth, thirst.

Tongue: Thin yellow coating.

Pulse: Rapid, floating.

Treatment Method: Course wind, clear heat, disperse swelling, relieve pain.

PRESCRIPTION

Mint and Forsythia Formula *bò hé lián qiào fāng*

jīn yín huā	lonicera [flower]	Lonicerae Flos	12 g.
lián qiáo	forsythia [fruit]	Forsythiae Fructus	12 g.
niú bàng zǐ	arctium [seed]	Arctii Fructus	9 g.
bò hé	mint (abbreviated decoction)	Menthae Herba	9 g.
zhú yè	black bamboo [leaf]	Bambusae Folium	9 g.
shēng dì huáng	rehmannia [root] dried/fresh	Rehmanniae Radix Exsiccata seu Recens	9 g.
zhī mǔ	anemarrhena [root]	Anemarrhenae Rhizoma	9 g.
lù dòu pí	mung bean [seed-coat]	Phaseoli Aurei Testa	6 g.

ACUPUNCTURE AND MOXIBUSTION

Main Points: Needle with draining.

LI-04	*hé gǔ*
ST-07	*xià guān*
ST-06	*jiá chē*
TB-05	*wài guān*
GB-20	*fēng chí*

Auxiliary points:

For toothache because of dental caries, add:

LI-02	*èr jiān*
SI-05	*yáng gǔ*

For swelling of the gums, add:

TB-20	*jiǎo sūn*
SI-08	*xiǎo hǎi*

For headache, add:

M-HN-9	*tài yáng* (Greater Yang)

2. STOMACH FIRE TOOTHACHE

Clinical Manifestations: Excruciating toothache, severe swelling of the gums, exudation of pus with bleeding in some cases, pain generally radiating to the cheeks, headache, fever, thirst, halitosis, constipation.

Tongue: Thick yellow coating.

Pulse: Surging.

Treatment Method: Drain stomach heat, cool the blood, disperse swelling, relieve pain.

PRESCRIPTION

Stomach-Clearing Powder *qīng wèi sǎn*

huáng lián	coptis [root]	Coptidis Rhizoma	9 g.
shēng dì huáng	rehmannia [root] dried/fresh	Rehmanniae Radix Exsiccata seu Recens	12 g.
mǔ dān pí	moutan [root bark]	Moutan Radicis Cortex	9 g.
shēng má	cimicifuga [root]	Cimicifugae Rhizoma	6 g.
dāng guī	tangkuei	Angelicae Sinensis Radix	3 g.

MODIFICATIONS

In cases with constipation, the prescription is modified to free the stool and drain heat.

Add:

dà huáng	rhubarb (abbreviated decoction)	Rhei Rhizoma	9 g.

In cases of swelling and pain of the gums with severe bleeding, the prescription is modified to clear heat, cool the blood, disperse swelling and relieve pain.

Select from and add:

shí gāo	gypsum (extended decoction)	Gypsum	30 g.
zhú yè	black bamboo [leaf]	Bambusae Folium	9 g.
xuán shēn	scrophularia [root]	Scrophulariae Radix	9 g.
bǎn lán gēn	isatis [root]	Isatidis Radix	9 g.
bái máo gēn	imperata [root]	Imperatae Rhizoma	15 g.

ACUPUNCTURE AND MOXIBUSTION

Main Points: Needle with draining.

LI-04	*hé gǔ*
ST-07	*xià guān*
ST-06	*jiá chē*
ST-44	*nèi tíng*
PC-08	*láo gōng*

Auxiliary points:

For toothache because of dental caries, add:

LI-02	*èr jiān*
SI-05	*yáng gǔ*

For swelling of the gums, add:

TE-20	*jiǎo sūn*
SI-08	*xiǎo hǎi*

For headache, add:

M-HN-9	*tài yáng* (Greater Yang)

3. VACUITY FIRE TOOTHACHE

Clinical Manifestations: Dull intermittent toothache, slight redness and swelling of the gums, atrophy of the gums, loosening of the teeth, loss of force in biting, increase in pain during the afternoon, no apparent foulness of the breath. Accompanying signs include weakness and aching of the lower back and knees, dizziness and vertigo, blurred vision and dryness of the mouth without desire for drink.

Tongue: Red, tender with little coating.

Pulse: Rapid, thready.

Treatment Method: Supplement kidney yin, drain fire, relieve pain.

PRESCRIPTION

Anemarrhena, Phellodendron and Rehmannia Decoction
zhī bǎi dì-huáng tāng

shú dì huáng	cooked rehmannia [root]	Rehmanniae Radix Conquita	24 g.
shān zhū yú	cornus [fruit]	Corni Fructus	12 g.
shān yào	dioscorea [root]	Dioscoreae Rhizoma	12 g.
zé xiè	alisma [tuber]	Alismatis Rhizoma	9 g.
fú líng	poria	Poria	9 g.
mǔ dān pí	moutan [root bark]	Moutan Radicis Cortex	9 g.
zhī mǔ	anemarrhena [root]	Anemarrhenae Rhizoma	9 g.
huáng bǎi	phellodendron [bark]	Phellodendri Cortex	9 g.

MODIFICATIONS

To strengthen the kidney and relieve toothache, add:

gǔ suì bǔ	drynaria [root]	Drynariae Rhizoma	12 g.

ACUPUNCTURE AND MOXIBUSTION

Main Points: Needle with even supplementation, even draining.

LI-04	*hé gǔ*
ST-07	*xià guān*
ST-06	*jiá chē*
KI-03	*tài xī*
LR-02	*xíng jiān*

Auxiliary points:

For toothache because of dental caries, add:

      LI-02　　　*èr jiān*
      SI-05　　　*yáng gǔ*

For swelling of the gums, add:

      TB-20　　　*jiǎo sūn*
      SI-08　　　*xiǎo hǎi*

For headache, add:

      M-HN-9　　*tài yáng* (Greater Yang)

ALTERNATE THERAPEUTIC METHODS

1. Ear Acupuncture

Auricular points: Maxilla, Mandibula, Tragic Apex, Adrenal, *Shén Mén.*

Method: Needle to elicit a strong sensation and retain needles for twenty to thirty minutes. Alternately, embed needles for two to three days.

REMARKS

In cases of toothache because of dental caries, apart from the use of these treatments to relieve pain, refer to a dentist for filling or pulling the affected tooth.

PART X

EMERGENTOLOGY

WIND STROKE

Zhòng Fēng

1. Channel-Connection Stroke - 1A. Depleted Channels and Connections Allowing Invasion by Wind - 1B. Liver and Kidney Yin Vacuity with Disturbance by Ascendant Wind-Yang - 2. Viscera-Bowel Stroke - 2A. Tension Pattern - 2B. Desertion Pattern - 3. Sequelae - 3A(i). Hemiplegia from Qi Vacuity and Blood Stasis with Obstruction of Channels and Connections - 3A(ii). Hemiplegia from Ascendant Hyperactivity of Liver Yang with Obstruction of Channels and Connections - 3B(i). Slurred Speech from Obstruction of the Connections by Wind-Phlegm - 3B(ii). Slurred Speech from Depletion of Kidney Essence - 3C. Facial Paralysis

Wind stroke refers to patterns typified by a sudden loss of consciousness or without an initial loss of consciousness but with facial paralysis, slurred speech or hemiplegia. In Chinese, these patterns are known as wind stroke because of two factors: the major etiological factor is external or internal wind; and the onset of the illness is abrupt with rapid and varied pathological changes that are analogous to the mobile and changeable characteristics of wind.

Cerebral hemorrhage, cerebral thrombosis, cerebral embolism, subarachnoid hemorrhage, cerebral angiospasm and Bell's palsy and their sequelae may all be treated according to the differential diagnosis and treatment found in this chapter.

ETIOLOGY AND PATHOGENESIS

The etiology and pathogenesis of wind stroke is complex, and may involve vacuity, fire, wind, phlegm, qi or blood. These include yin vacuity or qi vacuity; liver or heart fire; internal or external wind; wind-phlegm or phlegm-dampness; counterflow ascent of stomach qi; or blood stasis. In certain circumstances, all six of these factors may affect one another to bring about the sudden onset of wind stroke.

Cases caused by invasion of external wind are termed *wài fēng* (external wind) or *zhēn zhòng fēng* (true wind stroke). *Nèi fēng* (internal wind) or *lèi zhòng fēng* (wind-like stroke) are caused by disharmony of the yin, yang, qi and blood of the viscera and bowels, without the prior invasion of external evils. Stroke caused by internal etiological factors are more frequently encountered.

Cases of stroke vary in acuteness and severity. Mild cases involve pathological changes in the channels and connections, and have no apparent influence on the higher mental centers. Severe cases, affecting the related viscera and bowels, usually include clouding of mental clarity or loss of consciousness. According to the degree of severity, stroke is classified as either channel-connection stroke or viscera-bowel stroke.

On the basis of differing clinical manifestations, viscera and bowel stroke is further divided into tension stroke patterns and desertion stroke patterns. Tension strokes, characterized by the sealing of evils within the body, are classified as repletion patterns. They may be subdivided into yang tension stroke and yin tension stroke according to whether the evil involves internal wind complicated by phlegm-fire or external wind complicated by phlegm-dampness.

Desertion pattern strokes are characterized by the outward escape of yang qi and are classified as vacuity patterns. Viscera-bowel stroke is often followed by sequelae; these tend to have a vacuity root, but can manifest as patterns showing both repletion and vacuity.

1A. CHANNEL-CONNECTION STROKE – DEPLETED CHANNELS AND CONNECTIONS ALLOWING INVASION BY WIND

Clinical Manifestations: Numbness of the extremities, abrupt onset of facial paralysis, slurred speech, drooling from the corner of the mouth on the affected side, hemiplegia (in severe cases), aversion to cold, fever, muscle spasms in the limbs and, in some cases, sore aching joints.

Tongue: Thin white coating.

Pulse: Floating.

Treatment Method: Dispel wind, nourish the blood, clear the channels and connections.

PRESCRIPTION

Large Gentian Decoction *dà qín jiāo tāng*

qín jiāo	large gentian [root]	Gentianae Macrophyllae Radix	9 g.
qiāng huó	notopterygium [root]	Notopterygii Rhizoma	3 g.
fáng fēng	ledebouriella [root]	Ledebouriellae Radix	3 g.
xì xīn	asarum	Asiasari Herba cum Radice	1.5 g.
bái zhǐ	angelica [root]	Angelicae Dahuricae Radix	3 g.
dú huó	tuhuo [angelica root]	Angelicae Duhuo Radix	6 g.
shú dì huáng	cooked rehmannia [root]	Rehmanniae Radix Conquita	3 g.
dāng guī	tangkuei	Angelicae Sinensis Radix	6 g.
chuān xiōng	ligusticum [root]	Ligustici Rhizoma	6 g.
bái sháo yào	white peony [root]	Paeoniae Radix Alba	6 g.
shēng dì huáng	rehmannia [root] dried/fresh	Rehmanniae Radix Exsiccata seu Recens	3 g.
huáng qín	scutellaria [root]	Scutellariae Radix	3 g.
shí gāo	gypsum (extended decoction)	Gypsum	6 g.
bái zhú	ovate atractylodes [root]	Atractylodis Ovatae Rhizoma	3 g.
fú líng	poria	Poria	3 g.
zhì gān cǎo	licorice [root] (honey-fried)	Glycyrrhizae Radix	6 g.

MODIFICATIONS

In cases without internal heat, the prescription is modified to dispel wind and clear the channels and connections.

Delete:

shí gāo	gypsum	Gypsum
huáng qín	scutellaria [root]	Scutellariae Radix

Add:

| *bái fù zǐ* | aconite-typhonium [tuber] (processed) | Aconiti Coreani seu Typhonii Gigantei Tuber Praeparatum | 4.5 g. |
| *quán xiē* | scorpion | Buthus | 4.5 g. |

In cases presenting external patterns of wind heat, the prescription is modified to dispel wind and clear heat.

Delete the warm pungent medicines:

qiāng huó	notopterygium [root]	Notopterygii Rhizoma
fáng fēng	ledebouriella [root]	Ledebouriellae Radix
dāng guī	tangkuei	Angelicae Sinensis Radix

Add:

sāng yè	mulberry [leaf]	Mori Folium	9 g.
jú huā	chrysanthemum [flower]	Chrysanthemi Flos	9 g.
bò hé	mint (abbreviated decoction)	Menthae Herba	9 g.

In cases presenting copious phlegm, vomiting, slimy tongue coating and slippery pulse, the prescription is modified to expel phlegm and dry dampness.

Delete:

| *shēng dì huáng* | rehmannia [root] dried/fresh | Rehmanniae Radix Exsiccata seu Recens |

Add:

fǎ bàn xià	pinellia [tuber] (processed)	Pinelliae Tuber Praeparatum	9 g.
zhì tiān nán xīng	arisaema [root] (prepared)	Arisaematis Rhizoma Praeparatum	6 g.
jú hóng	red tangerine [peel]	Citri Exocarpium Rubrum	9 g.
fú líng	poria	Poria	9 g.

In cases of aged patients with weaker constitutions, the prescription is modified to boost qi and strengthen bodily resistance.

Add:

| *huáng qí* | astragalus [root] | Astragali (seu Hedysari) Radix | 12 g. |

ACUPUNCTURE AND MOXIBUSTION

Main Points: During the initial stages of the illness, needle only the affected side. In prolonged cases, apply both acupuncture and moxibustion bilaterally or alternate from left to right, beginning with the unaffected side. Needle with draining during the initial stages of illness and with supplementation in prolonged cases.

GV-20	*bǎi huì*
GB-20	*fēng chí*
GV-14	*dà zhuī*
LI-04	*hé gǔ*

Auxiliary points:

For hemiplegia on the upper limbs, add:

LI-15	*jiān yú*
LI-11	*qū chí*
TB-05	*wài guān*

For hemiplegia on the lower limbs, add:

GB-30	*huán tiào*
GB-34	*yáng líng quán*
ST-36	*zú sān lǐ*
ST-41	*jiě xī*
BL-60	*kūn lún*

For slurred speech, add:

CV-23	*lián quán*
HT-05	*tōng lǐ*

For facial paralysis, add:

ST-04	*dì cāng*
ST-06	*jiá chē*
GB-14	*yáng bái*
LI-20	*yíng xiāng*
BL-02	*zǎn zhú*
ST-01	*chéng qì*
BL-60	*kūn lún*

For drooling, add:

CV-24	*chéng jiāng*

1B. CHANNEL-CONNECTION STROKE – VACUITY OF LIVER AND KIDNEY YIN WITH DISTURBANCE BY ASCENDANT WIND-YANG

Clinical Manifestations: Prior history of vertigo or dizzy spells, headache, tinnitus, numbness of the extremities, irritability, insomnia or dream-disturbed sleep, weak aching lower back and knees, and hot flashes; abrupt onset of facial paralysis, slurred speech, sluggish movements and, in severe cases, hemiplegia.

Tongue: Red with little coating.

Pulse: Thready, rapid, wiry.

Treatment Method: Nourish liver and kidney yin, subdue yang, eradicate internal wind, clear the channels and connections.

PRESCRIPTION

Liver-Settling Wind-Extinguishing Decoction *zhèn gān xī fēng tāng*

huái niú xī	achyranthes [root]	Achyranthis Bidentatae Radix	30 g.
bái sháo yào	white peony [root]	Paeoniae Radix Alba	15 g.
dài zhě shí	hematite (extended decoction)	Haematitum	30 g.
lóng gǔ	dragon bone (extended decoction)	Mastodi Ossis Fossilia	15 g.
mǔ lì	oyster shell (extended decoction)	Ostreae Concha	15 g.
guī bǎn	tortoise plastron (extended decoction)	Testudinis Plastrum	15 g.
xuán shēn	scrophularia [root]	Scrophulariae Radix	15 g.
tiān mén dōng	asparagus [tuber]	Asparagi Tuber	15 g.
chuān liàn zǐ	toosendan [fruit]	Toosendan Fructus	6 g.
mài yá	barley sprout	Hordei Fructus Germinatus	6 g.
yīn chén hāo	capillaris	Artemisiae Capillaris Herba	6 g.
gān cǎo	licorice [root]	Glycyrrhizae Radix	4.5 g.

MODIFICATIONS

To reinforce the liver-subduing, wind-eradicating strength, add:

tiān má	gastrodia [root]	Gastrodiae Rhizoma	9 g.
gōu téng	uncaria [stem and thorn] (abbreviated decoction)	Uncariae Ramulus cum Unco	9 g.
jú huā	chrysanthemum [flower]	Chrysanthemi Flos	9 g.

In cases with phlegm-heat, the prescription is modified to clear heat and transform phlegm.
Add:

dǎn xīng	bile-processed arisaema [root]	Arisaematis Rhizoma cum Felle Bovis	4.5 g.
zhú lì	dried bamboo sap (stirred in)	Bambusae Succus Exsiccatus	40 g.
chuān bèi mǔ	Sichuan fritillaria [bulb]	Fritillariae Cirrhosae Bulbus	9 g.

In cases of vexing heat in the heart, the prescription is modified to clear heat and relieve vexation.
Add:

| *shān zhī zǐ* | gardenia [fruit] | Gardeniae Fructus | 9 g. |
| *huáng qín* | scutellaria [root] | Scutellariae Radix | 9 g. |

In cases of severe headache, the prescription is modified to subdue yang and relieve headache.
Add:

xià kū cǎo	prunella [spike]	Prunellae Spica	12 g.
líng yáng jiǎo	antelope horn (powdered and stirred in, 0.5 g. each time)	Antelopis Cornu	3 g.
shí jué míng	abalone shell (extended decoction)	Haliotidis Concha	15 g.

In cases of insomnia and dream-disturbed sleep, the prescription is modified to settle, tranquilize and quiet the spirit.
Add:

zhēn zhū mǔ	mother-of-pearl (extended decoction)	Concha Margaritifera	15 g.
lóng chǐ	dragon bone (extended decoction)	Mastodi Dentis Fossilia	15 g.
yè jiāo téng	flowery knotweed [stem]	Polygoni Multiflori Caulis	15 g.

ACUPUNCTURE AND MOXIBUSTION

Main Points: Needle with even supplementation, even draining.

BL-18	*gān shū*
BL-23	*shèn shū*
KI-03	*tài xī*
GB-20	*fēng chí*
LR-03	*tài chōng*
LI-04	*hé gǔ*

Auxiliary points: See above, 1A., "Depleted Channels and Connections Allowing Invasion by Wind."

2A. VISCERA-BOWEL STROKE – TENSION PATTERN

Clinical Manifestations: Sudden loss of consciousness, muscular spasm of the jaw, hands clenched tightly into fists, wheezing respiration, retention of urine and stool, muscular spasms and rigidity of the limbs. According to the manifestation of heat, tension stroke pattern is divided into yang tension stroke and yin tension stroke.

YANG TENSION STROKE: In addition to the general symptoms, patients also manifest flushed complexion, fever, heavy breathing, halitosis, red lips, agitation and restlessness.

YIN TENSION STROKE: In addition to the general symptoms of tension stroke, patients also manifest pale complexion, greyish lips, tranquil state without restlessness and cold extremities.

Tongue:

YANG TENSION STROKE: Red or yellow slimy coating.

YIN TENSION STROKE: White slimy coating.

Pulse:

YANG TENSION STROKE: Rapid, wiry, slippery.

YIN TENSION STROKE: Deep, tardy, slippery.

Treatment Method:

YANG TENSION STROKE: Open the orifices with cool pungent medicines, clear the liver, extinguish wind.

YIN TENSION STROKE: Open the orifices with warm pungent medicines, expel phlegm, extinguish wind.

PRESCRIPTION

YANG TENSION STROKE:

Combine Antelope Horn Decoction *(líng yáng jiǎo tāng)* with the prepared medicines SUPREME JEWEL ELIXIR *(zhì bǎo dān)* or PEACEFUL PALACE BOVINE BEZOAR PILL *(ān gōng niú huáng wán)*.

Antelope Horn Decoction *líng yáng jiǎo tāng*

líng yáng jiǎo	antelope horn (powdered and stirred in) (0.5 g. each time)	Antelopis Cornu	3 g.
guī bǎn	tortoise plastron (extended decoction)	Testudinis Plastrum	30 g.
shēng dì huáng	rehmannia [root] (dried/fresh)	Rehmanniae Radix Exsiccata seu Recens	15 g.
mǔ dān pí	moutan [root bark]	Moutan Radicis Cortex	12 g.
bái sháo yào	white peony [root]	Paeoniae Radix Alba	12 g.
chái hú	bupleurum [root]	Bupleuri Radix	6 g.
bò hé	mint (abbreviated decoction	Menthae Herba	6 g.
chán tuì	cicada molting	Cicadae Periostracum	6 g.
jú huā	chrysanthemum [flower]	Chrysanthemi Flos	12 g.
xià kū cǎo	prunella [spike]	Prunellae Spica	12 g.
shí jué míng	abalone shell (extended decoction)	Haliotidis Concha	30 g.

MODIFICATIONS

In cases of convulsions, the prescription is modified to extinguish wind and relieve convulsions.

Add:

quán xiē	scorpion (or, powdered and stirred in, 0.5 g. each time)	Buthus	4.5 g.
wú gōng	centipede	Scolopendra	3 g.
bái jiāng cán	silkworm	Bombyx Batryticatus	9 g.

In cases of copious phlegm, the prescription is modified to expel phlegm.

Add:

zhú lì	dried bamboo sap (stirred in)	Bambusae Succus Exsiccatus	40 g.
tiān zhú huáng	bamboo sugar	Bambusae Concretio Silicea	6 g.
dǎn xīng	arisaema [root] (bile-processed)	Arisaematis Rhizoma cum Felle Bovis	4.5 g.

In cases accompanied by constipation, halitosis and abdominal distention, the prescription is modified to free the stool and drain heat.
Add:

dà huáng	rhubarb (abbreviated decoction)	Rhei Rhizoma	9 g.
máng xiāo	mirabilite (stirred in)	Mirabilitum	9 g.
zhǐ shí	unripe bitter orange [fruit]	Aurantii Fructus Immaturus	9 g.

PRESCRIPTION

YIN TENSION STROKE:

Combine Phlegm-Flushing Decoction *(dí tán tāng)* with the prepared medicine, LIQUID STORAX PILL *(sū hé xiāng wán)*.

Phlegm-Flushing Decoction *dí tán tāng*

fǎ bàn xià	pinellia [tuber] (processed)	Pinelliae Tuber Praeparatum	9 g.
tiān nán xīng	arisaema [root]	Arisaematis Rhizoma	6 g
chén pí	tangerine peel	Citri Exocarpium	9 g.
zhǐ shí	unripe bitter orange	Aurantii Fructus Immaturus	9 g.
fú líng	poria	Poria	12 g.
rén shēn	ginseng	Ginseng Radix	6 g.
shí chāng pú	acorus [root]	Acori Rhizoma	9 g.
zhú rú	bamboo shavings	Bambusae Caulis in Taeniam	9 g.
shēng jiāng	fresh ginger [root]	Zingiberis Rhizoma Recens	6 g.
gān cǎo	licorice [root]	Glycyrrhizae Radix	3 g.

MODIFICATIONS

To settle the liver and extinguish wind, add:

tiān má	gastrodia [root]	Gastrodiae Rhizoma	9 g.
gōu téng	uncaria [stem and thorn] (abbreviated decoction)	Uncariae Ramulus cum Unco	9 g.
bái jiāng cán	silkworm	Bombyx Batryticatus	9 g.

ACUPUNCTURE AND MOXIBUSTION

Main points: Needle with draining.

GV-26	shuǐ gōu
ST-40	fēng lóng
KI-03	tài xī
LR-03	tài chōng

Auxiliary points:

For yang tension stroke, add:

PC-08	láo gōng

Bleed the hand jing-well points *(shí èr jǐng xué):*

LU-11	shào shāng
HT-09	shào chōng
PC-09	zhōng chōng
LI-01	shāng yáng
TB-01	guān chōng
SI-01	shào zé

For yin tension stroke, add:

GV-20	bǎi huì

For muscular spasm of the jaw, add:

ST-07	xià guān
ST-06	jiá chē
LI-04	hé gǔ

2B. VISCERA-BOWEL STROKE – DESERTION PATTERN

Clinical Manifestations: Sudden loss of consciousness, closed eyes and open mouth, snoring, shallow breathing, relaxed hands, cold extremities, copious persistent perspiration, incontinence of stool and urine, flaccid paralysis of the limbs.

Tongue: Flaccid.

Pulse: Thready, faint, barely palpable.

Treatment Method: Boost qi, revitalize yang, secure yang desertion.

PRESCRIPTION

Combine Ginseng and Aconite Decoction *(shēn fù tāng)* with Pulse-Engendering Beverage *(shēng mài yǐn)*.

Ginseng and Aconite Decoction *shēn fù tāng*

rén shēn	ginseng	Ginseng Radix	30 g.
zhì fù zǐ	aconite [accessory tuber] (processed)	Aconiti Tuber Laterale Praeparatum	15 g.

with:

Pulse-Engendering Beverage *shēng mài yǐn*

rén shēn	ginseng	Ginseng Radix	9 g.
mài mén dōng	ophiopogon [tuber]	Ophiopogonis Tuber	15 g.
wǔ wèi zǐ	schisandra [berry]	Schisandrae Fructus	6 g.

MODIFICATIONS

In cases of copious persistent perspiration, the prescription is modified to secure yang desertion and relieve sweating.

Add:

huáng qí	astragalus [root]	Astragali (seu Hedysari) Radix	15 g.
duàn lóng gǔ	dragon bone (calcined, extended decoction)	Mastodi Ossis Fossilia Calcinatum	15 g.
duàn mǔ lì	oyster shell (calcined, extended decoction)	Ostreae Concha Calcinatum	15 g.
shān zhū yú	cornus [fruit]	Corni Fructus	12 g.

ACUPUNCTURE AND MOXIBUSTION

Main Points: Employ moxibustion.

CV-04	*guān yuán*
CV-08	*shén què*
CV-06	*qì hǎi*
GV-20	*bǎi huì*

Indirect salt moxibustion with large moxa cones can be used at:

CV-08	*shén què*
CV-06	*qì hǎi*

Auxiliary points:

For persistent perspiration, add moxibustion to:

HT-06	*yīn xī*

For cases of snoring and somnolence, add moxibustion to:

BL-62	*shēn mài*

For incontinence of stool and urine, add moxibustion to:

ST-28	*shuǐ dào*
SP-06	*sān yīn jiāo*
ST-36	*zú sān lǐ*

3A(i). Sequelae – Hemiplegia from Qi Vacuity and Blood Stasis Obstruction of the Channels and Connections

Clinical Manifestations: Loss of conscious control of one side of the body; numbness of the affected side in some cases, complete loss of sensation of the affected side in more severe cases; sallow complexion, weakness and flaccidity of affected limbs.

Tongue: Purple, sometimes with stasis macules on the tongue.

Pulse: Thready, rough, forceless.

Treatment Method: Boost qi, quicken the blood, clear channels and connections.

PRESCRIPTION

Yang-Supplementing Five-Returning Decoction *bŭ yáng huán wŭ tāng*

huáng qí	astragalus [root]	Astragali (seu Hedysari) Radix	30-120 g.
	(Use 30 g. at the beginning and increase dosage gradually)		
dāng guī	tangkuei	Angelicae Sinensis Radix	6 g.
chì sháo yào	red peony [root]	Paeoniae Radix Rubra	6 g.
dì lóng	earthworm	Lumbricus	3 g.
chuān xiōng	ligusticum [root]	Ligustici Rhizoma	3 g.
hóng huā	carthamus [flower]	Carthami Flosa	3 g.
táo rén	peach [kernel]	Persicae Semen	3 g.

MODIFICATIONS

In cases of incontinence of urine the prescription is modified to warm the kidney and retain urine.
Add:

sāng piāo xiāo	mantis egg-case	Mantidis Oötheca	9 g.
yì zhì rén	alpinia [fruit]	Alpiniae Oxyphyllae Fructus	9 g.

In cases of disability of an upper limb the prescription is modified to clear the upper channels and connections.
Add:

sāng zhī	mulberry [twig]	Mori Ramulus	15 g.
guì zhī	cinnamon [twig]	Cinnamomi Ramulus	9 g.

In cases of flaccid paralysis of a lower limb, the prescription is modified to supplement the kidney and strengthen the bones and muscles.
Add:

sāng jì shēng	mistletoe	Loranthi seu Visci Ramus	12 g.
niú xī	achyranthes [root]	Achyranthis Bidentatae Radix	9 g.
xù duàn	dipsacus [root]	Dipsaci Radix	12 g.
dù zhòng	eucommia [bark]	Eucommiae Cortex	12 g.

In cases accompanied by slurred speech, the prescription is modified to expel phlegm and clear the orifices.
Add:

yù jīn	curcuma [tuber]	Curcumae Tuber	6 g.
shí chāng pú	acorus [root]	Acori Rhizoma	6 g.
yuǎn zhì	polygala [root]	Polygalae Radix	9 g.

In cases accompanied by facial paralysis, the prescription is modified to expel wind and free the connections.

Add:

zhì bái fù zǐ	aconite/typhonium [tuber] (processed)	Aconiti Coreani seu Typhonii Gigantei Tuber Praeparatum	4.5 g.
quán xiē	scorpion	Buthus	4.5 g.
bái jiāng cán	silkworm	Bombyx Batryticatus	9 g.

In cases of numbness of the limbs, the prescription is modified to dispel wind-phlegm.

Add:

chén pí	tangerine [peel]	Citri Exocarpium	9 g.
fǎ bàn xià	pinellia [tuber] (processed)	Pinelliae Tuber Praeparatum	9 g.
fú líng	poria	Poria	9 g.
dǎn xīng	bile-processed arisaema [root]	Arisaematis Rhizoma cum Felle Bovis	4.5 g.

In cases accompanied by constipation, the prescription is modified to moisten and free the stool.

Add:

yù lǐ rén	bush cherry [kernel]	Pruni Japonicae Semen	9 g.
huǒ má rén	hemp [seed]	Cannabis Semen	12 g.
ròu cōng róng	cistanche [stem]	Cistanches Caulis	12 g.

In persistent cases of hemiplegia, the prescription is modified to break stasis and free the connections.

Add:

shuǐ zhì	leech	Hirudo seu Whitmania	3 g.
méng chóng	tabanus	Tabanus	1.5 g.
chuān shān jiǎ	pangolin scales	Manitis Squama	9 g.
	(or, powdered and administered separately, 1.5 g. each time)		

ACUPUNCTURE AND MOXIBUSTION

Main Points: Needle with even supplementation, even draining; add moxibustion.

GV-20	*bǎi huì*
CV-06	*qì hǎi*
SP-10	*xuè hǎi*
SP-06	*sān yīn jiāo*
LI-15	*jiān yú*
LI-11	*qū chí*
TB-05	*wài guān*
LI-04	*hé gǔ*
GB-30	*huán tiào*
GB-34	*yáng líng quán*
ST-36	*zú sān lǐ*
ST-41	*jiě xī*
BL-60	*kūn lún*

Auxiliary points:

Auxiliary points on the upper limb might include:

TB-14	*jiān liáo*
TB-04	*yáng chí*
SI-03	*hòu xī*

Auxiliary points on the lower limb might include:

GB-31	*fēng shì*
ST-33	*yīn shì*
GB-39	*xuán zhōng*

For prolonged cases, select:

For the upper limb:

BL-11	*dà zhū*
SI-14	*jiān wài shū*

For the lower limb:

GV-03	*yāo yáng guān*
BL-30	*bái huán shū*

3A(ii). SEQUELAE – HEMIPLEGIA FROM ASCENDANT HYPERACTIVITY OF LIVER YANG WITH OBSTRUCTION OF CHANNELS AND CONNECTIONS

Clinical Manifestations: Spastic paralysis of affected side with rigidity of limbs and difficulty in flexion and extension, accompanied by headache, dizziness and vertigo, flushed complexion, tinnitus.

Tongue: Red or crimson with thin yellow coating.

Pulse: Wiry, forceful.

Treatment Method: Settle the liver, subdue yang, extinguish wind, clear the channels and connections.

PRESCRIPTION

Use Liver-Settling Wind-Extinguishing Decoction *(zhèn gān xī fēng tāng)* or Gastrodia and Uncaria Beverage *(tiān-má gōu-téng yǐn)*.

Liver-Settling Wind-Extinguishing Decoction *zhèn gān xī fēng tāng*

huái niú xī	achyranthes [root]	Achyranthis Radix	30 g.
bái sháo yào	white peony [root]	Paeoniae Radix Alba	15 g.
dài zhě shí	hematite (extended decoction)	Haematitum	30 g.
lóng gǔ	dragon bone (extended decoction)	Mastodi Ossis Fossilia	15 g.
mǔ lì	oyster shell (extended decoction)	Ostreae Concha	15 g.
guī bǎn	tortoise plastron (extended decoction)	Testudinis Plastrum	15 g.
xuán shēn	scrophularia [root]	Scrophulariae Radix	15 g.
tiān mén dōng	asparagus [tuber]	Asparagi Tuber	15 g.
chuān liàn zǐ	toosendan [fruit]	Toosendan Fructus	6 g.
mài yá	barley sprout	Hordei Fructus Germinatus	6 g.
yīn chén hāo	capillaris	Artemisiae Capillaris Herba	6 g.
gān cǎo	licorice [root]	Glycyrrhizae Radix	4.5 g.

or:

Gastrodia and Uncaria Beverage *tiān má gōu téng yǐn*

tiān má	gastrodia [root]	Gastrodiae Rhizoma	9 g.
gōu téng	uncaria [stem and thorn] (abbreviated decoction)	Uncariae Ramulus cum Unco	12 g.
shí jué míng	abalone shell (extended decoction)	Haliotidis Concha	12 g.
shān zhī zǐ	gardenia [fruit]	Gardeniae Fructus	9 g.
huáng qín	scutellaria [root]	Scutellariae Radix	9 g.
chuān niú xī	cyathula [root]	Cyathulae Radix	12 g.

dù zhòng	eucommia [bark]	Eucommiae Cortex	9 g.
yì mǔ cǎo	leonurus	Leonuri Herba	9 g.
sāng jì shēng	mistletoe	Loranthi seu Visci Ramus	9 g.
yè jiāo téng	flowery knotweed [stem]	Polygoni Multiflori Caulis	9 g.
fú shén	root poria	Poria cum Pini Radice	9 g.

MODIFICATIONS

Either of the above prescriptions can be reinforced in clearing channels and connections.

Add:

| *dì lóng* | earthworm | Lumbricus | 9 g. |
| *jī xuè téng* | millettia [root and stem] | Millettiae Radix et Caulis | 12 g. |

ACUPUNCTURE AND MOXIBUSTION:

Main Points: Needle with even supplementation, even draining.

BL-18	*gān shū*
BL-23	*shèn shū*
LR-03	*tài chōng*
KI-03	*tài xī*
LI-15	*jiān yú*
LI-11	*qū chí*
TB-05	*wài guān*
LI-04	*hé gǔ*
GB-30	*huán tiào*
GB-34	*yáng líng quán*
ST-36	*zú sān lǐ*
ST-41	*jiě xī*
BL-60	*kūn lún*

Auxiliary points:

For spasms in the elbow region, add:
    PC-03   *qū zé*
For spasms in the wrist region, add:
    PC-07   *dà líng*
For spasms in the ankle region, add:
    KI-03   *tài xī*
For spasms in the fingers, add:
    M-UE-22   *bā xié* (Eight Evils)
For spasms in the toes, add:
    M-LE-8   *bā fēng* (Eight Winds)
For the rest, see 3A(ii), Qi Vacuity and Blood Stasis Obstruction of Channels and Connections.

3B(i). SEQUELAE – SLURRED SPEECH FROM OBSTRUCTION
OF THE CONNECTIONS BY WIND-PHLEGM

Clinical Manifestations: Stiffness of the tongue, difficulty speaking, numbness of the limbs.

Tongue: White slimy coating.

Pulse: Slippery, wiry.

Treatment Method: Dispel wind, expel phlegm, clear the orifices and connections.

PRESCRIPTION

Slurred Speech Relieving Elixir *jiĕ yŭ dān*

zhì bái fù zĭ	aconite/typhonium [tuber] (processed)	Aconiti Coreani seu Typhonii Gigantei Tuber (prepared)	6 g.
shí chāng pú	acorus [root]	Acori Rhizoma	6 g.
yuǎn zhì	polygala [root]	Polygalae Radix	6 g.
tiān má	gastrodia [root]	Gastrodiae Rhizoma	9 g.
quán xiē	scorpion	Buthus	3 g.
qiāng huó	notopterygium [root]	Notopterygii Rhizoma	6 g.
tiān nán xīng	arisaema [root] (prepared)	Arisaematis Rhizoma	6 g.
mù xiāng	saussurea [root]	Saussureae (seu Vladimiriae) Radix	6 g.
gān cǎo	licorice [root]	Glycyrrhizae Radix	6 g.

MODIFICATIONS

In cases accompanied by ascension of liver yang, with headache and dizziness and vertigo, the prescription should be reinforced by the addition of Gastrodia and Uncaria Beverage *(tiān má gōu téng yǐn)* or Liver-Settling Wind-Extinguishing Decoction *(zhèn gān xī fēng tāng)*.
Add:

Gastrodia and Uncaria Beverage *tiān má gōu téng yǐn*

tiān má	gastrodia [root]	Gastrodiae Rhizoma	9 g.
gōu téng	uncaria [stem and thorn] (abbreviated decoction)	Uncariae Ramulus cum Unco	12 g.
shí jué míng	abalone shell (extended decoction)	Haliotidis Concha	12 g.
shān zhī zǐ	gardenia [fruit]	Gardeniae Fructus	9 g.
huáng qín	scutellaria [root]	Scutellariae Radix	9 g.
chuān niú xī	cyathula [root]	Cyathulae Radix	12 g.
dù zhòng	eucommia [bark]	Eucommiae Cortex	9 g.
yì mǔ cǎo	leonurus	Leonuri Herba	9 g.
sāng jì shēng	mistletoe	Loranthi seu Visci Ramus	9 g.
yè jiāo téng	flowery knotweed [stem]	Polygoni Multiflori Caulis	9 g.
fú shén	root poria	Poria cum Pini Radice	9 g.

or:

Liver-Settling Wind-Extinguishing Decoction *zhèn gān xī fēng tāng*

huái niú xī	achyranthes [root]	Achyranthis Radix	30 g.
bái sháo yào	white peony [root]	Paeoniae Radix Alba	15 g.
dài zhě shí	hematite (extended decoction)	Haematitum	30 g.
lóng gǔ	dragon bone (extended decoction)	Mastodi Ossis Fossilia	15 g.
mǔ lì	oyster shell (extended decoction)	Ostreae Concha	15 g.
guī bǎn	tortoise plastron (extended decoction)	Testudinis Plastrum	15 g.
xuán shēn	scrophularia [root]	Scrophulariae Radix	15 g.
tiān mén dōng	asparagus [tuber]	Asparagi Tuber	15 g.
chuān liàn zǐ	toosendan [fruit]	Toosendan Fructus	6 g.
mài yá	barley sprout	Hordei Fructus Germinatus	6 g.
yīn chén hāo	capillaris	Artemisiae Capillaris Herba	6 g.
gān cǎo	licorice [root]	Glycyrrhizae Radix	4.5 g.

ACUPUNCTURE AND MOXIBUSTION

Main Points: Needle with even supplementation, even draining.

GB-20	*fēng chí*
ST-40	*fēng lóng*
CV-23	*lián quán*
HT-05	*tōng lǐ*
GV-15	*yǎ mén*
TB-01	*guān chōng*
M-HN-20a	*yù yè* (Jade Humor) (bleed)
M-HN-20b	*jīn jīn* (Gold Liquid) (bleed)

Auxiliary points:

For cases accompanied by ascension of liver yang with headache and dizziness and vertigo, add:

M-HN-9   *tài yáng* (Greater Yang)

3B(ii). SEQUELAE – SLURRED SPEECH FROM DEPLETION OF KIDNEY ESSENCE

Clinical Manifestations: Slurred speech or aphasia, weak aching lower back and legs, palpitations, shortness of breath.

Tongue: Thin coating.

Pulse: Weak, thready.

Treatment Method: Supplement kidney essence, nourish yin, open the orifices.

PRESCRIPTION

Rehmannia Drink *dì huáng yǐn zǐ*

shú dì huáng	cooked rehmannia [root]	Rehmanniae Radix Conquita	15 g.
bā jǐ tiān	morinda [root]	Morindae Radix	9 g.
shān zhū yú	cornus [fruit]	Corni Fructus	9 g.
ròu cōng róng	cistanche [stem]	Cistanches Caulis	9 g.
shí hú	dendrobium [stem] (extended decoction)	Dendrobii Caulis	9 g.
wǔ wèi zǐ	schisandra [berry]	Schisandrae Fructus	3 g.
fú líng	poria	Poria	9 g.
mài mén dōng	ophiopogon [tuber]	Ophiopogonis Tuber	9 g.
shí chāng pú	acorus [root]	Acori Rhizoma	6 g.
yuǎn zhì	polygala [root]	Polygalae Radix	6 g.
shēng jiāng	fresh ginger [root]	Zingiberis Rhizoma Recens	3 g.
bò hé	mint (abbreviated decoction)	Menthae Herba	3 g.
zhì fù zǐ	aconite [accessory tuber] (processed) (extended decoction)	Aconiti Tuber Laterale Praeparatum	6 g.
ròu guì	cinnamon [bark] (abbreviated decoction)	Cinnamomi Cortex	3 g.
dà zǎo	jujube	Ziziphi Fructus	2 pc.

MODIFICATIONS

The prescription is often modified to benefit the voice and clear the orifices.

Delete:

zhì fù zǐ	aconite [accessory tuber] (processed)	Aconiti Tuber Laterale Praeparatum
ròu guì	cinnamon [bark]	Cinnamomi Cortex

Add:

xìng rén	apricot [kernel] (abbreviated decoction)	Armeniacae Semen	9 g.
jié gĕng	platycodon [root]	Platycodonis Radix	6 g.

ACUPUNCTURE AND MOXIBUSTION

Main Points: Needle with supplementation and moxibustion.

BL-23	*shèn shū*
KI-03	*tài xī*
CV-23	*lián quán*
HT-05	*tōng lĭ*
GV-15	*yă mén*
TB-01	*guān chōng*

Bleed:

M-HN-20a	*yù yè* (Jade Humor)
M-HN-20b	*jīn jīn* (Gold Liquid)

3C. SEQUELAE – FACIAL PARALYSIS

Clinical Manifestations: The affected side of the face presents numbness, flaccidity and weakness of the muscles; slanting of the features toward the unaffected side and drooling from the corner of the mouth; inability to wrinkle the forehead, knit the brow, expose the teeth or bulge the cheek; inability to fully close the eyelid, with tearing of the eye; disappearance of forehead wrinkles, shallowness or even disappearance of the nasolabial groove; difficulty in speech and, in severe cases, weakening or loss of the sense of taste on the anterior two-thirds of the tongue.

Treatment Method: Dispel wind, transform phlegm, quicken the blood and free the connections.

PRESCRIPTION

Pull Aright Powder *qiān zhèng sǎn*

zhì bái fù zĭ	aconite-typhonium [tuber] (processed)	Aconiti Coreani seu Typhonii Gigantei Tuber	9 g.
bái jiāng cán	silkworm	Bombyx Batryticatus	9 g.
quán xiē	scorpion	Buthus	9 g.

Grind the ingredients into a powder, in equal proportions. Take a 3 g. dosage with warm water or alcohol. Better therapeutic effects are achieved with powder than with decoction.

MODIFICATIONS

In cases presenting twitching of the eyelids and mouth, the prescription is modified to settle the liver and extinguish wind. Add:

tiān má	gastrodia [root]	Gastrodiae Rhizoma	9 g.
gōu téng	uncaria [stem and thorn] (abbreviated decoction)	Uncariae Ramulus cum Unco	9 g.
shí jué míng	abalone shell (extended decoction)	Haliotidis Concha	15 g.

ACUPUNCTURE AND MOXIBUSTION

Main Points: Acupoint connection method is often used. Needle bilaterally with even supplementation, even draining, and follow with moxibustion.

ST-04	*dì cāng*
ST-06	*jiá chē*
GB-14	*yáng bái*
ST-01	*chéng qì*
LI-20	*yíng xiāng*
LI-04	*hé gŭ*
BL-02	*zăn zhú*
ST-44	*nèi tíng*
SI-06	*yăng lăo*
BL-60	*kūn lún*

Auxiliary points:

SI-18	*quán liáo*
GB-01	*tóng zǐ liáo*
ST-07	*xià guān*

For drooling, add:

CV-24	*chéng jiāng*

For irritability, add:

LR-03	*tài chōng*

For pain in the region posterior to the ears, add:

TB-17	*yì fēng*

ALTERNATE THERAPEUTIC METHODS

1. Ear Acupuncture

Main Points: Adrenal, *Shén Mén*, Kidney, Spleen, Heart, Liver, Eye, Gallbladder, Brain, Auricular Apex, Hypotensive Groove. Also points corresponding to paralyzed areas.

Method: Select three to five points each session and needle bilaterally to elicit a moderate sensation. In cases of tension stroke, bleed at the auricular apex. For sequelae, treat once every two days, ten treatments per therapeutic course. Allow a five day interval between courses. The number of courses should be based on the rate of improvement in the patient's condition.

2. Scalp Acupuncture

Location: Motor region, moto-sensory region of the lower limb, speech region of the unaffected side.

Method: Insert needles horizontally under the surface of the skin to a depth of three to five mm. Rotate needles at high frequency, approximately two hundred rotations per minute, for two to three minutes. During needle manipulation, have patients move their limbs in various directions. After a short period of needle retention, repeat the manipulation one or two times, with a treatment lasting ten to twenty minutes. After withdrawal of needles, the points of entry should be pressed to prevent bleeding. Treat once daily or once every two days, ten sessions per therapeutic course. Scalp acupuncture is effective in the treatment of hemiplegia sequelae of stroke.

PREVENTION

In middle-aged or elderly people, attention should be paid to sensations of dizziness, vertigo, headache, numbness of the fingers or occasional stiffness of the tongue with slurring of speech, as these are often indications of impending stroke. Such people should maintain a tranquil emotional state, follow a light bland diet and set a regular sleeping schedule. Apply moxibustion frequently to prevent the occurrence of stroke.

Use:

ST-36	*zú sān lǐ*
GB-31	*fēng shì*
GB-39	*xuán zhōng*

REMARKS

Stroke symptoms are often critical. In addition to medicinals, various other therapies are beneficial, including acumoxa therapy, tuina massage, physical therapy and speech therapy. Since there is always a possibility for a repeated stroke, appropriate preventative measures should be taken in addition to remedial treatment.

Outstanding therapeutic effects have been achieved using acupuncture and moxibustion in the treatment of sequelae of stroke. Prompt treatment is important: treatment within the first three months yields relatively good effects; after six months the effectiveness is lower, and after one year, poor. In prolonged cases of stroke sequelae, since the patterns are generally complicated by both repletion and vacuity, the classical manipulations are often used to reinforce therapeutic effectiveness: reinforce the healthy side to supplement qi and blood of the whole body, and drain the affected side to dispel blood stasis and wind-phlegm.

INVERSION PATTERNS

Jué Zhèng

1. Repletion Qi Inversion - 2. Vacuity Qi Inversion - 3. Repletion Blood Inversion - 4. Vacuity Blood Inversion - 5. Phlegm Inversion - 6. Food Inversion - 7. Summerheat Inversion

Inversion describes patterns marked by loss of consciousness and coldness of the extremities. The loss of consciousness is usually brief, without the sequelae of hemiplegia, aphasia or facial paralysis. It thus corresponds to syncope. At its most severe, however, the patient will die having never regained consciousness. According to traditional Chinese medicine, *jué* has two definitions, the first being sudden loss of consciousness, and the second, coldness of the extremities. The Western medical diagnoses of shock, collapse, fainting, sunstroke, postural hypotension, hypoglycemic coma and hysterical syncope can be treated according to the differential diagnosis and treatment presented in this chapter.

ETIOLOGY AND PATHOGENESIS

A variety of etiological factors, including emotional upset, improper diet and eating habits, excessive fatigue, excessive loss of blood and summer-heat evil can all cause syncope. Psychological factors are commonly involved. The main pathogenic mechanism is abrupt inversion or confusion of the flow of qi, with subsequent disruption of qi and blood circulation.

Syncope can be categorized according to repletion and vacuity. The pathogenesis of repletion patterns involves upward surges of qi that counter the normal flow of qi and blood. This causes inversion of the blood flow, which temporarily blocks the sense orifices. In some instances, these blockages are further complicated by phlegm or food stasis.

Vacuity patterns involve one of two pathogenic mechanisms. The first is qi vacuity. The clear yang is unable to ascend. Subsequent lack of force in blood circulation then causes loss of proper nourishment to the brain, resulting in syncope. The second is excessive blood loss allowing qi desertion and leading to syncope.

On the basis of differing etiology, pathogenesis and clinical manifestations, inversion is generally classified as qi inversion, blood inversion, phlegm inversion, food inversion and summerheat inversion.

1. REPLETION QI INVERSION

Clinical Manifestations: Syncope brought on by radical changes in emotional state, characterized by sudden loss of consciousness, clenching of teeth, clenching of hands to fists, heavy respiration, coldness of the extremities.

Tongue: Thin white coating.

Pulse: Hidden or deep, wiry.

Treatment Method: Rectify qi, resolve stagnation.

PRESCRIPTION

Six Milled Ingredients Beverage *liù mò yǐn*

chén xiāng	aquilaria [wood] (powdered and stirred in)	Aquilariae Lignum	3 g.
bīng láng	areca [nut]	Arecae Semen	9 g.
mù xiāng	saussurea [root]	Saussureae (seu Vladimiriae) Radix	9 g.
wū yào	lindera [root]	Linderae Radix	9 g.
zhǐ shí	unripe bitter orange [fruit]	Aurantii Fructus Immaturus	9 g.
dà huáng	rhubarb (abbreviated decoction)	Rhei Rhizoma	9 g.

MODIFICATIONS

To rectify qi and soothe the chest, delete:

dà huáng	rhubarb	Rhei Rhizoma	

Add:

bái dòu kòu	cardamom (abbreviated decoction)	Amomi Cardamomi Fructus	6 g.
tán xiāng	sandalwood (abbreviated decoction)	Santali Lignum	3 g.
huò xiāng	agastache/patchouli	Agastaches seu Pogostemi Herba	9 g.

In cases of weak constitution, the prescription is modified to boost qi.
Add:

dǎng shēn	codonopsis [root]	Codonopsitis Radix	9 g.

In cases of profusion of liver yang, with symptoms of flushed complexion, dizziness and headache, the prescription is modified to clear the liver and subdue yang.
Add:

gōu téng	uncaria [stem and thorn] (abbreviated decoction)	Uncariae Ramulus cum Unco	12 g.
shí jué míng	abalone shell (extended decoction)	Haliotidis Concha	30 g.
xià kū cǎo	prunella [spike]	Prunellae Spica	12 g.

In cases exhibiting emotional outbursts upon regaining consciousness, or inability for peaceful sleep, the prescription is changed to nourish the heart and quiet the spirit.
Use:

Licorice, Wheat and Jujube Decoction *gān mài dà zǎo tāng*

gān cǎo	licorice [root]	Glycyrrhizae Radix	9 g.
fú xiǎo mài	light wheat [grain]	Tritici Semen Leve	30 g.
dà zǎo	jujube	Ziziphi Fructus	10 pc.

Add:

yuǎn zhì	polygala [root]	Polygalae Radix	9 g.
suān zǎo rén	spiny jujube [kernel]	Ziziphi Spinosi Semen	12 g.
shí chāng pú	acorus [root]	Acori Rhizoma	9 g.
yù jīn	curcuma [tuber]	Curcumae Tuber	9 g.
dān shēn	salvia [root]	Salviae Miltiorrhizae Radix	9 g.

ACUPUNCTURE AND MOXIBUSTION

Main points: Needle with draining.

GV-26	*rén zhōng*
PC-06	*nèi guān*
LR-03	*tài chōng*
PC-09	*zhōng chōng*

Auxiliary points:

For clenching of the teeth, add:

ST-06	*jiá chē*
LI-04	*hé gǔ*

For convulsions, add:

LI-04	*hé gǔ*
GB-43	*xiá xī*

For gurgling in the throat, add:

CV-22	*tiān tú*

For fever, add:

GV-14	*dà zhuī*
LI-11	*qu chí*

2. VACUITY QI INVERSION

Clinical Manifestations: Dizziness, vertigo and syncope following overwork, surprise or fright in patients with poor physical constitutions. Accompanying symptoms include pale complexion, feeble respiration, perspiration, coldness of the extremities.

Tongue: Pale.

Pulse: Faint, deep.

Treatment Method: Supplement qi, return yang.

PRESCRIPTION

Four-Ingredient Yang-Returning Beverage *sì wèi huí yáng yǐn*

rén shēn	ginseng	Ginseng Radix	9 g.
gān jiāng	dried ginger [root]	Zingiberis Rhizoma Exsiccatum	9 g.
zhì fù zǐ	aconite [accessory tuber] (processed) (extended decoction)	Aconiti Tuber Laterale Praeparatum	9 g.
zhì gān cǎo	licorice [root] (honey-fried)	Glycyrrhizae Radix	6 g.

MODIFICATIONS

In cases of spontaneous perspiration, the prescription is modified to boost qi and consolidate the body surface.
Add:

huáng qí	astragalus [root]	Astragali (seu Hedysari) Radix	12 g.
bái zhú	ovate atractylodes [root]	Atractylodis Ovatae Rhizoma	12 g.

If perspiration continues unabated, to consolidate retention and relieve sweating.
Add:

duàn lóng gǔ	dragon bone (calcined)	Mastodi Ossis Fossilia Calcinatum	15 g.
duàn mǔ lì	oyster shell (calcined)	Ostreae Concha Calcinatum	15 g.

In cases presenting palpitations, the prescription is modified to nourish the heart and quiet the spirit. Add:

dān shēn	salvia [root]	Salviae Miltiorrhizae Radix	9 g.
yuǎn zhì	polygala [root]	Polygalae Radix	6 g.
suān zǎo rén	spiny jujube [kernel]	Ziziphi Spinosi Semen	15 g.

In cases manifesting poor appetite and excessive phlegm, the prescription is modified to fortify the spleen and transform phlegm. Add:

bái zhú	ovate atractylodes [root]	Atractylodis Ovatae Rhizoma	9 g.
fú líng	poria	Poria	9 g.
chén pí	tangerine [peel]	Citri Exocarpium	9 g.

In cases where the tongue is red with little coating, the prescription is modified to nourish yin. Add:

mài mén dōng	ophiopogon [tuber]	Ophiopogonis Tuber	12 g.
wǔ wèi zǐ	schisandra [berry]	Schisandrae Fructus	6 g.

ACUPUNCTURE AND MOXIBUSTION

Main points: Needle with supplementation; add moxibustion.

GV-20	*bǎi huì*
CV-06	*qì hǎi*
ST-36	*zú sān lǐ*

Auxiliary points:

For excessive perspiration, add:

KI-07	*fù liū*

For undigested food matter in the stools, add:

ST-25	*tiān shū*

For greenish complexion and cold extremities, add moxibustion to:

CV-08	*shén què*
CV-04	*guān yuán*

3. REPLETION BLOOD INVERSION

Clinical Manifestations: Loss of consciousness following outbursts of rage, coldness of the extremities, clenching of teeth, flushed complexion, purplish complexion and lips.

Tongue: Purplish with white coating.

Pulse: Deep, wiry.

Treatment Method: Quicken the blood, rectify qi.

PRESCRIPTION

Stasis-Freeing Brew *tōng yū jiān*

dāng guī wěi	tangkuei tail	Angelicae Sinensis Radicis Extremitas	12 g.
shān zhā	crataegus [fruit]	Crataegi Fructus	12 g.
xiāng fù zǐ	cyperus [root]	Cyperi Rhizoma	9 g.
hóng huā	carthamus [flower]	Carthami Flosa	9 g.
wū yào	lindera [root]	Linderae Radix	9 g.
qīng pí	unripe tangerine [peel]	Citri Exocarpium Immaturum	9 g.
mù xiāng	saussurea [root]	Saussureae (seu Vladimiriae) Radix	9 g.
zé xiè	alisma [tuber]	Alismatis Rhizoma	6 g.

MODIFICATIONS

In cases of irritability, insomnia and dream-disturbed sleep, the prescription is modified to clear and soothe the liver, subdue yang and quiet the spirit.
Add:

gōu téng	uncaria [stem and thorn] (abbreviated decoction)	Uncariae Ramulus cum Unco	12 g.
shí jué míng	abalone shell (extended decoction)	Haliotidis Concha	30 g.
lóng dǎn cǎo	gentian [root]	Gentianae Radix	6 g.
mǔ dān pí	moutan [root bark]	Moutan Radicis Cortex	9 g.
yuǎn zhì	polygala [root]	Polygalae Radix	6 g.
shí chāng pú	acorus [root]	Acori Rhizoma	6 g.

In cases where liver yang remains exuberant, with dizziness, vertigo and headache, the prescription is modified to foster yin and subdue yang.
Add:

jú huā	chrysanthemum [flower]	Chrysanthemi Flos	9 g.
gǒu qǐ zǐ	lycium [berry]	Lycii Fructus	9 g.
zhēn zhū mǔ	mother-of-pearl (extended decoction)	Concha Margaritifera	30 g.

ACUPUNCTURE AND MOXIBUSTION

Main points: Needle with draining.

GV-26	*rén zhōng*
PC-09	*zhōng chōng*
LR-03	*tài chōng*
LI-04	*hé gǔ*
KI-01	*yǒng quán*

Auxiliary points:
For clenching of the teeth, add:
    ST-06   *jiá chē*
For convulsions, add:
    GB-43   *xiá xī*
For gurgling in the throat, add:
    CV-22   *tiān tú*
For fever, add:
    GV-14   *dà zhuī*
    LI-11   *qū chí*

4. VACUITY BLOOD INVERSION

Clinical Manifestations: Sudden loss of consciousness following excessive blood loss, coldness of the extremities, pale complexion, lack of luster of the lips, spasms of the limbs, sunken eyes, open mouth, perspiration, coolness of the skin, feeble respiration.
Tongue: Pale.
Pulse: Hollow or thready, rapid, forceless.
Treatment Method: Boost qi, supplement blood.

PRESCRIPTION

Immediately administer:
Pure Ginseng Decoction *dú shēn tāng*

rén shēn	ginseng	Ginseng Radix	30 g.

Decoct on a low fire and take as a single dose. Follow with:

Ginseng Construction-Nourishing Decoction (Pill)
rén shēn yǎng róng tāng (wán)

rén shēn	ginseng	Ginseng Radix	9 g.
bái zhú	ovate atractylodes [root]	Atractylodis Ovatae Rhizoma	9 g.
fú líng	poria	Poria	9 g.
huáng qí	astragalus [root]	Astragali (seu Hedysari) Radix	12 g.
shú dì huáng	cooked rehmannia [root]	Rehmanniae Radix Conquita	9 g.
dāng guī	tangkuei	Angelicae Sinensis Radix	9 g.
bái sháo yào	white peony [root]	Paeoniae Radix Alba	12 g.
chén pí	tangerine [peel]	Citri Exocarpium	9 g.
ròu guì	cinnamon [bark] (abbreviated decoction)	Cinnamomi Cortex	3 g.
wǔ wèi zǐ	schisandra [berry]	Schisandrae Fructus	6 g.
yuǎn zhì	polygala [root]	Polygalae Radix	6 g.
zhì gān cǎo	licorice [root] (honey-fried)	Glycyrrhizae Radix	6 g.
shēng jiāng	fresh ginger [root]	Zingiberis Rhizoma Recens	3 g.
dà zǎo	jujube	Ziziphi Fructus	3 pc.

MODIFICATIONS

In cases of uncontrolled bleeding, the prescription is modified to relieve bleeding. Add:

ē jiāo	ass hide glue (dissolved and stirred in)	Asini Corii Gelatinum	9 g.
xiān hè cǎo	agrimony	Agrimoniae Herba	12 g.
cè bǎi yè	biota [leaf]	Biotae Folium	12 g.

In cases presenting perspiration, coolness of the skin and feeble respiration, the prescription is modified to warm yang and re-establish the harmonious flow of qi. Add:

zhì fù zǐ	aconite [accessory tuber] (processed) (extended decoction)	Aconiti Tuber Laterale Praeparatum	9 g.
gān jiāng	dried ginger [root]	Zingiberis Rhizoma Exsiccatum	9 g.

In cases manifesting palpitations and insomnia, the prescription is modified to nourish the heart and quiet the spirit. Add:

yuǎn zhì	polygala [root]	Polygalae Radix	6 g.
lóng yǎn ròu	longan [flesh]	Longanae Arillus	15 g.
suān zǎo rén	spiny jujube [kernel]	Ziziphi Spinosi Semen	15 g.

In cases of dryness of the mouth and insufficient secretion of saliva, the prescription is modified to nourish the stomach and generate liquid. Add:

mài mén dōng	ophiopogon [tuber]	Ophiopogonis Tuber	12 g.
wǔ wèi zǐ	schisandra [berry]	Schisandrae Fructus	6 g.
běi shā shēn	glehnia [root]	Glehniae Radix	12 g.

ACUPUNCTURE AND MOXIBUSTION

Main points: Needle with supplementation; add moxibustion.

GV-20	*bǎi huì*
CV-06	*qì hǎi*
CV-04	*guān yuán*
SP-06	*sān yīn jaiō*
ST-36	*zú sān lǐ*

Auxiliary points:

For excessive perspiration, add:
      KI-07   *fù liū*

For undigested food matter in the stools, add:
      ST-25   *tiān shū*

For greenish complexion and cold extremities, add moxibustion to:
      CV-08   *shén què*

5. PHLEGM INVERSION

Clinical Manifestations: Sudden loss of consciousness, coldness of the extremities, gurgling sounds in the throat, vomiting of frothy fluid, heavy respiration.

Tongue: White slimy coating.

Pulse: Deep, slippery.

Treatment Method: Move qi, transform phlegm.

PRESCRIPTION

Phlegm-Abducting Decoction *dǎo tán tāng*

fǎ bàn xià	pinellia (processed)	Pinelliae Tuber Praeparatum	9 g.
zhì tiān nán xīng	arisaema [root] (processed)	Arisaematis Rhizoma Praeparatum	6 g.
fú líng	poria	Poria	12 g.
chén pí	tangerine [peel]	Citri Exocarpium	9 g.
zhǐ shí	unripe bitter orange [fruit]	Aurantii Fructus Immaturus	9 g.
gān cǎo	licorice [root]	Glycyrrhizae Radix	3 g.

MODIFICATIONS

To open the orifices and arouse the spirit, add:

yuǎn zhì	polygala [root]	Polygalae Radix	9 g.
shí chāng pú	acorus [root]	Acori Rhizoma	9 g.
yù jīn	curcuma [tuber]	Curcumae Tuber	9 g.

In cases of profuse phlegm, the prescription is modified to transform phlegm and downbear qi.

Add:

zǐ sū zǐ	perilla [fruit]	Perillae Fructus	9 g.
bái jiè zǐ	white mustard [seed]	Brassicae Albae Semen	9 g.

In cases presenting yellow sticky phlegm, dryness of the mouth, constipation, yellow slimy tongue coating and rapid slippery pulse, indications that the internal phlegm-heat is profuse, the prescription is modified to clear heat and transform phlegm.

Add:

huáng qín	scutellaria [root]	Scutellariae Radix	9 g.
yú xīng cǎo	houttuynia	Houttuyniae Herba cum Radice	12 g.
guā lóu	trichosanthes [fruit]	Trichosanthis Fructus	12 g.

In cases accompanied by constipation, the prescription is modified to clear heat, transform phlegm and promote elimination.

Add:

dà huáng	rhubarb (abbreviated decoction)	Rhei Rhizoma	9 g.
máng xiāo	mirabilite (stirred in)	Mirabilitum	9 g.

The prepared medicine, CHLORITE-MICA PHLEGM-SHIFTING PILL (*méng-shí gǔn tán wán*) may also be used to achieve the same result.

ACUPUNCTURE AND MOXIBUSTION

Main points: Needle with draining.

GV-26	*rén zhōng*
PC-09	*zhōng chōng*
PC-06	*nèi guān*
ST-40	*fēng lóng*
CV-12	*zhōng wǎn*

Auxiliary points:

For clenching of the teeth, add:

ST-06	*jiá chē*
LI-04	*hé gǔ*

For convulsions, add:

LI-04	*hé gǔ*
GB-43	*xiá xī*

For gurgling in the throat, add:

CV-22	*tiān tú*

For fever, add:

GV-14	*dà zhuī*
LI-11	*qū chí*

6. FOOD INVERSION

Clinical Manifestations: Sudden loss of consciousness following excessive eating or drinking coupled with a bout of rage; accompanied by congested, suffocating sensations in the chest, fullness and distention of the epigastrium and abdomen.

Tongue: Thick slimy coating.

Pulse: Forceful, slippery.

Treatment Method: Calm the stomach, disperse food.

PRESCRIPTION

Combine Wondrous Atractylodes Powder *(shén zhú sǎn)* with Harmony-Preserving Pill *(bǎo hé wán)*.

Wondrous Atractylodes Powder *shén zhú sǎn*

cāng zhú	atractylodes [root]	Atractylodis Rhizoma	9 g.
chén pí	tangerine [peel]	Citri Exocarpium	9 g.
hòu pò	magnolia [bark]	Magnoliae Cortex	9 g.
zhì gān cǎo	licorice [root] (honey-fried)	Glycyrrhizae Radix	3 g.
huò xiāng	agastache/patchouli	Agastaches seu Pogostemi Herba	9 g.
shā rén	amomum [fruit] (abbreviated decoction)	Amomi Semen seu Fructus	6 g.

with:

Harmony-Preserving Pill *bǎo hé wán*

shān zhā	crataegus [fruit]	Crataegi Fructus	18 g.
shén qū	medicated leaven	Massa Medicata Fermentata	9 g.
zhì bàn xià	pinellia [tuber] (processed)	Pinelliae Tuber Praeparatum	9 g.
fú líng	poria	Poria	9 g.
chén pí	tangerine [peel]	Citri Exocarpium	6 g.
lián qiào	forsythia [fruit]	Forsythiae Fructus	6 g.
lái fú zǐ	radish [seed]	Raphani Semen	6 g.

<u>MODIFICATIONS</u>

In cases of abdominal fullness and constipation, the prescription is changed to remove stagnation and promote elimination.
Use:

Minor Qi-Infusing Decoction *xiǎo chéng qì tāng*

dà huáng	rhubarb (abbreviated decoction)	Rhei Rhizoma	12 g.
zhǐ shí	unripe bitter orange [fruit]	Aurantii Fructus Immaturus	9 g.
hòu pò	magnolia [bark]	Magnoliae Cortex	6 g.

ACUPUNCTURE AND MOXIBUSTION

Main points: Needle with draining.

GV-26	*rén zhōng*
CV-12	*zhōng wǎn*
ST-36	*zú sān lǐ*
PC-06	*nèi guān*

Auxiliary points:

For constipation, add:

BL-25	*dà cháng shū*
LI-04	*hé gǔ*

For clenching of the teeth, add:

ST-06	*jiá chē*
LI-04	*hé gǔ*

For convulsions, add:

LI-04	*hé gǔ*
GB-43	*xiá xī*

For gurgling in the throat, add:

CV-22	*tiān tú*

For fever, add:

GV-14	*dà zhuī*
LI-11	*qū chí*

7. SUMMERHEAT INVERSION

Clinical Manifestations: Syncope occurring during the heat of the summer, generally preceded by dizziness, headache, oppression in the chest, fever, flushed complexion and hindered perspiration. Loss of consciousness follows, sometimes with delirium.

Tongue: Red and dry.

Pulse: Surging, rapid or empty, wiry, rapid.

Treatment Method: Resolve summerheat, boost qi, clear heart, open the orifices.

PRESCRIPTION

In unconscious patients, it is imperative that the heart be cleared and the orifices opened. Use the prepared medicines, BOVINE BEZOAR HEART-CLEARING PILL *(niú huáng qīng xīn wán)* or PURPLE SNOW ELIXIR *(zǐ xuě dān)*.

Afterward, to clear summerheat and boost qi, use:

White Tiger Decoction Plus Ginseng *bái hǔ jiā rén shēn tāng*

shí gāo	gypsum (extended decoction)	Gypsum	30 g.
zhī mǔ	anemarrhena [root]	Anemarrhenae Rhizoma	12 g.
rén shēn	ginseng	Ginseng Radix	9 g.
jīng mǐ	rice	Oryzae Semen	15 g.
zhì gān cǎo	licorice [root] (honey-fried)	Glycyrrhizae Radix	6 g.

or:

Summerheat-Clearing Qi-Boosting Decoction *qīng shǔ yì qì tāng*

xī yáng shēn	American ginseng	Panacis Quinquefolii Radix	6 g.
mài mén dōng	ophiopogon [tuber]	Ophiopogonis Tuber	9 g.
zhú yè	black bamboo [leaf]	Bambusae Folium	6 g.
shí hú	dendrobium [stem] (extended decoction)	Dendrobii Caulis	15 g.
huáng lián	coptis [root]	Coptidis Rhizoma	3 g.
hé yè gěng	lotus [leafstalk]	Nelumbinis Petiolus	15 g.
zhī mǔ	anemarrhena [root]	Anemarrhenae Rhizoma	6 g.
gān cǎo	licorice [root]	Glycyrrhizae Radix	3 g.
jīng mǐ	rice	Oryzae Semen	15 g.
xī guā cuì yī	watermelon [rind]	Citrulli Exocarpium	30 g.

<u>MODIFICATIONS</u>

In cases where summerheat has injured yin, allowing the activation of liver wind, with symptoms including spasms of the limbs, heavy perspiration, thirst, dizziness and vertigo, nausea and rapid wiry pulse, the prescription is changed to calm the liver, extinguish wind, nourish yin and clear summerheat. Use:

Antelope Horn and Uncaria Decoction *líng jiǎo gōu téng tāng*

líng yáng jiǎo	antelope horn (or, powdered and stirred in, 0.5 g. each time)	Antelopis Cornu	3 g.
gōu téng	uncaria [stem and thorn] (abbreviated decoction)	Uncariae Ramulus cum Unco	9 g.
sāng yè	mulberry [leaf]	Mori Folium	6 g.
jú huā	chrysanthemum [flower]	Chrysanthemi Flos	9 g.
chuān bèi mǔ	Sichuan fritillaria [bulb]	Fritillariae Cirrhosae Bulbus	12 g.
zhú rú	bamboo shavings	Bambusae Caulis in Taeniam	9 g.
shēng dì huáng	rehmannia [root] dried/fresh	Rehmanniae Radix Exsiccata seu Recens	15 g.
bái sháo yào	white peony [root]	Paeoniae Radix Alba	9 g.
fú shén	root poria	Poria cum Pini Radice	9 g.
gān cǎo	licorice [root]	Glycyrrhizae Radix	3 g.

Add:

xī guā cuì yī	watermelon [rind]	Citrulli Exocarpium	30 g.
hé yè	lotus [leaf]	Nelumbinis Folium	9 g.
zhú yè	black bamboo [leaf]	Bambusae Folium	9 g.

In cases of rapid onset of sunstroke, where excessive perspiration allows qi desertion, with accompanying symptoms of dizziness, palpitations, fatigue, pale complexion, heavy perspiration, cold extremities and abrupt onset of syncope, treatment should boost qi and control perspiration.

Use:

Ginseng, Aconite, Dragon Bone and Oystershell Decoction
shēn fù lóng mǔ tāng

rén shēn	ginseng	Ginseng Radix	9 g.
zhì fù zǐ	aconite [accessory tuber] (processed) (extended decoction)	Aconiti Tuber Laterale Praeparatum	9 g.
duàn lóng gǔ	dragon bone (calcined)	Mastodi Ossis Fossilia Calcinatum	30 g.
duàn mǔ lì	oyster shell (calcined)	Ostreae Concha Calcinatum	30 g.

ACUPUNCTURE AND MOXIBUSTION

Main points: Needle with draining.

GV-26	*rén zhōng*
LI-04	*hé gǔ*
LI-11	*qū chí*
M-UE-1-5	*shí xuān* (Ten Diffusing Points)

Auxiliary points:

For clenching of the teeth, add:

ST-06	*jiá chē*

For convulsions, add:

GB-43	*xiá xī*

For gurgling in the throat, add:

CV-22	*tiān tú*

For fever, add:

GV-14	*dà zhuī*

ALTERNATE THERAPEUTIC METHODS

1. Ear Acupuncture

Auricular points: Heart, Subcortex, *Shén Mén,* Brain, Sympathetic, Adrenal.

Method: Select two to three points each session, needle to elicit a strong sensation for repletion patterns, and a mild sensation for vacuity patterns. Apply manipulation every five minutes and retain needles a total of thirty minutes.

REMARKS

It is extremely important in differential diagnosis of syncope to understand the precipitating factors, so as to distinguish syncope from coma, stroke or epilepsy. Although coma can also occur suddenly, it is caused by conditions quite different from those of syncope. In coma, the loss of consciousness is generally extended, the patient's condition is more severe, and it is difficult to quickly revive patients from a coma. Also, in most cases, clinical symptoms that were seen before the onset of coma are still evident once consciousness is regained.

In stroke or apoplexy, the period of unconsciousness is longer than that in syncope. It is often followed by sequelae of hemiplegia, aphasia or facial paralysis.

In epilepsy, sudden loss of consciousness is often accompanied by spasms of the limbs, rolling back of the eyes, foaming at the mouth and, in some cases, bleating sounds. Loss of consciousness is brief, precipitating factors are not obvious and, upon regaining consciousness, there are no abnormal clinical manifestations. This makes epilepsy easily distinguishable from syncope.

Concerning the treatment of syncope, differentiate repletion from vacuity immediately and administer first aid.

Repletion patterns are marked by heavy respiration, stiffness of the limbs, clenching of the teeth and deep wiry or deep hidden pulse. To open the orifices and arouse the spirit in repletion patterns, use the prepared medicines, LIQUID STORAX PILL *(sū-hé-xiāng wán)* or JADE AXIS ELIXIR *(yù shū dān)*.

Yang vacuity patterns are marked by feeble respiration, an open mouth, spontaneous perspiration, coldness of the extremities and a thready deep faint pulse. Returning yang and securing qi can be effected through the administration of:

Ginseng and Aconite Decoction *shēn fù tāng*

rén shēn	ginseng	Ginseng Radix	30 g.
zhì fù zǐ	aconite [accessory tuber] (processed)	Aconiti Tuber Laterale Praeparatum	15 g.

Yin vacuity patterns are marked by pale complexion, feeble respiration, perspiration, fever, red tongue and thready rapid faint pulse. To boost qi and save yin, use:

Pulse-Engendering Beverage *shēng mài yǐn*

rén shēn	ginseng	Ginseng Radix	9 g.
mài mén dōng	ophiopogon [tuber]	Ophiopogonis Tuber	15 g.
wǔ wèi zǐ	schisandra [berry]	Schisandrae Fructus	6 g.

Acupuncture at points such as GV-26 *(rén zhōng)*, PC-09 *(zhōng chōng)*, and KI-01 *(yǒng quán)* is quite effective in reviving patients. When necessary, a comprehensive treatment combining both traditional and Western methods should be undertaken. Once consciousness is regained, differential diagnosis and treatment according to indications of qi, blood, phlegm, food stasis and summerheat can be undertaken.

TETANY PATTERNS

Jīng Zhèng

1. Obstruction of the Channels and Connections by Evils - 2. Liver Wind Stirring from Exuberant Heat - 3. Depletion of Yin and Blood

Tetany patterns *(jīng zhèng)* manifest in a variety of pathologies, presenting stiffness of the neck and spine, lockjaw, spasms or shaking of the limbs, and, in severe cases, opisthotonos. Refer to this chapter for tetany associated with the Western medical diseases of epidemic cerebrospinal meningitis, encephalitis, meningitis secondary to infectious diseases and convulsions related to high fever.

ETIOLOGY AND PATHOGENESIS

Overall, the etiology and pathogenesis of tetany patterns may be divided into external attack or internal disruption. External attack has one of two causes. The first is invasion of wind, cold and dampness, which obstruct the channels and connections, hindering the flow of qi and blood. The second involves profuse external heat, which scorches fluids and stirs internal wind.

Internal disruption begins with either a constitutional yin and blood vacuity, or the loss of a large amount of blood or other body fluid. Depletion of yin and blood allows vacuity wind to stir, with tetany arising from malnourishment of the sinews.

Although different in etiology, the basic pathogenic mechanism of tetany patterns is the same whether caused by external or internal factors: disruption in the balance of yin and yang and malnourishment of the sinews. Tetany patterns related to external attack are generally classified as repletion illness, while those caused by internal factors are classified as vacuity illness.

1. OBSTRUCTION OF THE CHANNELS AND CONNECTIONS BY EVILS

Clinical Manifestations: Stiffness of the neck and spine, accompanied by aversion to cold, fever, aching and heaviness of the body, headache.

Tongue: White slimy coating

Pulse: Tight, floating.

Treatment Method: Course wind and cold, dry dampness, clear the channels and connections.

PRESCRIPTION

Notopterygium Dampness-Overcoming Decoction
qiāng huó shèng shī tāng

qiāng huó	notopterygium [root]	Notopterygii Rhizoma	6 g.
dú huó	tuhuo [angelica root]	Angelicae Duhuo Radix	6 g.
gǎo běn	Chinese lovage [root]	Ligustici Sinensis Rhizoma et Radix	6 g.
fáng fēng	ledebouriella [root]	Ledebouriellae Radix	6 g.
màn jīng zǐ	vitex [fruit]	Viticis Fructus	6 g.
chuān xiōng	ligusticum [root]	Ligustici Rhizoma	6 g.
zhì gān cǎo	licorice [root] (honey-fried)	Glycyrrhizae Radix	3 g.

MODIFICATIONS

In cases where cold evil is severe, with symptoms of stiffness of the neck and spine, lockjaw, spasms of the limbs, strong aversion to cold, fever, headache, no perspiration, thin white tongue coating and tight floating pulse, the prescription is changed to relieve the body surface and promote perspiration.

Use:

Pueraria Decoction *gé gēn tāng*

gé gēn	pueraria [root]	Puerariae Radix	15 g.
má huáng	ephedra	Ephedrae Herba	6 g.
guì zhī	cinnamon [twig]	Cinnamomi Ramulus	9 g.
bái sháo yào	white peony [root]	Paeoniae Radix Alba	9 g.
zhì gān cǎo	licorice [root] (honey-fried)	Glycyrrhizae Radix	6 g.
shēng jiāng	fresh ginger [root]	Zingiberis Rhizoma Recens	6 g.
dà zǎo	jujube	Ziziphi Fructus	3 pc.

In cases of profusion of wind evil, with symptoms of stiffness of the neck and spine, fever without aversion to cold, headache, perspiration, thin white tongue coating and deep thready pulse, the prescription is changed to course wind, relieve the body surface, clear heat and generate liquid.

Use:

Trichosanthes and Cinnamon Twig Decoction *guā lóu guì zhī tāng*

guā lóu	trichosanthes [fruit]	Trichosanthis Fructus	9 g.
guì zhī	cinnamon [twig]	Cinnamomi Ramulus	9 g.
bái sháo yào	white peony [root]	Paeoniae Radix Alba	9 g.
zhì gān cǎo	licorice [root] (honey-fried)	Glycyrrhizae Radix	6 g.
shēng jiāng	fresh ginger [root]	Zingiberis Rhizoma Recens	9 g.
dà zǎo	jujube	Ziziphi Fructus	3 pc.

Add:

tiān huā fěn	trichosanthes [root]	Trichosanthis Radix	12 g.

In cases where damp-heat has invaded the connections, with symptoms of fever, convulsions, congestion and discomfort of the chest and epigastrium, thirst without the desire for drink, dark scanty urine, yellow slimy tongue coating and rapid slippery pulse, treatment should clear heat, transform dampness and clear the channels and connections.

Use:

Three Kernels Decoction *sān rén tāng*

xìng rén	apricot [kernel] (abbreviated decoction)	Armeniacae Semen	12 g.
huá shí	talcum (wrapped)	Talcum	15 g.
yì yǐ rén	coix [seed]	Coicis Semen	15 g.
bái dòu kòu	cardamom (abbreviated decoction)	Amomi Cardamomi Fructus	6 g.
hòu pò	magnolia [bark]	Magnoliae Cortex	6 g.
tōng cǎo	rice-paper plant pith	Tetrapanacis Medulla	6 g.
fǎ bàn xià	pinellia [tuber] (processed)	Pinelliae Tuber Praeparatum	6 g.
zhú yè	black bamboo [leaf]	Bambusae Folium	6 g.

Add:

dì lóng	earthworm	Lumbricus	9 g.
qín jiāo	large gentian [root]	Gentianae Macrophyllae Radix	9 g.
sī guā luò	loofah	Luffae Fasciculus Vascularis	9 g.

ACUPUNCTURE AND MOXIBUSTION

Main points: Needle with draining.

LI-04	*hé gǔ*
TB-05	*wài guān*
GV-14	*dà zhuī*
GB-20	*fēng chí*
BL-12	*fēng mén*

Auxiliary points:

For headache, add:

M-HN-3	*yìn táng* (Hall of Impression)
GV-20	*bǎi huì*

For stiffness of the neck and spine, add:

BL-11	*dà zhù*
SI-03	*hòu xī*

For invasion of the connections by damp-heat, add:

SP-09	*yīn líng quán*
LI-11	*qū chí*

2. LIVER WIND STIRRING FROM EXUBERANT HEAT

Clinical Manifestations: High fever, irritability, lockjaw, spasms of the limbs, stiffness of the neck and spine, dryness of the mouth and throat, abdominal distention and constipation in some cases. Opisthotonos, loss of consciousness and delirium in severe cases.

Tongue: Yellow slimy coating.

Pulse: Rapid, wiry.

Treatment Method: Calm the liver, extinguish wind, nourish yin, clear heat.

PRESCRIPTION

Antelope Horn and Uncaria Decoction *líng jiǎo gōu téng tāng*

líng yáng jiǎo	antelope horn (or, powdered and stirred in, each time 0.5 g.)	Antelopis Cornu	3 g.
gōu téng	uncaria [stem and thorn] (abbreviated decoction)	Uncariae Ramulus cum Unco	9 g.
sāng yè	mulberry [leaf]	Mori Folium	6 g.
jú huā	chrysanthemum [flower]	Chrysanthemi Flos	9 g.

chuān bèi mǔ	Sichuan fritillaria [bulb]	Fritillariae Cirrhosae Bulbus	12 g.
zhú rú	bamboo shavings	Bambusae Caulis in Taeniam	9 g.
shēng dì huáng	rehmannia [root] dried/fresh	Rehmanniae Radix Exsiccata seu Recens	15 g.
bái sháo yào	white peony [root]	Paeoniae Radix Alba	9 g.
fú shén	root poria	Poria cum Pini Radice	9 g.
gān cǎo	licorice [root]	Glycyrrhizae Radix	3 g.

MODIFICATIONS

In cases of abdominal distention and constipation, the prescription is modified to clear heat and free the stool.

Add:

| *dà huáng* | rhubarb (abbreviated decoction) | Rhei Rhizoma | 9 g. |
| *máng xiāo* | mirabilite (stirred in) | Mirabilitum | 9 g. |

In cases of delirium or coma, the prescription is changed to clear heat and open the orifices. Use the prepared medicines, PEACEFUL PALACE BOVINE BEZOAR PILL (*ān gōng niú-huáng wán*) or SUPREME JEWEL ELIXIR *(zhì bǎo dān)*.

In cases where the prolonged presence of heat has led to the scorching of yin, with symptoms of intermittent convulsions, dry tongue with little coating and thready rapid pulse, the prescription is changed to calm the liver, extinguish wind, nourish yin and relieve convulsions.

Use:

Major Wind-Stabilizing Pill *dà dìng fēng zhū*

bái sháo yào	white peony [root]	Paeoniae Radix Alba	18 g.
ē jiāo	ass hide glue (dissolved and stirred in)	Asini Corii Gelatinum	9 g.
guī bǎn	tortoise plastron (extended decoction)	Testudinis Plastrum	12 g.
shú dì huáng	cooked rehmannia [root]	Rehmanniae Radix Conquita	18 g.
huǒ má rén	hemp [seed]	Cannabis Semen	6 g.
wǔ wèi zǐ	schisandra [berry]	Schisandrae Fructus	6 g.
mǔ lì	oyster shell (extended decoction)	Ostreae Concha	12 g.
mài mén dōng	ophiopogon [tuber]	Ophiopogonis Tuber	18 g.
biē jiǎ	turtle shell (extended decoction)	Amydae Carapax	12 g.
zhì gān cǎo	licorice [root] (honey-fried)	Glycyrrhizae Radix	12 g.
jī zǐ huáng	egg yolk (stirred in while decoction cools)	Galli Vitellus	2 pc.

ACUPUNCTURE AND MOXIBUSTION

Main points: Needle with draining.

GV-14	*dà zhuī*
LI-11	*qū chí*
LI-04	*hé gǔ*
LR-03	*tài chōng*
GB-20	*fēng chí*

Auxiliary points:

For loss of consciousness and delirium, add:

| GV-26 | *rén zhōng* |
| M-UE-1-5 | *shí xuān* (Ten Diffusing Points) |

For lockjaw, add:

ST-06	*jiá chē*
TB-06	*zhī gōu*

For abdominal distention and constipation, add:

BL-25	*dà cháng shū*
ST-25	*tiān shū*

For profusion of phlegm, add:

PC-06	*nèi guān*
ST-40	*fēng lóng*

3. DEPLETION OF YIN AND BLOOD

Clinical Manifestations: Clinical history of constitutional yin vacuity, loss of blood or excessive perspiration, stiffness of the neck and spine, cramps in the limbs, dizzy spells, tiredness.

Tongue: Pale red.

Pulse: Thready, wiry.

Treatment Method: Moisten yin, nourish the blood, extinguish wind, relieve convulsions.

PRESCRIPTION

Combine Four Agents Decoction *(sì wù tāng)* with Major Wind-Stabilizing Pill *(dà dìng fēng zhū)*.

Four Agents Decoction *sì wù tāng*

shú dì huáng	cooked rehmannia [root]	Rehmanniae Radix Conquita	9 g.
dāng guī	tangkuei	Angelicae Sinensis Radix	9 g.
bái sháo yào	white peony [root]	Paeoniae Radix Alba	9 g.
chuān xiōng	ligusticum [root]	Ligustici Rhizoma	9 g.

with:

Major Wind-Stabilizing Pill *dà dìng fēng zhū*

bái sháo yào	white peony [root]	Paeoniae Radix Alba	18 g.
ē jiāo	ass hide glue (dissolved and stirred in)	Asini Corii Gelatinum	9 g.
guī bǎn	tortoise plastron (extended decoction)	Testudinis Plastrum	12 g.
shú dì huáng	cooked rehmannia [root]	Rehmanniae Radix Conquita	18 g.
huǒ má rén	hemp [seed]	Cannabis Semen	6 g.
wǔ wèi zǐ	schisandra [berry]	Schisandrae Fructus	6 g.
mǔ lì	oyster shell (extended decoction)	Ostreae Concha	12 g.
mài mén dōng	ophiopogon [tuber]	Ophiopogonis Tuber	18 g.
biē jiǎ	turtle shell (extended decoction)	Amydae Carapax	12 g.
zhì gān cǎo	licorice [root] (honey-fried)	Glycyrrhizae Radix	12 g.
jī zǐ huáng	egg yolk (stirred in while decoction cools)	Galli Vitellus	2 pc.

MODIFICATIONS

In cases presenting with dizziness and insomnia, the prescription is modified to settle, tranquilize and quiet the spirit.

Add:

zhēn zhū mŭ	mother-of-pearl (extended decoction)	Concha Margaritifera	30 g.
yè jiāo téng	flowery knotweed [stem]	Polygoni Multiflori Caulis	15 g.

In cases of loss of appetite and abdominal distention, the prescription is modified to rectify qi and harmonize the stomach.

Add:

shā rén	amomum [fruit] (abbreviated decoction)	Amomi Semen seu Fructus	6 g.
jī nèi jīn	gizzard lining	Galli Gigerii Endothelium	9 g.
chén pí	tangerine [peel]	Citri Exocarpium	9 g.

In cases with weakness of the limbs and loose stools, the prescription is modified to boost qi and fortify the spleen.

Add:

dăng shēn	codonopsis [root]	Codonopsitis Radix	9 g.
bái zhú	ovate atractylodes [root]	Atractylodis Ovatae Rhizoma	9 g.

ACUPUNCTURE AND MOXIBUSTION

Main points: Needle with supplementation.

GV-20	*băi huì*
ST-36	*zú sān lǐ*
SP-06	*sān yīn jiāo*
KI-01	*yŏng quán*
CV-04	*guān yuán*

Auxiliary points:

For cramps in the upper limbs, add:

LI-04	*hé gŭ*
PC-07	*dà líng*

For cramps in the lower limbs, add:

SP-09	*yīn líng quán*
BL-57	*chéng shān*

ALTERNATE THERAPEUTIC METHODS

1. Ear Acupuncture

Auricular points: Liver, Subcortex, *Shén Mén,* Brain Stem.

Method: Use draining manipulation in cases of repletion and supplementing manipulation in cases of vacuity. Retain the needles for twenty to thirty minutes.

REMARKS

Tetany patterns develop either from external attack or from internal disruption and patterns exhibit either repletion or vacuity. The treatment of repletion patterns is directed toward removing evils: dispelling wind, dispersing cold, transforming dampness and clearing heat. On the other hand, treatment of vacuity patterns calls for reinforcing correct qi, moistening yin, nourishing blood and relaxing sinews to alleviate tetany.

BLEEDING PATTERNS

Xuè Zhèng

1. Coughing Blood - 1a. Damage to the Lung by Wind, Heat and Dryness - 1b. Liver Fire Invading the Lung - 1c. Yin Vacuity Fire - 2. Vomiting Blood - 2a. Stomach Heat - 2b. Liver Fire Invading the Stomach - 2c. Spleen and Stomach Qi Vacuity - 3. Bloody Stools - 3a. Intestinal Damp-Heat - 3b. Spleen and Stomach Vacuity Cold - 4. Urinary Bleeding - 4a. Yin Vacuity with Effulgent Fire - 4b. Exuberant Heart Fire - 4c. Spleen and Kidney Qi Vacuity - 5. Subcutaneous Bleeding - 5a. Blood Heat - 5b. Yin Vacuity with Effulgent Fire - 5c. Qi Failing to Secure the Blood

Bleeding patterns (*xuè zhèng*) include any bleeding outside the proper courses, whether it runs from the nose or mouth, is passed with the feces or urine or extravasates into the skin. These patterns encompass a variety of both acute and chronic Western medical conditions. This chapter concentrates on the most common bleeding patterns: coughing blood, vomiting blood, bloody stools, urinary bleeding and subcutaneous bleeding.

ETIOLOGY AND PATHOGENESIS

The etiology of bleeding patterns can involve either external or internal factors. The basic pathogenic mechanisms are either fire evil or vacuous qi that cannot contain the blood. The involvement of different viscera and bowels is inferred according to the site of the bleeding.

In the pathogenesis of bleeding, fire can either be replete or vacuous. Repletion fire arises from one of two conditions. The first is from attack by external evils such as wind, heat or dryness. The second is from liver fire brought about by internal factors like emotional upset or dietary imbalances, especially over-consumption of alcohol or rich spicy foods.

Vacuity patterns involve vacuity fire, or qi vacuity unable to secure the blood. Vacuity fire is the result of the depletion of yin following a febrile or extended illness. Qi vacuity patterns can be caused by injury to spleen qi, by improper diet and eating habits or by an insufficiency of qi from physical and mental exertion or indulgent sexual activity. When qi is vacuous, one must also consider injury to yang and the presence of cold.

Bleeding can also result from blood stasis, which congests the vessels and ultimately leads to blood flow outside the normal courses.

Concerning repletion and vacuity in bleeding patterns, exuberant fire is considered repletion, while depletion of yin with frenetic vacuity fire and vacuity of qi are categorized as vacuity patterns. Patterns involving blood stasis are generally complicated by both repletion and vacuity. Regardless of the etiology, both repletion and vacuity patterns can result in depletion of qi and degeneration of yang because of the excessive loss of blood. Thus, repletion patterns have a high probability of transforming to vacuity patterns. At the same time, blood that has already escaped the vessels but not left the body adds to the extraneous factor of static blood, further complicating treatment and retarding recovery.

1A. COUGHING BLOOD – DAMAGE TO THE LUNG BY WIND, HEAT AND DRYNESS

Clinical Manifestations: Itchy throat, coughing, difficult expectoration, dry mouth and nose, fever or blood-streaked phlegm in some cases.

Tongue: Red, dry with thin yellow coating.

Pulse: Rapid, floating.

Treatment Method: Clear heat, moisten the lung, relieve bleeding.

PRESCRIPTION

Mulberry Leaf and Apricot Kernel Decoction *sāng xìng tāng*

sāng yè	mulberry [leaf]	Mori Folium	9 g.
xìng rén	apricot [kernel] (abbreviated decoction)	Armeniacae Semen	9 g.
shā shēn	glehnia [root]	Glehniae Radix	9 g.
zhè bèi mǔ	Zhejiang fritillaria [bulb]	Fritillariae Verticillatae Bulbus	9 g.
dàn dòu chǐ	fermented soybean (unsalted)	Glycines Semen Insulsum Fermentatum	9 g.
shān zhī zǐ	gardenia [fruit]	Gardeniae Fructus	6 g.
lí pí	pear [skin]	Pyri Exocarpium	6 g.

MODIFICATIONS

In cases of severe coughing of blood, the prescription is modified to cool the blood and relieve bleeding. Add:

bái máo gēn	imperata [root]	Imperatae Rhizoma	15 g.
ǒu jié	lotus [root node]	Nelumbinis Rhizomatis Nodus	9 g.
qiàn cǎo gēn	madder [root]	Rubiae Radix	9 g.
cè bǎi yè	biota [leaf]	Biotae Folium	12 g.

In cases of fever, headache and sore throat, the prescription is modified to clear heat and relieve external symptoms. Add:

jīn yín huā	lonicera [flower]	Lonicerae Flos	9 g.
lián qiào	forsythia [fruit]	Forsythiae Fructus	9 g.
jú huā	chrysanthemum [flower]	Chrysanthemi Flos	9 g.

In cases showing severe injury to fluids, the prescription is modified to nourish yin and moisten dryness. Add:

mài mén dōng	ophiopogon [tuber]	Ophiopogonis Tuber	9 g.
xuán shēn	scrophularia [root]	Scrophulariae Radix	9 g.
tiān huā fěn	trichosanthes [root]	Trichosanthis Radix	9 g.

ACUPUNCTURE AND MOXIBUSTION

Main points: Needle with draining.

BL-13	*fèi shū*
LI-04	*hé gǔ*
LU-06	*kǒng zuì*
LU-05	*chǐ zé*

Auxiliary points:

For fever, add:

GV-14	*dà zhuī*
LI-11	*qū chí*

For dry sore throat, add bloodletting at:

LU-11	*shào shāng*

1B. COUGHING BLOOD – LIVER FIRE INVADING THE LUNG

Clinical Manifestations: Recurrent cough, blood-streaked phlegm, pulling pain in the chest and hypochondrium when coughing and, in severe cases, spitting of large quantities of bright red or purplish blood. Accompanying symptoms include irritability, bitter taste in the mouth, dry stools and dark yellow urine.

Tongue: Red with thin yellow coating.

Pulse: Rapid, wiry.

Treatment Method: Clear the liver and lung, relieve bleeding.

PRESCRIPTION

Combine White-Draining Powder *(xiè bái sǎn)* with Indigo and Clamshell Powder *(dài gé sǎn)*

White-Draining Powder *xiè bái sǎn*

sāng bái pí	mulberry [root bark]	Mori Radicis Cortex	9 g.
dì gǔ pí	lycium [root bark]	Lycii Radicis Cortex	12 g.
jīng mǐ	rice	Oryzae Semen	15 g.
zhì gān cǎo	licorice [root] (honey-fried)	Glycyrrhizae Radix	6 g.

with:

Indigo and Clamshell Powder *dài gé sǎn*

qīng dài	indigo (stirred in)	Indigo Pulverata Levis	3 g.
hǎi gé ké	clamshell	Cyclinae (seu Meretricis) Concha	12 g.

MODIFICATIONS

To reinforce blood cooling and bleeding relief, add:

shēng dì huáng	rehmannia [root] dried/fresh	Rehmanniae Radix Exsiccata seu Recens	12 g.
hàn lián cǎo	eclipta	Ecliptae Herba	9 g.
bái máo gēn	imperata [root]	Imperatae Rhizoma	15 g.
dà jì	cirsium	Cirsii Herba seu Radix	12 g.
xiǎo jì	cephalanoplos	Cephalanoploris Herba seu Radix	12 g.

In cases of severe liver fire, the prescription is modified to clear the liver and drain fire.

Add:

mǔ dān pí	moutan [root bark]	Moutan Radicis Cortex	9 g.
shān zhī zǐ	gardenia [fruit]	Gardeniae Fructus	9 g.
huáng qín	scutellaria [root]	Scutellariae Radix	9 g.

In cases of coughing or expectoration of large quantities of bright red blood, the prescription is changed to clear heat, drain fire, cool the blood and relieve bleeding. Use:

Rhinoceros Horn and Rehmannia Decoction *xī jiǎo dì huáng tāng*

xī jiǎo	rhinoceros horn* (powdered and stirred in)	Rhinocerotis Cornu	3 g.
shēng dì huáng	rehmannia [root] dried/fresh	Rehmanniae Radix Exsiccata seu Recens	30 g.
bái sháo yào	white peony [root]	Paeoniae Radix Alba	12 g.
mǔ dān pí	moutan [root bark]	Moutan Radicis Cortex	9 g.

*Use of *xī jiǎo* (rhinoceros horn) is prohibited in North America by the endangered species law. Water Buffalo Horn *(shuǐ niú jiǎo)* may be substituted. Increase the dose to 15 g., extended decoction.)

Add:

sān qī	notoginseng [root] (or, powdered and stirred in, each time 1.5 g.)	Notoginseng Radix	9 g.

ACUPUNCTURE AND MOXIBUSTION

Main points: Needle with draining.

BL-13	*fèi shū*
LU-10	*yú jì*
PC-08	*láo gōng*
LR-02	*xíng jiān*

1C. COUGHING BLOOD – DEPLETION OF YIN WITH RISE OF FIRE

Clinical Manifestations: Coughing, expectoration of small quantities of blood-streaked phlegm or recurrent coughing of bright red blood accompanied by tidal fever, night sweating, fever in the five hearts, flushed cheeks, dryness of the mouth and throat, emaciation.

Tongue: Red with little coating.

Pulse: Thready, rapid.

Treatment Method: Nourish yin, moisten the lung, relieve bleeding.

PRESCRIPTION

Lily Bulb Metal-Securing Decoction *bǎi hé gù jīn tāng*

shēng dì huáng	rehmannia [root] dried/fresh	Rehmanniae Radix Exsiccata seu Recens	9 g.
shú dì huáng	cooked rehmannia [root]	Rehmanniae Radix Conquita	9 g.
mài mén dōng	ophiopogon [tuber]	Ophiopogonis Tuber	9 g.
bǎi hé	lily [bulb]	Lilii Bulbus	9 g.
bái sháo yào	white peony [root]	Paeoniae Radix Alba	9 g.
dāng guī	tangkuei	Angelicae Sinensis Radix	6 g.
chuān bèi mǔ	Sichuan fritillaria [bulb]	Fritillariae Cirrhosae Bulbus	9 g.
xuán shēn	scrophularia [root]	Scrophulariae Radix	9 g.
jié gěng	platycodon [root]	Platycodonis Radix	6 g.
gān cǎo	licorice [root]	Glycyrrhizae Radix	6 g.

MODIFICATIONS

Because of its ascending quality, delete:

jié gĕng	platycodon [root]	Platycodonis Radix	

To reinforce the bleeding relief, add:

bái jí	bletilla [tuber]	Bletillae Tuber	9 g.
ŏu jié	lotus [root node]	Nelumbinis Rhizomatis Nodus	9 g.
bái máo gēn	imperata [root]	Imperatae Rhizoma	15 g.

In cases of recurrent coughing of blood, as well as those where there is a large quantity of expectorated blood, the prescription is reinforced to relieve bleeding. Add:

ē jiāo	ass hide glue (dissolved)	Asini Corii Gelatinum	9 g.
sān qī	notoginseng [root]	Notoginseng Radix	9 g.
	(or, powdered and stirred in, each time 1.5 g.)		

In cases of vacuity fire, with tidal fever, fever in the five hearts and flushed cheeks, the prescription is modified by adding:

qīng hāo	sweet wormwood	Artemisiae Apiaceae	9 g.
	(abbreviated decoction)	seu Annuae Herba	
biē jiǎ	turtle shell (extended decoction)	Amydae Carapax	30 g.
dì gǔ pí	lycium [root bark]	Lycii Radicis Cortex	9 g.
bái wéi	baiwei [cynanchum root]	Cynanchi Baiwei Radix	9 g.

In cases of night sweating, the prescription is modified to strengthen retention functions and relief of sweating. Add:

fú xiǎo mài	light wheat [grain]	Tritici Semen Leve	15 g.
wǔ wèi zǐ	schisandra [berry]	Schisandrae Fructus	6 g.
duàn mǔ lì	oyster [shell] (calcined)	Ostreae Concha Calcinatum	15 g.

ACUPUNCTURE AND MOXIBUSTION

Main points: Needle with even supplementation, even draining.

LU-05	chǐ zé
LU-06	kǒng zuì
LU-10	yú jì
KI-02	rán gǔ
M-HN-30	bǎi láo (Hundred Taxations)

2A. VOMITING BLOOD – DEPRESSION OF STOMACH HEAT

Clinical Manifestations: Epigastric distention and congestion (or pain in more severe cases), vomiting of bright red or purplish blood that is often mixed with food matter, foul breath, constipation or black stools.

Tongue: Red with yellow slimy coating.

Pulse: Rapid, slippery.

Treatment Method: Clear stomach heat, relieve bleeding.

PRESCRIPTION

Combine Heart-Draining Decoction (*xiè xīn tāng*) with Ten Cinders Powder (Pill) (*shí huī săn [wán])*

Heart-Draining Decoction *xiè xīn tāng*

dà huáng	rhubarb	Rhei Rhizoma	12 g.
huáng lián	coptis [root]	Coptidis Rhizoma	9 g.
huáng qín	scutellaria [root]	Scutellariae Radix	9 g.

with:

Ten Cinders Powder (Pill) *shí huī săn (wán)*

dà jì	cirsium	Cirsii Herba seu Radix	9 g.
xiăo jì	cephalanoplos	Cephalanoploris Herba seu Radix	9 g.
hé yè	lotus [leaf]	Nelumbinis Folium	9 g.
cè băi yè	biota [leaf]	Biotae Folium	9 g.
bái máo gēn	imperata [root]	Imperatae Rhizoma	9 g.
qiàn căo gēn	madder [root]	Rubiae Radix	9 g.
shān zhī zĭ	gardenia [fruit]	Gardeniae Fructus	9 g.
dà huáng	rhubarb	Rhei Rhizoma	9 g.
mŭ dān pí	moutan [root bark]	Moutan Radicis Cortex	9 g.
zōng lŭ pí	trachycarpus [stipule fiber]	Trachycarpi Stipulae Fibra	9 g.

Char all the medicinals with "nature-preserving burning," i.e., not past the point that their shape is lost thus preserving their properties; dry-stir in a wok. Grind into a fine powder and administer in 9 g. doses. The prescription may also be administered as a simple decoction.

MODIFICATIONS

In cases manifesting an upward flow of stomach qi with nausea and vomiting, the prescription is modified to harmonize the stomach and move qi downward. Add:

dài zhĕ shí	hematite (extended decoction)	Haematitum	12 g.
xuán fù huā	inula flower (wrapped)	Inulae Flos	6 g.
zhú rú	bamboo shavings	Bambusae Caulis in Taeniam	6 g.

ACUPUNCTURE AND MOXIBUSTION

Main points: Needle with draining.

CV-13	*shàng wăn*
PC-04	*xī mén*
ST-44	*nèi tíng*

2B. VOMITING BLOOD – LIVER FIRE INVADING THE STOMACH

Clinical Manifestations: Vomiting of bright red or purplish blood, bitter taste in the mouth, costal pain, irritability, insomnia, dream-troubled sleep, dark scanty urine.

Tongue: Deep red.

Pulse: Rapid, wiry.

Treatment Method: Drain the liver, clear the stomach, relieve bleeding.

PRESCRIPTION

Gentian Liver-Draining Decoction *lóng dǎn xiè gān tāng*

lóng dǎn cǎo	gentian [root]	Gentianae Radix	6 g.
huáng qín	scutellaria [root]	Scutellariae Radix	9 g.
shān zhī zǐ	gardenia [fruit]	Gardeniae Fructus	9 g.
zé xiè	alisma [tuber]	Alismatis Rhizoma	12 g.
mù tōng	mutong [stem]	Mutong Caulis	9 g.
dāng guī	tangkuei	Angelicae Sinensis Radix	3 g.
chē qián zǐ	plantago [seed] (wrapped)	Plantaginis Semen	9 g.
shēng dì huáng	rehmannia [root]	Rehmanniae Radix	9 g.
	dried/fresh	Exsiccata seu Recens	
chái hú	bupleurum [root]	Bupleuri Radix	6 g.
gān cǎo	licorice [root]	Glycyrrhizae Radix	6 g.

MODIFICATIONS

To cool the blood and relieve bleeding, add:

bái máo gēn	imperata [root]	Imperatae Rhizoma	30 g.
ǒu jié	lotus [root node]	Nelumbinis Rhizomatis Nodus	12 g.
hàn lián cǎo	eclipta	Ecliptae Herba	9 g.

In cases where continual vomiting of blood – accompanied by fullness of the chest and epigastrium and thirst without the desire for drink – indicates blood stasis, the prescription is modified to dispel stasis and relieve bleeding.

huā ruǐ shí	ophicalcite	Ophicalcitum	12 g.
sān qī	notoginseng [root]	Notoginseng Radix	9 g.
	(or, powdered and stirred in, each time 1.5 g.)		

In cases where liver yin is vacuous, the prescription is modified to nourish liver yin.
Add:

gǒu qǐ zǐ	lycium [berry]	Lycii Fructus	9 g.
nǚ zhēn zǐ	ligustrum [fruit]	Ligustri Fructus	12 g.
bái sháo yào	white peony [root]	Paeoniae Radix Alba	12 g.

ACUPUNCTURE AND MOXIBUSTION

Main points: Needle with draining.

ST-19	*bù róng*
ST-34	*liáng qiū*
PC-08	*láo gōng*
LR-03	*tài chōng*
GB-42	*dì wǔ huì*

2C. VOMITING BLOOD – SPLEEN AND STOMACH QI VACUITY

Clinical Manifestations: Vomiting of blood of varying severity over a prolonged period where the vomited blood is pale in color, accompanied by epigastric pain that is alleviated by heat or pressure, loss of appetite, tiredness, fatigue, palpitations, shortness of breath, pale complexion.

Tongue: Pale with white coating.

Pulse: Thready, weak or thready, deep.

Treatment Method: Strengthen the spleen, benefit qi, relieve bleeding.

PRESCRIPTION

Spleen-Returning Decoction *guī pí tāng*

huáng qí	astragalus [root]	Astragali (seu Hedysari) Radix	9 g.
rén shēn	ginseng	Ginseng Radix	9 g.
bái zhú	ovate atractylodes [root]	Atractylodis Ovatae Rhizoma	9 g.
fú shén	root poria	Poria cum Pini Radice	9 g.
lóng yǎn ròu	longan [flesh]	Longanae Arillus	9 g.
suān zǎo rén	spiny jujube [kernel]	Ziziphi Spinosi Semen	9 g.
mù xiāng	saussurea [root]	Saussureae Radix (seu Vladimiriae)	6 g.
dāng guī	tangkuei	Angelicae Sinensis Radix	6 g.
yuǎn zhì	polygala [root]	Polygalae Radix	3 g.
zhì gān cǎo	licorice [root] (honey-fried)	Glycyrrhizae Radix	6 g.
shēng jiāng	fresh ginger [root]	Zingiberis Rhizoma Recens	3 g.
dà zǎo	jujube	Ziziphi Fructus	5 pc.

MODIFICATIONS

To warm the middle burner, strengthen retention and relieve bleeding, add:

xiān hè cǎo	agrimony	Agrimoniae Herba	9 g.
bái jí	bletilla [tuber]	Bletillae Tuber	9 g.
hǎi piāo xiāo	cuttlefish bone	Sepiae seu Sepiellae Os	9 g.
pào jiāng	blast-fried ginger [root]	Zingiberis Rhizoma Tostum	6 g.

In cases where injury to qi has led to injury to yang with symptoms of cold extremities and loose stools, the following prescription is used to warm and supplement spleen yang.

Use:

Center-Rectifying Decoction *lǐ zhōng tāng*

rén shēn	ginseng	Ginseng Radix	12 g.
bái zhú	ovate atractylodes [root]	Atractylodis Ovatae Rhizoma	9 g.
gān jiāng	dried ginger [root]	Zingiberis Rhizoma Exsiccatum	9 g.
zhì gān cǎo	licorice [root] (honey-fried)	Glycyrrhizae Radix	6 g.

plus:

cè bǎi yè	biota [leaf]	Biotae Folium	9 g.
ài yè tàn	mugwort [leaf] (charred)	Artemisiae Argyi Folium Carbonisata	9 g.

If cold is severe, to warm and supplement kidney yang, add:

zhì fù zǐ	aconite [accessory tuber] (processed) (extended decoction)	Aconiti Tuber Laterale Praeparatum	9 g.

ACUPUNCTURE AND MOXIBUSTION

Main points: Needle with supplementation; add moxibustion.

CV-12	*zhōng wǎn*
BL-20	*pí shū*
ST-36	*zú sān lǐ*
SP-01	*yǐn bái*

3A. BLOODY STOOLS – INTESTINAL DAMP-HEAT

Clinical Manifestations: Passage of bright red blood with the stools, difficult bowel movements or loose stools, intermittent abdominal pain, bitter taste in the mouth.

Tongue: Yellow slimy coating.

Pulse: Slippery, rapid.

Treatment Method: Clear heat, disinhibit dampness, relieve bleeding.

PRESCRIPTION
Sanguisorba Powder *dì yú sǎn*

dì yú	sanguisorba [root]	Sanguisorbae Radix	12 g.
qiàn cǎo gēn	madder [root]	Rubiae Radix	12 g.
huáng qín	scutellaria [root]	Scutellariae Radix	9 g.
huáng lián	coptis [root]	Coptidis Rhizoma	9 g.
shān zhī zǐ	gardenia [fruit]	Gardeniae Fructus	9 g.
fú líng	poria	Poria	12 g.

MODIFICATIONS

With the passage of a large quantity of bright red blood just preceding the stools, accompanied by swelling and pain of the anus, red tongue and rapid pulse, intestinal wind *(chàng fēng)* is indicated. The prescription is modified to dispel wind, clear heat, cool the blood and relieve bleeding.

Add:

Sophora Flower Powder *huái-huā sǎn*

huái huā	sophora [flower]	Sophorae Flos	12 g.
cè bǎi yè	biota [leaf]	Biotae Folium	9 g.
jīng jiè suì tàn	schizonepeta [spike] (charred)	Schizonepetae Flos Carbonisatum	9 g.
zhǐ ké	bitter orange [fruit]	Aurantii Fructus	9 g.

In cases where a large amount of blood has been lost, depleting both yin and blood, with damp-heat not completely dispelled, repletion and vacuity should be addressed simultaneously.

Use:

Carriage-Halting Pills *zhù chē wán*

huáng lián	coptis [root]	Coptidis Rhizoma	9 g.
dāng guī	tangkuei	Angelicae Sinensis Radix	6 g.
ē jiāo	ass hide glue (dissolved and stirred in)	Asini Corii Gelatinum	9 g.
pào jiāng	blast-fried ginger [root]	Zingiberis Rhizoma Tostum	1.5 g.

ACUPUNCTURE AND MOXIBUSTION

Main points: Needle with draining.

GV-01	*cháng qiáng*
BL-32	*cì liáo*
BL-57	*chéng shān*
ST-37	*shàng jù xū*
BL-25	*dà cháng shū*

3B. BLOODY STOOLS – SPLEEN AND STOMACH VACUITY COLD

Clinical Manifestations: Passage of dark purplish or even black-colored blood with the stools, dull abdominal pain, preference for warm liquids, lusterless complexion, tiredness, disinclination to speak, loose stools.

Tongue: Pale with white coating.

Pulse: Weak, thready.

Treatment Method: Strengthen the spleen, warm the middle burner, relieve bleeding.

PRESCRIPTION

Yellow Earth Decoction *huáng tǔ tāng*

fú lóng gān	oven earth (wrapped) (extended decoction)	Terra Flava Usta	30 g.
shú dì huáng	cooked rehmannia [root]	Rehmanniae Radix Conquita	9 g.
bái zhú	ovate atractylodes [root]	Atractylodis Ovatae Rhizoma	9 g.
zhì fù zǐ	aconite [accessory tuber] (processed) (extended decoction)	Aconiti Tuber Laterale Praeparatum	9 g.
ē jiāo	ass hide glue	Asini Corii Gelatinum	9 g.
huáng qín	scutellaria [root]	Scutellariae Radix	9 g.
gān cǎo	licorice [root]	Glycyrrhizae Radix	9 g.

MODIFICATIONS

To relieve bleeding, add astringent medicines such as:

bái jí	bletilla [tuber]	Bletillae Tuber	9 g.
hǎi piāo xiāo	cuttlefish [bone]	Sepiae seu Sepiellae Os	9 g.

In cases of uncontrolled bleeding with signs of blood stasis, the prescription is modified to dispel stasis and relieve bleeding.
Add:

sān qī	notoginseng [root] (or, powdered and stirred in, each time 1.5 g.)	Notoginseng Radix	9 g.
huā ruǐ shí	ophicalcite (extended decoction)	Ophicalcitum	12 g.

In cases of severe yang vacuity, with aversion to cold and cold extremities, the prescription is modified to warm yang and relieve bleeding.
Add:

pào jiāng	blast-fried ginger [root]	Zingiberis Rhizoma Tostum	6 g.
lù jiǎo shuāng	degelatinated deer antler	Cervi Cornu Degelatinum	9 g.
ài yè tàn	mugwort [leaf] (charred)	Artemisiae Argyi Folium Carbonisatus	9 g.

ACUPUNCTURE AND MOXIBUSTION

Main points: Needle with supplementation; add moxibustion.

CV-04	*guān yuán*
ST-36	*zú sān lǐ*
GV-20	*bǎi huì*
SP-03	*tài bái*
BL-35	*huì yáng*

4A. URINARY BLEEDING – YIN VACUITY WITH EFFULGENT FIRE

Clinical Manifestations: Dark scanty urine that contains blood, no apparent urethral pain, dizziness, tinnitus, tidal fever, night sweating, tiredness, flushed cheeks, weakness and aching of the lower back and knees.

Tongue: Red with little coating.

Pulse: Thready, rapid.

Treatment Method: Nourish yin, clear fire, cool the blood, relieve bleeding.

PRESCRIPTION

Anemarrhena, Phellodendron and Rehmannia Decoction (Pill)
zhī bǎi dì huáng tāng (wán)

shú dì huáng	cooked rehmannia [root]	Rehmanniae Radix Conquita	24 g.
shān zhū yú	cornus [fruit]	Corni Fructus	12 g.
shān yào	dioscorea [root]	Dioscoreae Rhizoma	12 g.
zé xiè	alisma [tuber]	Alismatis Rhizoma	9 g.
fú líng	poria	Poria	9 g.
mǔ dān pí	moutan [root bark]	Moutan Radicis Cortex	9 g.
zhī mǔ	anemarrhena [root]	Anemarrhenae Rhizoma	9 g.
huáng bǎi	phellodendron [bark]	Phellodendri Cortex	9 g.

MODIFICATIONS

To cool the blood and relieve bleeding, add:

hàn lián cǎo	eclipta	Ecliptae Herba	12 g.
dà jì	cirsium	Cirsii Herba seu Radix	9 g.
xiǎo jì	cephalanoplos	Cephalanoploris Herba seu Radix	9 g.
pú huáng	typha pollen (wrapped)	Typhae Pollen	9 g.

ACUPUNCTURE AND MOXIBUSTION

Main points: Needle with draining.

CV-04	*guān yuán*
KI-10	*yīn gǔ*
KI-03	*tài xī*
LR-01	*dà dūn*

4B. URINARY BLEEDING – EXUBERANT HEART FIRE

Clinical Manifestations: Dark yellow urine containing bright red blood that is generally not accompanied by pain (although a slight distending pain or burning pain may be present in some cases), irritability, thirst, oral ulcers, restless sleep.

Tongue: Redness of the tip.

Pulse: Rapid.

Treatment Method: Clear the heart, drain fire, cool the blood, relieve bleeding.

PRESCRIPTION

Cephalanoplos Drink *xiǎo jì yǐn zǐ*

shēng dì huáng	rehmannia [root] dried/fresh	Rehmanniae Radix Exsiccata seu Recens	30 g.
xiǎo jì	cephalanoplos	Cephalanoploris Herba seu Radix	15 g.
mù tōng	mutong [stem]	Mutong Caulis	6 g.
huá shí	talcum (wrapped)	Talcum	15 g.
chǎo pú huáng	typha pollen (charred)	Typhae Pollen Carbonisatum	9 g.
dàn zhú yè	bamboo [leaf]	Lophatheri Folium	9 g.
ǒu jié	lotus [root node]	Nelumbinis Rhizomatis Nodus	9 g.
dāng guī	tangkuei	Angelicae Sinensis Radix	9 g.
shān zhī zǐ	gardenia [fruit]	Gardeniae Fructus	9 g.
zhì gān cǎo	licorice [root] (honey-fried)	Glycyrrhizae Radix	6 g.

<u>**MODIFICATIONS**</u>

To dispel stasis and relieve bleeding, add:

hŭ pò mò	amber (powder) (stirred in)	Succinum Pulvis	3 g.

ACUPUNCTURE AND MOXIBUSTION

Main points: Needle with draining.

CV-04	*guān yuán*
HT-08	*shào fŭ*
PC-07	*dà líng*
SP-06	*sān yīn jiāo*
SP-10	*xuè hăi*

4C. URINARY BLEEDING – SPLEEN AND KIDNEY VACUITY

Clinical Manifestations: Frequent painless urination, passage of pale red urine, loss of appetite, tiredness, sallow complexion, lower backache, dizziness, tinnitus.

Tongue: Pale with white coating.

Pulse: Weak, forceless.

Treatment Method: Supplement the spleen and kidney, strengthen retention, relieve bleeding.

PRESCRIPTION

Combine Center-Supplementing Qi-Boosting Decoction (*bŭ zhōng yì qì tāng*) with Matchless Dioscorea Pill *(wú bǐ sān yào wán)*.

Center-Supplementing Qi-Boosting Decoction *bŭ zhōng yì qì tāng*

huáng qí	astragalus [root]	Astragali (seu Hedysari) Radix	15 g.
rén shēn	ginseng	Ginseng Radix	9 g.
bái zhú	ovate atractylodes [root]	Atractylodis Ovatae Rhizoma	9 g.
dāng guī	tangkuei	Angelicae Sinensis Radix	9 g.
chén pí	tangerine [peel]	Citri Exocarpium	6 g.
shēng má	cimicifuga [root]	Cimicifugae Rhizoma	3 g.
chái hú	bupleurum [root]	Bupleuri Radix	3 g.
zhì gān căo	licorice [root] (honey-fried)	Glycyrrhizae Radix	6 g.

with:

Matchless Dioscorea Pill *wú bǐ shān yào wán*

shān yào	dioscorea [root]	Dioscoreae Rhizoma	30 g.
ròu cōng róng	cistanche [stem]	Cistanches Caulis	15 g.
shú dì huáng	cooked rehmannia [root]	Rehmanniae Radix Conquita	12 g.
shān zhū yú	cornus [fruit]	Corni Fructus	12 g.
fú shén	root poria	Poria cum Pini Radice	9 g.
tù sī zǐ	cuscuta [seed]	Cuscutae Semen	9 g.
wŭ wèi zǐ	schisandra [berry]	Schisandrae Fructus	6 g.
chì shí zhī	halloysite (wrapped)	Halloysitum Rubrum	12 g.
bā jǐ tiān	morinda [root]	Morindae Radix	12 g.
zé xiè	alisma [tuber]	Alismatis Rhizoma	9 g.
dù zhòng	eucommia [bark]	Eucommiae Cortex	12 g.
niú xī	achyranthes [root]	Achyranthis Bidentatae Radix	9 g.

MODIFICATIONS

In cases of prolonged urinary bleeding, the prescription is modified to strengthen retention and relieve bleeding. Add:

duàn mǔ lì	oyster shell (calcined)	Ostreae Concha Calcinatum	15 g.
duàn lóng gǔ	dragon bone (calcined)	Mastodi Ossis Fossilia Calcinatum	15 g.
jīn yīng zǐ	Cherokee rose [fruit]	Rosae Laevigatae Fructus	9 g.

ACUPUNCTURE AND MOXIBUSTION

Main points: Needle with supplementation; add moxibustion.

BL-20	*pí shū*
BL-23	*shèn shū*
ST-36	*zú sān lǐ*
CV-04	*guān yuán*
SP-03	*tài bái*

5A. SUBCUTANEOUS BLEEDING – BLOOD HEAT

Clinical Manifestations: Presence of small dark purple points or patches on the skin that are sometimes accompanied by bleeding of the nose or gums, bloody stools or urinary bleeding. Accompanying symptoms can also include fever, thirst and constipation.

Tongue: Red with yellow coating.

Pulse: Rapid, wiry.

Treatment Method: Clear heat, resolve toxins, cool the blood, relieve bleeding.

PRESCRIPTION

Rhinoceros Horn and Rehmannia Decoction *xī jiǎo dì huáng tāng*

xī jiǎo	rhinoceros horn* (powdered and stirred in)	Rhinocerotis Cornu	3 g.
shēng dì huáng	rehmannia [root] dried/fresh	Rehmanniae Radix Exsiccata seu Recens	30 g.
bái sháo yào	white peony [root]	Paeoniae Radix Alba	12 g.
mǔ dān pí	moutan [root bark]	Moutan Radicis Cortex	9 g.

*Use of *xī jiǎo* (rhinoceros horn) is prohibited in North America by the endangered species law. Water Buffalo Horn *(shuǐ niú jiǎo)* may be substituted. Increase the dose to 15 g., extended decoction.)

MODIFICATIONS

In cases of exuberant heat-toxin accompanied by fever and extensive subcutaneous bleeding, the prescription is modified to clear heat, cool the blood and relieve bleeding. Add:

shí gāo	gypsum (extended decoction)	Gypsum	30 g.
lóng dǎn cǎo	gentian [root]	Gentianae Radix	9 g.
zǐ cǎo	puccoon	Lithospermi, Macrotomiae, seu Onosmatis Radix	9 g.

plus the prepared medicine, PURPLE SNOW ELIXIR *(zǐ xuě dān)*.

For a stronger hemostatic effect, simultaneously administer:

Ten Cinders Powder (Pill) *shí huī sǎn (wán)*

dà jì	cirsium	Cirsii Herba seu Radix	9 g.
xiǎo jì	cephalanoplos	Cephalanoploris Herba seu Radix	9 g.
hé yè	lotus [leaf]	Nelumbinis Folium	9 g.
cè bǎi yè	biota [leaf]	Biotae Folium	9 g.
bái máo gēn	imperata [root]	Imperatae Rhizoma	9 g.
qiàn cǎo gēn	madder [root]	Rubiae Radix	9 g.
shān zhī zǐ	gardenia [fruit]	Gardeniae Fructus	9 g.
dà huáng	rhubarb	Rhei Rhizoma	9 g.
mǔ dān pí	moutan [root bark]	Moutan Radicis Cortex	9 g.
zōng lǘ pí	trachycarpus	Trachycarpi Stipulae Fibra	9 g.

Char all the medicinals with nature-preserving burning, i.e., not past the point where their shape is lost to preserve their properties by dry-stirring in a wok. Grind into a fine powder and administer in 9 g. doses. The prescription may also be administered as a decoction.)

In cases where heat evil has obstructed the channels and connections causing pain and swelling of the joints, the prescription is modified to clear the channels and connections, disperse swelling and relieve pain.

Add:

qín jiāo	large gentian [root]	Gentianae Macrophyllae Radix	9 g.
mù guā	chaenomeles [fruit]	Chaenomelis Fructus	9 g.
sāng zhī	mulberry [twig]	Mori Ramulus	15 g.

ACUPUNCTURE AND MOXIBUSTION

Main points: Needle with draining.

GV-14	*dà zhuī*
LI-11	*qū chí*
SP-10	*xuè hǎi*
SP-06	*sān yīn jiāo*
BL-17	*gé shū*

5B. SUBCUTANEOUS BLEEDING – YIN VACUITY WITH EFFULGENT FIRE

Clinical Manifestations: Intermittent subcutaneous bleeding, often accompanied by bleeding of the nose and gums or heavy menstrual bleeding, flushed cheeks, vexing heat in the five hearts, tidal fever and night sweating in some cases.

Tongue: Red with little coating.

Pulse: Rapid, thready.

Treatment Method: Nourish yin, clear fire, cool the blood, relieve bleeding.

PRESCRIPTION

Madder Root Powder *qiàn gēn sǎn*

qiàn cǎo gēn	madder [root]	Rubiae Radix	12 g.
huáng qín	scutellaria [root]	Scutellariae Radix	9 g.
ē jiāo	ass hide glue (dissolved)	Asini Corii Gelatinum	9 g.
cè bǎi yè	biota [leaf]	Biotae Folium	12 g.
shēng dì huáng	rehmannia [root] dried/fresh	Rehmanniae Radix Exsiccata seu Recens	30 g.
gān cǎo	licorice [root]	Glycyrrhizae Radix	6 g.

MODIFICATIONS

In cases of severe yin vacuity, the prescription is modified to nourish yin and clear heat.

Add:

xuán shēn	scrophularia [root]	Scrophulariae Radix	9 g.
guī bǎn	tortoise plastron (extended decoction)	Testudinis Plastrum	30 g.
nǚ zhēn zǐ	ligustrum [fruit]	Ligustri Fructus	12 g.
hàn lián cǎo	eclipta	Ecliptae Herba	12 g.

In cases where kidney yin is vacuous but fire is not marked, with symptoms of weak aching lower back and knees, dizziness, fatigue, vexing heat in the five hearts, red tongue with little coating and thready deep rapid pulse, the prescription is changed to nourish yin, cool the blood and relieve bleeding.

Use:

Six-Ingredient Rehmannia Pill *liù wèi dì huáng wán*

shú dì huáng	cooked rehmannia [root]	Rehmanniae Radix Conquita	24 g.
shān zhū yú	cornus [fruit]	Corni Fructus	12 g.
shān yào	dioscorea [root]	Dioscoreae Rhizoma	12 g.
zé xiè	alisma [tuber]	Alismatis Rhizoma	9 g.
fú líng	poria	Poria	9 g.
mǔ dān pí	moutan [root bark]	Moutan Radicis Cortex	9 g.

Add:

qiàn cǎo gēn	madder [root]	Rubiae Radix	12 g.
zǐ cǎo	puccoon	Lithospermi, Macrotomiae, seu Onosmatis Radix	9 g.
xiān hè cǎo	agrimony	Agrimoniae Herba	9 g.

ACUPUNCTURE AND MOXIBUSTION

Main points: Needle with even supplementation, even draining.

CV-04	*guān yuán*
BL-23	*shèn shū*
SP-06	*sān yīn jiāo*
KI-02	*rán gǔ*
KI-03	*tài xī*

5C. SUBCUTANEOUS BLEEDING – QI FAILING TO SECURE THE BLOOD

Clinical Manifestations: Extended history of recurrent subcutaneous bleeding, tiredness, fatigue, dizziness, pale or sallow complexion, poor appetite.

Tongue: Pale.

Pulse: Weak, thready.

Treatment Method: Supplement qi, secure the blood.

PRESCRIPTION

Spleen-Returning Decoction *guī pí tāng*

huáng qí	astragalus [root]	Astragali (seu Hedysari) Radix	9 g.
rén shēn	ginseng	Ginseng Radix	9 g.
bái zhú	ovate atractylodes [root]	Atractylodis Ovatae Rhizoma	9 g.
fú shén	root poria	Poria cum Pini Radice	9 g.
lóng yǎn ròu	longan [flesh]	Longanae Arillus	9 g.
suān zǎo rén	spiny jujube [kernel]	Ziziphi Spinosi Semen	9 g.
mù xiāng	saussurea [root]	Saussureae Radix (seu Vladimiriae)	6 g.
dāng guī	tangkuei	Angelicae Sinensis Radix	6 g.
yuǎn zhì	polygala [root]	Polygalae Radix	3 g.
zhì gān cǎo	licorice [root] (honey-fried)	Glycyrrhizae Radix	6 g.
shēng jiāng	fresh ginger [root]	Zingiberis Rhizoma Recens	3 g.
dà zǎo	jujube	Ziziphi Fructus	5 pc.

MODIFICATIONS

To reinforce the hemostatic effect, add:

xiān hè cǎo	agrimony	Agrimoniae Herba	12 g.
dì yú	sanguisorba [root]	Sanguisorbae Radix	9 g.
pú huáng	typha pollen (wrapped)	Typhae Pollen	9 g.
qiàn cǎo gēn	madder [root]	Rubiae Radix	9 g.

In cases where kidney qi is insufficient, with weakness and aching of the lower back and knees, the prescription is modified to supplement kidney qi.

Add:

shān zhū yú	cornus [fruit]	Corni Fructus	12 g.
tù sī zǐ	cuscuta [seed]	Cuscutae Semen	12 g.
xù duàn	dipsacus [root]	Dipsaci Radix	12 g.

ACUPUNCTURE AND MOXIBUSTION

Main points: Needle with supplementation; add moxibustion.

BL-20	*pí shū*
BL-21	*wèi shū*
CV-04	*guān yuán*
ST-36	*zú sān lǐ*
BL-17	*gé shū*
SP-06	*sān yīn jiāo*
BL-31, BL-32, BL-33, BL-34	*bā liáo* (ginger moxibustion without needle)
GV-03	*yāo yáng guān* (ginger moxibustion without needle)

ALTERNATE THERAPEUTIC METHODS

1. Ear Acupuncture

Main points: Points corresponding to the viscera and bowels and sensory organs that are exhibiting pathological changes; plus Adrenal, Subcortex.

Method: Select two to three points per session and retain needles ten to twenty minutes. Treat once daily.

REMARKS

To differentiate bleeding patterns, the first emphasis should be on the site of the bleeding and the viscera and bowels involved. Then, a clear differentiation between repletion of heat evil and vacuity of yin or qi should be determined. From a clinical standpoint, patterns of heat are more frequent than those of cold. In addition to the site and etiology of the pathological change, treatment of bleeding patterns should be governed by the repletion and vacuity and severity of the patient's condition.

The treatment of bleeding patterns should exhibit the three fundamental principles inherent in "treatment of fire," "treatment of qi," and "treatment of blood." Treatment of fire includes clearing repletion heat and draining repletion fire, as well as moistening yin and reducing vacuity fire. Treatment of qi includes both clearing and rectifying the replete qi, plus supplementing and benefiting vacuous qi. The treatment of the blood involves controlling the bleeding, by cooling the blood to relieve bleeding, or containing the blood or quickening the blood to stop bleeding.

Concerning medicinals, those with ascending characteristics are contraindicated in cases of bleeding from the upper orifices when it is appropriate to add small amounts of downbearing medicinals such as achyranthes root *(tŭ niú xī)* or hematite *(dài zhě shí)* (with an extended decoction). Similarly, when the bleeding is from the lower orifices, medicinals with descending characteristics are contraindicated and small amounts of upbearing medicinals such as charred schizonepeta *(jīng jiè tàn)*, cimicifuga *(shēng má)* and astragalus *(huáng qí)* are appropriate.

When the bleeding is chronic, treat the root of illness, or treat the root and the branch simultaneously. In cases of acute bleeding, the loss of blood is a high priority and treatment should be focused on the branch symptoms. When qi is lost with the blood, supplementation of qi becomes primary to prevent the critical patterns of qi syncope.

As for cases of bleeding complicated by blood stasis, prescriptions should include blood-quickening stasis-transforming medicines to prevent further blood stasis caused by homeostatic medicinals.

GLOSSARY[1]

abdominal masses: *zhēng jiǎ*

acute fright wind: *jí jīng fēng*

acute jaundice: *jí huáng*

abduct stagnation: *dǎo zhì*

absorb qi: *nà qì*

acid regurgitation: fàn suān

arouse the spirit: *xǐng shén*

ascendant hyperactivity of liver yang: *gān yáng shàng kàng*

assist yang: *zhù yáng*

astringe the essence: *sè jīng*

aversion to cold: *wù hán*

binding depression of phlegm and qi: *tán qì yù jié*

binding depression of phlegm-fire: *tán huǒ yù jié*

blockage and obstruction by wind phlegm: *fēng tán bì zǔ*

blood dryness: *xuè zaò*

blood inversion: xuè jué

blood stasis: *xuè yū*

blood vacuity: *xuè xū*

blue-eye blindness: *qīng máng*

boost qi: *yì qì*

boost qi and secure desertion : *yì qì gù tuō*

boost the blood: *yì xuè*

boost the essence: *yì jīng*

boost the eyes: *yì mù*

boost the kidney: *yì shèn*

boost the stomach: *yì wèi*

branch: *biāo*

break qi: *pò qì*

break stasis: *pò yū*

brighten the eyes: *míng mù*

calm the liver: *píng gān*

calm wheezing: *píng chuǎn*

channel connection stroke: *zhòng jīng luò*

channels and connections: *jīng luò*

chronic fright wind: *màn jīng fēng*

clamoring stomach: *cáo zá*

clear fire: *qīng huǒ*

clear heat and disinhibit dampness: *qīng lì shī rè*

clear heat and resolve toxin: *qīng rè jiě dú*

clear summerheat and transform dampness: *qīng shǔ huà shī*

clear the heart: *qīng xīn*

clear the interior: *qīng lǐ*

clear the liver: *qīng gān*

clear the lung: *qīng fèi*

clear the pharynx: *qīng yān*

clear the stomach: *qīng wèi*

clear yang: *qīng yáng*

cold constipation: *hán bì*

cold-dampness: *hán shī*

cold-dampness dysentery: *hán shī lì*

cold evil: *hán xié*

cold malaria: *hán nüè*

cold-phlegm: *hán tán*

congealed cold: *hán níng*

congealed phlegm: *tán níng*

congestion by phlegm-turbidity: *tán zhuó yōng sè*

congestion of qi and phlegm: *tán qì yù jié*

complicated pattern: *nì zhèng*

construction aspect: *yín fèn*

construction qi: *yíng qì*

consume qi: *haò qì*

contain the blood: *shè xuè*

contain the essence: *shè jīng*

cool the blood: *liáng xuè*

correct qi: *zhèng qì*

counterflow ascent of lung qi: *fèi qì shàng nì*

---

[1]For additional reference, please refer to Wiseman, N. *Glossary of Chinese Medical Terms and Acupuncture Points.* Brookline, MA: Paradigm Publications, 1990. See also Wiseman, N. *English-Chinese Chinese-English Dictionary of Chinese Medicine.* Hunan: Hunan Science and Technology Press, 1995. See also Wiseman, N. *Clinical Dictionary of Chinese Medicine.* Brookline, MA: Paradigm Publications, 1997.

counterflow ascent of stomach qi: *wèi qì shàng nì*

course and free the channels and connections: *shū tōng jīng luò*

course the liver: *shū gān*

course wind: *shū fēng*

course wind and moisten dryness: *shū fēng rùn zaò*

crimson (tongue body): *jiàng*

damage the blood: *shāng xuè*

damage to liquid: *shāng jīn*

damp-heat: *shī rè*

damp-heat dysentery: *shī rè lì*

dampness: *shī*

dampness evil: *shī xié*

dark (tongue body): *àn*

dark purple (tongue body): *zǐ àn*

debilitation of life-gate fire: *mìng mén huǒ shuāi*

deep (pulse): *chén*

defense qi: *wèi qì*

depletion of yin: *yīn kuī*

desertion pattern: *tuō zhèng*

devitalization of yang: *yáng bú zhèn*

diffuse stagnation: *xuān zhì*

diffuse the lung: *xuān fèi*

disharmony of the liver and spleen: *gān pí bù hé*

disinclination to speak: *lǎn yán*

disinhibit dampness: *lì shī*

disinhibit the pharynx: *lì yān*

disinhibit the urine: *lì niaò*

disinhibit water and disperse swelling: *lì shuǐ xiāo zhǒng*

dispel cold: *qū hán*

dispel dampness: *qū shī*

dispel evil: *qū xié*

dispel jaundice: *qū huáng*

dispel phlegm: *qū tán*

dispel stasis: *qū yū*

dispel turbidity: *qū zhuó*

dispel water: *qū shuǐ*

dispel wind: *qū fēng*

disperse distension: *xiāo zhàng*

disperse food : *xiāo shí*

disperse stagnation: *xiāo zhì*

disperse swelling: *xiāo zhǒng*

disperse toxin: *xiāo dú*

disperse warts: *xiāo yóu*

disruption of the stomach by liver qi: *gān qì fàn wèi*

dissipate binds: *sàn jié*

dissipate cold: *sàn hán*

downbear fire: *jiàng huǒ*

downbear qi: *jiàng qì*

downpour of damp-heat: *shī rè xià zhù*

drain: *xiè*

drain fire: *xiè huǒ*

drain heat: *xiè rè*

drain heat and resolve toxin: *xiè rè jié dú*

drain the liver: *xiè gān*

drain the lung: *xiè fèi*

draining: *xiè fǎ*

dry dampness: *zaò shī*

dry evil: *zaò xié*

dryness heat: *zaò rè*

eclampsia: *zǐ xián*

effulgent fire: *huǒ wàng*

effuse the rash: *fā zhěn*

eliminate dampness: *chú shī*

eliminate heat: *chú rè*

eliminate phlegm: *chú tán*

eliminate vexation: *chú fán*

emotional depression: *qíng zhì yù jié*

enduring loss of voice: *jiǔ yīn*

enlarged (tongue body): *pàng dà*

epidemic dysentery: *yì dú lì*

essence: *jīng*

essential qi: *jīng qì*

even supplementation, even draining: *píng bǔ píng xiè*

evil: *xié*

exhaustion of kidney yang: *shèn yáng shuāi jié*

expel stones: *pái shí*

expel toxin: *pái dú*

expel wind: *qū fēng*

expel worms: *qū chóng*

expulsion of toxin: *pái dú*

external evil: *waì xié*

external evil attack: *waì gǎn*

external wind: *waì fēng*

extinguish wind: *xī fēng*

exuberance of liver fire: *gān huǒ kàng shèng*

exuberant fire: *huǒ shèng*

exuberant heat: *rè shèng*

exuberant lung heat congestion: *fèi rè yōng shèng*

faint (pulse): *wēi*

fasting dysentery: *jìn kǒu lì*

fearful throbbing: *zhēng chōng*

fire evil: *huǒ xié*

fire toxin: *huǒ dú*

flat wart: *biǎn píng yóu*

floating (pulse): *fú*

fluids: *jīn yè*

flush phlegm: *dí tán*

food accumulation and stagnation: *yīn shí jī zhì*

food collection and stagnation: *yīn shí tíng zhì*

food inversion: *shí jué*

food stasis: *shí yū*

forceful (pulse): *yǒu lì*

forceless (pulse): *wú lì*

fortify the spleen: *jiàn pí*

forty-eight hour malaria: *jiān rì nüè*

foster yin and subdue yang: *yù yīn qián yáng*

free and disinhibit the urine: *tōng lì xiǎo biàn*

free menstruation: *tōng jīng*

free the connections: *tōng luò*

free the milk: *tōng rǔ*

free the orifices: *tōng qiào*

free the stool: *tōng biàn*

free yang: *tōng yáng*

frenetic vacuity fire: *xū huǒ wàng dòng*

gangrene: *tuō gǔ jū*

generate liquid: *shēng jīn*

glossy (tongue coating): *huá*

gray (tongue coating): *huī*

grimy (tongue coating): *gòu*

half exterior, half interior: *bàn biǎo bàn lǐ*

harmonize the connections: *hé luò*

harmonize the stomach: *hé wèi*

heat brewing in the stomach and spleen: *pí wèi yùn rè*

heat constipation: *rè bì*

heat evil: *rè xié*

heat strangury: *rè lín*

heat-toxin: *rè dú*

hidden (pulse): *fú*

hindered passage gives rise to pain: *bù tōng zé tòng*

hollow (pulse): *kōu*

humor: *yè*

imbalance between construction and defense qi: *yín wèi bù hé*

infantile convulsions: *xiǎo ér jīng fēng*

Infantile Palsy: *xiǎo ér má bì zhèng*

infantile malnutrition: *xiǎo ér gān jī*

insufficient liver yin: *gān yīn bù zú*

intermittent chronic dysentery: *jiān xiē lì*

internal disruption: *nèi shāng*

internal exuberance of phlegm-fire: *tán huǒ nèi shèng*

internal wind: *nèi fēng*

intestinal abscess: *cháng yōng*

intestinal wind: *cháng fēng*

invigorate yang: *zhuàng yáng*

kill worms: *shā chóng*

large (pulse): *dà*

life-gate: *mìng mén*

life-gate fire: *mìng mén zhī huǒ*

liquid: *jīn*

little (tongue coating): *shǎo*

liver and stomach disharmony: *gān wèi bù hé*

liver depression transforming into fire: *gān yù huà huǒ*

liver wind stirring internally: *gān fēng nèi dòng*

malarial evils: *nüè xié*

mammary abscess: *rǔ yōng*

mental depression: *jīng shén yì yù*

miasmic malaria: *zhàng nüè*

moisten dryness: *rùn zào*

moisten the intestines: *rùn cháng*

moisten the lung: *rùn fèi*

moisten the throat: *rùn hóu*

mother of malaria: *nüè mǔ*

move dampness: *xíng shī*

move qi: *xíng qì*

move stagnation: *xíng zhì*

move the spleen: *yùn pí*

move water: *xíng shuǐ*

move water and disinhibit the orifices: *xíng shuǐ lì qiào*

nourish the blood: *yǎng xuè*

nourish the essence: *yǎng jīng*

nourish the heart: *yǎng xīn*

nourish the liver: *yǎng gān*

nourish the stomach: *yǎng wèi*

nourish yin: *yǎng yīn*

obstruction and stagnation of channels and connections: *jīng luò zǔ zhì*

obstruction by dampness: *shī zǔ*

offensive precipitation: *gōng xià*

open the orifices: *kāi qiaò*

open the voice: *kāi yīn*

oppression in the chest: *xiōng mèn*

outthrust the exterior: *tòu biǎo*

pale (tongue body): *cāng bái*

pattern, patterns: *zhèng*

pecled (tongue coating): *bō*

phlegm: *tán*

phlegm-dampness: *tán shī*

phlegm depression: *tán yù*

phlegm-fire: *tán huǒ*

phlegm-heat: *tán rè*

phlegm inversion: *tán jué*

phlegm-rheum: *tán yǐn*

phlegm stagnation: *tán zhì*

phlegm-turbidity: *tán zhuó*

postpartum syncope: *chǎn hòu xuè yùn*

purple (tongue body): *zǐ*

qi blockage: *qì bì*

qi constipation: *qǐ bǐ*

qi counterflow: *qì nì*

qi desertion: *qì tuō*

qi deserting with the blood: *qì suí xuè tuō*

qi failing to contain the blood: *qì bú shè xuè*

qi inversion: *qì jué*

qi stagnation: *qì zhì*

qi vacuity: *qì xū*

qi vacuity with prolapse: *qì xū xià xiàn*

quicken the blood: *huó xuè*

quicken the connections: *huó luò*

quiet roundworms: *ān huí*

quiet the fetus: *ān tāi*

quiet the spirit: *ān shén*

quiet the spirit and stabilize the mind: *ān shén dìng zhì*

raise the fallen: *shēng xiàn*

raise the yang and boost qi: *shēng yáng yì qì*

rapid (pulse): *shuò*

rapid, irregularly interrupted (pulse): *cù*

rectify qi: *lǐ qì*

rectify the spleen: *lǐ pí*

red (tongue body): *hóng*

regularly intermittent (pulse): *jié dai*

regulate and harmonize construction and defense: *tiáo hé yíng wèi*

regulate and rectify the chong and ren: *tiáo lǐ chōng rèn*

regulate menstruation: *tiáo jīng*

regulate qi: *tiáo qì*

relieve bleeding: *zhǐ xuè*

relieve cough: *zhǐ ké*

relieve diarrhea: *zhǐ xiè*

relieve dysentery: *zhǐ lì*

relieve hiccough: *zhǐ è*

relieve itching: *zhǐ yǎng*

relieve malaria: *zhǐ nüè*

relieve pain: *zhǐ tòng*

relieve sweating: *zhǐ hàn*

relieve tetany: *zhǐ*

relieve thirst: *zhǐ kě*

relieve vaginal discharge: *zhǐ dai*

relieve vomiting: *zhǐ ǒu*

replete (pulse): *shí*

repletion: *shí*

repletion fire: *shí huǒ*

repress the liver: *yì gān*

resolve depression: *jiě yù*

resolve summerheat: *jiě shǔ*

resolve the exterior: *jiě biǎo*

resolve toxin: *jiě dú*

restore the pulse: *fù mai*

restrain acid: *zhì suān*

return the milk: *huí rǔ*

return yang: *huí yáng*

rheum: *yǐn*

root: *běn*

root vacuity with branch repletion: *běn xū biāo shí*

rough (pulse): *sè*

roundworm inversion: *huí jué*

save yin: *jiù yīn*

sea of blood: *xuè hǎi*

seasonal heat-toxin: *shí xíng rè dú*

secure and astringe the urine: *gù sè xiǎo biàn*

secure the blood: *gù xuè*

secure the essence: *gù jīng*

secure the exterior: *gù biǎo*

secure the intestines: *gù cháng*

secure the kidney: *gù shèn*

secure qi and contain the blood: *gù qì shè xuè*

secure yang qi desertion: *gù tuō yáng qì*

settle the heart: *zhèn xīn*

settle the liver and extinguish wind: *zhèn gān xí fēng*

settle, tranquilize and quiet the spirit: *zhèn jìng ān shén*

seventy-two hour malaria: *sān rì nüè*

six depressions: *liù yù*

slimy (tongue coating): *nì*

slippery (pulse): *huá*

slow (pulse): *chí*

soft (tongue body): *nèn*

soft (pulse): *huá*

soften hardness: *ruǎn jiān*

soggy (pulse): *rú*

soothe the liver: *shū gān*

spirit: *shén*

spleen failing to manage the blood: *pí bù tǒng xuè*

spleen qi vacuity: *pí qì xū*

stabilize epilepsy: *dìng xián*

stagnation of liver qi: *gān qì yū jié*

stagnation of spleen qi and liver blood: *gān pí xuè yū*

stasis macules on the tongue (tongue body): *shé shàng yū bān*

static blood obstruction and stagnation: *yū xuè zǔ zhì*

static blood: *yū xuè*

static heat: *yū rè*

static qi: *qì yū*

stomach qi counterflow: *wèi qì shàng nì*

stone strangury: *shí lín*

subdue yang: *qián yáng*

sudden loss of voice: *baò yīn*

summerheat: *shǔ*

summerheat-dampness: *shǔ shī*

summerheat inversion: *shǔ jué*

supplement: *bǔ*

supplement and boost kidney yin: *bǔ yì shèn yīn*

supplement qi: *bǔ qì*

supplement the blood: *bǔ xuè*

supplement the kidney to promote qi absorption: *bǔ shèn nà qì*

supplement the kidney: *bǔ shèn*

supplement the spleen: *bǔ pí*

supplementation: *bǔ fǎ*

support the spleen: *fú pí*

surging (pulse): *hóng*

tardy (pulse): *huǎn*

taxation: *láo*

taxation malaria: *láo nüè*

taxation strangury: *láo lín*

tension pattern: *bì zhèng*

terminate malaria: *jié nüè*

thick (tongue coating): *hòu*

thin (tongue coating): *bó*

thready (pulse): *xì*

tight (pulse): *jǐn*

tongue with tooth marks: *chǐ hén shé*

transform dampness: *huà shī*

transform phlegm: *huà tán*

transform rheum: *huà yǐn*

transform turbidity: *huà zhuó*

transformation into fire: *huà huǒ*

transformation into heat: *huà rè*

triple burner: *sān jiāo*

twenty-four hour malaria: *rì nüè*

typical malaria: *zhèng nüè*

uncomplicated patterns: *shùn zhèng*

unctuous strangury: *gāo lín*

uterine network vessels: *bāo mài*

vacuity: *xū*

vacuity-cold: *xū hán*

vacuity-cold dysentery: *xū hán lì*

vacuity constipation: *xū bì*

vacuity-fire: *xū huǒ*

vacuity of yin and exuberance of yang: *yīn xū yáng kàng*

vacuity-repletion complex: *xū shí jiā zá zhèng*

vacuous (pulse): *xū*

vexation of the heart: *xīn fán*

vexing heat in the five hearts: *wǔ xīn fán rè*

viscera and bowels: *zàng fǔ*

warm qi: *wēn qì*

warm the channels: *wēn jīng*

warm the kidney: *wēn shèn*

warm the middle burner: *wēn zhōng*

warm the spleen: *wēn pí*

warm the stomach: *wēn wèi*

warm yang: *wēn yáng*

warm-heat epidemic toxins: *wēn rè yì dú*

warm malaria: *wēn nüè*

water-dampness: *shuǐ shī*

water qi intimidating the heart: *shuǐ qì líng xīn*

weak (pulse): *ruò*
white (tongue coating): *bái*
wind-cold: *fēng hán*
wind-dryness: *fēng zaò*
wind evil: *fēng xié*
wind evil damaging the connections: *fēng xié shāng luò*
wind-fire: *fēng huǒ*
wind-heat: *fēng rè*
wind-phlegm: *fēng tán*
wind rash: *fēng zhěn*
wiry (pulse): *xián*

yang edema: *yáng suǐ*
yang jaundice: *yáng huáng*
yellow (tongue coating): *huáng*
yin edema: *yīn suǐ*
yin fire: *yīn huǒ*
yin humor: *yīn yè*
yin jaundice: *yīn huáng*
yin vacuity: *yīn xū*
yin vacuity dysentery: *yīn xū lì*
yin vacuity fire effulgence: *yīn xū huǒ wàng*

BIBLIOGRAPHY

Cheng Xin-nong, ed. *Chinese Acupuncture and Moxibustion.* Beijing: Foreign Language Press, 1987

Compiling Commission for Medical Dictionary, ed. *Chinese-English Medical Dicitonary.* Beijing: People's Health Publishing House, 1987.

Guo Bo-Kang, ed. *Traditional Chinese Surgery: A Text for Medical Colleges and Universities.* Shanghai: Shanghai Science and Technology Publishing House, 1985.

Jiang Yu-ren, ed. *Traditional Chinese Paediatrics: A Text for Medical Colleges and Universities.* Shanghai: Shanghai Science and Technology Publishing House, 1985.

Liao Pin-zhang, ed. *Traditional Chinese Opthalmology: A Text for Medical Colleges and Universities.* Shanghai: Shanghai Science and Technology Publishing House, 1985.

Ling Yu-kui, ed. *Traditional Chinese Herbology: A Text for Medical Colleges and Universities.* Shanghai: Shanghai Science and Technology Publishing House, 1985.

Luo Yuan-kai, ed. *Traditional Chinese Gynecology: A Text for Medical Colleges and Universities.* Shanghai: Shanghai Science and Technology Publishing House, 1985.

Qiu Mao-liang, ed. *Traditional Chines Acu-moxaology: A Text for Medical Colleges and Universities.* Shanghai: Shanghai Science and Technology Publishing House, 1985.

Shanghai College of Traditional Chinese Medicine, ed. *Traditional Chinese Internal Medicine, Vol 1 & II, A Text for Medical Colleges and Universities.* Shanghai: Shanghai Science and Technology Publishing House, 1980.

Wang De-jian, ed. *Traditional Chinese Otorhinolaryngology: A Text for Medical Colleges and Universities.* Shanghai: Shanghai Science and Technology Publishing House, 1985.

Wiseman, Nigel and Ken Boss. *Glossary of Chinese Medical Terms and Acupuncture Points.* Brookline, MA: Paradigm Publications, 1990.

Xu Ji-qun, ed. *Traditional Chinese Pharmacology: A Text for Medical Colleges and Universities.* Shanghai: Shanghai Science and Technology Publishing House, 1984.

Yang Chang-sen, ed. *Traditional Chinese Acupuncture and Moxibustion Techniques: A Text for Medical Colleges and Universities.* Shanghai: Shanghai Science and Technology Publishing House, 1985.

Yang Jia-san, ed. *Traditional Chinese Acupointology: A Text for Medical Colleges and Universities.* Shanghai: Shanghai Science and Technology Publishing House, 1984.

Yeung Him-che. *Handbook of Chinese Herbs and Formulas, Vol 1 and II.* Los Angeles: Institute of Chinese Medicine, 1985.

Zhang Bo-yu, ed. *Traditional Chinese Internal Medicine, A Text for Medical Colleges and Universities.* Shanghai: Shanghai Science and Technology Publishing House, 1985.

INDEX